your
Pregnancy
week by week

WHAT TO EXPECT FROM CONCEPTION TO BIRTH

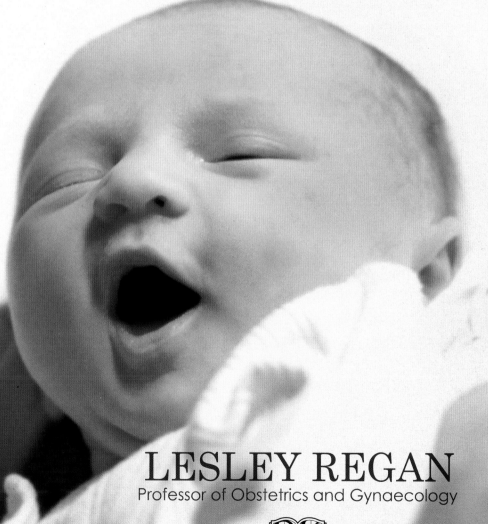

LESLEY REGAN
Professor of Obstetrics and Gynaecology

LONDON, NEW YORK, MUNICH, MELBOURNE, DELHI

Updated 2013 edition
Project editors Julia Halford, Elizabeth Yeates
Producer Andy Hilliard
Senior producer Jennifer Scothern
Creative technical support Sonia Charbonnier
Managing editor Dawn Henderson
Managing art editor Christine Keilty
Publishing Manager Anna Davidson
Publisher Peggy Vance

DK India
Senior editor Alicia Ingty
Assistant editor Aditi Batra
Art editors Anjan Dey, Ira Sharma
Managing editor Glenda Fernandes
Managing art editor Navidita Thapa
CTS Manager Sunil Sharma
DTP designers Satish Chandra Gaur,
Rajdeep Singh, Anurag Trivedi

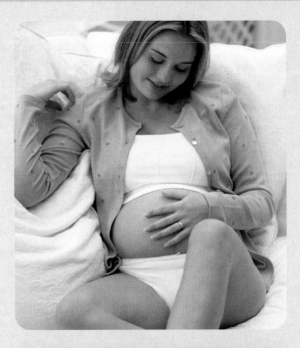

DISCLAIMER

Every effort has been made to ensure that the information in this
book is complete and accurate. However, neither the publisher nor
the author is engaged in rendering professional advice or services to
the individual reader. The ideas, procedures and suggestions contained
in this book are not intended as a substitute for consulting with your
healthcare provider. All matters regarding the health of you and
your baby require medical supervision. Neither the publishers nor the
author shall be liable or responsible for any loss or damage allegedly
arising from any information or suggestion in this book.

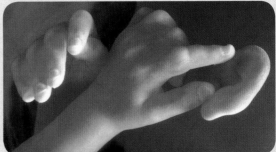

First published in Great Britain in 2005 by
Dorling Kindersley Limited,
80 Strand, London WC2R 0RL
A Penguin Company

Revised edition 2010, 2013

2 4 6 8 10 9 7 5 3 1
001-188209-May/13

A CIP catalogue record for this book is available
from the British Library

ISBN 978-1-4093-2666-3

Reproduced by Alta Image
Printed and bound by South China Printing Co. Ltd, China

see our complete catalogue at **www.dk.com**

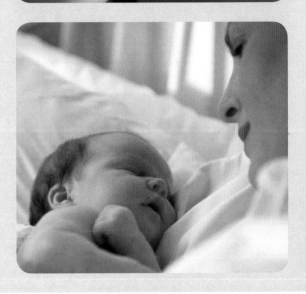

Contents

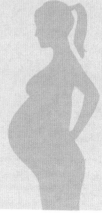

Introduction

There are plenty of pregnancy books on the market so why should I embark on writing another one? The reason is simple – the women I care for keep telling me that they would like more detailed answers to their questions about pregnancy and childbirth. Further, that they want a book that provides them with clear, comprehensive information, without any prescriptive or personal agenda.

I understand and sympathize with the request since, when I was expecting my twins, I remember feeling both astonished and intimidated by books that seem to suggest that there are right and wrong approaches to pregnancy and childbirth. I have no argument with the many different childbirth philosophies, but I do have a problem when they result in pregnant women feeling that they have failed in

About this book

Pregnancy is one of the most important journeys that you will ever embark upon. To help you understand as much as possible about this eventful and exciting period of your life, this book is arranged chronologically. It takes you from the moment you conceive, through each week of your pregnancy to the day of delivery, and then provides all the information you need to give birth and care for yourself and your baby afterwards. This chronological arrangement means that, as your journey through pregnancy progresses, you will be able to find your way around the relevant part of the book smoothly. I also hope that you will be able to find the answers to most – if not all – of your questions quickly and easily. Above all, I want to offer you clear, comprehensive and up-to-date information that should help you to understand the medical jargon and the experiences you may

encounter in the next few months.

The "journey" section of the book is divided into the three trimesters of pregnancy. Everyone seems to have their own idea about exactly which weeks fall in each trimester so I have allowed some overlap here. The only important thing is that each one corresponds to an important and quite distinct phase of your baby's development. At the beginning of each trimester, there is a broad overview of the major milestones that occur, then it is broken down into three more detailed "through the weeks" guides. Each of these covers what happens routinely in pregnancy, including a description of your baby's development, how your own body changes, how you may be feeling both physically and emotionally, together with a section on the antenatal care you can expect to be receiving and some common concerns linked to that particular time.

some way if they do not follow the advice to the last letter, or their pregnancy does not follow a textbook pattern.

So the agenda here is very simple – knowledge is key. My aim is to offer you a level of information about your antenatal care that is not always readily available. I want to ensure that you are fully aware of the extraordinary events in your baby's development and the remarkable adaptations your body will make. My belief is that the only way to be confident about the choices and decisions that you will need to make in pregnancy is to have a clear understanding of everything that may happen to you. I also believe that this is the best way to achieve the happiest outcome – a healthy mother and a beautiful take-home baby.

Lesley Ryan

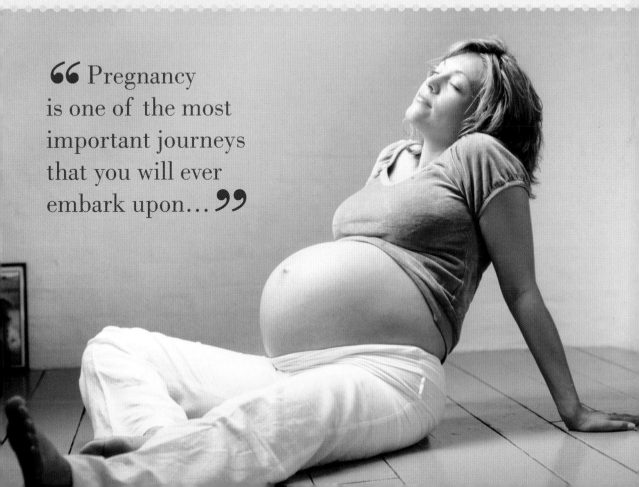

66 Pregnancy is one of the most important journeys that you will ever embark upon... **99**

66 The first trimester is the crucial period when all the organs, muscles, and bones of your baby are formed. 99

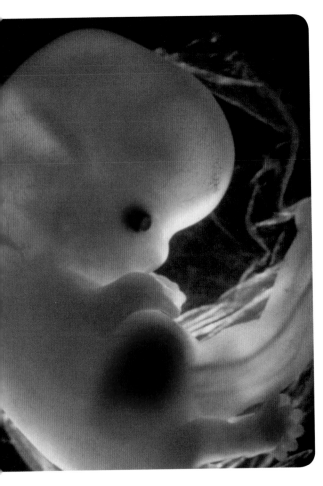

To keep things simple I am defining the age of your pregnancy and your baby as the number of weeks from your last period. The exact dates will vary depending on your menstrual cycle and when you conceived, so please don't worry about trying to tie down the details too precisely.

In this book, I have defined the first trimester of pregnancy as the period between 0 and 13 weeks for the practical reason that by the time you reach the 13th-week, milestone you will probably have been booked in for your pregnancy care at an antenatal clinic at your local hospital or birth centre, GP's surgery or at home. Broadly speaking, the first trimester is the crucial period when all the organs, muscles, and bones of your baby are formed. During the first eight weeks we refer to the baby as an embryo, which comes from the Greek word for "newborn", in recognition of the fact that this is the stage of organ formation, or organogenesis. By eight to nine weeks of pregnancy, the embryo becomes a fetus, which means "the young one", since organ formation is complete. The second trimester is taken up with consolidating all the basic structures that have

THE JOURNEY TIMELINE ··

The three trimesters are divided into 4–6 week sections offering detailed information that relates to your exact stage of pregnancy.

week 8   week 12   week 16   week 20

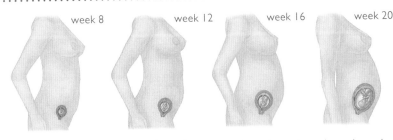

| 1 | 2 | 3 | 4 | 5 | 6 | 7 | 8 | 9 | 10 | 11 | 12 | 13 | 14 | 15 | 16 | 17 | 18 | 19 | 20 |

▶ WEEKS 0–6   ▶ WEEKS 6–10   ▶ WEEKS 10–13   ▶ WEEKS 13–17   ▶ WEEKS 17–21

▶ FIRST TRIMESTER   ▶ SECOND TRIMESTER

developed. During this period, the fetus grows rapidly and starts to make facial expressions, swallow, hear sounds, and can be felt kicking in the mother's womb. Until relatively recently, a fetus born before 28 weeks rarely survived. Happily, advances in neonatal medicine have enabled some babies born at 25 and 26 weeks to survive, which is why I have chosen to end the second trimester here. In the third trimester, the baby has an important final phase of growth and maturation in preparation for birth. Everything that happens in the third trimester is based on the building blocks that have been laid many months before. During these final weeks, your baby will double in weight and develop the maturity to cope with the journey into the world and life after birth.

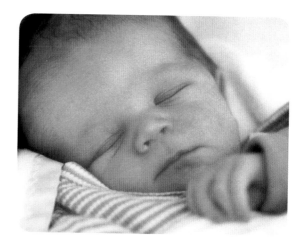

Although the vast majority of pregnancies are relatively problem-free, not every pregnancy is an entirely smooth journey. Whenever less common problems arise, you will be referred to the final section of the book, Concerns and Complications, where they are explained in greater detail.

No two labours are alike and the Labour and Birth chapter will help you prepare for most eventualities. The summary of how normal labour progresses and the various pain-relief options will be all that is needed for the majority of readers, but for those who may need more specialized

treatment there is detailed information and advice on topics such as Caesarean birth and premature delivery. My hope is that even if you find yourself caught up in unexpected events, you will be prepared for what is about to happen, aware of the choices available, and reassured that in the vast majority of cases all ends well.

The Life after Birth chapter looks at the potential highs and lows you may experience after your baby is born. This is always an emotional time; delight in your new baby will be intermingled with anxiety about minor problems and your ability to cope with your new role. Once again, I hope my advice will help ease you and your baby through these first important weeks together.

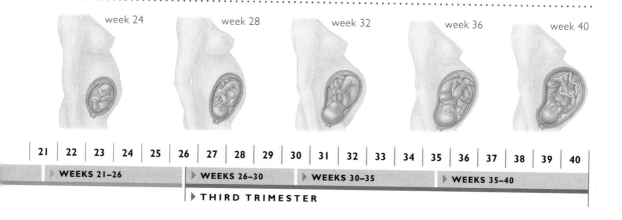

week 24   week 28   week 32   week 36   week 40

| 21 | 22 | 23 | 24 | 25 | 26 | 27 | 28 | 29 | 30 | 31 | 32 | 33 | 34 | 35 | 36 | 37 | 38 | 39 | 40 |

▶ **WEEKS 21–26**   ▶ **WEEKS 26–30**   ▶ **WEEKS 30–35**   ▶ **WEEKS 35–40**

▶ **THIRD TRIMESTER**

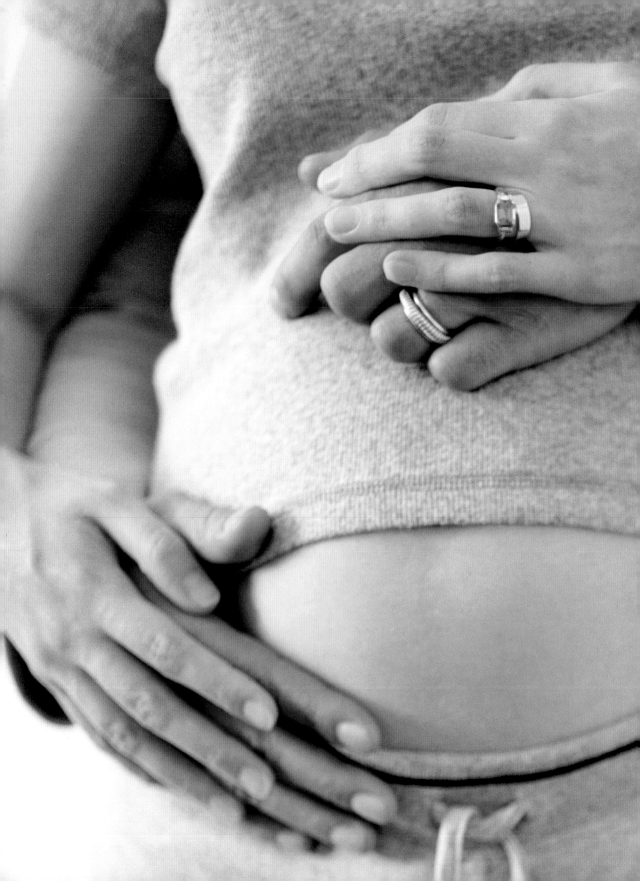

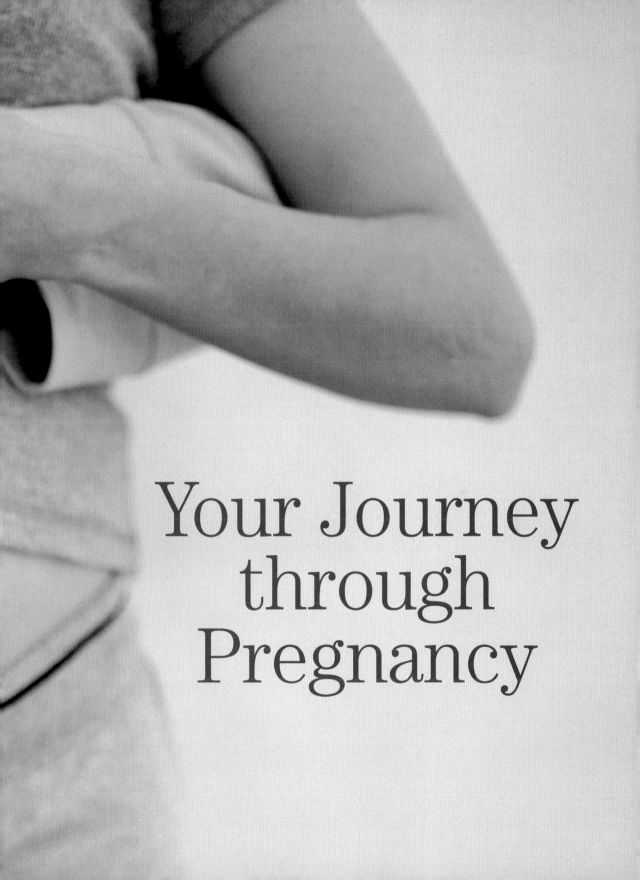

Your Journey through Pregnancy

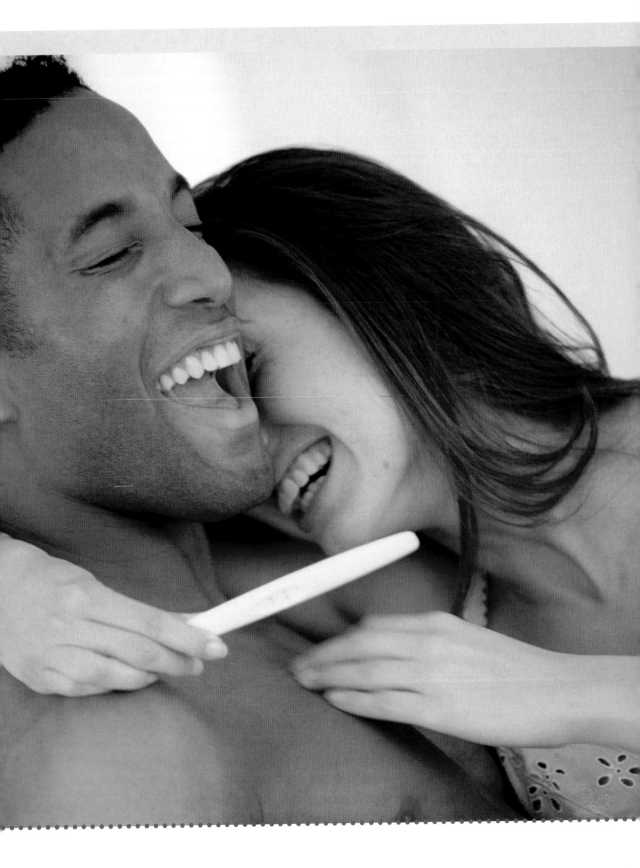

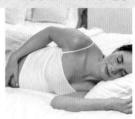

The very beginning

Whether you are pregnant already or have simply made the decision to have a baby soon, this is the beginning of one of life's most exciting and, occasionally, daunting experiences. This section helps you lay the foundation for an enjoyable pregnancy – offering insights into conception and answering questions about what is safe in pregnancy; the best foods to eat; how to stay fit over the coming weeks and how to negotiate your rights and benefits as a parent. These are your guidelines for the journey ahead…

CONTENTS

The origins of life

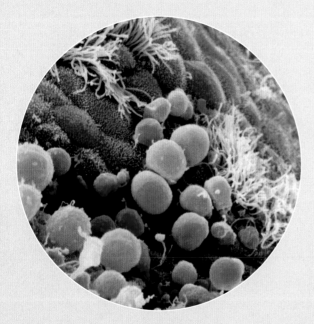

INSIDE THE UTERUS

The lining is perfectly primed for a life to begin. The granules of mucus (yellow) will provide nutrients for a newly fertilized egg.

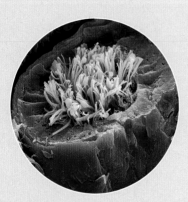

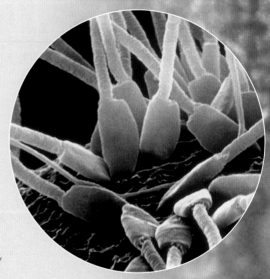

MATURING SPERM

As sperm pass slowly along the epididymis — a coiled tube that lies behind the testes — they mature until they are ready to be ejaculated.

JOURNEY'S END

A swarm of surviving sperm lock on to the thick, inviting surface of the egg after their long journey up the Fallopian tube.

" A mature egg drifts in the Fallopian tube... conditions are perfect for fertilization. "

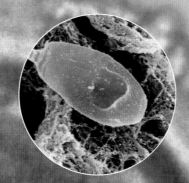

THE WINNER

Just one sperm penetrates the ovum's thick outer layer, and fertilization occurs.

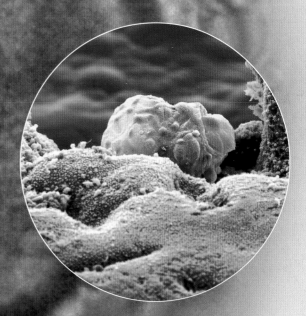

SIX DAYS OLD

The tiny cluster of cells, now known as a blastocyst, embeds in the wall of the uterus – a pregnancy begins.

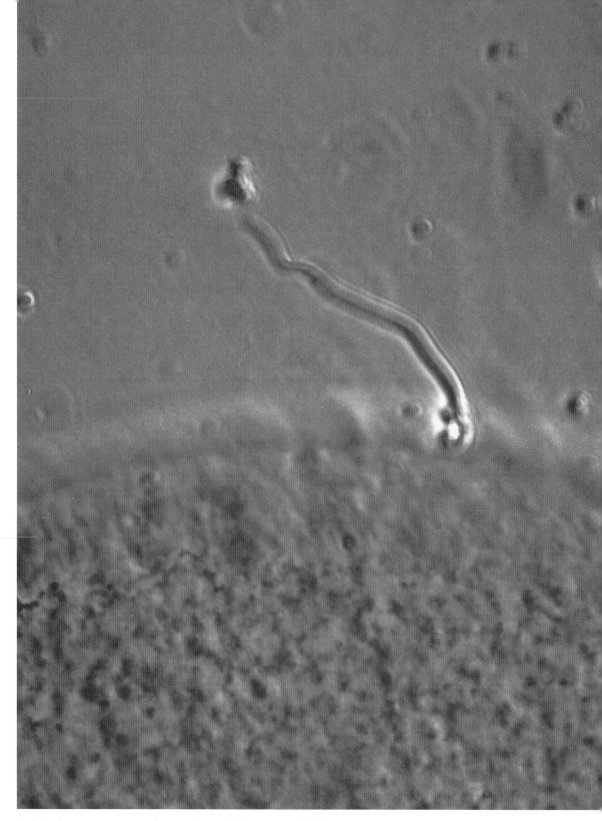

▲ A single sperm penetrates the outer layer of the comparatively huge ovum.

Conceiving a baby

WHEN YOU CONSIDER the complex sequences of hormonal events that are necessary for you to become pregnant, and the hoops that your partner's sperm have to go through to fertilize an egg, you will begin to realize why the expression "the miracle of conception" is not an overstatement.

The series of events that occur during your menstrual cycle need to be carefully orchestrated if a pregnancy is to occur. Conception is a bit like a jigsaw – it takes only one piece to be missing to prevent the puzzle from being completed.

As soon as your period ends, a hormone called follicle stimulating hormone (FSH) is secreted into your bloodstream by the pituitary gland, a small bean-sized gland that lies just behind your eyes in your brain. This hormone acts upon your ovaries, which sit at the end of your Fallopian tubes and contain many thousands of eggs. You were born with about three million eggs, but by puberty these will have degenerated to about 400,000. All of these eggs are exposed to FSH, and it is not clear why only a few are recruited to start developing. On average, a woman will release only 400 or fewer mature eggs during her reproductive lifespan.

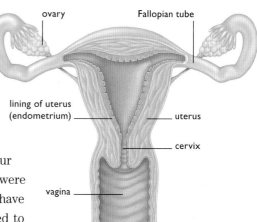

FEMALE REPRODUCTIVE SYSTEM The ovaries store and release eggs, which travel along the Fallopian tube into the uterus. The narrow cervix connects the uterus to the vagina.

Ovulation

Each ovary releases one egg (or occasionally more than one) in alternate menstrual cycles, so ovulation takes place from only one ovary at a time. Eggs that are selected to start to mature do so within a fluid-filled bubble called a follicle, which starts to enlarge under the influence of FSH. Every month about 20 eggs start this process, but usually only one "dominant" follicle becomes fully mature and ovulates; the others shrivel, and the eggs within them are lost. The egg grows to one side of the follicle, surrounded by special cells called granulosa cells, which feed it with nutrients and also produce oestrogen. This hormone stimulates the growth of the lining of the uterus (endometrium) as well as breast tissues, which is why breast tenderness is a common premenstrual symptom.

> " Conception is a bit like a jigsaw – it takes only one piece to be missing to prevent the puzzle from being completed. "

As the level of oestrogen in your blood rises, it feeds back a message to the hypothalamus (a control centre in the brain) telling it that the follicle is mature and ready to ovulate. In response, the hypothalamus informs the pituitary gland to release a short sharp burst of luteinizing hormone (LH), called a pulse, which triggers the release of the egg about 36 hours later. The egg bursts from the follicle, which has grown to about the size of a one pound coin. This is called ovulation and it usually occurs around the 14th day of the menstrual cycle.

The mature egg has developed several important features. It contains chromosomes (which carry genetic information) at the right stage for further development and it is capable of taking in a single sperm while blocking the entry of any other sperm surrounding it. The egg is wafted into your Fallopian tube by delicate wand-like projections called fimbria, which resemble the fronds of a sea anemone. Tiny hair-like strands, called cilia, line the Fallopian tube and these help the newly released egg to pass down the tube towards your uterus.

Meanwhile, the remaining cells in the ruptured follicle form a swelling in the ovary called the corpus luteum, which starts to produce the hormone progesterone. Like oestrogen, progesterone has an effect on your uterus, breasts, and the hypothalamus and pituitary glands in your brain. In the uterus, progesterone makes the cells receptive to a pregnancy by producing the nutrients needed to support a developing embryo and by thickening the lining of your uterus.

If the egg is not fertilized after ovulation, your production of luteinizing hormone begins to fall and the corpus luteum withers away. When the levels of both oestrogen and progesterone have fallen below the threshold needed to maintain the lining of the uterus in a receptive state for embryo implantation,

THE RACE TO THE EGG ···

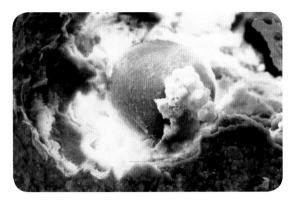

Ovulation occurs mid menstrual cycle when the mature ovum (egg) bursts from its follicle.

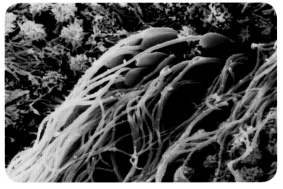

Cohorts of sperm stream through the narrow opening of the cervix and into the uterus.

the blood-filled lining starts to disintegrate and your period begins. In a normal cycle, this usually occurs around 14 days after ovulation. The onset of your period signals that a new cycle of follicle growth can begin again.

Your partner's role in conception

This may seem to be the simpler part of the proposition, but the statistical probability of your partner's sperm meeting your egg is astounding. On average a man ejaculates about 5ml (a teaspoonful) of semen containing 100 to 300 million sperm. Less than 100,000 make their way through the cervix; a mere 200 survive the journey up into the Fallopian tubes – and only one can fertilize the egg.

Boys are not born with a full complement of sperm. Production starts around puberty and from this time onwards, sperm are manufactured in the testes regularly at a rate of 1,500 per second. Each sperm has a lifespan of about 72 days. The testes deliver the sperm into the epididymis (a long coiled tube sitting at the top of each testis) and over the next two or three weeks they become capable of moving on their own and fertilizing an egg. From here the sperm move into the vas deferens. These tubes contract during male orgasm and transport the sperm out of the scrotum, past the seminal vesicles and the prostate gland (from which they collect seminal fluid), and into the urethra – the tube that travels between the bladder and the penis. During ejaculation, the opening to the bladder is shut off and the sperm are rapidly transported into the penis ready for their journey into the vagina.

Arriving in the vagina is not the end of the sperm's extraordinary obstacle race; they still need to navigate a considerable distance before they have an opportunity to fertilize an egg. The environment is fairly hostile to sperm:

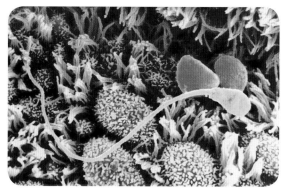

A sperm negotiates the frond-filled lining of the Fallopian tube on its way to the ovum.

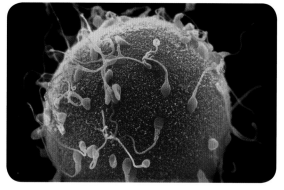

Mission accomplished – the successful surviving sperm swarm over the mature ovum.

> ❝ It is amazing to reflect that, even before you realize you are pregnant, the design of your baby's body is being programmed. ❞

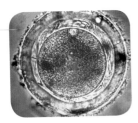

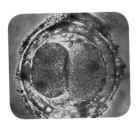

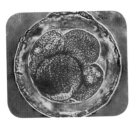

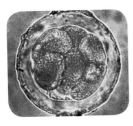

FIRST DIVISIONS After fertilization, the zygote divides rapidly. Within 36 hours it is made up of 12 separate cells.

vaginal secretions are quite acidic to prevent bacteria and other organisms reaching the uterus and Fallopian tubes and causing damaging infections. However, once in the vagina, the semen coagulates rapidly and this helps keep the sperm in the right place and protect them against vaginal fluids.

Within 5 to 10 minutes after ejaculation some sperm have entered the uterus and are heading towards the Fallopian tubes. During this journey the sperm become hyperactive and attain full fertilizing capacity so that when they get close to the egg they are able to shed their cap (acrosome) and fuse with the egg. For the next 72 hours, further sperm from the pool at the cervix continue to enter the uterus. Once in the Fallopian tubes, the remaining sperm (by now reduced to about 200) swim upwards aided by muscular contractions of the uterus and tubes. This in itself is an extraordinary feat, since at the same time the egg is being propelled downwards towards the uterine cavity.

Fertilization

The process during which the sperm enters the egg, fuses with it, and the egg starts dividing takes about 24 hours to complete and usually takes place while the egg is still travelling down the Fallopian tube.

Only the strongest cohort of sperm reaches the egg, but it seems that the "winner" in the race is entirely random. Several sperm may bind to the surface of the egg and this stimulates them to lose their caps, exposing enzymes that digest their way through the outer membrane (the zona). However, only one sperm penetrates the oocyte, the innermost part of the egg, and fertilization occurs. The sperm tail, which has been so vital in propelling it to this point, is left outside and eventually disintegrates. The newly formed single cell that results is called a zygote and it now forms a thick wall around itself to prevent penetration by any other sperm. Your pregnancy has begun!

The zygote now begins to divide into further cells, called blastomeres, which by the third day number around a dozen. This tiny cluster of new life then takes about 60 hours to make its way to the uterus by which time it is made up of about 50–60 cells and is called a blastocyst.

Already there are two distinct cell types – an outer layer of trophoblast cells, which will develop into the placenta, and an inner cell mass, which will eventually form the fetus. Two to three days later (about a week after fertilization) the blastocyst embeds itself in the lining of the uterus. It has now subdivided into approximately 100 cells and starts to produce the hormone human chorionic gonadotrophin (HCG), which sends a signal to the corpus luteum to carry on producing progesterone. If it failed to do so, the lining of the uterus would begin to break down and menstrual bleeding would begin.

In the second week after conception, the trophoblast cells continue to invade into the uterine lining and the inner cell mass develops into an embryo. It is only a dot, but has already started to differentiate into three different cell layers, called the germ layers, which will each become a different part of the baby's body. It is amazing to reflect that, even before you realize you are pregnant, the design of your baby's body is being programmed.

HOW TWINS ARE CONCEIVED

Twins and triplets are conceived in two different ways:
▶ When two or more eggs are released and fertilized, the result is non-identical twins.
▶ When one egg is fertilized by one sperm and then divides into two separate zygotes, the result is two separate embryos. These share identical genetic structures and will therefore become identical twins.

With both types of twin each baby develops surrounded by amniotic fluid, within its own amniotic sac. But because non-identical twins are conceived from two separate eggs, each has its own placenta. Identical twins share one placenta, but each twin has a separate umbilical cord.

The number of twin pregnancies has doubled compared to a generation ago. Twins now make up around 2 per cent of all

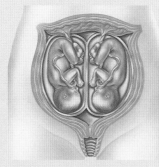

IDENTICAL TWINS share a placenta.

 one fertilized egg divides

pregnancies – partly because of medical advances, such as in vitro fertilization (IVF) and fertility drugs (both of which carry an increased risk of multiple pregnancy), and partly because women are having babies later in life. Women over 35

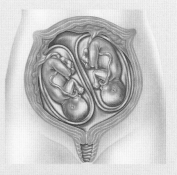

NON-IDENTICAL TWINS have two placentas.

 two separate eggs are fertilized

have a greater chance of conceiving non-identical twins because they are more likely to release more than one egg per cycle. Non-identical twins also run in families. However, there are no factors that increase the risk of conceiving identical twins.

Genes and inheritance

Genes control the growth and repair of our bodies and are also the code by which we pass on physical and mental characteristics to our children. At conception, your baby inherits a unique package of genes that will make him or her different from any other person.

The 40,000 or so genes that make up the human genome are arranged in pairs along chromosomes, long strands of genetic material that are found in the nucleus of virtually all body cells. Individual genes are single units of information inherited from the parents and occupy a specific position on the chromosome. Genes contain numerous small segments of DNA (the genetic blueprint), which provide codes for specific traits such as blood type and also dictate the specialized function of cells. In some cases, the presence or absence of a gene can predispose a person to a disease or protect against it. Genes are also either dominant or recessive. In a pair made up of one dominant and one recessive gene, the dominant gene prevails and this has effects on inherited traits such as eye colour (see opposite) and also in the development of some genetic diseases (see p.144).

When a baby is conceived, both the mother's egg and the father's sperm contribute a single set of 23 chromosomes to the embryo, making a total complement of 46. Each egg and sperm carries a different mix of genes, which is why, apart from identical twins (see p.21), every baby inherits a unique selection. However, because all cells are derived from this single fertilized egg, the same genetic material is duplicated in every cell of a baby's body.

BOY OR GIRL?

When an egg is fertilized by a sperm, the embryo that results has 23 pairs of chromosomes. The sex of your baby is determined by just one pair: chromosomes 45 and 46 (known as pair 23) are the sex chromosomes.

▶ The sex chromosomes are labelled the X (female) and Y (male) chromosomes. All eggs carry a single X chromosome, while sperm carry either a single X or a single Y in equal numbers. It is therefore the sperm that determines the sex of a child.

▶ When a sperm carrying the X chromosome fertilizes an egg, it forms an XX pair of chromosomes and the result is a girl.

▶ When a sperm carrying the Y chromosome fertilizes an egg, this results in an XY pair – a boy.

▶ Methods that claim to tip the balance in favour of a boy or girl rely on the fact that the Y-bearing sperm swim a little faster than the X-bearing sperm, but the latter survive a little longer. However, theories on the timing of conception to produce a boy or girl vary considerably. In spite of these methods, the ratio of boys to girls remains reassuringly normal.

BROWN EYES OR BLUE?

One of the most easily understood examples of inherited traits involving dominant and recessive genes concerns eye colour. Because the brown-eye gene is dominant and the blue-eye gene is recessive, the gene for brown eyes always prevails.

Both you and your partner carry a pair of genes for eye colour and this offers four possible combinations of genes in your own children. To work out your baby's chance of having blue or brown eyes you need to look at the eye-colour genes you have inherited from your own parents. Even if you both have brown eyes, you may each have a blue-eyed parent and so be carrying recessive blue-eye genes. If these recessive genes combine, your baby will have blue eyes.

If you both have blue eyes, neither of you possess dominant brown-eye genes, so together you cannot have a child with brown eyes. (The brown-eye gene also covers hazel eyes, and the blue-eye gene includes grey and light-green eyes.)

Two brown-eyed parents In this example, the dominant brown-eye gene masks the recessive blue-eye gene so all children have brown eyes.

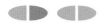 PARENTS BR/BL+BR/BR

CHILD
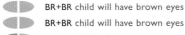
BR+BR child will have brown eyes
BR+BR child will have brown eyes
BL+BR child will have brown eyes
BL+BR child will have brown eyes

One brown-eyed parent; one blue-eyed parent The dominant brown-eye gene will prevail or two recessive blue-eye genes will combine to produce blue eyes.

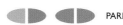 PARENTS BR/BL+BL/BL

CHILD
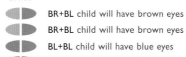
BR+BL child will have brown eyes
BR+BL child will have brown eyes
BL+BL child will have blue eyes
BL+BL child will have blue eyes

Two brown-eyed parents In this example, both parents carry a recessive blue-eye gene from their own parents so have a 1 in 4 chance of a blue-eyed child.

 PARENTS BR/BL+BR/BL

CHILD
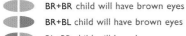
BR+BR child will have brown eyes
BR+BL child will have brown eyes
BL+BR child will have brown eyes
BL+BL child will have blue eyes

Two blue-eyed parents Blue-eyed parents both carry two copies of the recessive blue-eye gene so cannot have a brown-eyed child.

 PARENTS BL/BL+BL/BL

CHILD
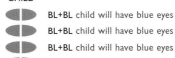
BL+BL child will have blue eyes
BL+BL child will have blue eyes
BL+BL child will have blue eyes
BL+BL child will have blue eyes

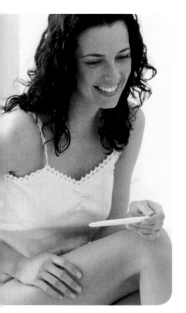

HOME PREGNANCY TEST Most kits are reliable and very easy to use.

Confirming that you are pregnant

As soon as you begin to suspect that you might be pregnant, you can find out with certainty. Nowadays, testing is quick and easy and can give you a reliable answer as soon as you have missed a period.

Most women opt for a urine test, which measures rising levels of the hormone human chorionic gonadotrophin (HCG), which is produced by the blastocyst about a week after fertilization has taken place. Your GP, pharmacist or family planning clinic can perform the test for you or you can choose to use a home pregnancy testing kit, available from your local pharmacy. These are accurate and simple to perform and offer the great advantages of speed, privacy, and convenience. The test strip or wand is packaged in a plastic container that looks like a tampon applicator; before you use it check the sell-by date and read the instructions carefully. Most kits advise you to perform the test several days after your first missed period, although it may be positive earlier. The result may be negative if you take the test too early and there is too little HCG in your urine.

Using a pregnancy testing kit

To use a kit all you have to do is sit on the loo and pass some fresh urine over the strip. The concentration of HCG is always highest in your early morning urine, but newer test kits are sensitive enough to be used later in the day. When the HCG in your urine comes into contact with the test strip it produces a colour change. At first a blue line or pink circle appears in the test window to confirm that the test kit is working, followed in a matter of minutes by a second blue line or a pink circle in the results window if you are pregnant. The kits always provide a second test strip, so it is a good idea to check a borderline positive result with a follow-up test a week or so later. Sadly, some positive tests become negative later on because the embryo has not been able to implant successfully and will be followed shortly by your menstrual period.

Other ways of testing

In one or two special circumstances, you may be offered a blood test to detect and quantify the exact level of HCG hormone in your body. If, for example, you have been undergoing fertility treatment, you may want to know if it has been successful even before your period is expected. Accurate regular measuring of HCG is also needed if an ectopic pregnancy (a pregnancy that develops outside the uterus, usually in the Fallopian tube) is suspected (see p.81).

Another method of diagnosing a pregnancy is using an ultrasound scan. Scans are not performed routinely in very early pregnancy, but they can be useful if you are unsure of your dates, have a history of miscarriage or if you have symptoms or signs to suggest that you may have an ectopic pregnancy. Although there is little to see on the scan until about 10 days after your missed period, after this time it is usually possible to see the pregnancy sac in the uterus with a tiny fetal pole (a definite rectangular blob within the sac), and sometimes even a beating fetal heart.

Before the days of home pregnancy testing kits, most women had their pregnancy confirmed with an internal examination performed by their GP after they had missed one or two periods. An experienced doctor can diagnose a pregnancy by noting the bluish tinge of the vaginal skin and cervix, the fact that the uterus and cervix are softer than normal and, by six weeks, the uterus is slightly larger. These changes are due to the increased blood supply to all the pelvic organs. Internal examinations are not performed routinely nowadays, but every now and again an unsuspected pregnancy is diagnosed this way.

YOUR EMOTIONAL RESPONSE

I have had many conversations with women who have just discovered they are pregnant and their reactions range from elation to mild panic. Here is a selection of the feelings that are expressed most frequently:

▶ I don't believe it.
▶ It's wonderful.
▶ I'm ecstatic.
▶ Help – I hadn't thought it would happen this quickly.
▶ What have I let myself in for?
▶ Can I afford a baby?
▶ I shouldn't have had that glass of wine after work.
▶ Will my job be safe?

▶ Why didn't I stop smoking last month, the way I planned to?
▶ Where will I have my baby?
▶ What can I do to help my baby?
▶ Will my baby be normal?

Not all of these are positive reactions and this is entirely normal, so don't feel guilty about any negative thoughts that you may be having. Even if you have been planning your pregnancy for some time, you may feel daunted as the consequences begin to sink in. Adding to the reaction is a cocktail of pregnancy hormones coursing through your bloodstream, which

is enough to make anyone feel emotionally unpredictable. There is no doubt that being pregnant and bringing a baby into the world will be one of the most eventful and unpredictable periods of your life and there will be times when the sheer magnitude of it leaves you feeling overwhelmed.

However, like every other important life event, pregnancy will be much more enjoyable if you feel confident and in control of the situation. The only way to achieve this is to find out everything you can about it – I hope this book will help you to do just that.

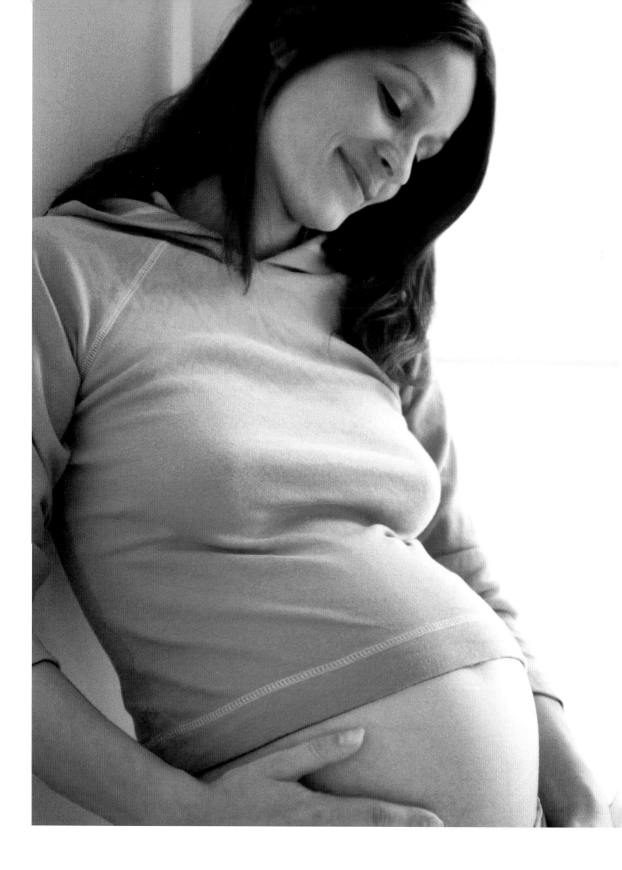

Staying safe in pregnancy

EVERY WORRYING PREGNANCY STATISTIC and media horror story comes into sharp focus as soon as you are pregnant, and you may be wondering just how much of your everyday life needs to be re-evaluated. This section looks at some common concerns and will, I hope, help you weed out the myths and scares from the more sensible pregnancy precautions.

Of course, it is impossible to eliminate risk from life, and pregnancy is no exception. In case you are feeling overwhelmed by worry, let's begin by getting things into perspective. About 4 in every 100 babies have an abnormality at birth (congenital abnormality). Most are due to genetic causes (see pp.144–5 and pp.416–9), with only a small proportion resulting from factors such as drugs, infections, and environmental hazards. Even if you are concerned that you have been exposed to something that may have harmed your baby (known as a teratogen), do remember that you are more likely to be knocked down by the proverbial bus than to have a baby affected by one of these hazards in pregnancy.

> " ...it is impossible to eliminate risk from life, and pregnancy is no exception. "

An unexpected event

If you find yourself pregnant unexpectedly or were not as prepared for it as you hoped you might be, you may be feeling a mixture of shock and disbelief coupled with anxiety about the kind of start your pregnancy might have had in the days and weeks when you were totally unaware of what was going on.

My first piece of advice to you is to stop worrying. Instead of dwelling on what you were meaning to do or might have done to prepare for a future pregnancy, start focusing on adopting a healthier lifestyle now. Promise yourself that you will eat a well-balanced daily diet (see pp.43–9). Ideally avoid alcohol and keep caffeine intake to a minimum. If you are a cigarette smoker, stop today.

If you are still in the first trimester of your pregnancy then start taking folic acid supplements (see p.51) immediately, because these will help protect your baby from neural tube defects such as spina bifida (see p.146 and p.418). Although women are advised to begin taking the supplement while they are trying to conceive, starting them now and continuing them until the 13th week is definitely worthwhile – so don't think that it's too late.

Another possible concern is that this unexpected baby may have been exposed to all sorts of potential damage when you did not know that you were pregnant. You might be worried, for example, that you had too much to drink at a party, or that you were taking medical drugs before you knew that you were pregnant. In practice, the most commonly prescribed drugs are antibiotics and fortunately there are very few that harm a developing embryo (see p.35). There is also the possibility that you were using contraception around the time of conception and you may now be wondering if this has the potential to cause problems. I've addressed these concerns below, but let me begin with some reassurance: the reality is that most tiny embryos destined to make it through pregnancy and become a live take-home baby are really very resilient.

IF YOUR CONTRACEPTION FAILED...

If you conceived your baby while you were using contraception, you are probably wondering if this is going to cause problems. In most cases, there is nothing to worry about.

▶ **If you were taking hormonal contraception**, such as the combined pill or the minipill, simply stop taking them because they are no longer useful. The combined pill contains oestrogen to inhibit ovulation, and progesterone, which makes the cervical mucus less penetrable by sperm, and cells in the lining of the uterus less receptive to implantation of the tiny embryo. Progesterone-only contraceptives, such as the mini-pill and three-monthly injections, such as depoprovera, have similar effects on the cervical mucus and lining of the uterus. Now that you have become pregnant these effects are no longer a consideration. There

is no evidence that the hormones in modern-day preparations cause problems for the developing embryo and fetus.

▶ **Barrier methods of contraception** that involve spermicides are not harmful to a developing embryo, so there is no need to worry about them.

▶ **If you used postcoital contraception** such as the morning-after pill and are nonetheless pregnant, you may be distressed that the method has failed you, but again no harm will have come to the developing baby.

▶ **When pregnancy occurs with an intrauterine contraceptive device (IUD) in place** there is an increased risk of miscarriage because of the presence of a foreign body in the uterus; the inflammatory response that it causes; and the increasing risk of infection ascending along

the IUD strings in the vagina. If the strings or the device are visible on vaginal examination, it is best to remove the IUD. This does not further increase the risk of miscarriage but does reduce the risk of miscarriage at a later stage in the pregnancy due to infection.

However, if neither strings nor IUD are visible, then it is best left where it is. It is unlikely to cause problems in a pregnancy that progresses to term since the baby develops within the fluid-filled amniotic sac. The IUD will be outside the sac and is usually delivered with the placenta.

▶ **If you have been sterilized** (tubal ligation) and find that you are pregnant, you should consult your doctor promptly. Your tubes will have been damaged mechanically by the procedure putting you at risk of an ectopic pregnancy (see p.81 and p.423).

Smoking

If you are still smoking now that you are pregnant, you need to be aware of the problems that this can cause for your growing baby. During the first three months of pregnancy, smoking can directly reduce the ability of the developing placenta to invade the wall of the uterus and grow. If you continue to smoke in later pregnancy, you will be reducing the supply of oxygen and nutrients to your baby and increasing your risk of premature delivery, placental abruption (see p.428), and fetal growth restriction (see p.429). Give up now, and if your partner smokes, encourage him to give up. Your GP and midwife can help by referring you both to smoking cessation services. Be aware that if you are exposed regularly to cigarette smoke you become a passive smoker, with similar risks to your baby's health. Try to avoid very smoky places, such as the areas outside train stations or pubs and bars.

Alcohol

Any pregnant woman who has a heavy regular alcohol intake is at increased risk of experiencing pregnancy complications. During the first few months of pregnancy, large quantities of alcohol can cause a distinctive pattern of abnormalities in the baby, known as fetal alcohol syndrome (see p.435): these include failure to thrive after the birth, damage to the nervous system, and poor childhood growth. Regular heavy consumption throughout pregnancy can have further toxic effects on the fetus. New research also suggests that even small amounts of alcohol can affect your baby. Try to cut out alcohol altogether now that you are pregnant, particularly in the first few crucial months of development. If there were one or two occasions when you drank a bit too much in the weeks before you knew that you were pregnant, try not to worry unduly – but please make sure that you stop drinking straight away.

> 66
> ...the reality is that most tiny embryos destined to become a live, take-home baby are very resilient.
> 99

Recreational drugs

I have no intention of preaching about the rights and wrongs of taking recreational drugs, but I do want to pass on some facts: drugs such as cocaine, heroine, and ecstasy have the potential to be a serious problem for a developing fetus. They all cross the placenta and enter the baby's bloodstream, increasing the risk of miscarriage (see p.431), placental abruption, and premature delivery of a baby that is usually growth restricted (see p.429). After delivery, the baby may suffer serious withdrawal symptoms and possible brain damage, and will therefore inevitably be kept in hospital under close observation for several weeks. So, if you want to have a trouble-free pregnancy and a healthy baby, avoid all recreational drugs.

ENVIRONMENTAL HAZARDS

Potential hazards in the environment are of particular concern in early pregnancy when your baby's major organs and body systems are developing rapidly. Much of what you hear on this topic will be anecdotal, so I've included below evidence-based information on some of the most common concerns.

Although many environmental factors are blamed anecdotally for causing miscarriages and fetal abnormalities, most of them are not based on specific evidence. A brief summary of those that cause most anxiety is included here.

CONTACT WITH CHEMICALS

It is almost impossible to avoid all contact with chemicals in daily life, but you can try to minimize your exposure to them.

▶ **In your home** Avoid inhaling vapours from petrol, glue, cleaning fluids, volatile paints, household aerosols, and oven cleaners. Read the labels on any chemicals that you are thinking of using and if you are unsure about safety, don't use them. If you are stripping old paint and redecorating your house, keep the rooms well ventilated. If you think that the paint you are removing is so old that it may contain lead, delegate the decorating to someone else.

▶ **In the workplace** A wide variety of solvents used in manufacturing industries can be the cause of problems to pregnant women who are overly exposed to them during their work. Fat-soluble organic solvents, found in paints, pesticides, adhesives, lacquers, and cleaning agents, can cross the placenta and inhaling these compounds may lead to complications.

Women at risk are those working in factories, dry cleaners, pharmacies, laboratories, garages, funeral parlours, carpentry workshops, and artists' studios, to name but a few. However, a recent study concluded that potential damage can be avoided if employers provide well-ventilated working premises and pregnant women are vigilant about wearing protective clothing and avoiding fume-filled areas.

One last point about chemicals: if your partner uses any of the above chemicals and/or vinyl chloride (found in plaster) in his work, avoid handling his overalls while you are pregnant. The same applies to clothes contaminated by pesticides.

X-RAYS

Large doses of ionizing radiation are known to cause problems in the fetus, and as a result, doctors are rightly concerned about the potential problems of X-rays during pregnancy. However, it is important to know that modern X-ray machines emit much less radiation than they used to and focus much more accurately on the part of the body being investigated.

The only risk of fetal abnormality would occur if you had undergone a series of abdominal or pelvic X-rays (at least eight) before week eight of pregnancy, and even then, the risk is only 0.1 per cent (one in 1,000 cases). A single chest or abdominal X-ray will cause no harm, so even if you unwittingly had one when you were pregnant, rest assured that it will not have damaged your baby.

The other point to mention is that there are some problems in pregnancy that really do need to be investigated with X-rays. If this proves to be the case, it is highly unlikely that they will cause harm.

If you work in a hospital you will be required to wear a protective lead jacket whenever you are in contact with X-rays. Female radiographers are usually moved to other duties in their department while pregnant, although the risks to their baby are negligible because of the strict safety rules that apply at all times.

VIDEO DISPLAY TERMINALS

Even if your job demands that you work in front of a VDT screen for long periods of time each day, your baby is not at risk. Similarly, equipment that produces ultraviolet and infrared radiation, such as laser printers and photocopiers (and the microwave in the kitchen), is safe to use in pregnancy. There is also nothing to support the allegation that miscarriage and pregnancy problems are more common in women who live near electrical substations, electromagnetic fields, radio stations, and telephone masts. Ignore scare stories about them.

MOBILE TELEPHONES

Our use of mobile telephone technology has exploded over recent years, giving rise to concerns that it may lead to various health problems. Fortunately, the fears that exposure to radiofrequency radiation in the part of the head closest to the phone may result in an increase in brain tumours have been unfounded. Similarly, the suggestion that the babies of mothers who are regular mobile phone users during their pregnancies have more behavioural problems and hyperactivity syndrome in infancy and are more likely to develop childhood cancers is weak.

The specific absorption rate (SAR) value of your phone is the amount of radiation that your body absorbs when you are using the phone. The amount of energy emitted by your phone depends on how strong the signal is. The more powerful the signal the less energy your phone needs to work and the lower the SAR value. So only using your phone when you have a strong signal is one way to reduce the level of radiation you are exposed to.

SAFETY OF ULTRASOUND

One of the questions I am asked most frequently by my patients is whether they should be concerned about ultrasound, particularly if they have early pregnancy problems that require repeated ultrasound examinations. Happily, I feel confident in stating that ultrasound causes no problems for mother or baby, thanks to several studies that have looked carefully at this issue.

Although it has been suggested that ultrasound waves might cause changes in the membranes of cells, theoretically affecting the development of the embryo and later growth of the fetus, there is no scientific evidence to support this claim. A Swedish study found no association between repeated pregnancy scans and childhood leukaemia. Several other large studies followed up babies who had been scanned on many occasions during pregnancy and found no serious developmental abnormalities.

On a more functional level, many women worry that the vaginal ultrasound probes used to scan in early pregnancy may cause them to bleed, or aggravate a pregnancy that is threatening to miscarry. This is not the case, and avoiding a vaginal scan may mean missing out on vital information about your pregnancy.

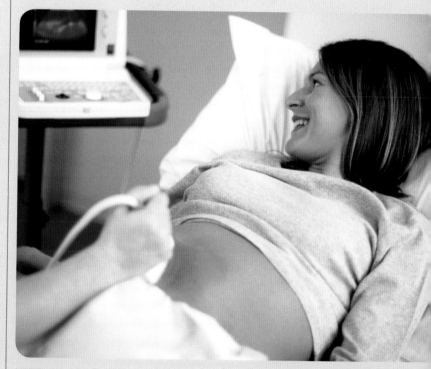

ULTRASOUND Even if you need repeated scans, they will not harm your baby.

Illness during pregnancy

Staying well can never be entirely within your control, but while you are pregnant, you need to be even more cautious than usual about avoiding infections – especially in the first three months.

Of course, this is much easier said than done and as many as 1 in 20 pregnant women contract an infection during pregnancy. This may seem an alarming figure, but the majority of these infections are completely harmless. Only a small number are capable of causing damage to the fetus or the newborn baby.

Since the majority of viral infections are caught from other people, the only way to avoid them completely is to become a hermit – not a practical solution. Young children are one of the commonest reservoirs of infection, so it is sensible to minimize your contact with any child who has a rash or unexplained fever. If you work with young children, the very least you can do is insist that any child with a fever is sent home promptly.

Childhood infections

The two serious viral infections for pregnant women are common childhood infections – chickenpox (see p.412) and rubella, also known as German measles (see p.412). Chickenpox increases the risk of miscarriage in the first eight weeks of pregnancy and if it is contracted between eight and 20 weeks, carries a 1–2 per cent risk of congenital varicella syndrome – abnormalities affecting the limbs, eyes, skin, and brain, together with growth problems in later pregnancy.

If you are infected by the rubella virus for the first time when you are in early pregnancy, you are at risk of miscarrying; if the pregnancy continues, there can be severe effects on the fetus, including deafness, blindness, heart defects, and mental retardation. Fortunately, this is now rare, since almost all women and men in the UK have either had the infection or been immunized against it. Even so, your rubella status will be one of your first antenatal blood tests. If you are not immune, you will be advised to have a rubella vaccination as soon as you have delivered your baby. Meanwhile, you will need to take extra care to reduce your chances of becoming infected. Although rubella is a live vaccine and best administered to women before they become pregnant, I have met several patients who have become pregnant almost immediately after having the vaccination. Happily, I can tell you that there is a UK registry of women who have conceived close to a rubella vaccination, and no abnormalities

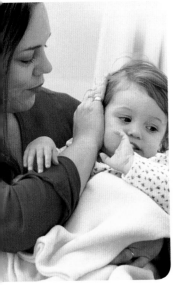

AVOIDING INFECTIONS
It is impossible to avoid all contact with infections, especially if you already have a child.

have been detected in their babies. Mumps, measles, and polio are unlikely to be a problem for pregnant women due to the UK's vaccination programmes.

Whooping cough (pertussis) is a serious bacterial infection, which usually begins as an ordinary cold with a cough and then deteriorates into spasmodic bouts of severe coughing and wheezing, making it difficult to breathe. The characteristic "whoop" sound comes from the effort of trying to draw air over the swollen vocal cords. The highest rate of infection is among babies and teenagers, who are also at greatest risk of serious complications, which is why routine vaccination is recommended at two, three, and 24 months of life, followed by a booster jab in the teenage years. In the UK, all pregnant women are now strongly encouraged to be vaccinated between 28 and 38 weeks to protect their newborn babies who are unable to mount an immune response until they are eight weeks old. The mother is given the vaccine so that she will make antibodies, which cross the placenta and protect her baby until the first vaccination can be given.

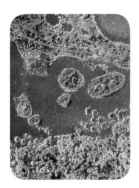

RUBELLA Virus particles are visible as pink spots in this blood sample.

Colds, flu, and stomach bugs

If you catch a cough or a cold, it is highly unlikely that your baby will be affected unless you develop a very high fever, which is a recognized cause of miscarriage in early pregnancy. Your doctor will advise you about safe drugs to help you reduce the fever quickly. Pregnant women who develop seasonal flu in pregnancy are at risk of severe illness, which is why the UK recommendation is that all pregnant women should be actively encouraged to undergo vaccination. However, I am conscious of the fact that immunization rates among pregnant women tend to be low because of fears about the safety of the vaccine during pregnancy. Happily, I can reassure you that the vaccine is inactivated and poses very little risk to the baby; indeed the benefits of vaccination far outweigh any possible risks. If you suffer from medical problems such as diabetes or a heart condition, you are in a high-risk group for catching influenza and it is particularly important that you have your annual flu vaccination, to protect you and your baby.

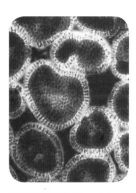

INFLUENZA The pink fringe around the core of each virus attaches to host cells.

The recent epidemic of swine flu in the UK has clearly shown that pregnant women and their babies are particularly vulnerable to serious complications from this respiratory virus if they become infected. This is why we now recommend all pregnant women to get vaccinated against swine flu, too. The drug Pandemrix is advised for pregnant women because only one dose of vaccine is required, which means that you will be protected more quickly, whereas the other brand requires two doses at least three weeks apart. Swine flu vaccine can be given at the same time as other vaccines. It cannot give you swine flu because it does not contain the live virus, although some women will experience a mild fever, headache, and muscle aches for up to 48 hours as their immune system responds to the vaccine.

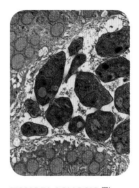

TOXOPLASMOSIS The single-cell, green parasites invade liver tissue (pink).

An upset stomach or gastroenteritis during pregnancy is best treated with rest and plenty of clear fluids, and is unlikely to cause problems to the baby.

Toxoplasmosis and brucellosis

Good hygiene around pets and other animals is especially important during the first trimester of pregnancy. The most serious potential problem is of contracting toxoplasmosis, a parasitic infection that is carried in the faeces of infected animals, most commonly cats. About 80 per cent of the population have already been infected but may not be aware of it because its flu-like symptoms are usually mild. As a result, most women develop an immunity that also protects their fetus. However, if you become infected for the first time during pregnancy, there is a risk that the baby could miscarry or develop mental retardation and blindness. Most people catch toxoplasmosis because they have inhaled eggs from cat faeces or have eaten unwashed vegetables or salads or poorly cooked, infected meat. Even though there is a good chance that you are immune to the parasite (particularly if you have a cat), always wash your hands carefully after handling a pet.

If you work on a farm or in a veterinary surgery, take precautions to reduce your risk of catching the bacterial infection brucellosis, which can be the cause of miscarriage. Avoid work that involves lambing/calving or milking animals that have recenty given birth, and wash your hands frequently.

> " Good hygiene around pets and other animals is especially important during the first trimester of pregnancy. "

Other medical conditions

If you have an existing medical or mental health condition (see pp.408–411), such as a heart problem, diabetes or bipolar disease, you will need special care during your pregnancy and should see your doctor as soon as you know that you are pregnant (ideally, you should do this before you start trying to conceive). Do not on any account take it upon yourself to discontinue taking any prescribed medication – see your doctor. If you underwent a surgical procedure before you discovered you were pregnant, you may be concerned about the effect of the anaesthetic or the procedure on your baby. In the very early weeks, the risk of miscarriage is quite high, particularly if you have a laparoscopy or similar procedure that involves placing instruments into the uterine cavity or abdomen. This is why fertility specialists always take particular care to ensure that the woman is not pregnant when performing invasive tests or diagnostic procedures. An emergency appendectomy also increases the risk of miscarriage. That said, I have cared for many women who discovered they were pregnant after undergoing surgery and suffered no ill effects. If your pregnancy survived the operation, rest assured that your baby will not have been harmed by the anaesthetic.

TAKING MEDICINES IN PREGNANCY

The information below can be used as a guide for treating a minor problem, but keep all medicines to a minimum and see your doctor if a problem does not respond to treatment promptly.

ANTIEMETICS If you need to take an antiemetic due to severe morning sickness, your doctor will advise on the safest types available.

ANTIHISTAMINES Some prescribed and common over-the-counter types are contraindicated in pregnancy. If you suffer from hay fever, skin itching or another form of allergy, consult your doctor before taking antihistamines. Most over-the-counter preparations are safe, as are nasal steroid sprays.

ANTIDEPRESSANTS Do not stop taking antidepressants before talking to your doctor, who may advise you that you should continue to take them during pregnancy to avoid a relapse.

PAINKILLERS Paracetamol is probably the best option during pregnancy. Avoid aspirin (unless your doctor prescribes it for a specific reason), ibuprofen (or other non-steroidal anti-inflammatory drugs), and ergotamine (migraine remedy).

ANTIBIOTICS If you are prescribed antibiotics for an infection, the penicillin, cephalosporin, ciprofloxacin, and Metronidazole family of drugs will not endanger your baby. If you are allergic to penicillin, erythromycin is a safe alternative. The antibiotics below should be avoided because they can cause problems in early pregnancy.

▶ **Tetracyclines** can cause discolouration and deformity of a baby's teeth and bones.

▶ **Trimethoprim** is dangerous in early pregnancy because it blocks the action of folate and may cause poor growth in later pregnancy.

▶ **Chloramphenicol** is used to treat typhoid fever, and can cause potential abnormal blood reactions in the baby. The chloramphenicol contained in eye drops or ointment will not harm your pregnancy.

▶ **Streptomycin** can cause hearing loss in the fetus.

▶ **Sulphonamides** are broad spectrum antibiotics that can cause jaundice in newborn babies and severe allergic reactions in the mother.

ANTACIDS Most antacids are effective and safe to use to treat heartburn and indigestion (see p.187). If you need iron tablets (see p.48) take them separately because antacids reduce their absorption.

ANTIHYPERTENSIVES If you are taking medication for high blood pressure, ask your doctor whether you should change your drugs, ideally before you become pregnant. Never stop your drugs without seeking advice.

LAXATIVES Constipation can be treated by adding fibre to your diet and by drinking plenty of water (see p.187). If you need to take a laxative, opt for the bulk-forming cellulose types such as Fybogel. Avoid senna-based laxatives: they irritate the gut, which has the potential to trigger uterine contractions.

DIURETICS Some fluid retention is to be expected in pregnancy and you should not take diuretics, including "natural" herbal types, in an attempt to deal with it. If your legs, feet or fingers become very swollen this can be a sign of pre-eclampsia (see p.426) – see your doctor straight away.

COLD AND FLU REMEDIES Read the labels carefully because most contain antihistamines and caffeine, which should be avoided in pregnancy. Taking paracetamol and a hot drink is usually just as effective.

STEROIDS Creams containing steroids for skin disorders should be used sparingly but are unlikely to cause problems. Steroid inhalers for asthma (see p.409) are trouble-free. If you are taking oral steroids for a disorder such as Crohn's disease (see p.409), see your doctor for advice. Anabolic (body-building) steroids should never be used in pregnancy as they can have a masculinizing effect on a female fetus.

COMPLEMENTARY THERAPIES If you decide to use a complementary therapy to treat some of the side effects of pregnancy, make sure that you see a qualified practitioner (see pp.437–8).

TROUBLE-FREE TRAVEL

Judging by the number of questions I am asked about the safety of travelling when pregnant, this is an issue that is at the top of most women's list of concerns. However, there is no evidence to suggest that travel increases your own or your baby's risk of potential complications.

Whenever and however you travel, it makes sense to plan your trips. Long car journeys can be tiring, so arrange regular stops to stretch your legs and get some fresh air.

Driving should not be a problem as long as you feel comfortable behind the wheel. Do not listen to scare stories about seat belts pressing on your uterus and unborn baby: you are both much safer behind a seat belt than not. However, three-point seat belts with the straps placed above and below your "bump" are best. Your journey to and from work can sometimes turn out to be the most stressful of all, especially if you commute. If you have to stand during a long bus or train journey, ask for a seat. Even in early pregnancy, you may feel tired and nauseous and just as desperate to sit down as you will be later on in pregnancy.

AIR TRAVEL

Freak accidents and terrorist attacks aside, I do not think that air travel needs to be avoided in normal pregnancies. However, long-haul flights do increase the risk of deep vein thrombosis. Fitted compression stockings are effective at reducing this risk. You may have heard that reduced cabin pressure can adversely affect a pregnancy, but this notion is difficult to explain scientifically. Your baby is surrounded by a thick muscular uterine wall and a pool of amniotic fluid, which protects it from any physical damage. Furthermore, the changes in your blood circulation and respiratory systems will ensure that your baby receives enough oxygen and nutrients, even if the oxygen supply in the outside world is a little lower than usual.

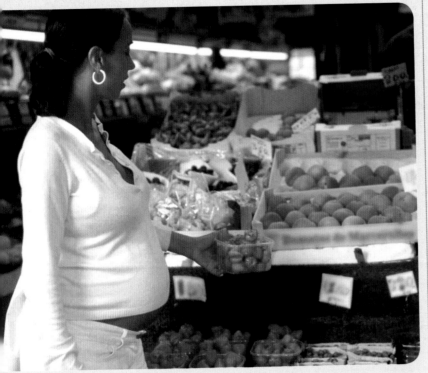

BUYING FRUIT Even the most enticing market fruits should be peeled or washed.

However, if you have had previous miscarriages, there are considerations about travel in general, and particularly air travel, to think about. Travelling by air will not cause you to miscarry, but you may not want to expose yourself to a situation where you would worry that you might be to blame should something go wrong. Miscarrying in the middle of a transatlantic flight, or in a foreign country where you do not speak the language, is something that needs to be avoided whenever possible. Most airlines do not accept pregnant women after the 34th week of pregnancy, but not, as is often assumed, because the mother's lower oxygen levels are likely to induce labour. It is because some 10 per cent of women deliver prematurely, and airlines wish to avoid the risk of dealing with this mid flight. (For more advice on travel in the third trimester see p.251.)

FOREIGN TRIPS

If you are planning a trip abroad, make sure you have valid medical insurance and find out where to seek medical help while you are away. Check on Foreign Office websites and helplines (see p.437) or ask your doctor whether or not you are at risk of endemic infections. If at all possible, avoid travelling to countries where malaria is rife because the high fever that accompanies the infection increases the risk of miscarriage. During pregnancy, you are more likely to catch malaria, which will often be more severe and unpredictable than is normal. This is because your immune response alters in pregnancy.

If your trip to a malarial zone is unavoidable, make sure that you take anti-malarial tablets and continue taking them after you leave the country and for as long as is recommended after your trip. New anti-malarial drugs are continually coming onto the market so talk to your doctor about which drugs are safe in pregnancy. As a general rule of thumb:

▶ Chloroquine will not harm your baby, nor will Proguanil if you take folate supplements at the same time.
▶ Mefloquin and Maloprim should be avoided in the first 12 weeks of pregnancy, but if you have taken these drugs already, do not panic. The most important thing to remember is that a malarial infection is far more likely

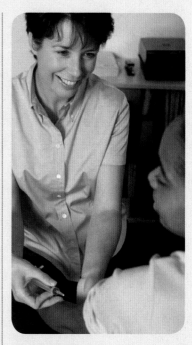

IMMUNIZATION Your doctor will advise which travel vaccines are safe.

to cause problems in pregnancy than the drugs you have taken to prevent infection.

TRAVEL IMMUNIZATION

You also need to check which, if any, immunizations are recommended for your destination and whether any of them are contraindicated in pregnancy. Your altered immune response in pregnancy makes immunization more unpredictable: vaccines prepared with live viruses are best avoided. Cholera, polio, rabies, and tetanus vaccinations are safe, but the safety of yellow fever and typhoid vaccinations is unclear.

For the latest advice on anti-malarial drugs and immunization contact the Hospital for Tropical Diseases (see p.438).

TIPS FOR STAYING WELL ABROAD

▶ Be meticulous about washing your hands before you eat.
▶ Drink plenty of bottled water, particularly in hot climates.
▶ Avoid unpasteurized foods and shellfish.
▶ Resist the temptation to buy delicacies from market stalls (they may have been recycled or reheated, and may contain harmful bacteria).
▶ Peel fruit and avoid watermelons, which are often spiked and then immersed in water to make them larger and juicier.
▶ Refuse ice in drinks – it may be made from contaminated water.

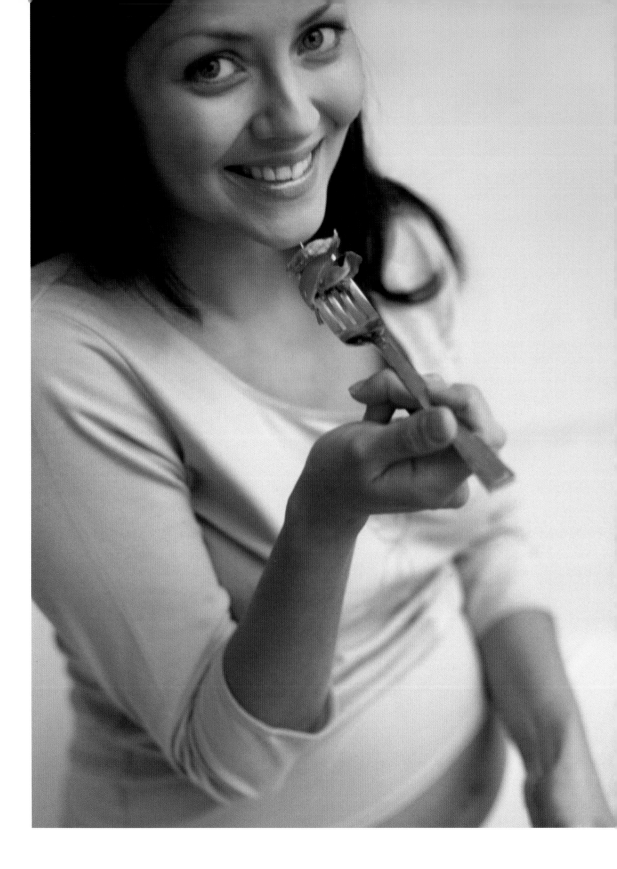

Diet and exercise

LIKE MANY WOMEN NOWADAYS, you probably started to improve your diet and fitness levels while you were trying to conceive – but if that is not the case, this is the time to start. Both you and your baby will reap the benefits. Most of the information you need is included here, but there are also additional features on diet and exercise specific to your particular stage of pregnancy in the sections covering each trimester.

From the moment you conceive, your body provides all your baby's nutrients. From now until the birth, everything you eat will be broken down into molecules that pass from your own bloodstream into your baby's via the placenta. Until after the birth, you will breathe and eat for your baby so it is important that you try to do the very best that you can. This is a major responsibility and I am well aware that the topic of what you should be eating during your pregnancy can be a source of anxiety. Without becoming obsessive about amounts and portions, you need to know what to eat to meet all those basic requirements, as well as which foods are better avoided. You should find most of the answers that you need in this section.

Being pregnant also raises a host of new questions about fitness. Whether you have an established exercise regime or whether you are not quite as committed to going to the gym or walking to work as you hoped that you might be, you are likely to be wondering what sort of physical activity you should be doing now. All sorts of myths suddenly crawl out of the woodwork: don't get too hot – it harms the baby; don't jump around – you'll miscarry; don't do sit-ups – you'll cramp your baby's growth. Ideas such as these, based on a mixture of anecdote and misconception, used to be passed down through the generations without much questioning of the wisdom behind them. However, we are fortunate that our knowledge and thinking on the subject of exercise in the first trimester has evolved considerably in recent decades. So while in your mother's day, the idea of playing a game of tennis during early pregnancy would have raised eyebrows, nowadays, doctors advise the majority of pregnant women that moderate exercise throughout the nine months is of positive benefit. However, you should avoid high-impact sports, contact sports, and scuba diving.

> 66
> ...all sorts of myths about diet and exercise suddenly crawl out of the woodwork. 99

Your pregnancy weight

As with all pregnancy topics, well-meaning but unsought advice on diet will be given to you in bucketfuls – much of it conflicting and confusing. The one thing that is certain is that this is a time in your life when you really do need to eat sensibly and healthily.

The first thing to understand is that the old adage of "eating for two" is a sure recipe for problems. You really do not need to eat more than 2,000 calories a day (the same as any non-pregnant woman) in the first trimester of pregnancy, the reason being that as soon as your body recognizes you are pregnant, your metabolism changes in order to make the most efficient use of the food that you eat. Extra calories will not benefit your developing baby and will simply be deposited as fat, which may prove hard to get rid of after your baby is born. In the last trimester you may need to increase your calorie intake, but by no more than 200–300 calories per day, which is the equivalent of a banana and a glass of milk.

At the other end of the scale, women who have spent most of their adult lives watching their weight and continually dieting may require a major shift in their psychology during pregnancy. The Western obsession with body image can make it difficult for some women to accept that they will be putting on around 14kg (two stones) in weight over the next few months. Now that you are pregnant, cranky faddish diets are out, and proper meals and healthy portions of food are definitely in. Studies of women with malnutrition during pregnancy and while breastfeeding in Africa have shown that babies born in these circumstances have an IQ that is significantly lower than normal. The evidence is enough to convince anyone that there is no place for vanity dieting in pregnancy. Let me reassure you: if you eat sensibly and exercise regularly, you can have your former body back very quickly after your baby is born.

Now that you are pregnant, faddish diets are out, and proper meals and healthy portions are definitely in.

Your ideal starting weight

Ideally, you should be of normal weight when you are trying to conceive, because being significantly under- or overweight can affect fertility. If a woman's body mass index (see right) falls below 17, her periods usually become irregular or cease altogether, which often leads to delays in conceiving. There are also good reasons for addressing a weight problem now that you are pregnant. An underweight pregnant woman is at risk of becoming anaemic (see p.424), delivering prematurely or having a small-for-dates baby (see p.429). So if your BMI is less than 18.5, please consult your doctor who will advise you on how to reduce these risks (see p.42).

Obesity

In the developed world, the problem of obesity has now reached epidemic proportions and is having a major adverse impact on our general health and wellbeing. In the UK, the increased prevalence of obesity has resulted in more than 50 per cent of women of reproductive age becoming overweight (BMI 25–29.9) or obese (BMI 30 or greater). There is no doubt that obesity increases the risk of immediate obstetric and fetal complications at every stage of pregnancy, delivery, and the postnatal period. However, obesity also leads to an increased risk of long-term health problems for both the mother and her baby.

If you are significantly overweight or obese, you may have experienced conception delays and will definitely be at greater risk of miscarriage, fetal abnormalities, and less accurate antenatal assessments of your baby's growth and wellbeing, for example on an ultrasound scan. Later complications such as high blood pressure and pre-eclampsia (see p.426), gestational diabetes (see p.427), and thrombosis (blood clots in your legs) are also more likely and as pregnancy progresses you will become increasingly uncomfortable and unnecessarily tired. All of these antenatal problems, together with the fact that your baby is more likely to be larger than average, may lead to an increased risk of complications at the time of delivery. Obese women have higher rates of induction, failed induction, and poor progress in labour, and are more likely to experience anaesthetic complications, require a Caesarean section or instrumental vaginal delivery, or suffer an extensive perineal tear when compared to lean women.

After the birth, obese women are at greater risk of haemorrhage, endometritis (see p.433), wound infections and breakdown (see p.433), prolonged hospital stay, and deep vein thrombosis (see p.424). Their babies are very likely to be overweight, which increases the risk of shoulder dystocia and other birth injuries, low apgar scores, and the need for admission to a neonatal unit. In addition, these infants are at greater risk of stillbirth and neonatal death.

Obesity results in a disordered metabolic state. Body fat is not inert padding – it is an organ that is actively producing many chemicals and breakdown products which cause all sorts of short- and long-term damage to our bodies. The more overweight you are the greater the risks, which is why any interventions that reduce an overweight woman's pre-pregnancy BMI and limit her weight gain during pregnancy should be actively encouraged. So if you are overweight, taking care with your diet from this point onwards can really help to improve the situation and will have no adverse effects on your baby's nutritional intake.

YOUR BODY MASS INDEX

The best way of knowing if you are either underweight or overweight at the beginning of your pregnancy is to work out your body mass index (BMI).

▶ **This is calculated using a simple equation:** your weight in kilograms divided by your height in metres squared (the power of 2, or times itself).

▶ **Most doctors use the following BMI ranges:**
Underweight: below 18.5
Normal: 18.5–24.9
Overweight: 25–29.9
Obese: over 30
Dangerously obese: over 40.

▶ **Here is the calculation** for a woman who is 1.7m (5'7") tall, weighing 65kg (9st 11lb):
$1.7 \times 1.7 = 2.89$
65kg divided by 2.89 = 22.5
This woman's BMI of 22.5 is within the normal range.

YOUR WEIGHT GAIN OVER 40 WEEKS

Although every woman's pregnancy is different, these guidelines for the amount and rate of weight gain over a normal pregnancy will help you keep a check on whether you are putting on weight too slowly or too fast in each trimester.

Your total weight gain should be dictated by your pre-pregnancy BMI. If your BMI is normal, you should gain 11–16kg (25–35lb) during pregnancy. If overweight, you should gain no more than 7–11kg. If you are obese your weight gain should be 5–9kg only. As you can see from the chart, there will be times when you put on weight faster than others. In the first trimester, your weight should change very little, and most of your weight gain will take place from the second trimester onwards. The chart is only a rough guide: allowances need to be made for individual women and their pregnancies. For example, if you are expecting twins, you are likely to gain in the region of 16–18kg (35–40lb).

WHAT MAKES UP THE WEIGHT?

Your overall weight gain is roughly divided into two different strands:
▶ **the weight of your baby**, the placenta, and amniotic fluid.
▶ **your own increased body weight** to support the pregnancy. This includes the increasing weight of the uterus, breasts, blood volume, and fat stores, together with a variable amount of water retention.

EXCESS WEIGHT

Most of the weight gain mentioned is governed by the natural needs of the pregnancy. However, the amount of fat that a pregnant woman deposits on her body depends on what and how much fat and carbohydrate she eats. Gaining 3kg (6lb) in body fat is to be expected – 90 per cent of this will occur during the first 30 weeks and most of it will be shed during breastfeeding. However, if you lay down excess fat during pregnancy, breastfeeding will not shift it – it will continue to sit there, storing up trouble for the future.

AVERAGE WEIGHT GAIN

Baby	3–4kg/7–9lb
Placenta	0.7kg/1½lb
Amniotic fluid	1kg/2lb
Maternal fat	2.5kg/5½lb
Increased blood + fluid	1.5kg/3lb
Water retention	2.5kg/5½lb
Breasts	0.5kg/1lb
Uterus	1kg/2lb
Total	**11.5–16kg/25–35lb**

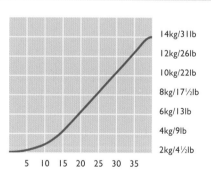

14kg/31lb
12kg/26lb
10kg/22lb
8kg/17½lb
6kg/13lb
4kg/9lb
2kg/4½lb

5 10 15 20 25 30 35

Weight gain over 40 weeks In a normal pregnancy, there is little gain in the first trimester. Most women then gain about 0.7–1kg (1½–2lb) a week until the last 1 or 2 weeks, when little further weight gain occurs.

The perfect pregnancy diet

The first thing to make clear is that there are two sorts of pregnancy diet – the textbook diet and the realistic diet that reflects your everyday life. This section is all about the second sort.

A healthy diet in pregnancy contains the right balance of carbohydrates, protein, fats, vitamins, and minerals. In this section I have listed the foods that are the best source of these essentials and explained why they are important in building your baby's body and helping to keep yours healthy. Having said that, I know that there will be times when there is some discrepancy between the ideal diet and what you actually eat, particularly in the early months when nausea and sickness can make well-planned eating nigh on impossible. Pregnant women are sometimes made to feel guilty and obsessive about diet and it is not my intention to fuel those sentiments. Women are led to believe that they will be harming the health and intelligence of their unborn child if they eat too much chocolate or have a day when the most they can face is a scone, a prawn cocktail sandwich, and a few pickled onions. I want to stress that if you try to eat as varied a diet as possible, you will be doing all that is necessary.

Protein

From the very early weeks of pregnancy, your protein requirement will increase by 15–20 per cent. Proteins are the essential building blocks for your own muscles, bones, connective tissues, and internal body organs and have the same key role in the healthy growth of your baby. They are made up of 20 different amino acids, 12 of which are produced within the body and so are termed non-essential amino acids. The other eight amino acids are referred to as essential amino acids because they have to be supplied from food. These are found in the right proportions in first-class proteins – such as meat, poultry, fish, eggs, and dairy products. Amino acids are also found in nuts, grains and pulses, soya, and tofu; these are known as second-class proteins because they need to be eaten in combinations to supply the necessary amino acids. If you are vegan or lactose intolerant you will need plenty of these.

Not all protein-rich foods have the same nutritional value: some are higher in fat than others and some have additional vitamins and minerals. So while red meat may be a first-class source of protein, it contains much more fat than chicken and fish. Fish is low in fat and high in vitamins, and oily fish, such as

> 66
> Pregnant women are sometimes made to feel guilty and obsessive about what they eat.
> 99

salmon and sardines, contains essential omega 3 fatty acids, which are especially beneficial for your baby's brain. Oily fish does contain pollutants, however, so you are advised to eat no more than two portions a week and to avoid shark, marlin, and swordfish, which may contain mercury. Cod liver oil supplements are also unsuitable in pregnancy because they contain high levels of vitamin A.

You need 2–3 servings of protein-rich foods each day, a typical serving being 85g (3oz) of red meat or poultry; 150g (5oz) of fish; 30–60g (1–2oz) of hard cheese; or 125g (4oz) of pulses, grains or cereals.

Carbohydrates

There are two types of carbohydrates, simple and complex. Generally speaking, simple carbohydrates, as found in cakes, biscuits, and sweet fizzy drinks are high in sugar (sucrose) and of little nutritional value. They give you a quick burst of energy because they are absorbed quickly into your bloodstream, but are only of short-term benefit. The only real exception is fructose in fruit. Since fruits are a good source of vitamins, minerals, and fibre, you should make sure you eat around five portions a day. Complex carbohydrates are found in starchy foods such as pasta, wholemeal bread, brown rice, potatoes, and pulses. They are the mainstay of a healthy diet, providing a slow and steady release of energy over a longer period because their starch has to be broken down into simple carbohydrates before it can be absorbed into your bloodstream. Unrefined wholemeal flour, rice, and pasta are good sources because they retain valuable vitamins and minerals and have a high fibre content to help prevent constipation. Include 4–6 servings a day of any of the following: one slice of wholemeal bread; 60–125g (2–4oz) of wholewheat pasta, brown rice or potatoes; 60g (2oz) of cereal.

RECOMMENDED PREGNANCY FOODS: HOW MUCH TO EAT EACH DAY ·······························

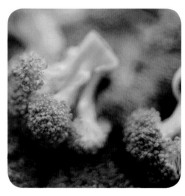

3–4 servings of vegetables such as broccoli and salad

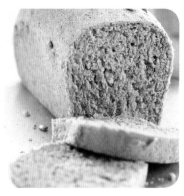

4–6 servings of carbohydrates such as wholemeal bread

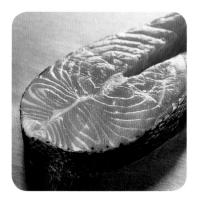

2–3 portions of protein – fish, chicken, red meat, and pulses

Fats

Although you should aim to limit your fat intake when you are pregnant, don't cut fat out completely. Fats have nutritional value in that they help to build cell walls in the body and supply important vitamins needed by your growing baby. Broadly speaking, dietary fats divide into less healthy saturated fats, which come from animal sources, and healthier unsaturated fats, sourced from vegetable oils and fish, which are important for the development of your baby's nervous system. Typically, fried foods and fatty meats and meat products such as sausages and pastries are loaded with unhealthy saturated fats. Eat too many of these and you will pile on extra pounds as well as encourage the build-up of fat deposits on the lining of your blood vessels, which increases your risk of heart disease later in life. For a healthy fat intake, trim the fat off meat, use butter sparingly, and choose low-fat varieties of dairy products and half-fat hard cheeses. Wherever possible choose foods that are rich in unsaturated fats.

Dairy products

Eating dairy products provides you with a balanced mixture of protein, fats, calcium, and vitamins A, B and D. Milk is a great standby in pregnancy so if you enjoy milk-based drinks include plenty of the semi-skimmed variety, which contains the same amount of calcium and vitamins as full-fat milk. Low-fat dairy products are preferable to the full-fat varieties, but some of the virtually no-fat varieties of yogurt and fromage frais are loaded with sugar and as a result are high in calories. Aim for 2–4 servings of dairy foods each day; typical portions are 30–60g (1–2oz) of hard cheese or 200ml (⅓ pint) of semi-skimmed milk.

> " Some virtually no-fat varieties of yogurt and fromage frais are loaded with sugar... "

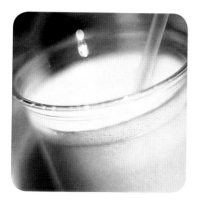

2–4 servings of low-fat dairy products such as milk

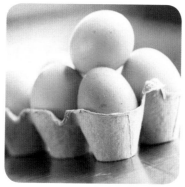

1–2 servings of iron-rich foods such as eggs and fortified cereals

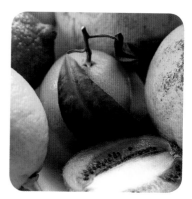

5 portions of fruit to provide fibre and vitamins

ESSENTIAL VITAMINS AND MINERALS

Your own health and that of your developing baby relies on a regular supply of vitamins and minerals, most of which have to be obtained from the food you eat. The chart below is a guide to the best sources. Vitamins and minerals tend to break down during cooking and processing so choose food that is as fresh as possible.

	BEST SOURCES	BENEFITS
VITAMIN A	orange fruit and vegetables – peaches, melons, mangoes, apricots, carrots, and peppers; green vegetables; egg yolk; oily fish such as herring	antioxidants; important for eyes, hair, skin, and bones; help fight infections; but, can be toxic in excess (do not eat offal or take supplements, which may harm the fetus)
B VITAMINS	poultry, pork, beef, and lamb; cod; dairy products; eggs; brewer's yeast; green vegetables, such as Brussels sprouts and cabbage; nuts, especially pecan nuts, peanuts, and walnuts; fortified cereals; wholemeal bread and pasta; oranges; mangoes; bananas; avocados; figs; sesame seeds	helps energy production and protein release from food; maintains healthy skin, hair and nails; essential for nervous system and brain function; assists in the production of antibodies to fight infection and red oxygen-carrying haemoglobin in the blood (B12 supplements may be needed if you don't eat meat or dairy food)
FOLIC ACID	green vegetables such as broccoli, spinach, and green beans; fortified cereals, pulses (peas and chick peas), and yeast extract such as Marmite	helps prevent neural tube defects in the fetus; aids red blood cell formation and protein break down in the body (400 mcg supplement recommended daily)
VITAMIN C	kiwi fruit, citrus fruit, sweet peppers, blackcurrants, potatoes (especially the skins), and tomatoes	assists growth and repair of tissues (skin, teeth and bones); aids iron absorption; antioxidant properties

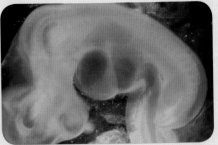

Folic acid Early in pregnancy, eat foods rich in folic acid such as green beans and pulses.

Fetus Folic acid helps prevent neural defects at a very early stage of fetal development.

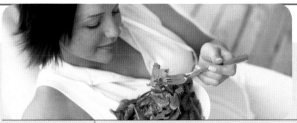

Food sources Vitamins and minerals are absorbed most effectively from food with little danger of overdose – any excess is eliminated naturally.

	BEST SOURCES	BENEFITS
VITAMIN D	eggs; oily fish such as herring, salmon, and sardines; butter; margarine; cheese; also provided through exposure to natural light	enhances calcium absorption; increases mineral deposition in bone. Women who have reduced sun exposure, and those with a BMI of over 30 should take a supplement
VITAMIN E	eggs; nuts, such as hazelnuts, pine nuts, and almonds; sunflower seeds; green vegetables such as broccoli and spinach; avocado; vegetable oils	maintains healthy skin, nerves, muscles, red blood cells, and heart; important antioxidant – protects against free radicals, which can damage body tissues
IRON	red meat; eggs; apricots, raisins, and prunes; tinned sardines, crab and tuna in oil; fortified cereals; sesame seeds (offal such as liver and kidneys is rich in iron but should be avoided in pregnancy)	essential for oxygen-carrying haemoglobin production in red blood cells of mother and fetus; builds and maintains muscles
CALCIUM	dairy products; eggs; small bony fish such as sardines; soya products; most nuts; fortified cereals; leafy green vegetables, especially broccoli	essential for healthy bones, teeth, and muscles in mother and fetus; also helps with conduction of nerve impulses
ZINC	beef; seafood; nuts; onions; sweetcorn; bananas; wholegrain foods (iron-rich foods block absorption)	necessary for growth and energy; aids healing of wounds; supports the immune system

Calcium Boost your intake of calcium-rich foods such as cheese in pregnancy.

Fetal skeleton Calcium builds fetal bones and teeth and preserves the health of your own.

Vitamins

Vitamins are vital for good health, both yours and your baby's. There are five of them in total – vitamins A, B, C, D, and E and, with the exception of vitamin D, all have to be obtained from the food we eat. We need about 40 minutes of light (not necessarily sunlight) per day to produce sufficient vitamin D. Vitamins A, C, and E are antioxidants, which have an important role in protecting the body from the damaging effects of free radicals – chemicals produced from the waste products of the oxygen that we breathe. Antioxidants help to mop up the chemicals and stop them injuring our body cells.

Some vitamins such as the B and C vitamins are not stored by the body, so you need to make a particular effort to ensure that you have an adequate daily intake when you are pregnant. Furthermore some vitamins, such as vitamin C, break down quickly when exposed to air and heat, which is why raw fruits or vegetables are preferable to the cooked variety in many instances. Similarly, frozen vegetables contain more vitamins than the canned variety, which lose most of their vitamins during processing.

Minerals

> When it comes to minerals, your baby will behave like a parasite, taking everything it needs...

Your diet also needs to include sufficient amounts of minerals and trace elements, the most important of which are iron, calcium, and zinc. These chemicals make an important contribution to the way our bodies function, but like vitamins, cannot be synthesized by the body, so have to be supplied from food. High levels of iron and calcium are particularly important during pregnancy because they help to support your baby's development. When it comes to minerals, your baby will behave like a parasite, taking everything it needs from your body's reserves, so don't leave yourself feeling tired and unwell because they have been depleted by the demands of your developing baby.

Iron is essential for oxygen-carrying haemoglobin in red blood cells and also helps to maintain healthy muscles. It clears from your body very quickly, so you need to eat iron-rich foods (see table, p.47) on a daily basis. Although requirements vary from woman to woman (and the best way to boost iron supplies is a matter of debate), what is absolutely certain is that your blood volume will double during pregnancy, so you will need more than your usual level of iron to protect yourself from anaemia (see p.424).

Animal sources of iron are better absorbed than the iron found in fruit and vegetables, although iron-rich food such as apricots and prunes have the advantage that they are also a good source of fibre, which helps prevent constipation. Pregnant women used to be advised to eat large amounts of liver because it is rich in iron, but it is now known that the high levels of vitamin A may cause birth defects. So avoid offal and liver products such as liver sausage and pâté.

An important point is that iron absorption is improved when iron is taken with acidic drinks that contain vitamin C, such as orange juice. On the other hand, both milk and antacid drugs reduce the uptake of iron, so have a glass of milk between meals and increase your intake of iron-rich foods if you need to take antacids for indigestion.

You do not need to take over-the-counter or prescribed iron supplements unless you are anaemic when you start your pregnancy or you develop iron deficiency during it. There is really no need to expose yourself to the common side effects of iron – constipation or stomach upsets – unless a blood test establishes that you have a low blood count.

Zinc is a mineral that helps to encourage growth and is also important in the immune system, wound healing, and digestion. Zinc absorption can be blocked by iron, especially supplements, so if you have to take these, try not to take them at the same time as zinc-rich foods (see table, p.47).

Calcium supplies are important for your bones and teeth and, while you are pregnant, your baby will be drawing all its calcium from you. This process starts very early on – your baby's bones begin to develop from the fourth to sixth week – so ideally you should make sure that your calcium intake is high before pregnancy and remains so throughout. The old saying that "for every pregnancy, a mother loses a tooth" has its origins in the fact that low levels of calcium led to poor teeth in later years. Even if you think you are eating enough calcium, do see your dentist. All dairy products are good sources of calcium, as are nuts and leafy vegetables, particularly broccoli (see table, p.47). An increasing variety of cereals and juices are now fortified with calcium and you might consider switching to these while you are pregnant.

Salt is used in high quantities in many processed and prepared foods, as it acts as a natural flavour enhancer and preservative. You can add a little salt to your food when you cook, but remember that too much salt can be harmful as it encourages fluid retention, which in turn may lead to high blood pressure.

VEGETARIANS & VEGANS

If you are vegetarian, vegan or allergic to dairy products, you need to discuss with your doctor the best way for you to obtain adequate levels of iron, calcium, and vitamin B12, in particular, as you may well be deficient in one or all of these elements. Vitamin B12 exists naturally only in animal products, although it is found in yeast extract spreads and fortified cereals. If you are a vegan, you may need to take supplements during pregnancy and while you are breastfeeding.

▶ **For a vegan diet** you can combine different plant proteins in order to receive your full complement of essential amino acids. For example, a handful of nuts or a portion of peas can be combined with a serving of rice or sweetcorn. To ensure you have enough iron, eat extra portions of haricot beans, cereals, and dried fruits such as apricots, raisins, and prunes.

▶ **If you are vegetarian**, you should eat more dairy products and eggs to ensure you keep up your intake of proteins, vitamin B12, calcium, and iron.

AVOIDING FOOD POISONING

When cooking involves little more than a ready meal and a microwave, it is easy to become relaxed about hygiene. In pregnancy you are more vulnerable to infections and need to be more careful about what you eat and how you prepare it.

Much of what follows may seem excessively cautious and I do want to emphasize that if you follow the basic rules of hygiene, such as always checking sell-by dates on labels and throwing away any suspect food, you would be very unlucky to be infected by any troublesome or potentially dangerous bacteria.

Having said that, some foods are known to carry bacteria that can be harmful to you, and sometimes to your baby as well. A severe episode of food poisoning can trigger a first-trimester miscarriage so it is worth being extra vigilant, especially during the first three months. As well as the precautions below, avoid eating raw shellfish.

SALMONELLA BACTERIA

These bacteria are found primarily in eggs and chicken. Infection causes vomiting, nausea, diarrhoea, and fever – effects that usually kick in within 12–48 hours of eating the affected food. Your baby will not be affected, as the bacteria do not cross the placenta, but see a doctor as soon as you suspect an infection.

Salmonella bacteria are killed by heat, so cook chicken right through and avoid dishes containing undercooked or raw eggs such as mayonnaise, ice cream, cheesecake, and chocolate mousse. When you cook eggs, make sure the whites and the yolks are both solid.

Note that free-range chicken and eggs are not free of salmonella, but a smaller percentage of them carry the bacteria than battery hens.

LISTERIA INFECTION

Although listeria infection is rare, it can have fatal effects on your unborn baby (see p.413). It is found occasionally in pâtés, unpasteurized soft cheeses such as brie and camembert, and blue cheeses. It can also be found in other chilled foods and ready-prepared meals that have not been stored to very high standards. Avoid these foods in pregnancy and stick to hard cheeses and those made from pasteurized milk (the pasturization process kills the bacteria). Cottage cheese and mozzarella are also safe. Drink only pasteurized or UHT milk. If you are in any doubt, boil milk before you drink it. Avoid unpasteurized goat's or sheep's milk and products.

E-COLI

This is another relatively rare bacteria that can be extremely dangerous to anyone who contracts it, as it can ultimately lead to kidney failure and death. It is primarily found in cooked meats and pâtés that have been stored at the wrong temperature. Again, I would advise you to avoid pâtés and to make sure that you buy cooked meats from hygienically proven sources. Always check sell-by dates, and if you are in any doubt about the freshness of a particular food, throw it in the bin.

TOXOPLASMOSIS

This is a relatively common infection, which produces only mild flu-like symptoms but which can be highly dangerous for your unborn baby (see p.413). It is derived from a parasite that is present in animal faeces, particularly cats' faeces, and is also found in raw or undercooked meat. While you are pregnant, make sure that you cook your meat right through and wash your hands thoroughly after preparing it. You should also wash all vegetables and fruit thoroughly (see opposite).

Should I take vitamin supplements?

The only vitamin supplement that you should be taking routinely during pregnancy is folic acid – one of the B vitamins that is particularly important during the first trimester of pregnancy because it reduces the risk of the fetus developing neural tube defects, such as spina bifida (see p.146 and p.419). There is some evidence that folic acid may also reduce the risk of other types of congenital abnormality and birth defects. Start taking 400mcg tablets of folic acid (available from your pharmacist) as soon as you know you are pregnant; if your pregnancy was planned, you may have been taking this dose for three months or more. A normal diet of folate-rich foods (see table, p.46) will provide you with a further 200mcg of folate, bringing your total daily intake up to 600mcg. If you have had a previous pregnancy affected by a neural tube defect, are taking anti-epileptic drugs or have a BMI greater than 30, you should be advised to take a higher dose of 5mg while you are trying to conceive and for the first 12 weeks of your pregnancy. This dose is only available on prescription.

Two other supplements that you might take (but only on the advice of your doctor) are calcium and iron. Under no circumstances should you rush off and buy other vitamin and mineral supplements "just to make sure". If you eat a healthy diet you will be getting all you need. I should add that your body absorbs vitamins and minerals more effectively from food – folic acid being the only exception. Also, by taking supplements you may overdose on certain vitamins, such as vitamin A, which can be harmful to the fetus in high doses.

> 66
> If you eat a healthy diet you will be getting all the vitamins and minerals that you need.
> 99

FOOD HYGIENE BASICS

▶ **Wash your hands** before and after handling food; take extra care with raw meat and poultry.
▶ **Make sure that raw food**, especially raw meat, is stored separately from prepared food to avoid contamination.
▶ **Use separate chopping boards** and knives for raw meats and wash both with very hot water and detergent afterwards.
▶ **Wash fruit carefully before eating**. Most fruit is treated with pesticides and ethylene oxide,

which is used to ripen fruit, has been shown to cause miscarriages.
▶ **Thoroughly wash** all vegetables and salads, peeling and topping carrots to remove all traces of soil. Wash your hands after picking fruit or gathering vegetables.
▶ **Take care to defrost frozen food**. In the microwave, turn the food around a few times so it is defrosted right through.
▶ **When you are reheating** previously cooked food in the microwave, ensure that it is really

piping hot everywhere. Do not reheat a frozen dish a second time round.

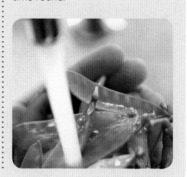

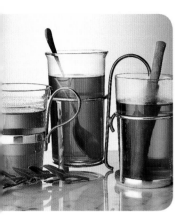

HERBAL TEAS These teas do not contain caffeine, which is best avoided in pregnancy, and many women find that they prefer the taste of them.

What to drink

Pregnant women need to drink eight large glasses of water – the equivalent of 1 litre (2 pints) – every day. If you cannot bear the thought of drinking so much water, try herbal teas instead. Fruit juice and milk are also good but not as effective as water. The better hydrated you are, the less tired you will be, since dehydration causes muscle fatigue, which in turn leads to a general feeling of tiredness. You are also less likely to suffer from constipation. Think of your kidneys as a waterfall – the more water you flush down them the better.

Caffeine in tea, coffee, and soft drinks is now on the list of substances "to be avoided in pregnancy", even though studies linking a moderate intake of caffeine to problems during pregnancy are, at best, inconclusive. However, a recent Italian study reported that more than six cups of coffee a day was accompanied by a higher rate of miscarriage. That said, so many women go off coffee during their first trimester, they rarely need any encouragement to cut down their intake. The problem with caffeine is that it acts as a diuretic, draining you of much-needed fluid. It also interferes with the absorption of iron, calcium, and vitamin C, thus negating all your healthy eating habits. Chocolate also contains caffeine, and however much you tell yourself that it also contains high levels of brain-boosting magnesium, it also contains too much sugar and fats to make it a food you should eat in anything other than small quantities.

How much alcohol?

Many of us drink alcohol – albeit in small amounts – and one of the most common questions I am asked is whether it is safe to drink in pregnancy and, if so, how much? There is no known safe level of alcohol use in pregnancy. New research suggests that even small amounts of alcohol can have a harmful effect on the fetus, so I would advise you to avoid alcohol consumption completely during pregnancy.

There is no doubt that drinking large quantities of alcohol during this period can cause fetal abnormalities. Alcoholic mothers put their babies at risk of fetal alcohol syndrome (see p.435), the effects of which are numerous and severe: the main ones include intrauterine growth restriction (see p.429), followed by failure to thrive after birth. When the child is a little older, other neurological and behavioural problems come to light. This syndrome is more common than people think and serves to illustrate the point that alcohol and pregnancy (particularly in the first trimester) do not mix. Not surprisingly, nature has an unerring way of pointing us in the right direction in early pregnancy, and many women cannot face the taste or smell of alcohol.

Exercise in pregnancy

There are particular reasons why being fit during pregnancy is a good idea. The next nine months are going to be a testing time for you physically so if you can boost your general fitness now, you are likely to cope much better with pregnancy, labour, and birth.

Why do we now advise women to keep fit during pregnancy and in what way do you and your developing baby benefit? It used to be thought that during exercise, blood flow to the uterus was reduced and this put the baby at risk, but many studies have shown that even strenuous exercise is of no risk to the baby, especially in the first half of pregnancy. Sufficient uterine blood flow is directed to the placenta during exercise and the uterine circulation is also able to increase the amount of oxygen it extracts from the mother's blood to compensate for the exercise requirements.

Female professional athletes who undertake endurance training at a high level during their pregnancy tend to have poor weight gain and small-for-dates babies. They are usually advised to reduce their training schedules in later pregnancy. Studies that involve monitoring the fetal heart rate show that usually there is a short period after exercise when the fetal heart rate and temperature rise, but that in neither instance is this a danger to the baby. The conclusion is that in pregnancy you can exercise at up to 70 per cent of your capacity (see box) without putting your baby's growth at risk.

Many women I meet are worried that if they continue to exercise in early pregnancy, they may precipitate a miscarriage. This concern has deep-rooted origins in the Western world: in the past it was generally assumed that strenuous exercise might disturb the implantation of a young embryo. The reality is that a pregnancy that is at risk of miscarrying will miscarry, even if the mother wraps herself in cotton wool or retires to her bed. Similarly, a healthy pregnancy that is destined to be successful will continue to be so and it will take a lot more than a few bursts of physical exertion to dislodge it. So do remember that exercise is very unlikely to cause problems in the development of

A SAFE HEART RATE

▶ **To calculate your personal safe heart rate** when exercising subtract your age from 220 and then work out 70 per cent of that figure. This will give you the rate of heartbeats per minute that you should be aiming for during exercise.
▶ **So, for example, if you are 30**, you will calculate 70 per cent of 190 (220 – 30), giving you an exercising heart rate of 133 beats per minute.
▶ **To find your heart rate during exercise**, take your pulse for 20 seconds, then multiply by three. Alternatively, consider buying a heart-rate monitor, available from good sports shops.

early pregnancy. If you doubt these words, then just reflect on the fact that, worldwide, most pregnant women are exposed to much more physical exertion in their day-to-day lives than the majority of Western women. Furthermore, the population explosion continues in countries where pregnant women are expected to undertake hard physical labour in early pregnancy.

> " *Worldwide, pregnant women are exposed to much more physical exertion in their day-to-day lives than the majority of Western women.* "

Benefits of exercise

As for the benefits of exercise in pregnancy, they are unquestionable. Doing any form of aerobic exercise, such as swimming, cycling or brisk walking, makes the heart pump faster than normal and so increases stamina. This means that your heart muscle is able to pump blood round your body more efficiently and work less hard at times of physical stress. This will be of particular value in late pregnancy when you find yourself climbing stairs with a great deal of extra weight around your middle and also during labour.

Anaerobic activity, such as pilates, yoga, isometrics or working with weights, is more resistance-based and is designed to exercise the muscles as well as improve flexibility. If you exercise in a gym, you probably do a mixture of aerobic and anaerobic exercises. The golden rule is that any sport you are already doing on a regular basis is safe to continue for the first three months, as long as there are no pregnancy complications such as pain or bleeding. You should aim to exercise regularly rather than in fits and starts, and make sure you warm up and cool down gradually and stop exercising if you experience any pain or discomfort. You are best placed to know how hard you can push your body and will instinctively know what your limits are. If you are feeling exhausted, it is your body's way of telling you to slow down.

What kind of exercise?

If you normally come out in a rash at the very thought of doing any exercise, but feel that for once in your life you are prepared to give it a try, then do not be over-ambitious. If you stick to activities you will a) enjoy b) not become bored with after two months, and c) be able to fit into your weekly schedule, you cannot go far wrong. Be realistic and you will be much more likely to succeed. Obviously, you would not be advised to take up a strenuous or difficult sport at this stage, so consider some of the activities below, all of which are safe to pursue throughout pregnancy. Whether you exercise regularly or not, you should think about including one of them in your fitness schedule.

Yoga is excellent for flexibility and general wellbeing (see opposite page). Choose a class that focuses on antenatal exercises rather than a general class. You will find yoga is a wonderful form of exercise in the latter stages

YOGA IN PREGNANCY

Many of my patients extol the virtues of yoga for its
all-round effects on strength and flexibility. Before you
start, ensure that the yoga class or book you choose
is suitable for pregnant women. Relaxation techniques
are quite safe to do.

One of the core components of all forms of antenatal exercise is relaxation. Learning a variety of comfortable positions and breathing exercises will enable you to recover your equilibrium when you feel overwhelmed by your pregnant state and give you some strategies to help you deal with the more testing times during labour and birth.

The key elements of any form of relaxation exercise are these:

▶ Find a time and place where you will not be disturbed, and lie down in a position in which you can remain comfortable for 5–10 minutes.

▶ Close your eyes, keep your head straight and your neck relaxed, and drop your lower jaw.

▶ Breathe evenly and effortlessly.

▶ Clear your mind of worrying thoughts or lists of things to do – this will take practice.

▶ Before you resume your activities, take a few deep breaths, roll on to your side and get up slowly.

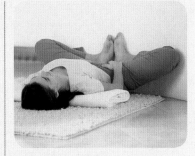

BUTTERFLY POSE Put your feet together against the wall and drop your knees to each side without straining, as wide as feels comfortable.

BREATHING TOGETHER

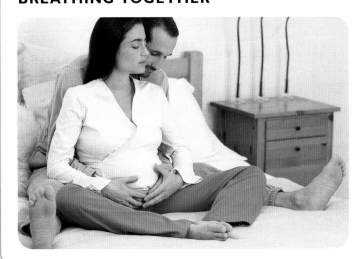

The belief that different types of breathing can help women deal with the pain of labour is central to many childbirth philosophies (see pp.248–9).

Joined breathing (shown left) is a yoga exercise designed to foster harmony between you, your partner, and your growing baby. Sit in a position where you can both place your hands comfortably over your baby and uterus. As you breathe together deeply and slowly, focus on the muscles of your uterus, taking care not to tense the muscles in the rest of your body.

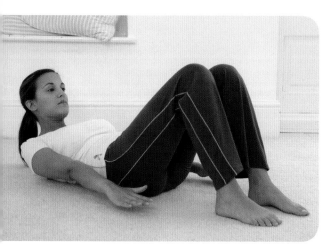

GENTLE LIFTS Head and shoulder lifts can be a good alternative to sit-ups during pregnancy.

of pregnancy when the delivery begins to loom ever closer and you are in need of relaxation. Yoga has the added benefit that it teaches you to control your breathing – a useful technique for the big day itself.

Swimming is the perfect three-in-one exercise, enabling you to develop your stamina, flexibility, and muscle tone all at once. Like most women, you are likely to find swimming wonderfully relaxing in pregnancy, especially in the later stages when all your extra weight is supported by water. Exercise in water has the added bonus of eliminating the possibility of overstraining any part of your body. The hardest bit is getting back up the steps and on to dry land and feeling the full force of your pregnant weight again.

Walking is easy to fit in as part of your daily routine – walking an extra 10 minutes on your way to or from work, or walking to the shops rather than automatically jumping into your car are good ways to start. You will find that your ability to walk longer distances reduces later on in your pregnancy.

Cycling is useful because your leg joints are not under excessive strain from your increased weight. It develops stamina and tones your lower body, so it is an activity that can be continued right through to the birth.

Adapting your exercise regime

During the first trimester, you are safe to do sit-ups, especially if you are used to doing them on a regular basis, although you should not do any more than usual. If you are not used to doing them, try gentle head and shoulder lifts:
• Lie flat on your back with your legs bent at the knees and your feet flat on the ground, shoulder-width apart. Your arms should be alongside your body.
• Raise your arms towards your knees while at the same time lifting your head and shoulders about 15cm (6in) off the ground. Do this exercise 10 times. If you have toned abdominal muscles they will help to support your bump, taking pressure off your back muscles and spine. The most usual advice is that you should stop sit-ups in the fourth month of pregnancy when your waistline begins to expand and the exercise may start to feel uncomfortable.

When you become pregnant, the level of the hormone relaxin begins to rise. The purpose of this hormone is to relax the ligaments, especially those in the pelvic area, in preparation for childbirth. Consequently, all your ligaments become looser, but this leaves you more prone to injury, should you put too much strain on them. Unlike muscles, which do regain their shape after the birth, your ligaments do not recover if you stretch them excessively. Bear this in mind if you do any exercise that involves lifting weights. After the first trimester, you should reduce the weights you lift to protect your pelvis and your lower spine from overwork and to avoid putting any strain on your abdominal area. This advice also applies to any form of heavy lifting, be it of grocery bags or toddlers. Of course, at times this will be unavoidable, so make sure you adopt a safe way of doing it (see p.193).

As your pregnancy advances

There are certain activities, such as squash, skiing, and horse riding, which are not particularly advisable for women to continue beyond the sixth month of pregnancy, largely because they carry the risk of high-impact injuries. However, if you are used to these sports and do not have a history of miscarriage, there is no reason why you shouldn't continue to do them during the first three months.

You can carry on playing sports such as tennis and golf as far into the pregnancy as comfort allows; you may have to stop when your tummy starts getting in the way, but it won't be because of a potential risk to your baby.

Your ability to withstand the biggest physical upheaval that your body is ever likely to know – labour and childbirth – is certain to be enhanced if you are reasonably fit, as will your ability to return to your pre-pregnancy shape. I hope you will not now rush to the gym and work out until you are red in the face and aching all over, but rather will make a vow to keep active and fit in the months ahead. Remember, too, that although moderation and regularity are key principles, so is your enjoyment.

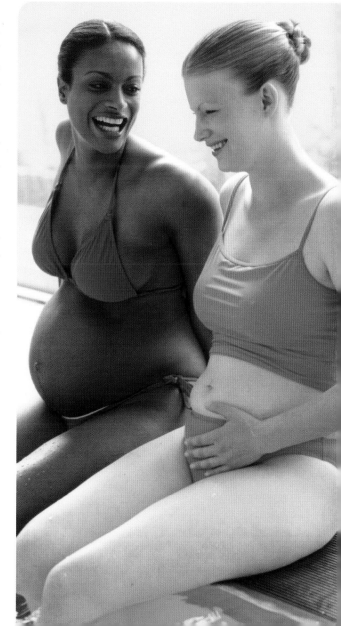

SWIMMING Whether you exercise in the water, swim lengths or float and relax, your buoyancy supports your extra weight and prevents damage to your ligaments and muscles.

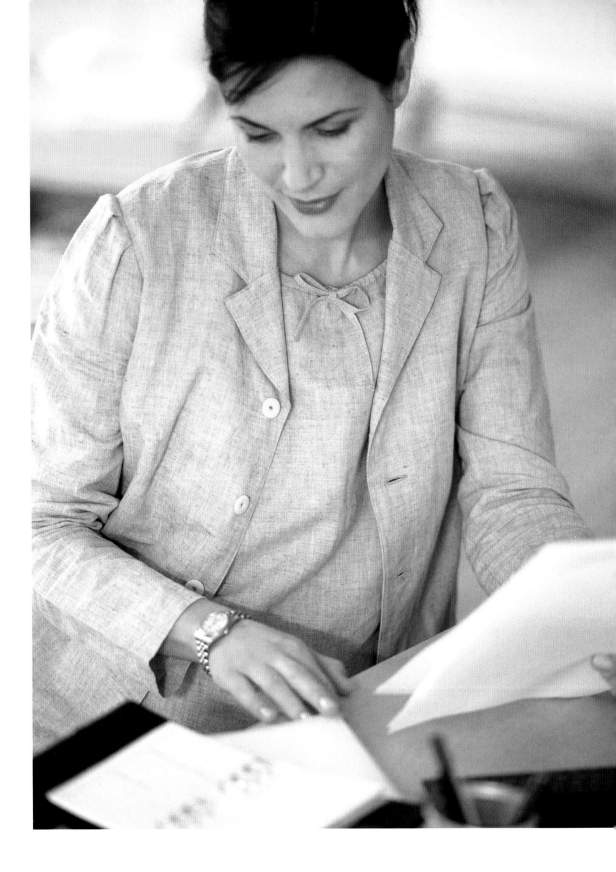

Work and maternity rights

BEFORE YOU GET ROUND TO TELLING your employer and colleagues at work that you are pregnant, you need to give some careful thought to the issue of your maternity rights. Now is the time to find out what benefits are available to you and make plans for working during pregnancy, timing your departure, and adapting your life after your baby is born.

Many women are justifiably worried that they will be perceived differently at work from the moment they announce they are pregnant, whether this is a first or a subsequent pregnancy. Some employers assume that you will be less committed to your career from this point onwards and so caught up in the exciting developments of your pregnancy that you will end up being less able to focus on your job. As a result, you may have serious concerns about your current job security and about your future career.

Rest assured that it is illegal to make a woman redundant while she is pregnant or to demote her after she returns from maternity leave. However, we have all heard tales of women who return to work and find themselves so sidelined and devalued that they feel under considerable pressure to quit their job. Fortunately, cases like these have become less common as the legal position of working pregnant women and mothers has improved.

Making plans

If you are aiming to return to your job after the birth, work out some clear ideas about what you want to do and explain your plans to your employers or colleagues. It is entirely within your rights to say that you intend to return to work after a certain period of maternity leave and subsequently change your mind. However, try not to vacillate between the two options – it won't inspire your employer to have long-term confidence in you.

Think through how long you would like to take off (you can always change the exact dates later on) and what you would like to happen to your job while you are away. There may be an established procedure in your workplace for maternity cover, but if there is not, you can help by suggesting how best to achieve this cover. Does an additional outside individual need to be hired? Can an existing colleague switch roles for a while? Don't undersell yourself

YOUR RIGHTS AND BENEFITS

Rights for parents have improved in recent years and
are changing all the time – this is a summary of the
current situation. However, your employer may offer
a better deal, so find out what maternity and paternity
packages are available.

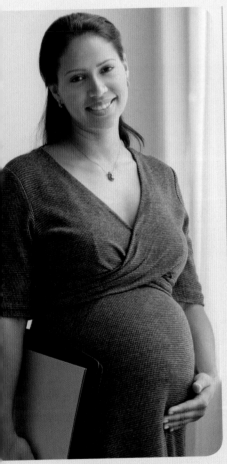

HOLDING ON You can work right up
until your due date, if you wish. But
if you are off sick with a pregnancy
problem in the last four weeks, your
boss can insist you start your leave.

STATUTORY MATERNITY PAY

If you have been employed full time,
part time or on a fixed-term contract
for more than six months, you will
qualify for up to 39 weeks of statutory
maternity pay (SMP).

▶ **You will need to have worked**
for the same company for 26 weeks
by the end of the qualifying week,
which is the 15th week before the
expected week of birth – about
the 26th week of pregnancy.

▶ **To qualify you must earn**
on average as much as the lower
earnings limit for National Insurance.
If you don't qualify for maternity pay,
you may be able to claim maternity
allowance (see right).

▶ **Your statutory maternity
pay** will be 90 per cent of your
average weekly pay for the first six
weeks, followed by the basic SMP
(or 90 per cent of your earnings if
they are less than this figure) for
the remaining 33 weeks.

▶ **Normally, your employer
pays** SMP in the same way as salary,
deducting National Insurance
contributions and tax in advance.
Your employer then reclaims most
of your pay from the Inland Revenue.
If you have more than one job you

may qualify for SMP from more
than one employer.

▶ **You can claim SMP** even if
you don't plan to go back to work.
If you plan to return but then change
your mind, you do not have to
repay it.

▶ **Women who are unfortunate**
enough to have a stillbirth have the
same entitlement.

MATERNITY ALLOWANCE

This benefit is for women who have
changed their jobs, are self-employed
or have had spells of unemployment
during their pregnancy. It is paid
directly by the Inland Revenue.

▶ **You will qualify for 39 weeks**
of maternity allowance if you have
been employed or self-employed for
at least 26 weeks during the 66 weeks
ending with the week before your
expected delivery date.

▶ **The maternity allowance**
you receive depends on your average
earnings: if these are at least equal
to the lower earnings limit you will
receive the standard rate of maternity
allowance per week, which is tax free.
If your earnings are below the lower
earnings limit, the allowance will be
90 per cent of your earnings.

▶ **The earliest you can begin** to claim maternity allowance is the 11th week before your baby is due. The latest date to start claiming the allowance is the day after your baby is born. Ask your local Job Centre or Social Security office for a claim form.

EMPLOYMENT AND SUPPORT ALLOWANCE

If you don't qualify for statutory maternity pay or allowance, but have paid National Insurance contributions in recent years, you may qualify for employment and support allowance for up to six weeks before your baby is due and up to 14 days after the birth. Ask your Social Security office or Job Centre for advice.

MATERNITY LEAVE

All women employees (regardless of length of service and salary) can

---

EXTRA BENEFITS

▶ From the start of your pregnancy and for 12 months after you have given birth, you are entitled to free prescriptions and free NHS dental care.

For details on how to receive your Exemption Certificate, speak to your midwife or GP.

▶ You also have the right to take reasonable time off for antenatal appointments and antenatal classes without loss of pay.

▶ After the birth, you may be able to claim child benefit.

---

take 26 weeks of ordinary maternity leave plus 26 weeks of additional maternity leave – a year in total.

▶ **If you qualify for SMP**, you will be paid for the first 39 weeks; the remaining weeks of additional maternity leave will be unpaid.

▶ **You can start** your maternity leave at any time from 11 weeks before your baby is due. However, you can choose to work right up until the date the baby is due, unless you have a pregnancy-related illness or absence in the four weeks before your expected delivery date. Even if you are only absent for one day, your employer is entitled to start your maternity leave.

If your baby is born before the day you were planning to start your leave, your maternity leave starts on the day of the birth.

▶ **You must by law** take a period of maternity leave of two weeks following your baby's birth or four weeks if you work in a factory or if there is another legal requirement for your leave to last longer.

▶ **Your employer is legally obliged** to give you exactly the same job after maternity leave or offer a job at a similar level and salary. If this does not happen, you can sue for unfair dismissal or sex discrimination. In addition, your employer is not allowed to treat you unfairly, dismiss you or select you for redundancy for any reason connected with pregnancy, childbirth or maternity leave. You have special rights if you are made redundant while on maternity leave.

PATERNITY LEAVE AND PAY

If your partner has been employed and earning as much as the lower earnings limit for National Insurance for more than 26 weeks by the 15th week before your baby is due, he is entitled to one or two weeks' paid paternity leave.

▶ **Ordinary statutory paternity pay (OSPP)** Husbands, biological fathers, adoptive fathers, same-sex partners or anyone with responsibility for the child qualify.

▶ **The two weeks of paid leave** have to be taken together within eight weeks of the baby's birth. Your partner could also qualify for additional paternity leave of up to 26 weeks.

▶ **Some companies offer more** generous paternity leave packages.

PARENTAL LEAVE

Parents have the right to take time off work to look after a child, make arrangements for the child's welfare or just strike a better balance between work and family life. Parents who have worked for at least a year with one employer are each entitled to take up to 13 weeks' unpaid parental leave per child, up until a child's fifth birthday.

REGULAR UPDATES

Rights and benefits are constantly changing. For updates, contact Maternity Action (see p.438), the directgov website or your local Citizen's Advice Bureau.

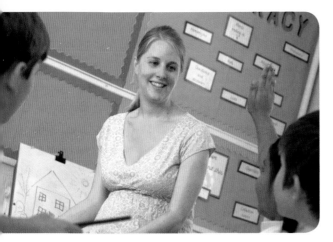

MAKING PLANS
Exploring options for your future working life will make you feel more secure and give your colleagues confidence in you.

by suggesting that someone can fill in for a couple of days a week or a few hours a day while you are away. First, this begs the question of what on earth you are doing for a full five days. Second, you do not want to return after your leave to find an overflowing in-tray or a catalogue of things that have not been done.

If you are self-employed, the ground rules are much the same as they are for an employed woman: be clear about your future plans; tell people how long you are taking off; and inform them of any maternity cover that will be arranged.

Part-time and flexible work

You may have already started to think about whether you want to work full time, part time or flexi time after your baby is born. Employers are obliged by law to give proper consideration to your request to work part time or flexibly and to try to accommodate your wishes, but you do not have an automatic right to these arrangements. Both parents of a child under six years old can formally request a change in their working hours, called "flexible time", and the firm must decide whether to agree to this within six weeks. If the answer is no, the reason must be given in writing. You can appeal and, if necessary, go to arbitration.

You may find that a precedent for part-time or flexible work has already been established in your workplace, but even if your preferred working option has never been tried before, it does not mean that it is not practical. Present all the arguments in favour of your suggestion and make sure you have ready solutions for any problems that might be raised. You may end up being a trailblazer for other women in your company.

When work is a hazard

Although some women worry that their work is potentially harmful to their unborn child, hard evidence showing the link between certain occupations and a risk to an unborn child is scant. The few types of work that are potentially hazardous are strenuous jobs involving long hours; shift work; jobs that require a lot of lifting or standing for long periods of time; and work that exposes women to certain chemicals or harmful environmental factors (see pp.30–1).

• If your job involves a great deal of standing, look for ways to reduce this in the second half of the pregnancy. This is not because long periods of standing will harm your baby, but they will exacerbate common pregnancy problems such as tiredness, backache, varicose veins, and swollen legs and ankles.

• If your work involves heavy lifting, you should first of all make sure that you always lift correctly by bending your knees and keeping your back straight (see p.193). After the second trimester, try to reduce the weight of what you lift and the frequency. If that is not possible, it is within your right to ask to switch to a less strenuous role until you stop work to have the baby.

• Working long hours or shift work is not dangerous to either you or your baby, but both become increasingly tiring, which can affect you both. You need to conserve your energy, particularly in the third trimester, so if there is no alternative to your current job, consider stopping work a little earlier.

• Some jobs, such as those in dentistry, medicine, and certain industries, involve exposure to chemicals, X-rays or other toxic substances. If you are in these sectors, your doctor or employer should be able to clarify whether your work is putting your baby at risk in any way. It is now standard for medical staff such as radiologists to switch to alternative work while they are pregnant. Similarly, airlines often ground their staff as soon as they become pregnant because of the slightly higher amounts of radiation they are routinely exposed to as a result of frequent flying. By this I mean long-haul journeys two times a week, rather than a few short flights, which are not harmful (see p.36).

RETURNING TO WORK   Q&A

▶ **Do I need to give notice to return to work after maternity leave?**
No, your employer must assume that you are taking your full maternity leave (including additional maternity leave). However, if you plan to return to work earlier you need to give eight weeks' notice before you return.

▶ **What happens if I need more time off work?**
You cannot stay off work after your maternity leave has ended or you will lose your right to return. But you can ask your employers if they will agree to a further period (you need this to be confirmed in writing). You may add any holidays you have accrued during your leave; use parental leave; or take sick leave if you are unwell.

▶ **I have decided not to go back to work. What should I do?**
Resign in the normal way, giving the notice required on your contract. If you do not have a contract, you should give a week's notice. You can work your notice as part of your maternity leave – you do not have to go back to work, nor do you have to repay any of the maternity pay you received during your maternity leave.

▶ **What dates do I need to be aware of to claim maternity benefits and leave?**
From 20 weeks of pregnancy you can give your employer a MAT B1 form (available from your doctor or midwife).

At least 15 weeks before your due date, tell your employer when you want to start maternity leave. To claim SMP, tell your employer at least 28 days before you intend to stop work to have your baby.

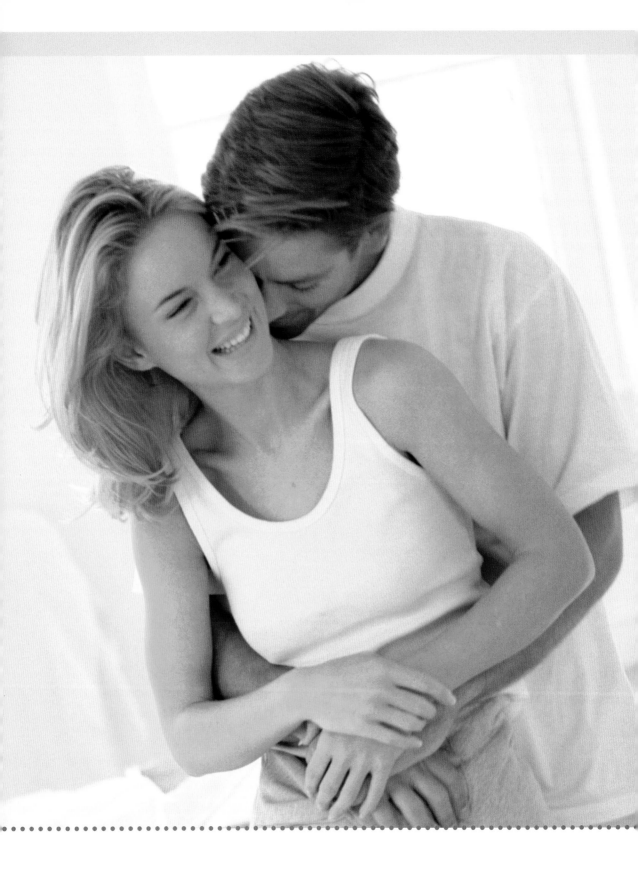

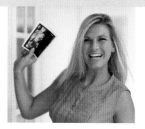

▶ **WEEKS 0–13**

The first trimester

During the first trimester, your baby will evolve from a cluster of cells into a recognizable fetus measuring about 80mm (3in). All the major organs, muscles, and bones will be formed. Until the placenta becomes mature enough to take over, your pregnancy is supported by maternal hormones, which also contribute to early symptoms such as nausea and tiredness. Although you may not look pregnant in the first trimester, you will almost certainly feel pregnant.

CONTENTS

Your baby

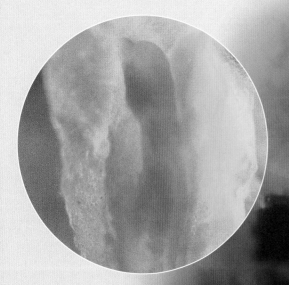

WEEKS 3–4

The brain develops from separate vesicles – within days these will close together.

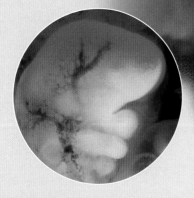

WEEK 5

The embryo has the beginnings of a profile with a bulging nasal region and a primitive cavity for a mouth.

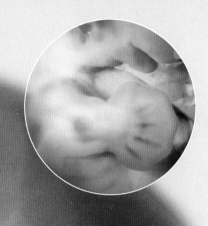

WEEKS 6–7

The fetal hand is a simple paddle with rays of cartilage where fingers will form.

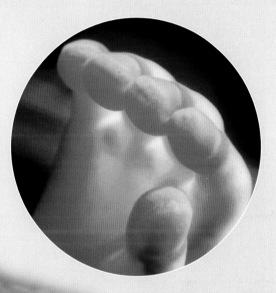

WEEK 12

The fingers are separating into individual digits and tiny nails are visible.

“ The embryo has tiny limb buds, which will develop into arms and legs. A balloon-like yolk sac (foreground) sustains its growth. ”

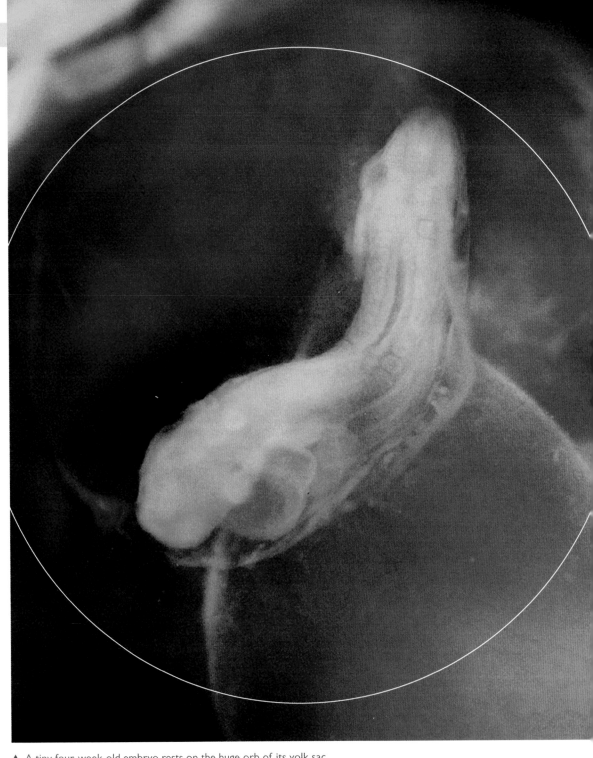

▲ A tiny four-week-old embryo rests on the huge orb of its yolk sac.

| 1 | 2 | 3 | 4 | 5 | 6 | 7 | 8 | 9 | 10 | 11 | 12 | 13 | 14 | 15 | 16 | 17 | 18 | 19 | 20 |

▶ WEEKS 0–6   ▶ WEEKS 6–10   ▶ WEEKS 10–13   ▶ WEEKS 13–17   ▶ WEEKS 17–21

▶ FIRST TRIMESTER   ▶ SECOND TRIMESTER

▶ **WEEKS 0–6**
The developing baby

THE FIRST SIX WEEKS OF PREGNANCY are an extremely creative time. Just three weeks after your last period, the newly fertilized egg starts to divide repeatedly to form a cluster of cells called a blastocyst. It floats down into the uterus and embeds itself in the lining.

At this early stage when you do not even know that you are pregnant, many of the foundations of your pregnancy are being laid down. This tiny blastocyst produces chemical messengers that will send signals to your body to prevent your menstrual period starting and prepare itself for the journey to come. At about the time of implantation, the clustered cells that will become your future baby have already become more specialized and have somehow acquired the capacity to know which part of the body they have been assigned to.

Three different layers of cell develop and each type will create different parts of your baby's body. The outer layer, or ectoderm, forms the skin, hair, nails, nipples, and tooth enamel together with the lenses of the eyes, the nervous system, and the brain. The middle layer, or mesoderm, will become the skeleton and muscles, the heart and blood vessels, together with the reproductive organs. The innermost layer, the endoderm, gives rise to the respiratory and digestive systems including the liver, pancreas, stomach and bowel together with the urinary tract and bladder. Once a cell has been directed or programmed to have a specific function, it cannot change to become another type of cell.

By the beginning of week five, the cluster of cells is just recognizable as an embryo and is visible as a tiny nubbin of tissue on the ultrasound scan. Although little bigger than a nailhead, all the building blocks for your baby's vital organs are already in place. The primitive heart begins to form and starts to circulate blood. At this early stage it is a simple tube-like structure. The position of the spinal cord has been decided and a row of dark cells appears down the back of the embryo. These cells then fold lengthwise and as they close together, they become the neural tube. At the top of the row, two large lobes of tissue become

10 x life size

At four weeks, the embryo measures about 2mm, roughly the size of this dash –. By the end of this six-week period it will double to 4mm in length.

visible, which will become the brain. A digestive system is in place, although it will be many months before it is capable of functioning. A tube now extends from the mouth to the tail of the embryo and from this tube the stomach, liver, pancreas, and bowels will develop. All of the above organs and tissues are covered by a thin layer of translucent skin.

What does the embryo look like?

This is the question that most women ask, and thanks to modern ultrasound scan techniques it is now possible to see the tiny embryo on screen and describe it. By week six, the ball of cells has changed dramatically and now resembles a tadpole or a rather odd-looking prawn. At the large head end, gill-like folds are visible, which will later become the face and jaw. The embryo's rudimentary heart bulges out of the mid portion of the body and by the sixth week it can be seen beating, or rather fluttering, on a vaginal ultrasound scan, although it is not always possible to see this if you have an abdominal ultrasound performed. Little bud-like protuberances start to appear on each side of the embryo, and these will become legs and arms. Very soon these limb buds will develop nodules at their ends and these will become the hands and feet.

The support system

As soon as the blastocyst starts to implant into your uterine wall, a support system for the embryo begins to develop. At this early stage, all its needs are met by the yolk sac, a balloon-like structure attached to the embryo by a stalk, which will continue to supply sustenance until the placenta is fully developed. The embryo floats in a fluid-filled bubble called the amniotic sac, which is covered by an outer protective sac called the chorion. The outer layer of the

EMBRYO AT SIX WEEKS ··············· · ········· · ···················· · ···············

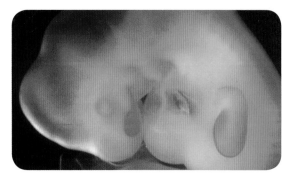

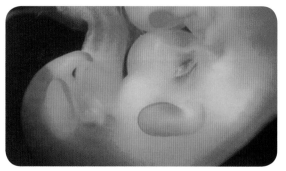

By week six, the beginnings of a nose can be seen on a head that nods over the bulging heart.

Two sets of limb buds will later develop into arms and legs. The body ends with a prominent tail.

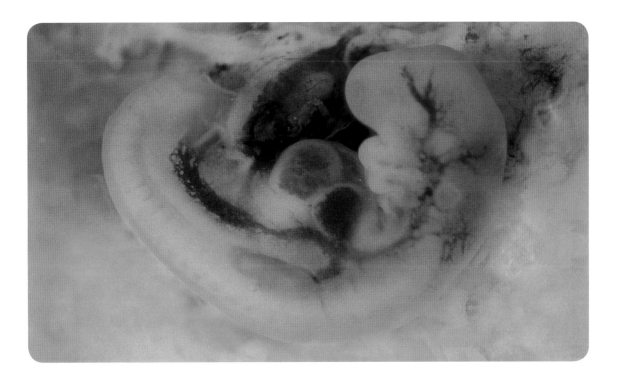

chorion will become the early placenta, and already little fingers of tissue called chorionic villi are starting to sprout and set up their future access to your circulation. Later on they will transfer nutrients and oxygen to your baby from your blood supply.

FIVE WEEKS
The embryo looks rather like an oddly shaped prawn, floating in a fluid-filled bubble called the amniotic sac.

Your changing body

In the first six weeks of your pregnancy you will not look pregnant and you may not be feeling pregnant, yet your body is already undergoing major changes in response to a massive surge in pregnancy hormones that started immediately after conception.

Even when your period is not due for another seven days or so and you are unlikely to have realized that you are pregnant, several changes are taking place inside you. Your body is producing a flood of pregnancy hormones. In particular, the levels of oestrogen hormone are higher than normal to help thicken the uterine lining and provide a rich environment for the tiny implanting embryo. The hormones human chorionic gonadotrophin (HCG) and progesterone help to keep the embryo embedded, and progesterone also ensures that your cervical mucus thickens and forms a protective plug, which will seal the uterus off from vaginal infections for the duration of the pregnancy. The overall size of your uterus is enlarging. When you are not pregnant, your uterus is roughly the size of a large plum, but during the course of your pregnancy it will expand to between 500 and 1,000 times its normal size. By the end of the sixth week of pregnancy, it will be the size of an apple, and although you will not feel any change, a doctor examining you internally would be able to feel the difference. However, it will not be possible to feel the uterus through your abdominal wall until the end of this trimester, when it rises above the pelvic brim and enters the abdominal cavity.

A boost in metabolism

> Some women are so sensitive to changes in their body, they know they are pregnant even before their period is due...

Not surprisingly, these early pregnancy developments are accompanied by significant changes in the way your body functions. Virtually every organ system in your body needs to adapt to cope with the increasing demands that your pregnancy will make upon it. Your metabolic rate rises by as much as 10 to 25 per cent during pregnancy to allow sufficient oxygen to reach the tissues of all the organs that are increasing in size and in their level of activity. To achieve this, the amount of blood being pumped through the heart every minute – the cardiac output – must increase by a total of 40 per cent before 20 weeks, and this adjustment starts early in the first trimester. This boost in blood flow to almost every organ in your body is already underway. The blood supply to your uterus has doubled and the increased blood supply to the vagina, cervix, and vulva results in these tissues taking on a blue/purple coloration, distinctive of pregnancy. This change in colour used to be one of the most common methods used by doctors to diagnose a pregnancy before more sensitive pregnancy tests were available. The blood flow to your uterus, kidneys, skin, and breasts will continue to increase until the very end of pregnancy.

To ensure that no area of the body is deprived of blood, the total volume has to increase from approximately 5 litres (8¾ pints) before pregnancy to around 7 or 8 litres (12¼ or 14 pints) at term. This process takes place gradually throughout pregnancy, but the volume of plasma, the watery component of the blood, starts to rise in the first six weeks to fill the newly formed blood vessels in the placenta and other growing organs. The volume of red blood cells also needs to rise to prevent the blood becoming too dilute and ensure that it has sufficient oxygen-carrying capacity, but this increase is slower and will not be noticeable until the beginning of the second trimester.

How you may feel physically

Some women are so sensitive to changes in their body that they know they are pregnant even before their period is due – and well before it is late or they have taken a pregnancy test. So you may know you are pregnant simply because you "feel" pregnant.

The sensation has been described as a strange and rather overwhelming sense of calm and fullness. For others it is a feeling of tenderness and tingling in the breasts that is much more pronounced than the usual symptoms that occur before their period starts. You will soon start to notice further changes in your breasts: they will feel heavier and look noticeably larger. Your nipples will continue to tingle, and you may see a change in the colour of the areola around the nipple, and the appearance of visible veins on the surface of your breasts. These changes are due to the high levels of oestrogen that are needed to provide a nurturing environment for the embryo.

You may notice that your bladder has gone wild and that you need to pass urine more frequently both day and night – this symptom usually continues until the end of the first trimester. The reasons for this are two-fold. First, the blood supply to the kidneys increases by about 30 per cent and results in more blood being filtered, which produces more urine. Secondly, the enlarging uterus presses on the bladder, which effectively reduces the amount of urine that can be stored because the bladder is prompted to empty itself at an earlier stage.

Tiredness and a tendency to feel over-emotional and tearful are common. These symptoms are entirely normal and merely reflect the fact that your body is dealing with a flood of pregnancy hormones to prepare it for the months ahead.

A heightened sense of smell

Many women tell me that a heightened awareness of smell is the first sign that suggests to them that something has changed in their body and that they are pregnant. It is not just that smells are stronger – they are also different. Similarly, you may experience a strange metallic taste in your mouth, develop cravings for certain foods and find yourself unable to stomach some others. I cannot explain these symptoms scientifically and can only hazard a guess that this is one way in which our bodies try to protect the tiny embryo from foods, drinks, and other substances in our environments that are slightly suspect, since this change in our perception of certain smells is often linked to a distaste for alcohol and tobacco, coffee, tea, and fried foods.

> " For many women a heightened awareness of smell is the first sign that suggests something has changed in their body and that they are pregnant. "

No early signs

Although some women know that they are pregnant even before their period is due, many others do not experience any early signs of pregnancy. Furthermore, if their periods are very irregular, they may not realize that they are pregnant for weeks or even months. When the embryo embeds further into the lining of the uterus between the eighth and tenth day after ovulation, there is sometimes a little bleeding; this can mislead a woman into thinking she is having a light period and is therefore not pregnant. The same is true for those women who, for reasons that we do not fully understand, continue to have light periods throughout their pregnancy. I know that many women worry if they do not experience clearly recognizable symptoms of pregnancy in the first few weeks and think this means that their pregnancy is weaker or at risk. This is not the case. There is no right or wrong way to feel at this stage of pregnancy and no one symptom – or lack of it – will have any bearing on your ability to carry a healthy baby to term. Signs and symptoms of pregnancy are very individual and, just as no two women will have an identical labour, no two women will have the same start to pregnancy or an identical journey through it.

PREGNANCY AFTER IVF TREATMENT

If you are undergoing in vitro fertilization (IVF), the treatment cycle begins by stimulating your ovaries with hormones to produce multiple eggs. These eggs are collected on or around Day 13

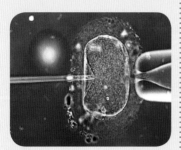

FERTILIZATION Intra-ctyoplasmic sperm injection (ICSI) involves injecting a single sperm into an egg.

and mixed with sperm in the laboratory (hence – in vitro). If fertilization is successful during the next 48 hours, two embryos will be transferred back into your uterus on about Day 16.

A blood test on Day 27 will check for raised levels of human chorionic gonadotrophin (HCG) – the first sign that the IVF treatment may have been successful. However, it is possible to have a positive test, only to discover, in a few days time, that the HCG levels have fallen because the embryo has not implanted successfully.

Your first ultrasound scan usually takes place 5–6 weeks after the start of the treatment.

All being well, there will be a small pregnancy sac visible in the uterine cavity. If no sac is present there is a risk that you have an ectopic pregnancy (see p.81 and p.423). Sometimes the scan reveals several sacs, suggesting twins or triplets, but quite frequently the extra sac(s) disappears (vanishing twin syndrome). Multiple pregnancies are at greater risk of miscarriage, congenital abnormalities, and prematurity, which is why IVF clinics are concerned to keep the number of embryos they transfer to the minimum.

A further scan at 6–7 weeks should show a fetal pole and beating fetal heart. Your pregnancy is under way!

Your emotional response

Undoubtedly your feelings at the beginning of pregnancy are very much dictated by your personal circumstances but if, like many women, you are feeling emotionally unpredictable, your surging pregnancy hormones are almost certainly playing a part.

As I described in my chapter on conception, the mix of panic and elation that you may be feeling from one moment to the next may not be simply a reaction to the new future that is about to unfold. Most pregnancy books explain that fragile emotions and tearfulness gradually settle down and become less troublesome, but I am increasingly of the view that they continue, since they are hormonally linked. Basically, we get used to them and, practical creatures that we are, we learn to ignore or accommodate them.

If your pregnancy was planned or has been difficult to achieve, you may feel on an almost permanent high in these early days and bursting to pass on your exciting news. However, for some women the knowledge that they are pregnant is something very private that they want to share only with their partner, or closest family and friends in the early weeks. Others, particularly those who have miscarried in the past, do not want to tempt fate by declaring to the world at large that they are pregnant, just in case something goes wrong, and prefer to wait until the pregnancy has progressed to the second trimester before announcing their news.

Deciding whether you want to tell other people about your pregnancy at this stage is a very individual issue and there is no right or wrong way to deal with it. As we all know, family dynamics are complex and only you will know the best way to break the news to your partner, mother, sister, in-laws or friends. The only piece of reassurance I can offer is that, by and large, most family members and friends will be thrilled by your news and the fact that you want to share it with them. Indeed, the only significant problem you are likely to meet, in my experience, is a deluge of well-meaning advice and offers of help.

Many women in early pregnancy tell me that they are concerned they will upset friends and family members who are having fertility problems, have lost a baby or experienced a pregnancy complication in the past. I think it is practically impossible to protect everyone you know from their own raw emotions and sad memories. In any event, they will have to come to terms with the situation sooner or later. However, I must add here that I am repeatedly impressed by patients in my miscarriage clinic and how generous they can be

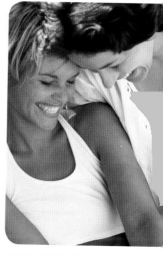

HIGH EMOTION
Some women are bursting to pass on their exciting news; others want to hug their secret to themselves for a little longer.

towards other women who announce they are pregnant, even when the news must bring them personal heartache. On balance, I think it is best to be open about the news that you are pregnant. I suspect that you will feel pleasantly surprised by the warmth of the response that you receive.

How your partner may feel

Whatever your decision about when and how to reveal your pregnancy, if you are part of a couple, your partner is likely to be the first to share your news. Remember that it is not only women who have a mass of conflicting emotions at this time – many men feel much the same. Although most will be pleased at the thought of becoming a father, I think there is a fundamental difference in how men and women feel about pregnancy in the early stages. For a start, men have nothing tangible to relate to in the first few weeks. Until a baby can be visualized on an ultrasound scan or can be felt and seen moving inside you, your partner may find it hard to feel as involved as you might want him to be. Women on the other hand are already conscious of the fact that a live baby is growing inside their body, they feel physically and emotionally different and soon they will start to look different too.

YOUR PARTNER
Becoming a father may be the best news possible or something that he needs time to come to terms with.

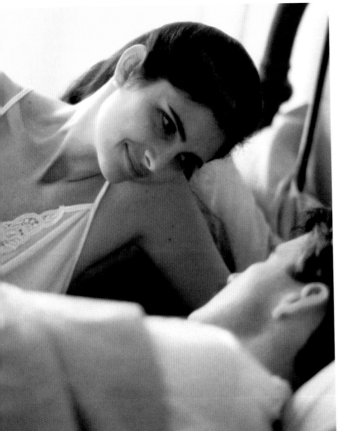

I do feel it is important to talk to your partner about how you are feeling, but it is all too easy to make your pregnancy the sole topic of conversation. Try not to feel disappointed or resentful if you find he is less than fascinated by your early symptoms and prefers to settle down with a crime novel rather than the pregnancy book that you are finding irresistible.

Just like you, he may need time to come to terms with the news and how it will impact on your lives. Remember he may be feeling very apprehensive about the responsibility that looms ahead, especially if you are considering living on his salary for a while. Although there are likely to be few noticeable changes in the next few months, he will be acutely aware that he is moving into another phase of life. Calm, relaxed discussions during which he can talk openly about his feelings will help to prevent any misunderstandings building up (on either side). So much of the focus during pregnancy is on the mother-to-be that your partner's opinions can end up being overlooked. For example, it is generally assumed nowadays that fathers should be, and will want to be, present at the birth. For some men, nothing could be further from the truth. Similarly, partners are often actively encouraged to attend antenatal classes. Great, if he wants to be included and is keen to join you, but pressurizing him to do things a certain way, or making him feel that he is letting you down if he does not immediately adopt the role of ideal prospective father, is likely to be the source of future conflicts. Having said that, don't worry if at this stage he swears blind that he is not coming to any antenatal classes and that you won't catch him anywhere near the delivery room. Believe me, most men do change their mind.

Having a baby on your own

Inevitably, much of the discussion in this book relates to women with partners with the general assumption that their partner is a man, but I'm conscious of the fact that society is a good deal more complex than this. Many readers will be embarking on their pregnancy alone and it is not my intention to make them feel excluded from this journey. If you have chosen to be a single parent, you have probably given plenty of thought to the way you will handle the next nine months and life with a baby. If lone parenting is something that has been forced on you by circumstances, you may be feeling overwhelmed by the prospect as well as by practical and financial considerations. The only general advice I can offer is that you should start to put in place a network of support now. Ask a relative or friend to share your pregnancy and to be with you for key events, such as the first scan, and for the birth. If this is difficult, find out about local antenatal classes for single mothers and single-parent support groups (see Useful Contacts, pp.437–8). Having close friends who share similar experiences can make all the difference.

WHAT IS HE THINKING?

The thoughts going through your partner's head may well include some of the following:
▶ Will our relationship stay the same?
▶ Will I still be able to go out with my mates/watch football/play cricket?
▶ What happens if one of us has to give up work?
▶ How much do I want to be involved in the pregnancy?
▶ Is she more fragile than she was before?
▶ What happens if something goes wrong?
▶ Do I want to be at the birth and what will I be expected to do?
▶ Will she give the baby all the attention?
▶ Will I be a good father?

66 Until a baby can be visualized on an ultrasound scan or can be felt and seen moving inside you, your partner may find it hard to feel as involved as you might want him to be. 99

Your antenatal care

As soon as you know that you are pregnant, make an appointment with your GP or midwife. It's a good idea to get to know your doctor at the beginning of your pregnancy, especially if, like most healthy women, you rarely see him or her normally.

Ideally, your first contact visit with your GP or midwife will be at 6–8 weeks (see p.161 for the recommended schedule of antenatal visits). The first thing he or she will ask you for is the date of your last menstrual period so that your estimated date of delivery (EDD) can be calculated. An average pregnancy lasts from 37 to 40 weeks from the first day of your last period, so your doctor will add 40 weeks on to that date using a chart or a pregnancy wheel. Much confusion and potential distress can be avoided if you always use weeks, rather than months, to measure the stage that your pregnancy has reached. The accuracy of the EDD calculated in this way will depend on whether you have a regular 28-day cycle. If yours is shorter, longer or irregular, the doctor or midwife will aim to adjust the EDD accordingly and may well suggest that you do not rely on this date until you have had your first scan, when the age of your pregnancy and your future EDD can be decided very precisely.

Your doctor or midwife may also carry out a few basic tests, such as testing your urine for the presence of protein and measuring your blood pressure. More detailed tests will be performed at your formal antenatal booking visit towards the end of the first trimester (usually at 10–12 weeks).

> Unless you have a specific problem, you will probably receive most of your antenatal care in the community.

Organizing your booking visit

This first contact with your GP or midwife will also give you the opportunity to discuss the options for care during your pregnancy. If you have had a baby before or have strongly held views on childbirth, you may know exactly what type of antenatal care you want and where you want to receive it. However, if this is your first baby, you will probably welcome a detailed explanation of what is available and some guidance as to which option is best suited to your individual needs. For this reason, I have included a comprehensive section on antenatal care and birth choices at the end of this section (see pp.84–91).

Your first formal antenatal booking visit will happen towards the end of the first trimester. This may take place in the community or hospital if you are high risk. You will be able to discuss your pregnancy with midwives and doctors, who will be able to offer you valuable advice as to how you can best achieve your aim.

YOUR ESTIMATED DELIVERY DATE

Look on the chart for the month and then the first day of your last menstrual period (printed in bold type). Directly below it is the date that your baby is due – your estimated delivery date.

January	1	2	3	4	5	6	7	8	9	10	11	12	13	14	15	16	17	18	19	20	21	22	23	24	25	26	27	28	29	30	31
Oct/Nov	8	9	10	11	12	13	14	15	16	17	18	19	20	21	22	23	24	25	26	27	28	29	30	31	1	2	3	4	5	6	7
February	1	2	3	4	5	6	7	8	9	10	11	12	13	14	15	16	17	18	19	20	21	22	23	24	25	26	27	28			
Nov/Dec	8	9	10	11	12	13	14	15	16	17	18	19	20	21	22	23	24	25	26	27	28	29	30	1	2	3	4	5			
March	1	2	3	4	5	6	7	8	9	10	11	12	13	14	15	16	17	18	19	20	21	22	23	24	25	26	27	28	29	30	31
Dec/Jan	6	7	8	9	10	11	12	13	14	15	16	17	18	19	20	21	22	23	24	25	26	27	28	29	30	31	1	2	3	4	5
April	1	2	3	4	5	6	7	8	9	10	11	12	13	14	15	16	17	18	19	20	21	22	23	24	25	26	27	28	29	30	
Jan/Feb	6	7	8	9	10	11	12	13	14	15	16	17	18	19	20	21	22	23	24	25	26	27	28	29	30	31	1	2	3	4	
May	1	2	3	4	5	6	7	8	9	10	11	12	13	14	15	16	17	18	19	20	21	22	23	24	25	26	27	28	29	30	31
Feb/Mar	5	6	7	8	9	10	11	12	13	14	15	16	17	18	19	20	21	22	23	24	25	26	27	28	1	2	3	4	5	6	7
June	1	2	3	4	5	6	7	8	9	10	11	12	13	14	15	16	17	18	19	20	21	22	23	24	25	26	27	28	29	30	
Mar/Apr	8	9	10	11	12	13	14	15	16	17	18	19	20	21	22	23	24	25	26	27	28	29	30	31	1	2	3	4	5	6	
July	1	2	3	4	5	6	7	8	9	10	11	12	13	14	15	16	17	18	19	20	21	22	23	24	25	26	27	28	29	30	31
Apr/May	7	8	9	10	11	12	13	14	15	16	17	18	19	20	21	22	23	24	25	26	27	28	29	30	1	2	3	4	5	6	7
August	1	2	3	4	5	6	7	8	9	10	11	12	13	14	15	16	17	18	19	20	21	22	23	24	25	26	27	28	29	30	31
May/Jun	8	9	10	11	12	13	14	15	16	17	18	19	20	21	22	23	24	25	26	27	28	29	30	31	1	2	3	4	5	6	7
September	1	2	3	4	5	6	7	8	9	10	11	12	13	14	15	16	17	18	19	20	21	22	23	24	25	26	27	28	29	30	
Jun/Jul	8	9	10	11	12	13	14	15	16	17	18	19	20	21	22	23	24	25	26	27	28	29	30	1	2	3	4	5	6	7	
October	1	2	3	4	5	6	7	8	9	10	11	12	13	14	15	16	17	18	19	20	21	22	23	24	25	26	27	28	29	30	31
Jul/Aug	8	9	10	11	12	13	14	15	16	17	18	19	20	21	22	23	24	25	26	27	28	29	30	31	1	2	3	4	5	6	7
November	1	2	3	4	5	6	7	8	9	10	11	12	13	14	15	16	17	18	19	20	21	22	23	24	25	26	27	28	29	30	
Aug/Sep	8	9	10	11	12	13	14	15	16	17	18	19	20	21	22	23	24	25	26	27	28	29	30	31	1	2	3	4	5	6	
December	1	2	3	4	5	6	7	8	9	10	11	12	13	14	15	16	17	18	19	20	21	22	23	24	25	26	27	28	29	30	31
Sep/Oct	7	8	9	10	11	12	13	14	15	16	17	18	19	20	21	22	23	24	25	26	27	28	29	30	1	2	3	4	5	6	7

It is often presumed (wrongly) that all obstetricians and hospital midwives are against home births. On the contrary, all they want to ensure is that both mother and baby are safe and that the mother knows what action needs to be taken should problems arise. There are good transfer systems in place if you need to be transferred from your home to a hospital during your labour.

Unless you have a specific problem that needs urgent attention, you will probably receive most of your antenatal care in the community. Indeed, most women will only need to visit the hospital for scan appointments. The exceptions are women who have been unlucky enough to experience a previous pregnancy problem, such as repeated miscarriages or a later pregnancy complication. If this is the case for you, your doctor or midwife will arrange an immediate antenatal visit and possibly an early scan. If you have an existing medical condition, such as diabetes, your hospital antenatal care is also likely to start sooner rather than later.

Many women used to feel disappointed that no one seemed very interested in their pregnancy until they attended their booking visit. They felt bewildered because there was no one to talk to about what to do and where to go to find out more about being pregnant. As one first-time mother told me: "I am very grateful that I am just a normal pregnant woman with no medical problems, but this is all new to me. This is a special time for me and I am out of my depth." This is why, ideally, most women are now offered a first-contact visit by eight weeks.

It is also one of the reasons why it is very important for pregnant women to be able to access as much information as possible both to reassure them and help them understand what is going to happen next. In an ideal world with limitless health-care resources, we would be able to offer women instant access to the antenatal care they choose at the moment that their pregnancy test is positive. In the real world, the best solution I can offer is an informative book.

Common concerns

You may already have a few queries about the early stages of your pregnancy and about your general health. These are definitely worth discussing with your doctor at your first consultation.

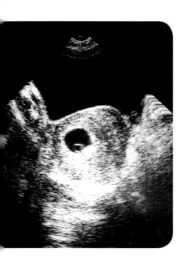

FETAL POLE The tiny embryo is just visible as a white speck on the yolk sac, which is floating in the dark circle of the amniotic sac.

I've included some common early pregnancy concerns below, but if you cannot find your particular problem here, check the further examples in the next two sections of the first trimester: weeks 6–10 and weeks 10–13. Do not hesitate to bring up any others you may have with your doctor; it is always better to have advice on them sooner rather than later. It is important that you have all the reassurance you need to make the next few weeks as enjoyable as possible.

Previous pregnancy problems

If you had previous pregnancy problems, such as a miscarriage, an ectopic pregnancy (see opposite and p.423) or complications in later pregnancy such as pre-eclampsia (see p.426), then your GP or midwife will probably arrange for you to have an early ultrasound scan and/or an early appointment to see an obstetrician. For women who have experienced miscarriages, a scan is often very helpful in allaying fears that history is repeating itself.

But do remember that all you need to see at this stage is a healthy sac in the uterine cavity. While a sophisticated scanner may detect a tiny fetal heartbeat at 5–6 weeks, every pregnancy is unique and as long as a pregnancy sac can be seen in the uterus, the absence of a fetal pole (a tiny rectangular blob within the sac) or a heartbeat at this early stage, is not uncommon. The most likely explanation is that your embryo implanted a few days later than you had calculated or expected and so a little more time is needed to see these landmarks in your pregnancy. This may well be the case if your menstrual cycle is irregular, or you are not sure exactly when you conceived.

Early ultrasound scans are also particularly valuable for women who have had a previous ectopic pregnancy, in which the embryo develops outside the uterus. The most common site is in the Fallopian tube, although ectopic pregnancies are also found on an ovary or in the abdominal cavity. A scan establishes whether there is an early pregnancy sac in the right place inside the uterus. If there is no evidence of this, you will probably undergo a series of blood tests to establish your blood levels of HCG hormone. If these are raised and yet there is still no sign of an intrauterine sac on the scan, you may need to undergo laparoscopy or drug treatment to stop the ectopic pregnancy continuing and prevent further damage to the Fallopian tube.

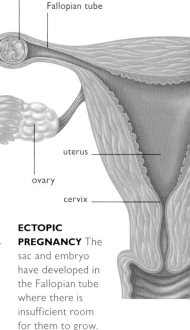

pregnancy sac with embryo

Fallopian tube

uterus

ovary

cervix

ECTOPIC PREGNANCY The sac and embryo have developed in the Fallopian tube where there is insufficient room for them to grow.

DIET AND EXERCISE

I am all too aware that nausea and tiredness in the first trimester can be a setback to your best-laid plans to eat the healthiest diet possible and stay fit and supple during pregnancy.

In the first trimester, what you eat is particularly important because, during these weeks, your baby's vital organs will be formed. The early development of the heart, liver, brain, and nervous system, for example, takes place in this period. Having said that, I know from personal experience that nausea

and sickness in the early months of pregnancy can make it impossible to follow your ideal diet.

▶ **Eat little and often**. Small meals and snacks are easier on the stomach than three large meals per day. Try nibbling on a piece of bread or some dry biscuits early in the day.

▶ **Keep healthy snack foods** such as fruit, nuts, and pieces of cheese easily available, so that your blood sugar level never gets too low.

▶ **However little solid food** you can cope with, try to remember to drink plenty of fluids regularly.

If you feel happier skipping your daily exercise now that you are pregnant, that's fine, but do remember that exercise is very unlikely to cause any problems in early pregnancy and, if you maintain your exercise programme, it will help you keep fit and healthy.

I can guarantee you that once the first three months are over, you are likely to feel a renewed vigour that will propel you back, if not to the badminton court, at least to the pool for some wonderfully relaxing and beneficial swimming sessions.

Urinary infections

Although it is normal for pregnant women to experience urinary frequency in the early weeks of pregnancy, the possibility of a urine infection should not be overlooked. If you feel tingling when you pass urine, urgency, lower abdominal pain or discomfort, or notice blood in the urine, you may well have an infection and need prompt treatment with antibiotics.

Urine infections are very common in pregnancy because progesterone makes the urinary tract more relaxed. This makes it easier for bacteria to enter the urethra and reach the bladder, where they cause inflammation or cystitis. Because the bladder is also relaxed in pregnancy, the infection can spread easily up the ureters and infect the kidneys, a condition known as pyelonephritis. Symptoms usually develop suddenly, and include a high temperature and shivering, and pain over the bladder and kidneys, with severe discomfort in the loin region, which may radiate down to the groin. Antibiotics will resolve the infection promptly. Left untreated, the infection can cause permanent scarring and damage to the kidney. The bacteria are present in 2–5 per cent of pregnant women without causing symptoms, but screening and treatment reduce the risk of pyelonephritis.

An existing condition

If you have a general medical problem, however minor, you should discuss this with your doctor or midwife as soon as you know that you are pregnant. They will help you to decide on the best type of care for your needs. If you are taking any medication, you will be advised on whether the dosage needs to be altered. On no account should you stop taking prescribed drugs without first seeking advice.

On pages 408–11 you will find details about existing medical conditions, such as diabetes, epilepsy, high blood pressure, thyroid disease, renal disease, heart disease, and inflammatory bowel disorders, which need specialist care. If you suffer from one of these (or a disorder that is not included in this list), your community midwife or GP will probably refer you directly to an obstetrician in a hospital that offers specialist expertise for your condition. You will be seen as quickly as possible, particularly if you are taking medications that may need to be altered. Throughout your pregnancy, you will be monitored by consultant obstetricians and, quite possibly, a consultant physician with specialist knowledge of your particular condition. Your part of the bargain is to try to stay healthy and to follow their advice.

❝ I can guarantee you that, once the first three months of pregnancy are over, you are likely to feel a renewed vigour… ❞

OLDER MUMS-TO-BE

Over recent years there have been very significant societal changes in our reproductive patterns. The average age of a woman giving birth for the first time has continued to rise steadily and the number of babies born to mothers aged 35 years or over has increased dramatically.

One in five of all births are currently to women over 35, and the number of babies born to women over the age of 40 is at an all time high, having doubled in the space of ten years. If you are over 35 years of age and this is your first pregnancy, you may well have heard someone describe you as an "elderly primigravida" or read in your maternity notes that your age is considered to be a risk factor. Although many women who are able to become pregnant at this age will go on to have a successful outcome, there is no doubt that women over 35 years of age are more likely to experience problems conceiving a baby, staying pregnant, and suffering later pregnancy complications than younger women.

That said, many of these complications can be identified or predicted to minimize the consequences. So there is no reason why your pregnancy should not have a successful outcome as long as you have regular antenatal care.

A woman's fertility starts to decline rapidly during her thirties because the quality of her eggs deteriorates with advancing age. Not only are her older eggs less likely to be fertilized, but they also have a greater chance of carrying a genetic or chromosomal abnormality. This may prevent her becoming pregnant or lead to an early miscarriage, because the resulting embryo is so abnormal that it cannot develop any further: for example Trisomy 16, the commonest abnormality found in miscarriage tissues, which is incompatible with life.

Importantly, some genetic abnormalities are not always fatal and the best known of these is Down's syndrome or Trisomy 21 (see p.147), the incidence of which increases sharply after 35 years of age. For this reason, older pregnant women are routinely offered antenatal tests to diagnose possible fetal genetic and physical abnormalities (see pp.134–43). Recent evidence suggests that advanced paternal age also increases the risk of chromosomal abnormalities and miscarriage.

Many important antenatal complications such as high blood pressure, pre-eclampsia, gestational diabetes, premature labour, placenta praevia, and poor fetal growth are more common in older mothers. And the older the woman, the more likely she is to have pre-existing medical problems such as high blood pressure, diabetes, heart disease, or obesity to further complicate the picture. Lastly, women giving birth over the age of 35 have a higher chance of requiring medical interventions during labour (particularly if this is a first birth) and of developing complications in the postnatal period: for example, they are more likely to be induced, to require a Caesarean section, or to have an episode of postnatal depression. I hope you will use this information to take the best possible care of yourself, in the knowledge that good antenatal care and support from family and friends will minimize the chances of these things happening to you.

As an older mother of twins myself, I am conscious of the fact that much of what I have said above may sound very negative, but my own experience was consistent with the increased risks of becoming pregnant in my late thirties. My twin daughters were born early at 33 weeks, delivered by emergency Caesarean section, needed help with breathing and feeding, and spent the first four weeks of their lives in a special care baby unit. They were vulnerable premature babies at birth – but happily are now completely healthy young adults.

ANTENATAL CARE AND BIRTH CHOICES

Most of your antenatal care will take place in the community, either at your GP's surgery or a birth centre. If you need more specialist care, your antenatal visits will be hospital-based. Getting the right kind of care goes a long way towards making your pregnancy a pleasurable time in your life.

An open-minded approach

When I was pregnant and looking for a book to read that would help me understand my special condition, I was struck by how polarized most

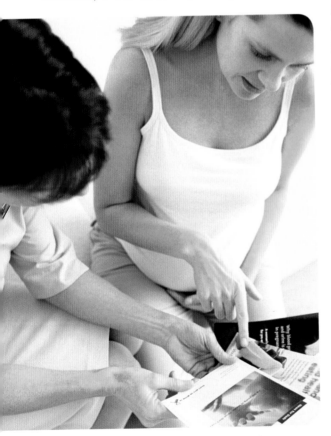

GOOD ADVICE Your antenatal carers look after your health in pregnancy and also offer advice and information.

books are on the particular issue of where I should have my baby. They divided roughly into two camps: those written by obstetricians who seemed to believe that the only place to have a baby is in a specialist hospital unit, and those written by vehement supporters of natural childbirth and home births who suggest that hospital units are designed to make women feel lost and vulnerable by taking away control of their own bodies during childbirth. Like most readers, I was left with the feeling that I would have failed as a mother, missed out or been cheated of something special if medical interventions were required. I concluded that both types of book were unrealistic and unhelpful because they did nothing to make me feel calm and confident about the potentially unpredictable journey I had just embarked upon. On reflection, that is when I decided another type of book was needed and that I should sit down and write it.

Before you decide

The main aim of antenatal care is to maintain your health and wellbeing and help you produce a healthy baby, and this involves detecting any condition that may adversely affect either of you as early as possible. During your antenatal care, you will be offered information and health education that will prepare you and your partner for labour and

TYPES OF ANTENATAL CARE

CASELOAD AND TEAM MIDWIFERY

This system is popular with women who have low-risk pregnancies because it enables them to develop a rapport with their midwife.

Most areas have caseload and team midwifery in which community midwives work individually and in teams to provide antenatal care. Caseload midwifery involves a midwife looking after a "caseload" of women, usually in a specific geographical area. This essentially means that you will be assigned a primary midwife, giving you continuity of care throughout your pregnancy and birth.

With team midwifery, the midwives take turns to be on call, attending the births of the women under their care either at home, or in a birth centre or hospital maternity unit.

SHARED CARE

Your care is shared, with some antenatal appointments at the hospital (for example for scans or to investigate problems) and the rest at the GP surgery or health centre. At about 10–12 weeks, you will have a detailed booking visit, and tests at your local hospital. Then, as long as no problems arise, your community midwife or GP will carry out most of your antenatal check-ups at your local surgery or health centre.

You will only need to attend a hospital clinic for ultrasound scans or blood tests and one or two visits late in pregnancy. In a GP group practice, there is usually one doctor who specializes in antenatal care.

Your care will be transferred to the hospital for the birth of your baby, and then back to your GP or midwife when you go home.

HOSPITAL-BASED CARE

If you have had or develop gynaecological, medical or obstetric complications or if a problem is identified in your baby, you will probably be advised to have all your antenatal care and to give birth at a local hospital. Your clinic appointments will be with your specialist doctors (either a high risk obstetrician, fetal medicine expert, obstetric physician or a combination of these) supported by midwives.

Your GP or community midwife will make arrangements for you to be referred as soon as possible and the remainder of your pregnancy check-ups and contacts will take place at the maternity hospital where you will deliver.

BIRTHING CENTRE

Many NHS hospitals now have a birthing centre on the premises or located close by. This option is for women who expect to have a straightforward pregnancy and birth. Care is provided in a homely, woman-centred environment before, during, and after the birth. The centres offer antenatal care, preparation classes for labour and birth, breastfeeding classes, and postnatal care for new mothers. Birth centres have multipurpose, comfortable rooms with facilities such as birthing pools, ensuite bathrooms, and gas and air piped in. There is a sitting room and kitchen for preparing meals, and consultation and meeting rooms. As this is a midwife-led service, there are no obstetricians, paediatricians or anaesthetists on site, therefore only women at low risk of complications in labour are suitable to have their babies at a birth centre. If an emergency arises, the woman is transferred to the care of an obstetrician at the local hospital maternity unit.

INDEPENDENT MIDWIFERY CARE

One way of ensuring complete continuity of care is to pay for the services of an independent midwife who will carry out all your antenatal checks (in your home at a time to suit you). She will be with you during the labour and delivery – whether at home or in hospital – and then care for you afterwards. Employing an independent midwife is becoming a popular option with women who wish to have a home birth.

> 66 Birth centres have comfortable rooms, with facilities such as birthing pools... 99

A CHANGE IN APPROACH

The issue of choice in childbirth has been a matter of fierce debate over the years, much of it prompted by the dissatisfaction many pregnant women began to feel with the more traditional hospital-based patterns of care.

What is nowadays perceived as a "medicalized" approach to childbirth developed over the last 50 years as a by-product of advances in the way labour and birth could be managed. Women protested that they were being treated as part of a baby production machine, rather than informed participants. These feelings prompted a government commission on maternity services, which led to the publication of "Changing Childbirth" in 1993 and a further updated publication in 2007 called "Maternity Matters". These recommended changes to the way maternity services are provided based on the following conclusions:

▶ It was no longer justified on the grounds of safety to encourage all women to give birth in hospital.
▶ Many women wished to have continuity of care throughout pregnancy and childbirth, and midwives were likely to be best placed to provide this.
▶ Greater choice in the type of care for pregnant women was needed.

▶ Provision for home birth or birth in a small maternity unit was largely unavailable in the UK, despite increasing demand.
▶ Some traditional interventions during labour and delivery such as continuous fetal monitoring, epidurals, and episiotomy were unnecessary or not evidence-based.
▶ The hospital environment was leaving some women feeling that they had lost control of their bodies and disappointed by their labour and birthing experience.
▶ GP surgeries and community-based antenatal clinics should replace hospital antenatal care, providing there is easy access to more specialist assessment.
▶ Within hospital, women should be able to exercise choice in the personnel who care for them.
▶ The relationship between the woman and her caregiver was of fundamental importance and needed to be recognized.

The reports and the NICE guidelines (see opposite and p.161) did much to raise public awareness of these issues with the result that hospital maternity units have become friendlier, more comfortable, and less clinical places in which to give birth. Although the number of home deliveries has not increased dramatically, there has been a very significant change in the way that hospital units provide care for women at the time of delivery. The emphasis is now on flexibility, one-to-one midwifery care, and minimizing medical interventions wherever possible.

However, considerable financial and educational resources are needed if we are to put other key resolutions into practice, not least of which is that we need many more experienced midwives. I believe that in the majority of cases, obstetricians should work in partnership with the midwife and only become the principal provider of care when a woman is at risk of medical and obstetric complications. The key to this is finding better ways of identifying the women who are at greatest risk and require medical intervention.

❝ ...hospital maternity units have become friendlier, more comfortable, and less clinical places in which to give birth. ❞

parenthood. These two major principles will be followed through wherever care is provided. Most women now follow the antenatal care pathway as recommended by the National Institute for Health and Clinical Excellence (NICE), which covers the routine care that all healthy women can expect to receive throughout their pregnancy (see p.161).

Even if you feel it is too early at this stage for you to know whether you would prefer to deliver your baby in hospital, in a birth centre or at home, your choice of antenatal care is a more pressing issue because your booking appointment will take place before the end of the first trimester. So take some time to read through the various options on page 85 to see what might suit you best.

Explore different sources of information before coming to a decision – talk to friends and neighbours, pick up the information leaflets in your GP's surgery, and contact your local Community Health Council for information, the National Childbirth Trust, midwivesonline or The Association for Improvements in the Maternity Services (see pp.437–8 for contact details). There is a bottomless pit of information on the internet, but remember that much of this is not backed with professional expertise. Lastly, remember you can always change your mind later on.

Childbirth in the UK

Today in the UK, most babies are born in hospital or birth centres – over 97 per cent according to recent maternity statistics – with just 2.7 per cent born at home. By contrast, in 1954, approximately 35 per cent of babies were born at home. This major swing in the choice of place of birth followed the Peel report of 1970, which concluded that hospital delivery was a safer option than home birth for both mother and baby. The report recommended that all women should be delivered in hospital and by 1985, as a direct result, less than one per cent of all babies were born at home.

More recently, it has been noted that the Peel report was not based on medical evidence that a hospital birth was safer, but simply on the fact that perinatal mortality rates had fallen dramatically in recent years. Undoubtedly, the major reason for this fall was an overall improvement in antenatal care and general living standards. As a result, in the last 10 years or so, a different approach to pregnancy and childbirth has started to develop.

Now that women are so well informed about pregnancy and their general health and living standards are so improved, there is the opportunity to offer greater choice in their antenatal care and place of birth. Although there will always be women who need high-tech medical care, the majority are likely to have straightforward pregnancies and a normal vaginal delivery. In view of this, many women and their carers now feel that the option of a home delivery should at least be considered for low-risk pregnancies. Indeed, a recent study concluded that home births and birth centres are safe options, although you are more likely to be transferred to hospital if you are a first-time mother.

Choosing a birthplace

Your choice of where to have your baby is likely to come down to one of the following options: in a hospital, in a midwifery-led birthing unit, or in your own home. The two important factors to take into account when you make your decision are your personal preference and the safety of both you and your baby. Sometimes a problem that arises in the pregnancy or a previous complication makes these factors incompatible, but it is usually possible to reach a compromise, as long as time is spent discussing the practicalities rather than sticking to a previously held bottom line.

In hospital

If this is your first pregnancy, a home birth is an option, but your GP or midwife is likely to suggest a hospital delivery. They may also recommend a hospital birth if you have current medical problems or if you had complications in a previous pregnancy.

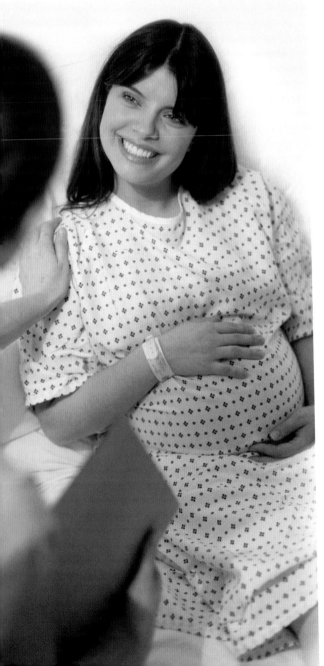

However, it is likely that you can still have shared antenatal care, with some appointments at the hospital and some with community midwives or your GP at the local surgery. There may be more than one hospital in your area and if you can choose which to go to, find out about the facilities and antenatal care options on offer at each one. Teams of midwives who share your care are available at some hospitals (see p.85).

Many hospitals nowadays have birthing rooms, which are designed to be much less clinical, with soft lighting, music, comfortable chairs, and large floor cushions, birthing balls, and stools. Some also provide a birthing pool.

In a midwifery-led birthing centre

Many maternity services now have a midwifery-led birthing centre, located either within the main hospital maternity unit or as a stand-alone unit in the local district or community hospital. Staffed by midwives who can offer continuity of care throughout pregnancy, labour, and delivery, these centres are designed to deal with normal pregnancies and deliveries in a low-tech and informal environment. Hospital maternity units that include a birthing centre probably offer pregnant women the best of both worlds in that the surroundings are less formal and continuity of care can be maintained, but expert medical help is just around the corner if any problems that need specialist expertise arise during the birth.

At home

If you are considering a home birth, the first thing to do is talk to your community midwife. If this is your first baby, some will have concerns about the

HOSPITAL BIRTH If this is your first baby, your carers may recommend a hospital birth.

safety of a home birth. No matter how well your pregnancy goes, no one can predict what will actually happen during your labour. They will have similar concerns if you have had medical problems or complications in a previous pregnancy.

While all women are entitled to a home birth, it is likely to be most suitable if you have had one or more previous pregnancies that were free of complications and that ended in straightforward vaginal deliveries. Even then, no two pregnancies can be guaranteed to follow the same pattern, so be prepared to change your plans if this pregnancy turns out differently.

If you are planning a home birth, your antenatal care will be provided by community midwives attached to the local hospital. In some areas, a midwife will visit you at home towards the end of your pregnancy to discuss preparations for the birth and the intended place for the delivery. Once you are in established labour, your midwife will stay with you and, as you near delivery, a second midwife will also come to your home to provide further support until the baby is born. If complications arise, they will accompany you into hospital. The UK has a good transfer system in place should you need to be referred to hospital. However, an important consideration when planning a home birth is the length of time it would take to transfer to hospital should any complications develop.

There are also midwives who work independently of the NHS. Independent Midwives UK (see Useful Contacts, pp.437–8) can put you in touch with a midwife who will follow you through your antenatal care and deliver your baby at home.

Finding out more

Before you reach a final decision about the place of birth, ask other parents, midwives, and doctors

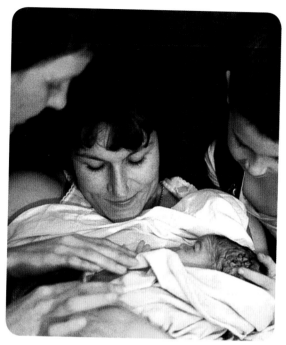

HOME BIRTH You may want to consider having your baby at home in the heart of your family if you have had a previous labour and delivery that was straightforward.

about the reputation of the hospitals available to you. Then arrange a visit to one or two local units so that you can see for yourself and get a feel for whether you will be comfortable and relaxed there. Remember that feeling comfortable in labour is not just about physical issues such as the facilities and decoration of the rooms, it is also about the friendliness of the staff and the attitude they have towards birthing. I know that many women feel nervous about going into hospitals because they associate them with illness or possibly sad or unpleasant memories. But delivery suites and antenatal clinics have a totally different atmosphere from any other hospital department. The women are fit and healthy, in fact they are positively blooming, and all the staff involved are participating in helping you to have a happy and successful ending to your pregnancy.

QUESTIONS TO ASK ON A VISIT TO A MATERNITY UNIT

The very best way to find out what is on offer in your local maternity hospital is to arrange a visit. The following questions will help you decide on your preferred type of maternity care and delivery.

GENERAL ISSUES

▶ Does the maternity department or birth centre have particular interests or offer specialist services?
▶ What is the hospital's policy on different types of antenatal and delivery care? Does it, for example, offer shared care with your GP and caseload midwifery teams?
▶ Is there the option to be seen by a woman doctor if preferred? This issue is usually dependent on the number of staff and the on-call rota.

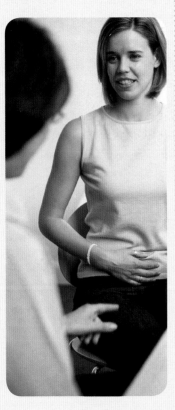

▶ Is there a 24-hour anaesthetic service available?
▶ Is there a special-care baby unit?
▶ Does the hospital antenatal clinic run an appointments system?
▶ Does it offer antenatal classes and tours of the labour ward and postnatal facilities?
▶ What is their view on birth plans?

LABOUR AND DELIVERY ISSUES

▶ Are midwives flexible about special requests and different types of delivery, for example, willing to encourage women to give birth in any position that feels comfortable, be it lying, standing or squatting?
▶ How long are the midwives' shifts? A 12-hour shift system gives you a better chance of being cared for by the same midwife throughout.
▶ What is the hospital policy on induction, rupturing the membranes, pain relief, and electronic monitoring during labour?
▶ Are partners, friends, and family welcome in the delivery room? Are the numbers limited?
▶ Is there a 24-hour epidural service and are mobile epidurals available?
▶ Is there a birthing pool or the facility to bring a hired one with you?
▶ What are the forceps, ventouse, and Caesarean section rates?

Remember that a specialist or teaching hospital will have a higher number of these than a small general hospital, because they will be caring for women who are more likely to experience complications in labour.
▶ Is there a hospital policy on episiotomy and repair of vaginal tears? Midwives usually suture, but occasionally some rely on their on-call doctors if the tear is severe.

AFTER THE BIRTH

▶ Are amenity beds (single rooms) available? If so, how many and what do they cost? Do they have private bathrooms? Are they reserved for women who have had difficult births? What size are the general maternity wards and how many beds per room?
▶ What is the usual length of stay after the birth? (This will probably be longer after a first baby than for subsequent births.)
▶ Will your baby be with you at all times or is there a separate nursery?
▶ Are specialist breastfeeding counsellors available? This can be enormously helpful when trying to establish breastfeeding.
▶ What are the visiting hours?
▶ Are special diets, such as kosher or vegetarian, available?
▶ Will you need to bring into hospital with you items such as pillows, towels, and nappies?

The who's who of maternity care

You will meet a variety of health-care professionals during your pregnancy, labour, and birth and also during the postnatal period. The following is a brief description of the role each person plays.

Midwives are the key players in our maternity care system working within a hospital, in the community or both. Some have trained directly as midwives but some also trained as nurses. They are qualified to take responsibility for you and your baby before, during, and after a normal birth and if complications arise, will seek advice from an obstetrician. Some hospital-based midwives have developed specialist skills in the management and care of pregnant women with specific problems such as diabetes, high blood pressure, infection, and other medical complications of pregnancy. If you are having a home birth, a midwife will come to your home when labour starts and accompany you to the hospital if necessary.

Independent midwives are self-employed and will charge you for their services. They offer continuity of care and individual attention and will undertake to look after you antenatally and during your labour whether in hospital or at home.

Your General Practitioner may arrange your booking into a hospital maternity unit if you are deemed potentially high risk, otherwise you will be put in touch with your local midwife. Your GP may see you during your pregnancy and for your six-week postnatal visit.

Obstetricians are doctors who are specialists in the care of pregnant women. If you are a high-risk case, you will be assigned to a consultant obstetrician whose name will appear on your antenatal notes. The consultant obstetrician heads a team of junior obstetricians and is sometimes linked to a team of midwives. You may only meet him or her occasionally if your pregnancy runs smoothly. If it is more complicated, you will see your consultant more often.

Obstetric physicians work in teams caring jointly for pregnant women with complex medical problems with obstetricians, anaesthetists, and midwives.

Paediatricians are doctors who are specially trained in the health of babies and young children. Every maternity unit works hand in hand with paediatricians to ensure that the babies they deliver are healthy and receive any medical help they need. A paediatrician is present at the delivery of twins and higher multiple births, most instrumental deliveries (such as forceps), and Caesarean sections. Every baby is checked by a paediatrician or a specialist midwife before she or he is taken home.

Neonatologists are paediatricians with specialist skills in the care of newborn babies with problems. They run the neonatal intensive care and Special Care Baby Units (SCBUs). If your baby is born prematurely or is found to have a problem, a neonatologist will be involved in your baby's care.

Health Visitors are usually nurses or midwives with special training in child health, who will visit you at home after the delivery of your baby.

Anaesthetists are doctors trained to give anaesthetics and pain relief including general anaesthesia, spinal and epidural regional blocks. Many maternity units have specialist obstetric anaesthetists who have made pregnant women their particular interest.

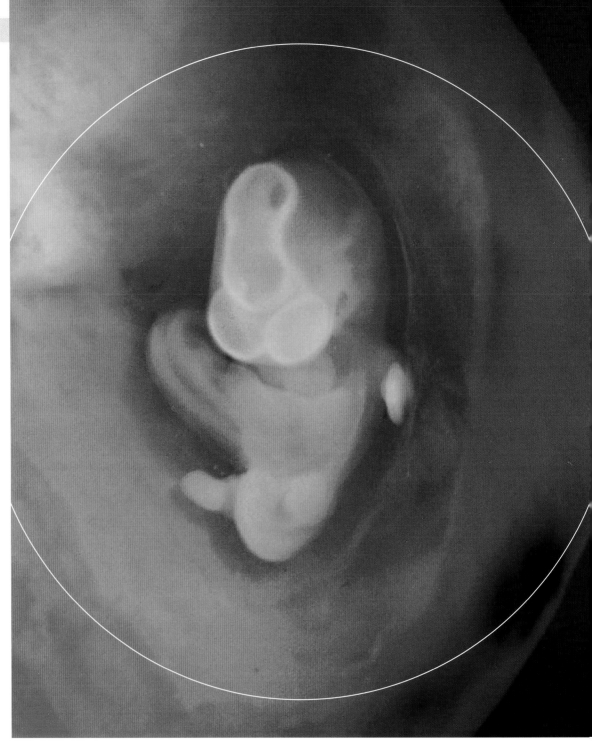

▲ A six-week-old embryo nested in the uterus.

| 1 | 2 | 3 | 4 | 5 | 6 | 7 | 8 | 9 | 10 | 11 | 12 | 13 | 14 | 15 | 16 | 17 | 18 | 19 | 20 |

▶ WEEKS 0–6   ▶ WEEKS 6–10   ▶ WEEKS 10–13   ▶ WEEKS 13–17   ▶ WEEKS 17–21

▶ FIRST TRIMESTER   ▶ SECOND TRIMESTER

▶ WEEKS 6–10
The developing baby

DURING THE NEXT FOUR WEEKS, your developing baby will quadruple in size and undergo dramatic changes in appearance. By week 10, the embryo has become a fetus and is starting to resemble a human being.

Several facial features can now be recognized on ultrasound and the body is straightening and the limbs developing. The head continues to grow more rapidly than any other part of the body in order to accommodate the developing brain. The back of the head grows at a faster rate than the front; as a result the embryo is curled over the front of the body and appears to be nodding at its bulging heart. However, the body has started to lose its earlier comma-like shape. A neck is appearing, the back is straighter, and the tail is disappearing.

The head now has a high forehead and, as the primitive facial bones develop and fuse together, eyes, nose, ears, and a mouth become recognizable. The primitive eyes and ears, which were mere swellings on the head at six weeks, are developing rapidly. By the end of the eighth week, the eyes have grown in size and already contain some pigment. By the 10th week, they are easily recognizable but will continue to be hidden behind sealed lids and cannot function until later in the second trimester, when the nervous system is fully formed. At each side of the head the depressions that will become ear canals have deepened and the inner ear starts to form. By the eighth week, the middle ear, which will become responsible for both balance and hearing, is formed and by 10 weeks, the external part of the ear (the pinna) has started to grow low down on the fetal head. The nostrils and upper lip can now be seen and inside the mouth there is a tiny tongue, which already has taste buds. Tooth buds for all the future milk teeth are in place within the developing jawbones.

Future limbs

Further miraculous changes are happening as your baby's limbs take shape. The folds of skin making up the limb buds condense and form cartilage, which will later develop into hard bones. These cartilaginous limb buds grow rapidly

2 x life size

By the end of the sixth week, the embryo is 4mm in length and weighs less than 1g (0.03oz). By week 10, the fetus will measure 30mm (1¼in) from the top of its head to its bottom (crown to rump) and weigh 3–5g (0.1oz).

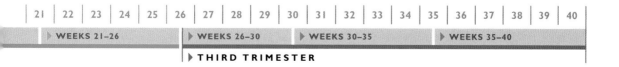

| 21 | 22 | 23 | 24 | 25 | 26 | 27 | 28 | 29 | 30 | 31 | 32 | 33 | 34 | 35 | 36 | 37 | 38 | 39 | 40 |

▶ WEEKS 21–26　　　▶ WEEKS 26–30　　　▶ WEEKS 30–35　　　▶ WEEKS 35–40

▶ **THIRD TRIMESTER**

and wrists and paddle-shaped hands can soon be identified. The arms lengthen and, by eight weeks, shoulders and elbows are present, making the upper limbs project forwards. The webbed hands now develop separate fingers and by week 10, touch pads have appeared at the end of the stubby fingertips. The lower limb buds start to go through the same process, but the distinction between thighs, knees, calves, ankles, and toes progresses more slowly. Most of the muscles are now in place, and small, jerky movements can be seen on an ultrasound scan.

Inside the body

Inside the body, the central neural tube is now differentiating into the brain and spinal cord. The nerve cells multiply rapidly, aided by support cells called glial cells, and migrate along pathways into the brain, where they connect with each other and become active. This is the beginning of the neural network that will later transmit messages from the brain to the body. The fetus has also developed some very basic sensory perceptions. It can respond to touch although it is still too early for you to be able to feel movements.

By week 10, the embryonic heart has developed into the definitive four-chambered heart. The two atria receive blood from the fetal circulation, while the ventricles pump blood out to the lungs and the rest of the baby's body. Valves develop at the exit of all four chambers to ensure that the blood is always pumped in one direction and cannot leak back into the heart. The heart is beating at a rate of 180 beats per minute – twice the speed of your own heart.

Although the digestive system is developing rapidly, it will be some time before it is functioning properly. The stomach, liver and spleen are all

FETUS AT 10 WEEKS ··

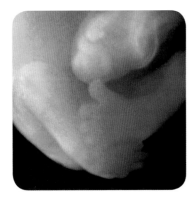

The fetal intestines still protrude from the abdominal wall.

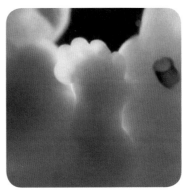

Shoulders and elbows develop and the arms project forwards.

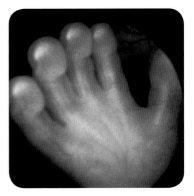

The webbed hands now develop fingers with touchpads.

THE AMNIOTIC SAC

The fetus continues to float within the amniotic sac, which is surrounded by an inner layer called the amnion and an outer layer called the chorion. These two layers are separated by a space (the extracoelomic cavity), which contains the yolk sac.

The small fingers of tissue called chorionic villi that sprout from the chorion are becoming concentrated in one circular area on the wall of the uterus; this will soon develop into the placenta. At this site, the villi are developing blood vessels and burrowing into the lining of the uterus, setting up their future access to your circulation.

Elsewhere, the chorionic villi are disappearing and the smooth chorion (known as the chorion laeve) is forming; this will fuse with the wall of the uterus in the second trimester, when the growing fetus has further distended the uterine cavity. The umbilical cord is now formed and blood is circulating through it, although the fetus is still receiving most nourishment from the yolk sac.

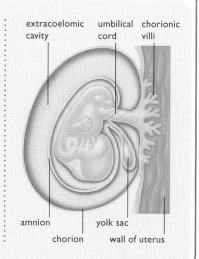

extracoelomic cavity · umbilical cord · chorionic villi · amnion · chorion · yolk sac · wall of uterus

in place and the intestines grow so fast that loops are formed and for a time, some of these actually protrude through the baby's abdominal wall.

By the end of the embryonic period, the new fetus has all its major organs and body systems, although the brain and spinal cord will continue to develop throughout your pregnancy. During this critical period of structural development, the fetus is highly susceptible to the damaging effects of a variety of drugs, viruses, and environmental factors (see pp.29–33). It is very rare for congenital fetal abnormalities to develop after this time.

Your changing body

During the next few weeks, your uterus will grow significantly in size. By eight weeks it is the size of a medium orange and by 10 weeks the size of a small grapefruit. However, it cannot be felt through your abdominal wall because it is still behind your pubic bone.

This growth in the uterus can only be achieved by increasing the blood flow to it. In the non-pregnant state, the uterus receives about 2 per cent of the total amount of blood that is pumped through the heart per minute (the cardiac output). Very early in pregnancy, this percentage increases dramatically and by the end of this trimester, 25 per cent of your cardiac output will be directed to the uterus to cope with the demands of the placenta and baby. This increase in cardiac output is mainly due to the volume of blood pumped with each heartbeat (the stroke volume) since your heart rate (the number of times the heart beats per minute) increases only slightly during pregnancy. The thick muscular walls of the heart are relaxed by pregnancy hormones and this allows the heart to increase the volume of blood it contains each time it fills (diastole) without having to increase the force with which it pumps the blood during contractions (systole). To ensure that your blood pressure does not become too high as a result of the rise in cardiac output and blood volume, the blood vessels throughout your body also develop an increased capacity to hold larger blood volumes – once again due to the increase in pregnancy hormones, especially progesterone. This is why your systolic blood pressure falls only slightly during pregnancy, but your diastolic blood pressure is markedly reduced, a change that occurs early in the first trimester and only returns to normal non-pregnant levels near to the time of delivery.

Noticeable effects

As a result of these dramatic changes in your circulatory system, you will start to become aware of differences in the way your body is functioning. You will already have noticed that you need to pass urine more frequently because your kidneys are working much harder to filter your blood more efficiently and also because your enlarging womb places pressure on your bladder. If your breasts had not begun to change earlier, they will almost certainly be larger, heavier, and more tender now, because the milk ducts are already beginning to swell in preparation for lactation, and the areola surrounding your nipples will be larger and darker in colour. The sweat glands (called Montgomery's tubercles) in the areola, which look like little pimples around the nipples, have also enlarged and start to secrete a fluid to lubricate the nipples. This is one of the most reliable signs of a first pregnancy, but since they do not shrink completely after pregnancy this cannot be depended on as a diagnostic sign for subsequent pregnancies. An outer ring of lighter-coloured tissue called the secondary areola starts to appear on the breasts, together with more visible veins, as a result of the increased blood flow.

Changes in your skin

One of the first things you may notice is that your skin is either spottier or drier than usual, due to your high progesterone levels. Many women also develop spidery red lines called spider naevi on their legs and across their

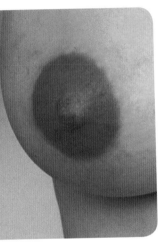

DARKENING AREOLA
The area around the nipples becomes larger and darker in colour.

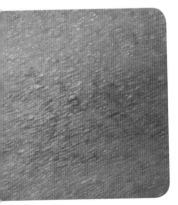

SPIDER NAEVI These tiny, spidery red lines on the skin are due to high levels of oestrogen.

upper chest. These are small blood vessels in the skin that have expanded due to the increased production of oestrogen. They usually fade away after pregnancy and are nothing to be alarmed about. The blood supply to your skin has increased and because the veins are now much more dilated, you are better able to eliminate heat from your body surface. However annoying you may find your sudden intolerance of only moderately warm temperatures, this adaptation is essential because you need to be able to dispose of the rising heat that you generate from your increased metabolic rate and blood flow.

The skin of your genital area will start to darken and you will probably have noticed that your vaginal discharge has increased. This is due to the secretion of a watery substance, which mixes with cells that are being shed from the vaginal walls. Normally this discharge is mucus-like and is usually clear or sometimes milky coloured. It may stain your underwear but it should not be the source of any discomfort. If the discharge becomes yellow, develops an offensive odour or causes you symptoms of itching or soreness, see your GP (see p.215).

> 66
> ...the reality is that many women are not physically sick, but they do feel very nauseous.
> 99

How you may feel physically

Some women sail through the first trimester feeling neither tired nor sick – indeed some will not even realize that they are pregnant. For the majority of women, however, the first three months are usually dominated by unpleasant symptoms – nausea, vomiting, and exhaustion.

No one can predict how you will feel during these early weeks of pregnancy because symptoms vary considerably from one woman to another and in each pregnancy that a woman has. Nor is there an accepted time for these common symptoms to start or finish. Some women feel exhausted from the time of the positive pregnancy test until they reach the second trimester, whereas others will only be troubled for a short time. Similarly, nausea may hit you hard briefly and then disappear or be troublesome for many weeks.

Nausea and vomiting in pregnancy (NVP)

Nausea and vomiting are, without doubt, the best known and most talked about side effects of early pregnancy – as many as 70 to 80 per cent of all pregnant women will experience them to some degree. I have always thought "morning sickness" a poor description of the problem, since many women are not physically sick, but they do feel very nauseous. What is more, this feeling is rarely confined to the mornings – it can continue throughout the day or only be a problem in the evening. However, I do want to stress that it is also perfectly normal not to feel any nausea and if you happen to be one of these fortunate women, then count your lucky stars. Many women I meet in the early pregnancy clinic worry that this is a warning sign that their pregnancy may be less robust or at greater risk of miscarriage. I promise you that you do not have to experience the misery of throwing up like clockwork every day in order to have a successful pregnancy.

No one has come up with the definitive answer as to why nausea and vomiting occur in pregnancy, but there are several plausible theories. Like most baffling medical problems, nausea is probably the result of a combination of a number of different factors. One suggested cause is the high levels of the hormone human chorionic gonadotrophin (HCG), which are present during the first trimester and which then tail off at about 13 weeks. This would explain why nausea usually resolves spontaneously between 16 and 20 weeks of pregnancy, although some women continue to feel sick for much longer.

Another theory is that nausea is linked to low blood sugar levels, since it often occurs first thing in the morning after many hours without food, or at the end of the day when you are likely to be tired and in need of rest and food.

Another possible explanation is that the flood of progesterone hormone in pregnancy relaxes the smooth muscles in the digestive tract and slows down the passage of food through it. As a result, the food you eat and the digestive acids that are produced to process it remain in your stomach for longer periods of time. This is why you may feel sick and may occasionally vomit as well.

> " ...there is a wide spectrum of foods that women either crave or develop a violent aversion to in early pregnancy. "

HOW TO RELIEVE NAUSEA AND VOMITING

There is no magic cure, just a variety of remedies to try in different combinations to see which work for you. I frequently quiz women about the individual remedies that helped them cope with their nausea and have included some of their recommendations here.

▶ **Eat small, easily digestible meals** at regular intervals rather than just one or two large meals during the day. Dry toast, rich tea biscuits, rice cakes, and savoury crackers are good standbys when you cannot stomach anything else. Cut down on the snacks when you start eating regular meals again or you will soon find that you are putting on unwanted pounds.

▶ **Stay clear of fatty food** because it can be particularly troublesome.

▶ **Bland foods** such as mushy cornflakes with skimmed milk are a well-tolerated favourite and have the advantage that they are fortified with iron and vitamins. They are a good substitute for a meal when you can't cope with anything else.

Whatever the cause, I know from personal experience how distressing and uncomfortable, not to mention inconvenient, nausea can be while it lasts. Added to which, you may start to worry that your inability to keep any food or fluids down may be putting your baby at risk. I must reassure you that this is not the case. However little you are eating or drinking, your baby will be creaming off everything it needs to develop normally. You may be feeling terrible, but your baby is fine.

More serious vomiting

Occasionally, women vomit so regularly and for such long periods of time (by which I mean weeks, not days) that they become dehydrated and weak because they cannot keep down fluids or food of any sort. This condition is called hyperemesis gravidarum and fortunately occurs only in about 1 in 200–500 pregnancies. However, if you do develop this problem, you will probably need to be admitted to hospital for a short while in order to have an intravenous drip to give you the necessary fluids, glucose, and minerals to help rehydrate you and stop you feeling so weak and ill. If you do need to be hospitalized, you will probably be advised to take some anti-sickness medication (called antiemetics), either in pill form or via your IV drip. These drugs are known to be safe in early pregnancy and will not have any harmful effect on your baby. Ever since the thalidomide disaster during the 1950s and '60s, doctors are extremely careful about what they prescribe to pregnant women to combat nausea. The antiemetic drugs that are now used have an excellent safety record, so do take them if you are advised to, as they will help you to get over a difficult period.

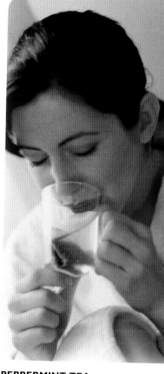

PEPPERMINT TEA
The refreshing taste of peppermint tea seems to combat the metallic taste that often accompanies feelings of nausea.

▶ **If you feel particularly nauseous** when you wake up in the morning, try nibbling on a plain biscuit before you get out of bed.
▶ **Some women swear by acupressure wristbands** (normally used to prevent travel sickness). These work by pressing on the acupuncture point known as P6.
▶ **Herbal teas** are also regularly recommended by my patients, especially peppermint tea, which has a refreshing taste that seems to help combat that horrible metallic taste in the mouth that so frequently develops when you feel sick. For the same reason, brushing your teeth at regular intervals during the day can also be a source of relief.
▶ **Try taking small amounts of ginger** either as ginger beer, ginger tea, ginger capsules, crystallized or root ginger or ginger biscuits.

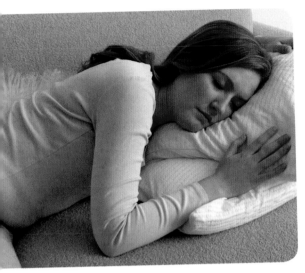

CATNAPPING No one knows why women feel inordinately tired in the early weeks of pregnancy, but while you feel this way, take a nap whenever the chance presents itself.

Food aversions and cravings

These often go hand in hand with nausea and vomiting in pregnancy, although they can also occur on their own. Again, we don't know why they happen, nor why there is such a wide spectrum of foods that women either crave or develop a violent aversion to in early pregnancy. I remember how puzzled I felt when I was suddenly unable to drink my usual daily quota of coffee, when orange juice seemed so heavy that I found it undrinkable, and when a sip from a glass of wine in the evening made me feel ill. The smell of roasted meat of any colour was repellent to me and, although a cheese lover since childhood, I could not look the smallest morsel in the eye without feeling seriously nauseous. I worried that the only sustenance I was offering my babies was grapefruit juice diluted with bubbly water, together with the occasional Marmite sandwich accompanied by an apple or a tinned asparagus spear. Mind you, compared to some of the stories about food cravings that my patients have shared with me these food oddities seem quite mild.

Coffee and alcohol appear to be one of the first things most women eliminate from their diet as a result of early pregnancy sickness or food aversion. Cravings for salty food such as Marmite, or pickles such as onions or gherkins at strange times of the day or night are also common. Perhaps this is our bodies' way of telling us that we need salt, but no one really knows. Similarly, we have all heard about pregnant women who develop a pica: a desire to eat an unusual substance such as chalk, coal or grass or to smell substances such as mothballs. I have no practical experience of these, but I can reassure you that I know of no data to suggest that they have ever caused any harm to a pregnancy. There are only a few foods in pregnancy – such as liver and unpasteurized cheeses for example – that are potentially dangerous and you will find more information about these in the diet section of this book (see p.50).

Feeling tired

I suspect that the time-honoured phrase "tiredness is the female condition" was first coined to describe a woman in early pregnancy. The feelings of exhaustion in the first few months can be quite overwhelming. I can remember finishing an ordinary day at work, reaching home and being just about capable of putting my key in the lock before collapsing in a heap at the bottom of the stairs. There was nothing wrong; I simply couldn't overcome my exhaustion and climb to the top. No one has so far been able to give a good scientific explanation for this tiredness, although theories abound. Some doctors believe that it is caused by the soporific effects of the high levels of progesterone hormone, while others attribute it to the huge physiological changes that are taking place – the raised cardiac output, blood volume, and oxygen consumption. The speed at which the tiny embryo is growing is another explanation, but you may find it difficult to understand how a baby that is small enough to fit into the palm of your closed hand can bring about such a dramatic change in your energy levels.

Like every experience in pregnancy, tiredness passes, but I am giving it a special mention here because it often raises concerns in partners and other family members. They see a woman who is usually full of energy flaked out and reduced to a wet rag and, since tiredness is so often equated with illness, they feel worried. Rest assured that after a couple of months of needing extra sleep and catnaps, tiredness lifts, so for the time being just go along with what your body is telling you to do.

> ❝
> The feelings of exhaustion that many women experience in the first few months can be quite overwhelming.
> ❞

Your emotional response

If you are suffering from wild fluctuations in mood, these are undoubtedly the result of the major hormonal changes occurring in early pregnancy. One minute you may be talking excitedly about the future, and a few minutes later you find yourself weeping like an overflowing bathtub about some trivial issue.

You may also find yourself lashing out verbally at a harmless comment your partner makes and accusing him of not understanding how you are feeling. Since you yourself may not know how you are feeling, or why you are so emotionally fragile, you can recognize how difficult it is for him at this time. The only practical thing to do is talk to him about how confused you feel and reassure him (and yourself) that you have not undergone a permanent character change. Although your mood swings can be very intense, leaving you feeling helpless and out of control, keep in mind that they are temporary and just one of the many side effects of a completely normal pregnancy.

You may also be feeling anxious about the future, the birth, and your ability to be a good parent. However well you are adjusting to the important changes that this new baby will bring to your life, when you are feeling tired and nauseous you may still be daunted by the prospect of it.

Common concerns

The most common concern at this stage of pregnancy is about miscarriage, the majority of which occur in the early weeks. But not every worrying symptom means miscarriage is inevitable, and with each week that passes your pregnancy is becoming more secure.

As many as one in three women have some sort of bleeding during the first trimester, ranging from brown to bright red spotting to large blood clots. In the majority of cases, it settles down and does not mean that there is any serious problem, since most women go on to have healthy babies. Having said that, I do understand how alarming bleeding can be.

As a safety measure you may be offered an early ultrasound scan, during which it may be possible to identify the pregnancy sac in the uterine cavity and the fetal pole and yolk sac developing. This will be very reassuring. Some women are frightened that a scan may increase the bleeding (it will not) or confirm their fears that the pregnancy has been lost. These feelings are understandable, but it is always the best plan to establish what is happening at the earliest opportunity.

I will never forget how distressed I felt when I experienced a heavy bleed at eight weeks into my pregnancy. I was sitting quietly in a meeting of a large number of medical colleagues and suddenly, without warning, I realized that

DECLINING RISK OF MISCARRIAGE

▶ **Miscarriage is the commonest complication** of pregnancy and by definition can occur at any gestational age up until 24 weeks (see p.431). However, the vast majority of miscarriages occur very early on, even before the pregnancy can be recognized on an ultrasound scan.
▶ **If you are six weeks from your last period**, the risk of miscarriage has fallen to approximately 15 per cent

or 1 in 6 pregnancies. At this stage it is usually possible to see the yolk sac in your uterus and the fetal pole inside it on an ultrasound scan.
▶ **By eight weeks, the risk is much smaller** and if a fetal heartbeat can be seen on the scan at this stage, your risk of miscarriage has fallen to 3 per cent. Looked at more positively, this means that 97 per cent of pregnant women with a fetal heartbeat at eight weeks can

expect their pregnancy to continue and to take home a baby at the end of it.
▶ **After 12 weeks**, the risk of miscarriage is no more than 1 per cent. So the message here is that, as pregnancy progresses, the risk of miscarriage falls dramatically, and by the time you reach the end of this trimester, you are very unlikely to experience this distressing event.

> 66 Bleeding in early pregnancy is always worth investigating and, even if it is heavy, does not necessarily mean that the pregnancy is over. 99

my seat was warm and wet and that I was bleeding. There was no pain and no forewarning – it just happened. I immediately assumed that I was miscarrying and after leaving the meeting as discreetly as possible for a woman with blood all over her clothes, I went home and cried. I nearly cancelled my scan the next day, but my husband (who is always practical and optimistic) persuaded me to go and find out exactly what the situation was. Happily, the scan showed two little embryos who appeared quite unruffled by the bleeding of the day before. Bleeding in early pregnancy is always worth investigating and, even if it is heavy, does not necessarily mean that the pregnancy is over.

Abdominal pain

Most pregnant women experience some abdominal aches and pains in early pregnancy. They are always a source of worry, but do try to remember that most of the time they simply reflect that enormous changes are occurring in your pelvic organs, particularly your growing uterus. All this growth occurs at the end of the same ligaments and muscles that were attached to your uterus in its non-pregnant state. So it is hardly surprising that the inevitable stretching of these ligaments results in some twinges and discomfort.

On the other hand, if your abdominal pains become constant or very severe, tell your doctor immediately, since they may be a sign that you have an ectopic pregnancy, which needs to be investigated and treated as a matter of urgency. Most ectopic pregnancies declare themselves during this stage of pregnancy, and if you develop severe abdominal pain, your doctor will arrange for you to have an ultrasound scan to see if the pregnancy sac is in the uterine cavity. If there is no sac in the uterus, you will need further investigative tests, which may include a laparoscopic examination under a general anaesthetic.

Feeling dizzy

Dizziness and feeling faint or light-headed are also quite common symptoms in early pregnancy. Most of the time these symptoms are harmless, but if they keep occurring they can become a cause for concern. If you feel faint or light-headed while sitting down, one of the likeliest explanations is that your blood sugar levels are low. This is quite common in the first trimester when many women find it very difficult to eat properly; you can solve it by making sure that you keep a supply of small carbohydrate snacks with you and eating them regularly. If you find yourself feeling faint or dizzy when you stand up suddenly or have been standing up for a long period, this is because there is insufficient blood reaching your brain at that moment. Your blood supply has increased, but when you are upright, it pools in your legs and feet. When you stand up suddenly, the blood rushes into your legs and the supply to your brain is reduced.

Things to consider

At this stage of pregnancy there are rarely any pressing concerns – just a period of gentle adjustment to the idea that you are carrying a new life and a few strategies that will help lay a good foundation for the months ahead.

Visiting the dentist

Dental treatment is free for pregnant women in the UK but I am all too aware of the current difficulty in finding dentists that offer NHS treatment. Please do not make this an excuse for not bothering – there are several good reasons why you should visit a dentist regularly over the next 40 weeks. In pregnancy, your gums become softened by pregnancy hormones and are more likely to bleed and become infected. Thorough toothbrushing and flossing, together with cleaning and plaque removal by your dentist, will ensure that you limit your chances of tooth decay and gum disease during your pregnancy.

Your dentist will always try to avoid performing any tooth or jaw X-rays when you are pregnant, but if your dental problems are serious and causing you pain, let me reassure you that your mouth is a long way (in X-ray terms) from your tiny embryo, and that there are lots of gadgets to help ensure that the rays do not spread anywhere else. Local anaesthetics are perfectly safe, so you do not have to endure dental procedures without pain relief.

A pregnancy bra

Your breasts will have begun to increase in size and for some women they may have become very uncomfortable, even painful. Now is the time to invest in a couple of good pregnancy bras because sagging breasts will be the source of physical discomfort and backache, not to mention distress at your own appearance. I remember thinking that there was no point in buying a new set of bras at this stage, because I wrongly assumed that I would grow out of them in a month or so and then need to invest in another set. The reality is that your

> **❝**
> You will love this new baby every bit as passionately as you do your other child.
> **❞**

breasts enlarge during the first three months of pregnancy and then do not change much until after the birth when you start breastfeeding, at which point you need a completely different type of breast support. The best way to be sure that you buy the right type of bra is to find a shop or department store that has specialist salespeople. A pregnancy bra has good support all the way round, including the underarm and back sections. Underwired bras are not a good option; the wiring will dig into your breasts and may harm the later development of breast milk ducts. If your breasts were full before you became pregnant, you may want to wear a bra to bed at night.

Women who have had cosmetic breast implants may be feeling especially tender now that their own breast tissue is growing. The skin over the breasts may feel taut and uncomfortable, too. You may be wondering if you will be able to breastfeed, and this largely depends on where the incisions were made to insert your implants. If cuts were made around the areola of your nipples, milk ducts and nerves that are essential to breastfeeding may have been severed. If incisions were made under your breasts, there is a good chance these are unaffected.

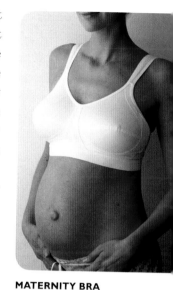

MATERNITY BRA
It is never too early to be fitted for a good supportive bra since your breast size increases right from the start and will not change much during the pregnancy.

Telling the rest of the family

If you have other children, you may well be anxious about how this new pregnancy will affect them and how they will react to their new sibling. There is no doubt that, while many older children are thrilled to learn that there will be a new baby arriving in the family, some younger children will not be so delighted. At this early stage I think it is probably best to wait a little before telling your existing children that you are pregnant.

However, if you have experienced early pregnancy problems and needed to go into hospital to resolve them, your young toddler may be extremely upset by your sudden disappearance and "illness". In the world of a young child, mummies are meant to be reliably available, rock-solid figures, and disappearing at short notice can be disturbing. If you find yourself in this situation, my advice is to explain that you have been unwell and be as honest as possible. The details you share with your children will depend on their ability to comprehend, but whatever you say to them, emphasize that you are going to get better quickly.

How can I love another child?

Some women worry that they will not love their new baby as much as their existing child and they can't imagine how this new addition will fit into their family set-up. I can assure you that such thoughts will seem ridiculous in a year's time. You will look back and not be able to imagine what life was like before this birth and love this baby every bit as passionately as you do your other child.

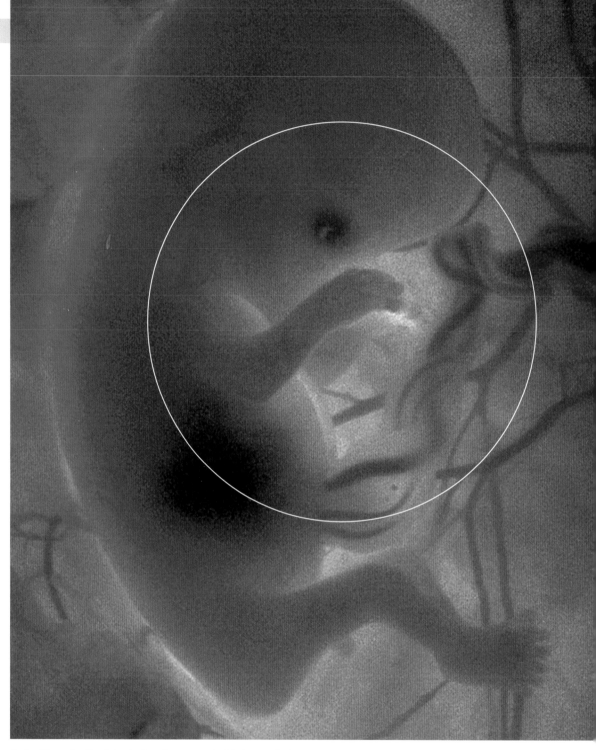

▲ By 10 weeks, the fetus is already a recognizable human being.

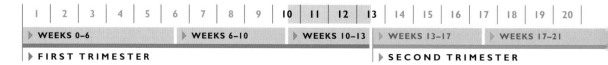

| 1 | 2 | 3 | 4 | 5 | 6 | 7 | 8 | 9 | **10** | **11** | **12** | **13** | 14 | 15 | 16 | 17 | 18 | 19 | 20 |

▶ WEEKS 0–6   ▶ WEEKS 6–10   ▶ WEEKS 10–13   ▶ WEEKS 13–17   ▶ WEEKS 17–21

▶ **FIRST TRIMESTER**   ▶ **SECOND TRIMESTER**

▶ **WEEKS 10–13**

The developing baby

THE FETAL STAGE HAS BEGUN and all of your baby's vital body organs are now in place. From this time onwards, your baby's development will be concerned entirely with the growth and maturation of these major body systems.

During the next few weeks the fetus will grow rapidly and steadily, at a rate of about 10mm (½in) per week and its weight will increase five-fold. If you have an ultrasound scan at this stage, you will be amazed by how easy it is to recognize the various parts of your baby's body and that it is already starting to look more and more like a tiny human.

The fetal head is still relatively large, accounting for approximately one-third of its length from the crown of its head to its bottom (the crown rump length or CRL), but the growth of the rest of the body is starting to catch up. The head is now supported by a recognizable neck and the features on the face are better defined, since all of the facial bones are completely formed. The forehead is still high, but there is now an obvious jaw line and chin and the nose is more pronounced; 32 tooth buds are in place. The eyes are fully developed and although still quite widely spaced, now appear closer to the front of the face. The eyelids are still developing and remain tightly closed. The external ears (pinna) become more clearly visible as they enlarge and assume their adult shape. They have now moved from the base of the skull to a higher position on the sides of the fetal head. The inner ear and middle ear are completely developed. The fetal skin is still thin, transparent, and permeable to the amniotic fluid and a layer of fine hairs now covers most of the body.

Your baby's limbs

The fetal body appears much straighter than it was just a few weeks ago. The limbs are growing rapidly, and shoulders, elbows, wrists, and fingers can be clearly seen. The lower limbs are developing too, but their growth will be at a slower pace for some time. The fingers and toes are separating into individual

life size

At 10 weeks, the fetus measures 30mm (1¼in) and weighs 3–5g (0.1oz). By the 13th week, it is 80mm (3in) long and weighs 25g (about 1oz).

21	22	23	24	25	26	27	28	29	30	31	32	33	34	35	36	37	38	39	40

▶ **WEEKS 21–26**   ▶ **WEEKS 26–30**   ▶ **WEEKS 30–35**   ▶ **WEEKS 35–40**

▶ **THIRD TRIMESTER**

66 The fetus is now moving around quite vigorously inside the amniotic sac, producing small jerky movements… **99**

digits and tiny nails are now present. At about 12 weeks, hard bone centres develop in the cartilage of the fetal bones, a process called ossification. As calcium continues to be deposited in these centres, the skeleton will gradually calcify and harden. This formation of hard bone continues long after your baby is born and will not be complete until adolescence. The fetus is now moving around quite vigorously inside the amniotic sac, producing small jerky movements of its body and upper limbs rather than simply free-floating. However, you are still quite unaware of its movements. The muscles of the chest wall are starting to develop and practice breathing movements along with the occasional hiccough, and swallowing movements can be seen on the ultrasound. Even more excitingly, your baby is starting to make reflex responses to external stimuli. For example, if your abdomen is prodded, the baby will try to wriggle away from the intruding finger. If a hand or foot happens to brush against the baby's mouth, the lips purse and the forehead may wrinkle – this is the very first sign of the future sucking reflex. Similarly, if the eyelids are touched, an early blinking reflex can be seen. However, these are only reflex movements and it is generally accepted that the fetus does not have the ability to feel pain until about 24 weeks of gestation.

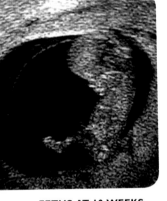

FETUS AT 10 WEEKS
A 2-D ultrasound reveals the fetus free-floating in the black circle of the amniotic sac. The faint white line is the sac's outer layer, called the chorion, which is still separate from the uterine wall.

Inside your baby's body

Inside your baby's body, the ovaries or testes have fully formed, and the external genitalia are developing from a small swelling between the fetal legs into a recognizable penis or clitoris. In theory, an experienced ultrasound scanner may be able to determine the sex of your baby at this early stage, but if you rely on the diagnosis now you might be in for a surprise at the birth.

The heart is now fully functional and pumping blood to all parts of the fetal body at a rate of 110–160 beats per minute. This is slower than it was a few weeks ago and will continue to slow down as the fetus becomes more mature. It may be possible to hear the heartbeat with a sonicaid machine placed over your lower abdomen, just above the pubic bone. This device uses Doppler ultrasound waves and is completely harmless to your baby. During the early weeks of pregnancy, the embryo's blood cells were manufactured in the yolk sac, but by 12 to 13 weeks the sac is fast disappearing, and this essential task is taken over by the fetal liver. Later in the second trimester, the fetal bone marrow and spleen will make important contributions to the production of fetal blood.

The chest and abdomen are gradually straightening out, and the intestines, which a few weeks ago were coiled around the umbilical cord in the amniotic cavity, are now firmly behind a closed abdominal wall. The fetal stomach is now linked to the mouth and the intestines – an important development because the fetus now begins to swallow small amounts of amniotic fluid. This will later be excreted as urine when the fetal kidneys start to function.

The volume of amniotic fluid at 12 weeks is about 30ml – less than an egg cup full. The amniotic fluid has many protective functions, not the least of which is to provide a sterile swimming pool maintained at a constant temperature (slightly higher than your own) in which the baby moves freely. Later on, waste products excreted in the fetal urine will be absorbed from the amniotic fluid back into the maternal blood by passing through the placental membranes.

FETUS AT 13 WEEKS
The fetal arms have developed rapidly – elbows, wrists, and hands with fingers are clearly visible on this 3-D ultrasound. The fetus makes reflex responses when its hand brushes its face.

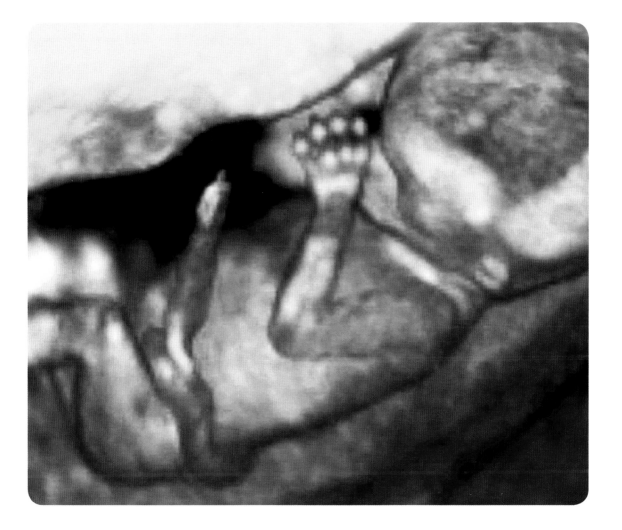

THE PLACENTA

Your fully-formed placenta is now your baby's life support system. It is a complex piece of biological engineering that supplies all your baby's needs via your bloodstream, yet also acts as a barrier against infections and harmful substances.

The placenta has been developing rapidly and by 12–13 weeks its structure is complete, although it will continue to grow in size throughout the remainder of pregnancy. By the end of the first trimester, it is fully established and performs a variety of essential functions for the rest of the pregnancy. In essence, the placenta is a sophisticated filtering system that allows your baby to breathe, eat, and excrete. It also acts as a protective barrier that shields your baby from most infections and potentially harmful substances. In addition, the placenta is responsible for producing increasing quantities of hormones that help to maintain the pregnancy and prepare your body for birth and breastfeeding.

All of this placental activity uses up a considerable amount of energy, and the metabolic rate of the placenta is similar to that of the adult liver or kidney. Furthermore, the successful functioning of the placenta depends upon a good maternal blood supply to the spiral arteries in the uterine wall. This is why smoking and disorders such as high blood pressure and pre-eclampsia (see p.426) that reduce the blood flow to the placenta, have a dramatic effect on its function and on the growth of the fetus.

A NETWORK OF TREES

The placenta is best understood by imagining a network of branching trees made up of about 200 trunks. These divide into limbs, branches, and twigs, which are covered with an extensive network of chorionic villi, the majority of which float in a lake of maternal blood called the intervillous space. Some of the longest branches grow down into the decidual lining of the uterus. A few travel even further, penetrating the deeper layers of the uterine wall to access the maternal blood vessels. These anchoring villi help to form the lower boundary of the intervillous space.

THE UMBILICAL CORD

The umbilical cord is now fully formed and consists of three blood vessels: a single large vein, which carries oxygen-rich blood and nutrients from the uterus to the fetus, via the placenta; and two small arteries, which transport waste products and oxygen-depleted blood from the fetus back to the mother for recharging. The three vessels are coiled like a spring to ensure that the growing baby can move around easily within the amniotic sac and are covered by a thick protective coating called Wharton's jelly.

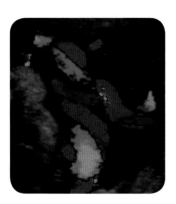

Doppler scan of the umbilical cord shows blood flow via a single large vein (red) and two arteries (blue).

THE LIFE SUPPORT SYSTEM

The extensive network of chorionic villi are bathed in maternal blood inside the intervillous space. Although nutrients and waste products can pass freely through the chorion (a thin membrane that surrounds the villi), the chorion acts as a barrier, too, protecting the fetus from infections and environmental poisons.

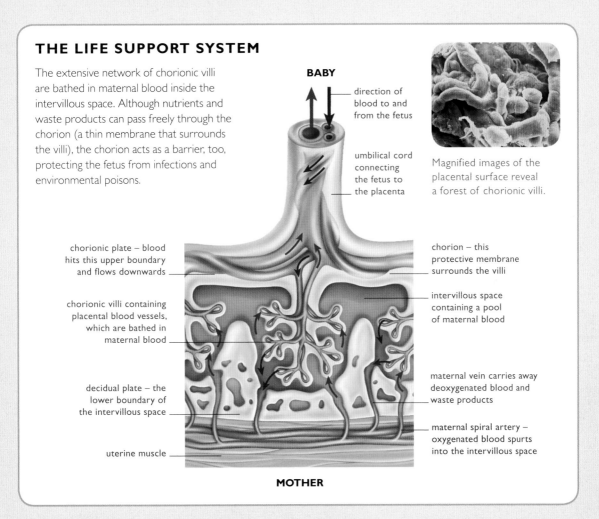

BABY

direction of blood to and from the fetus

umbilical cord connecting the fetus to the placenta

Magnified images of the placental surface reveal a forest of chorionic villi.

chorionic plate – blood hits this upper boundary and flows downwards

chorionic villi containing placental blood vessels, which are bathed in maternal blood

decidual plate – the lower boundary of the intervillous space

uterine muscle

chorion – this protective membrane surrounds the villi

intervillous space containing a pool of maternal blood

maternal vein carries away deoxygenated blood and waste products

maternal spiral artery – oxygenated blood spurts into the intervillous space

MOTHER

TRANSFER OF OXYGEN AND NUTRIENTS

With every beat of your heart, blood from your arteries in the lower boundary of the intervillous space (the decidual plate) spurts into the intervillous space like a fountain. The blood hits the upper boundary (the chorionic plate) and then flows downwards bathing the chorionic villi before seeping away through the veins in the decidual plate. The large number of blood vessels in the chorionic villi and the relatively sluggish flow of your blood through the intervillous space gives ample opportunity for oxygen and nutrients to pass to the fetal circulation. At the same time, carbon dioxide and other waste products from the fetus are transferred into the intervillous space and carried away in your blood.

SEPARATE CIRCULATIONS

Despite their very close proximity in the intervillous space, the maternal and fetal circulations remain entirely separate and never mix. They are separated by a thin membrane, in places as little as only one cell thick. This protects the developing fetus from infections, and other damaging substances such as pesticides, alcohol, and some drugs. Furthermore, any bleeding in pregnancy always originates from the pool of maternal blood, not from the fetus. The fetal circulation is protected, even if the placenta is damaged.

Your changing body

By the end of this trimester your waist will probably have thickened slightly and you will have put on a little weight. Your tummy may be starting to swell too, but this is more likely to be due to mild bloating and sluggish bowels than to your growing baby.

> By 12 weeks your uterus will be the size of a large grapefruit... by 14 weeks it will be the size of a small melon.

At 10 weeks, the size of your uterus will be equivalent to a large orange. By 12 weeks it will have reached the size of a large grapefruit and by 14 weeks it will be the size of a small melon. Sometime between 11 and 14 weeks, depending on your body weight and the size of your pelvis, your doctor or midwife will be able to feel the enlarging uterus through your abdominal wall just above the pubic bone. Of course, if you are expecting twins or triplets, the enlarging uterus rises above the pelvic brim at an earlier stage. Indeed, before the days of ultrasound scans, this was one of the first signs of a multiple pregnancy.

Your breasts will have continued to develop under the influence of progesterone and several other hormones, the production of which has been steadily increasing during this first trimester. Some previously small-chested women are alarmed to find themselves going up three or four bra cup sizes in the first 12 weeks of pregnancy. If this is the case with you, don't panic, you will probably find that your breasts stop filling out fairly soon and then will increase only a little more in the last month or so before the birth. If your breasts were full before you became pregnant, you may want to wear a bra to bed at night now for support. If they feel very tender, try using a soothing massage cream such as camomile or calendula on the breast tissue and nipples.

Increasing your oxygen supply

Many women notice that they occasionally feel breathless by the end of the first trimester; a symptom that sometimes continues throughout pregnancy. The major changes that have occurred in your heart and blood vessels mean that almost every organ in your body is now working much harder, demanding a dramatic increase in your oxygen supplies. Your oxygen requirements rise by 15–20 per cent during pregnancy, and half of this is used by the growing uterus, placenta, and baby. The other half is needed to fuel the work of the heart and kidneys, although some is directed to the respiratory muscles, breasts, and skin.

To achieve this extra supply, your lungs need to make a special adaptation to take in an increased volume of oxygen and expel an increased amount of waste carbon dioxide with every breath that you take. This is called the tidal volume of air and it increases by 40 per cent during pregnancy. When you exercise or exert yourself, your tidal volume and oxygen consumption increase way above their pre-pregnancy levels. Although the exact mechanisms for achieving this are not understood, we do know that progesterone makes an important contribution. It effectively allows your lungs to hyperventilate or overbreathe and that is why you experience feelings of breathlessness.

How you may feel physically

By the end of the first trimester, you are likely to be getting back into your stride and feeling more like your old self. However, every pregnancy is different – there are no hard and fast rules governing how you should or should not feel.

For many women, the nausea and vomiting that so often dominate the first 10–12 weeks of pregnancy has started to settle down, but for the less fortunate it may persist for longer. No one can predict a pregnancy experience exactly. However, as the nausea improves, you will be able to start eating normally once again, and if you have been worrying about how little nourishment you and your baby have been receiving, this is a welcome change.

Your uterus has already enlarged considerably, and as the ligaments attaching it to the sides of your pelvis have been stretched, it is quite normal to experience the odd twinge or muscular ache. Of course, if the pain continues or becomes severe, seek advice from your doctor as soon as possible. Now that the uterus is moving up into the abdominal cavity, there should be less pressure on your bladder, giving you some respite from the constant calls to pass water.

You may still be experiencing bouts of severe tiredness, but in general, the complete exhaustion so characteristic of the first 10–12 weeks of pregnancy is beginning to lift and you should be feeling more energetic. Doubtless there will still be days when you feel dreadful but these are becoming less frequent now, and after a bad day you will be pleasantly surprised at how quickly you are able to bounce back. Indeed, some women feel physically exhilarated at this stage in pregnancy. Whatever is the case for you, take this period of transition at your own pace and aim to deal with life one day at a time.

> ...after a bad day you will be pleasantly surprised at how quickly you are able to bounce back.

Your emotional response

If you have been troubled by mood swings, these are likely to be settling down now that you have had time to make some physical and mental adjustments to being pregnant. That said, there may still be times when you feel inexplicably anxious or irritable.

Just getting to the end of the first trimester eliminates an important source of worry because from now onwards you are extremely unlikely to suffer a miscarriage or later pregnancy loss. The reality is that the vast majority of miscarriages have occurred well before 10 weeks of gestation, and after 12 weeks, the risk of losing a pregnancy is no more than one per cent.

Many women tell me this was the point in their pregnancy when their partner first started to come to terms with the idea that he was going to become a father, and that there was going to be a baby in the house in the not too distant future. Even if his reaction is not exactly what you had hoped for, it is a relief that someone else is at least sharing the realization of what being pregnant is all about. Up until now, there have probably been days when it has been difficult for both of you to believe that you are pregnant, but from now on, there will be no doubt in your mind, particularly after you have had your antenatal booking visit and enjoyed the excitement of seeing your tiny baby on an ultrasound scan for the first time (see p.124). Like so many other important things in life, dealing with certainty is much easier than dealing with uncertainty.

Some women are able to relate to their unborn baby from a very early stage in the pregnancy, whereas others find it virtually impossible to do so until much later in pregnancy, particularly when it is a first pregnancy. I want to say here that there is nothing odd about talking to your baby and generally including this new person in your everyday life, if that feels right for you. Nor is it odd if you cannot begin to imagine that the tiny fetus growing inside you is going to develop into a real human being. What you do and how you feel is in no way an indication of how good or bad a mother you will turn out to be; it is just another example of how individual we human beings are.

> ❝ ...the first ultrasound scan may be the point when your partner starts to come to terms with the idea that he is going to be a father. ❞

Telling people your news

Now that you feel more secure about your pregnancy and no doubt convinced that everyone around you must have noticed that you are beginning to change shape, you will probably decide to tell people that you are pregnant. Sharing your news with friends and family is usually a cause for celebration, although inevitably there will be at least one person for whom the subject of pregnancy is difficult. Only you can know who to tell and how to handle the situation, but it is worth remembering that, a bit like deciding on a guest list for a wedding, there will always be someone who feels left out or upset by your news.

This is a good point to refer back to the section on work and maternity rights (see pp.58–63) because this is a subject that you should start thinking about sooner rather than later. You need to be clearly aware of your employment rights before you tell your boss or head of personnel your news.

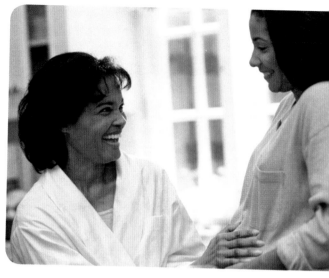

EXCITING NEWS Most women begin to feel more secure about their pregnancy as they come to the end of the first trimester – and are ready to share their news.

Your antenatal care

Your first detailed antenatal or booking visit usually takes place in the next few weeks. The purpose of this visit is to identify potential problems and create a set of individual antenatal case notes that detail all your current and past medical and social history.

If you are deemed to be high risk, your booking appointment will be at the hospital. If you are not in this category, you are likely to meet the community midwife at the GP's surgery, local birth centre or in your home. This visit provides an opportunity to discuss your antenatal care with your midwife or doctor and make arrangements for any tests that you may wish to have performed (see pp.134–43). You will need to set aside 45 minutes to an hour during which you will be asked detailed questions about your general health, your diet and lifestyle, and your previous medical and gynaecological history. Your responses will form the basis of your personal hand-held notes, which you will carry for the duration of your pregnancy so that you always have them to hand wherever and whenever you may need medical or midwifery assistance. For the majority of pregnant women, these notes will record the fact that you are at low risk of any complications and can be reassured of a trouble-free pregnancy. During this visit, it is very important that you discuss every aspect of your medical history, lifestyle, and social circumstances with your maternity carers. Sadly, 1 in 4 women suffer domestic violence during pregnancy, which is why your midwife will enquire sensitively when you are alone whether you need help or support.

Your previous pregnancies

Your past obstetric history (if any) is important because the outcome of previous pregnancies and any problems that you may have had will help your carers to assess whether you can be classified as low risk or high risk in your current pregnancy and the type of antenatal care you require. For every past pregnancy you will be asked about the gestation in weeks at the time of delivery, the weight of your baby, whether the labour was spontaneous or induced, the method of delivery, and any complications that arose antenatally, during the delivery and postnatally. If your previous pregnancy was complicated and you were cared for at another hospital, your midwife and doctor will ask the hospital concerned for a detailed summary of your notes.

QUESTIONS AT YOUR ANTENATAL BOOKING VISIT

The following list is not exhaustive but should give you a feel for the sort of information that your maternity carers need to know.

▶ **What is the date of your last period?** Your Estimated Date of Delivery (EDD) will be calculated according to this date (see p.79) so try to work it out before your visit.

▶ **Have you had problems becoming pregnant and if so, how was this pregnancy achieved?** Assisted fertility treatments such as IVF increase the chances of a multiple pregnancy, which needs specialist care.

▶ **Have you had any problems in this pregnancy so far?** This includes major concerns such as bleeding and abdominal pain, but you should also mention minor problems such as vaginal discharge.

Your midwife can then arrange for you to have appropriate investigations and treatment.

▶ **Do you smoke cigarettes or use recreational drugs?** If you haven't managed to give these up yet, this is an opportunity to ask for help to do so.

▶ **Do you have a medical illness?** If you have an illness such as diabetes, asthma, high blood pressure, thrombosis (blood clots), kidney or heart disease, you may need to see a specialist doctor during your pregnancy, and the type and dosage of drugs that you are taking may need to be altered.

▶ **Are you taking any medications?** Do make sure that you mention any medicines and preparations that you are taking, whether they are

prescription drugs, over-the-counter medicines or complementary remedies.

▶ **Do you suffer from any allergies?** It is important to record any allergies such as hay fever, asthma, as well as any allergic response you may have to drugs, foods, plasters, and iodine.

▶ **Have you ever suffered from a psychiatric illness?** You may feel that this is an intrusive question, but pregnancy can have a profound effect on some psychiatric disorders. It is important that you discuss any problems that you may have had in the past, so that your carers can help you minimize future problems. Postnatal depression, for example, is very likely to recur but it can be treated effectively if it is recognized quickly. The best way to do this is

Some women feel sensitive about a previous termination of pregnancy and would prefer not to have this information recorded in their hand-held notes, which theoretically could be picked up and read by anyone. You may have similar concerns if you had assisted fertility treatment to achieve this pregnancy (believing this to be a private matter between you and your partner). I can understand these feelings, but you do need to discuss every part of your history at the booking visit to ensure that any potential future complications can be identified and prevented. However, you can ask that this information is not recorded in your hand-held notes, and your midwife will honour this request.

Your first physical examination

How detailed a physical examination you undergo at your antenatal booking visit varies between different hospitals and local surgeries. When I was a junior trainee in obstetrics, a thorough physical examination of the heart, lungs, abdomen, legs, skin, and breasts, together with a routine pelvic and vaginal examination and cervical smear test were performed routinely by a doctor,

to identify those women who are at risk before it develops.

▶ **Have you undergone abdominal or pelvic surgery?** Previous surgical procedures may determine how you should deliver your baby. An elective Caesarean section is sometimes the preferred option if you have had, for example, surgery to remove a fibroid from your uterus. On the other hand, a vaginal delivery may be a better option if you have lesions or scar tissue as a result of a gastrointestinal or bladder operation. Always mention previous surgery, however minor you think it may have been.

▶ **Have you ever had a blood transfusion?** A previous blood transfusion will alert your carers to the possibility that you may have developed atypical antibodies in your blood or be at risk of a blood-borne infection such as hepatitis or HIV. These are extremely unlikely complications in the UK because our transfusion service is carefully monitored and is considered the safest in the world. However, this may not be the case if you had a transfusion in some European countries or American states.

▶ **Do you have a history of infection, particularly a sexually transmitted disease?** All maternity carers in the UK will screen you for immunity to rubella and possible infection with syphilis. You will also be offered screening for HIV infection and, if you live in an inner-city area, you may be offered screening for Hepatitis B and Hepatitis C. I strongly advise you to give full information about your possible exposure to infections and to undergo any screening tests that you are offered. The implications of these tests are discussed later in this section. Ignorance is not bliss for pregnant women. Knowledge will provide you and your unborn baby with an opportunity to reduce the damage the infection can cause.

▶ **Do you have a family history of twins, diabetes, high blood pressure, thrombosis, tuberculosis, congenital abnormalities or blood disorders?** If there is one or more of these in your family history, this does not necessarily mean that you will suffer from them during your pregnancy, but it does alert your carers to watch for signs that a potential problem is developing.

either at the time the midwife took down all the booking details or a week or so later. Nowadays, the physical examination tends to be much less intrusive, partly because most pregnant women are generally fit and well, but also because we are conscious that antenatal care providers are not general physicians and specific medical problems are best dealt with by a referral to a specialist.

If you have never had a medical problem and this is your first pregnancy, the physical examination will probably be confined to measuring your height, weight, and blood pressure, taking a urine sample, and examining your hands, legs, and abdomen. If you are high risk, your heart and lungs may be examined also.

Height

If you are less than 1.5m (5ft) tall, you may be concerned that your pelvis is also smaller than average and that this may lead to problems at the time of delivery. For the same reason, your shoe size used to be recorded in your notes because small feet can indicate a narrow pelvis. However, the reality is that your height and shoe size are not conclusive measures of the capacity of your pelvis; your ability to deliver a baby cannot be accurately assessed until you are in full-blown labour. So I think that worrying about your height at this stage in pregnancy is not helpful. I have seen plenty of very short women deliver big babies and seen some small babies experience problems negotiating an ample pelvis in a tall woman.

BOOKING VISIT Being candid about any previous pregnancies and your past medical history will help your carers to tailor your antenatal care.

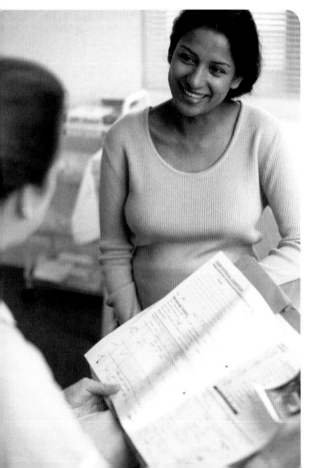

Weight

Your weight at the booking visit is a more useful measurement, since you are more likely to experience problems in pregnancy and at the time of delivery if you are significantly under- or overweight (see p.41). In days gone by, pregnant women were weighed at every antenatal visit, in the belief that putting on too much or too little weight in pregnancy could identify babies that were at risk of complications. This is simply not true, and maternity units no longer weigh women routinely. Having said that, if you start your pregnancy significantly under- or overweight, and if you have diabetes or develop gestational diabetes, your carers will monitor your weight and eating habits and will probably suggest that you follow a healthy diet and calorie-controlled eating programme.

WHY YOU MAY NEED SPECIAL CARE

The following factors may mean that you need specialist antenatal care:
▶ Previous preterm delivery (before 37 weeks)
▶ Recurrent miscarriages
▶ Baby with a congenital abnormality
▶ Pre-eclampsia or high blood pressure in previous pregnancy
▶ Diabetes or gestational diabetes
▶ Previous thrombosis (blood clot)

▶ Previous birth of baby weighing more than 4kg (9lb) or less than 2.5kg (5½lb)
▶ Pregnancy with identical twins (see p.123)

These risk factors may mean that you need extra care during delivery:
▶ Previous long labour and instrumental delivery (forceps or ventouse)

▶ Previous Caesarean section
▶ Previous failed induction of labour
▶ Previous birth of baby weighing more than 4kg (9lb) or less than 2.5kg (5½lb)
▶ Excessive bleeding after a birth (postpartum haemorrhage)
▶ Problems with an anaesthetic
▶ Urinary or bowel problems after a delivery
▶ Current twin pregnancy

Legs and hands

The appearance of your legs and hands is another useful baseline measurement at your booking visit and some midwives and doctors keep a regular check on this during pregnancy. The colour and state of your fingernails is a useful factor when assessing your general health since they can reflect your diet and whether you are anaemic. Spider naevi (small broken veins with a spider-like appearance) and reddening of the palms and soles are to be expected in pregnant women, but the sudden appearance of lots of broken veins or areas of bruising suggests that you need investigations, including blood clotting tests.

The other sign that will be looked for is swelling or puffiness of your fingers, feet, ankles, and lower legs, which may indicate problems with fluid retention. In later pregnancy, a degree of swelling in these areas is quite common, especially at the end of a busy day, but any sudden swelling or progressive increase in swelling needs to be taken seriously since it suggests that you are at risk of developing pre-eclampsia (see p.426).

Abdomen

Your midwife or doctor will examine the size of your expanding uterus at the booking visit and will also want to see whether you have any scars from previous operations and exactly where these are positioned. Provide as much detail as you can about previous abdominal or pelvic surgery, because this can influence decisions about how your baby would be best delivered. For example, having your appendix out could have been a simple uncomplicated operation leaving you with a small scar on your right side. But if your appendix burst and you developed peritonitis, you may well have undergone a major abdominal

66
...the reality is that your height and shoe size are not reliable measures of the capacity of your pelvis...
99

> Your blood pressure will be checked at every antenatal visit.

operation as an emergency and have been left with a scar that extends all the way down your abdomen and dense adhesions inside your abdominal cavity. For similar reasons, whether the scar is smooth, puckered or tethered to underlying tissues is also useful information to note. So, too, are details about any post-operative complications, such as a wound infection.

Later on in pregnancy, it is perfectly normal to notice stretch marks, or striae, appearing on your abdomen. However, if you suddenly develop livid stretch marks at this early stage in pregnancy it can be due to steroid medication or be a sign that you have an underlying hormonal problem. Your midwife or doctor will arrange for you to see a specialist promptly.

Vaginal and pelvic examinations

Routine vaginal examinations in the booking clinic and at later antenatal visits are no longer considered necessary, but if you have a discharge or have experienced some bleeding, your midwife may examine your cervix, take a swab to identify any infection and, sometimes, take a cervical smear for testing.

We now recognize that trying to judge the capacity of your pelvis at this early stage does not really contribute very much to the planning of your antenatal care. However, there are situations when it may be helpful for you to be examined internally at this visit – for example, if you have had a previous Caesarean section because you failed to progress in labour and the cause was attributed to the ischial spines of your pelvis being too prominent or your pubic arch being too narrow to let the baby through.

Breasts

Breast examination is not performed at booking visits, but in my view it should be. Breast cancer is uncommon in women under 40, but when it does affect this age group, the tumour is usually oestrogen dependent, which means that pregnancy can greatly accelerate both the local growth and distant spread of the abnormal cells. Midwives and obstetricians may not be the best clinicians to identify every suspicious breast lump, but it is probably better that they identify some rather than none at all, since early diagnosis and treatment may greatly improve prognosis. Advice and information about breast changes and self examination during pregnancy should be offered to all pregnant women.

Urine tests

At your booking and all of your subsequent antenatal visits a urine sample will be tested with a specially treated dipstick to identify sugar, protein, and ketones in your urine. Normally, our kidneys filter out all of the sugar and protein from our urine. However, during pregnancy the increase in blood flow (see p.156) places a further load on a woman's kidneys, and as a result, the urine of pregnant women sometimes contains a small amount of sugar or protein. This always needs to be investigated further. Ketones (chemicals produced when fat is metabolized) are typically found in the urine of diabetic people, but in healthy pregnant women they are sometimes present if your metabolism is upset, such as when you have not been eating enough or have been vomiting. Your urine will be checked for ketones if you are unwell, unusually thirsty, or urinating more frequently than usual.

Glycosuria – sugar in the urine

It is common for pregnant women to have a small quantity of sugar in their urine (glycosuria) during the second or third trimester, but finding sugar in the urine this early in pregnancy is unusual. If it persists at subsequent antenatal visits it suggests that you may be developing gestational diabetes, a condition that affects around 5 per cent of pregnant women (see p.427) and needs careful monitoring to minimize fetal complications. The UK guidelines no longer recommend urine testing for glycosuria before the glucose tolerance test is undertaken routinely at the end of the second trimester between 24 and

MONITORING BLOOD PRESSURE

Checking and recording your blood pressure using the correct size of cuff is important because this first measurement will be used as the baseline reading against which all subsequent readings are compared during your pregnancy. Your blood pressure will then be measured at every antenatal visit regardless of where it takes place.

▶ **A reading of around 120/70mm Hg** is usual for most women. The first figure (120) refers to your systolic blood pressure, which means the pressure in the main blood vessels as your heart pumps blood around your body. The second figure (70) is the diastolic blood pressure – the pressure in your arteries when the heart is at rest. Both the systolic and diastolic readings are important, but if you have a diastolic blood pressure reading of 90 or more, your carers will suggest that you need to be seen by a specialist team for advice and attend an antenatal day unit.

▶ **A persistent increase of 15–20** to either or both of your baseline figures is usually a cause of concern since it suggests that you may be at risk of developing problems such as pre-eclampsia (see p.426). Of course, blood pressures vary a great deal between different women during pregnancy, so this figure should be regarded simply as a useful rule of thumb.

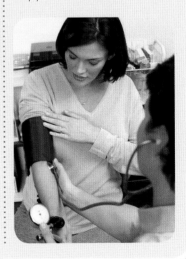

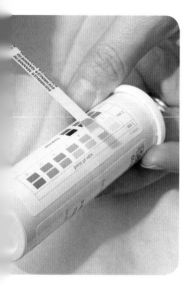

URINE TEST A dipstick is used to detect sugar in the urine. The chemically treated tip changes colour according to the amount of glucose that is present.

28 weeks (see p.212). However, your midwife will be checking your urine for protein at each visit, and if sugar is present you will be strongly advised to limit your intake of sweet foods, particularly cakes, biscuits, candy and chocolates, fruit juices, and whole fruits with high sugar content (bananas, pineapples, and melons). If the glycosuria persists; your BMI is over 35; you have a family history of diabetes or had gestational diabetes or a large baby in a previous pregnancy; or if you belong to a high-risk ethnic group (including South Asian, Black Caribbean, and Chinese), you may be advised to have an early glucose tolerance test to see whether you have really developed gestational diabetes or have simply eaten too much sugar-rich food just before your urine test.

Proteinuria – protein in the urine

There are several important causes of proteinuria in pregnancy, so your doctor or midwife will want to investigate you thoroughly on any occasion that it is found. If you are found to have protein in your urine at your booking visit, you will be asked to produce a clean midstream sample of urine. To do this you will be given a sterile urine collection pot. You need to pass the first few drops of urine into the toilet and then collect a midstream sample of your urine in the pot to be sent off to the laboratory for testing.

The most common cause of proteinuria is an infection in your kidneys or urinary tract. You are more prone to these infections in pregnancy because the tubes that connect your kidneys to your bladder and your bladder to your urethra are relaxed under the influence of pregnancy hormones. This makes it much easier for infective organisms to gain access to your bladder and kidneys. Most importantly, the usual early sign of a urine infection – pain or discomfort when passing urine, called cystitis – is often missing in pregnancy, which means that you can develop a full-blown infection of your kidneys (pyelonephritis) with very little warning. This is a potentially serious problem, because urine infections can cause the uterus to become irritable. If they are left untreated, they may lead to miscarriage or premature labour. Furthermore, repeated urine infections can cause permanent scarring of the kidneys. If an infection is diagnosed, you will be given appropriate antibiotic treatment and a further test will be performed approximately one week after completing the course of tablets to ensure that the infection has cleared. Most antenatal clinics suggest that you have a midstream sample test as a routine part of your booking visit to avoid missing a silent urine infection that has not produced symptoms.

More rarely, protein in the urine at your booking visit can be a sign that you have underlying kidney disease, in which case you will probably be under the care of a specialist kidney (renal) doctor already. Occasionally, however, underlying renal disease is identified for the first time during regular urine tests in pregnancy. In later pregnancy, proteinuria is one of the important signs of pre-eclampsia (see p.426). If at this early stage you have protein in your urine that is not caused by an infection or a previous history of renal problems, this will alert your midwife and doctors to the fact that you are a high-risk pregnancy and may develop pre-eclampsia or other complications at a later stage.

Your first ultrasound scan

All maternity units now offer pregnant women a dating ultrasound scan around 12 weeks (see pp.124–5) to measure the baby's size. You may also be offered a Nuchal Fold Translucency Scan (see p.136) between 11 and 14 weeks for the early detection of Down's syndrome, although this scan is not yet routinely available to all women in the UK.

If you are carrying twins, a scan at 12 weeks or earlier will identify which type of twins you are carrying (see p.125). This is an important detail to establish early on because it has implications for your antenatal care: identical twins are at greater risk of congenital abnormalities and complications such as intrauterine growth restriction (IUGR) and will therefore need specialist care. In fact, 70 per cent have serious problems and only 30 per cent are uncomplicated. If you are pregnant with non-identical twins, normal antenatal care is often all that is needed, although you are more likely to deliver early because of the extra size and weight of the babies inside your uterus.

All women are offered an anatomy scan at 18–20 weeks, which used to be referred to somewhat alarmingly as the fetal anomaly scan (see pp.173–6). By this stage, it is possible to get a clear picture of the development of your baby's organs and body systems, and the majority of structural abnormalities can be detected during this scan. If a problem is found you will probably have further specialist scans, but the majority of women will not need further scans.

ULTRASOUND SCANNING
An early scan is a valuable baseline because it can be used to establish the exact stage of your pregnancy.

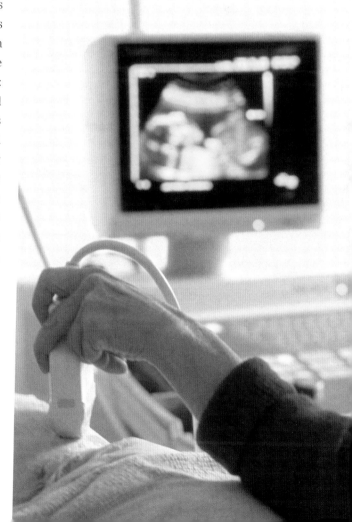

DATING ULTRASOUND SCAN

The dating ultrasound scan between 10 and 14 weeks measures the size of the fetus so that future antenatal care can be organized around your baby's gestational age – the earlier the scan, the more accurate the dating measurements will be.

HOW SCANS ARE USED

▶ **5–8 weeks** Pregnancy viability scan shows sac in uterus; after six weeks fetal pole and heartbeat detectable; dating using CRL measurement

▶ **10–14 weeks** Dating of pregnancy using CRL and BPD. Scan confirms growth, heartbeat, and brain formation

▶ **11–14 weeks** Nuchal Fold Translucency Scan screens for Down's syndrome; dates pregnancy

▶ **20 weeks** Detailed anatomy or anomaly scan examines baby for heart, kidney, bladder, spine, brain, and limb abnormalities; checks growth of head, body, and limbs; checks the position of the placenta

▶ **30 weeks plus** Detailed scans to detect placental problems, intra-uterine growth restriction, and volume of amniotic fluid

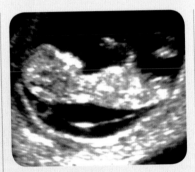

SCAN AT 10 WEEKS The fetal arms and hands are developing. A yolk sac is visible below the baby's head.

▶ **Ultrasound scans**, as their name implies, work by emitting high-frequency soundwaves, which are sent through a pregnant woman's body using a handpiece called a transducer. These soundwaves are reflected back from the solid tissues of the developing baby and translated into images on a computer screen. There is no radiation involved in ultrasound, only soundwaves.

▶ **During the hour before an abdominal ultrasound scan**, you will be asked to drink several pints of water and to avoid emptying your bladder. You may find this a little uncomfortable but there is a good reason for it. When your bladder is full, the ultrasound waves are reflected through this water-filled window lying immediately over the uterus and tiny baby, producing much clearer images.

You will be asked to lie down and lubricating gel is smeared onto the lower part of your abdomen to ensure good contact with the transducer. The sonographer or specially trained doctor or midwife moves the transducer smoothly forwards and backwards to produce ultrasound images on a computer screen.

▶ **For a vaginal scan** a tubular probe is introduced into your vagina. You will probably need to empty your bladder so that the probe is close enough to your uterus to produce clear pictures. Many women worry that a vaginal scan may be painful or will damage their pregnancy, but this is not the case. If you do have any bleeding afterwards, it was going to happen anyway and was not caused by the vaginal probe.

▶ **The key measurements** taken at the 12-week dating scan are the crown-rump length (CRL) – the distance between the top of your baby's head (crown) and bottom (rump) – and the biparietal diameter

(BPD), which is the distance between the two parietal bones on each side of the baby's head. The size of the limbs cannot be measured accurately while the baby is still in a curled position, so the length of the thigh bone or femur (FL) will not be used to assess fetal size until the middle of the second trimester.

Your baby's heartbeat will also be monitored – an extraordinary sight, as it beats fast and furiously. If your dates don't tally with the measurements, it may be because your dates are wrong or there is a problem with the pregnancy. You will probably be asked to come back for another scan at a later date to ensure that all is progressing well.

▶ **Twin pregnancies** are often diagnosed during the 12-week scan, although they can be detected as early as a six-week scan when two pregnancy sacs are usually clearly visible in the uterus. At 12 weeks the sonographer will be able to detect whether you are carrying identical (monochorionic) or non-identical (dichorionic) twins by examining the thickness of the membranes that separate the two amniotic sacs in the uterus. If only two thin layers of amnion (the sac's inner layer) separate the cavities, the twins are identical. If a thicker membrane made up of two layers of amnion and two layers of chorion (the sac's outer layer) separates the twins, they are non-identical.

DATING SCAN AT 12 WEEKS

skull bones   nasal bone   placenta   umbilical cord

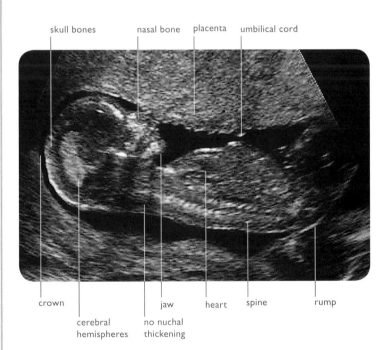

crown   cerebral hemispheres   no nuchal thickening   jaw   heart   spine   rump

INTERPRETING A SCAN Dense tissues such as bone appear white, while fluid-filled areas are dark. At 12 weeks, this fetus has well-formed skull bones and a clearly defined spine. The heart is visible as a small dense area mid-chest that pulsates on screen. The placenta is visualized as a spongy mass connected to the blood-filled umbilical cord, which appears white because blood cells reflect soundwaves.

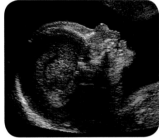

IN PROFILE The cerebral hemispheres are clearly visualized. The sharp profile shows that the nasal bone has formed.

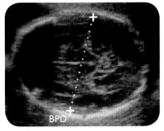

BPD

BIPARIETAL HEAD DIAMETER This is one of the baseline measurements plotted on a graph to monitor fetal growth.

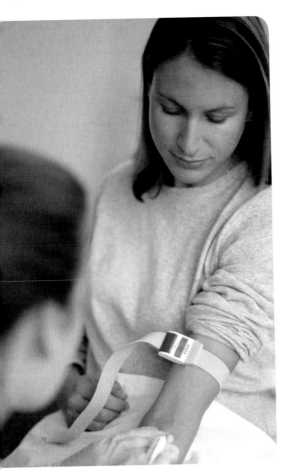

BLOOD TESTING
You are usually asked to provide blood samples for several blood tests at your antenatal booking visit.

Blood tests

You will be asked for permission to perform a variety of blood tests at your booking visit. Some are routine for all pregnant women, but you may be offered additional tests depending on your medical and obstetric history.

Your blood group

This will be one of the four types found in humans: either A, B, AB or O. The most common is O, followed by A and B, and then the rarer AB. For each of these combinations, the individual is either Rhesus positive or negative, the most common type being Rhesus positive. So your blood identity card reads – O Rhesus positive or negative, A Rhesus positive or negative and so on for each blood group. Rhesus status is especially significant in pregnancy because an Rh-negative mother who carries an Rh-positive baby can develop damaging antibodies to her baby's blood (see p.128 and p.425).

Establishing your blood group early in pregnancy is very important. The journey through pregnancy is one of the few times in your life when you are at increased risk of catastrophic bleeding requiring a blood transfusion, so it is essential that your exact blood group is known, included in your maternity notes and available at any time of the day or night. Until very recently, the most important cause of maternal death in the Western world was haemorrhage or blood loss, and in countries that do not have access to blood transfusion services, it remains so. We should never forget these facts or take them for granted. Of course, most women do not experience any bleeding in pregnancy and have no need of a blood transfusion. But for the few that do, knowledge of their blood group can save valuable time for the laboratory staff who are trying to cross-match stored samples of blood with the exact group of the pregnant woman. This is why you will have a blood sample taken if ever you are admitted to a maternity hospital with a problem that could result in a blood transfusion.

Haemoglobin level and blood count

The haemoglobin level in your blood is a measure of the oxygen-carrying pigment in your red blood cells. The normal range for women is 10.5 to 15.0 grammes per litre of blood in your body. If the level is low, this means that you are anaemic and you will be advised to eat foods with a high iron content (see p.47) and may be prescribed iron tablets as well. Anaemia (see p.424) can cause you to feel very tired and may also lead to problems if you have excessive bleeding at the time of delivery.

The full blood count also analyzes numbers of red blood cells, white blood cells, and platelets to provide further information about your general health. For example, it may suggest that your anaemia is not due to a lack of iron alone but other factors, such as vitamin deficiencies, which can be identified and treated.

Immunity to rubella

Every pregnant woman in the UK is tested to see whether she is immune to rubella. The fetal damage that a first infection with rubella can cause during early pregnancy has already been discussed (see p.32 and p.412). If you are found to be non-immune at your booking visit, you will be given advice as to how you can best avoid exposure to infection during your pregnancy and offered immunization as soon as your baby has been delivered. Some women may also need to be offered screening for toxoplasmosis (see p.413), recent chickenpox exposure (see p.412), and other less common infections such as hepatitis (see p.129 and p.117) and Human Immunodeficiency Virus (HIV, see p.130 and p.415).

Sexually transmitted diseases

Pregnant women are routinely screened for syphilis infection (see p.415) and offered prompt treatment with penicillin if they are found to be infected. Because syphilis is relatively uncommon nowadays, some clinicians have suggested that screening should be discontinued and the resources used to search for other infections. However, it is important to remember that undetected infection with syphilis during pregnancy can be the cause of severe congenital and developmental problems in the baby. Since syphilis can be treated so swiftly and easily, I believe that we should continue to screen for it routinely during pregnancy. Sadly, the incidence of syphilis is increasing in Eastern Europe, Russia, and Africa. If you have lived in any of these countries and are now receiving antenatal care in the UK, it is especially important that you are screened to prevent damage to yourself and your baby.

Infection with chlamydia and gonorrhoea (see p.414), two other sexually transmitted diseases, is more likely to cause problems with fertility. However, chlamydia infections are also the cause of serious eye infections in newborns, so if you think you may be at risk, do tell your midwife and doctor so that they can help you to prevent problems developing.

RHESUS NEGATIVE PREGNANCIES

▶ **If your blood group is Rhesus negative**, problems can arise in pregnancy if your baby inherits Rh-positive status from your partner. Rhesus status is rarely a problem in a first pregnancy, but if you are Rh-negative and exposed to some of your baby's Rh-positive blood during childbirth, you may develop anti-D antibodies that could cause problems in a subsequent pregnancy. The anti-D antibodies attack the next baby's blood, causing anaemia and distress for the baby in the uterus and anaemia and jaundice (see p.435) after the birth.

▶ **All mothers (both Rh-positive and negative)** are checked for anti-D antibodies during their booking-visit blood tests. The blood tests are repeated at 28 weeks.

▶ **If you have developed antibodies**, you will be offered

further blood tests every four weeks, and your baby will be carefully monitored for signs of anaemia or heart failure.

▶ **Even if you have not developed antibodies (but are Rh-negative)**, maternity units now offer a routine preventative anti-D injection at 28 weeks, which mops up Rh-positive fetal blood cells and prevents the development of destructive maternal antibodies. The exception is if the father is also Rh-negative, in which case there is no risk that the baby's blood will be incompatible. This anti-D programme in the UK has made rhesus haemolytic disease of the newborn relatively rare.

▶ **All Rh-negative mothers who give birth to a Rh-positive baby** are given an anti-D injection within 72 hours of delivery. A blood test establishes

the level of fetal cells present in her circulation, and if the concentration is high, another dose of anti-D may be needed.

▶ **Rh-negative women who have amniocentesis** (see pp.140–3), chorionic villus sampling (see p.140), external cephalic version (see p.271) or who have vaginal bleeding or abdominal trauma during pregnancy are given an injection of anti-D within 72 hours. Those who miscarry and require surgical evacuation of the uterus or who undergo termination of pregnancy or who have an ectopic pregnancy are also treated with anti-D.

KEY
− mother's blood
+ baby's blood
▲ antibodies

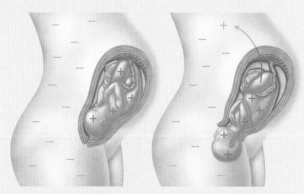

FIRST PREGNANCY Maternal and fetal circulations do not usually mix during pregnancy, but during birth the mother may be exposed to her baby's blood.

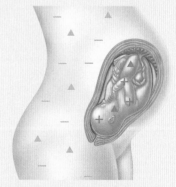

SUBSEQUENT PREGNANCY If the mother has developed antibodies to her baby's red blood cells they may cause problems in a future pregnancy.

Sickle cell anaemia and thalassaemia

A haemoglobin test is offered to all pregnant women to determine whether they have sickle cell or thalassaemia trait – inherited blood conditions that are more commonly found in people of Mediterranean or African origin. Haemoglobin is produced in different forms depending on your genetic background. These different forms are a result of evolutionary diversity and, in simple terms, some varieties of haemoglobins protect you from life-threatening diseases. For example, for people in countries where malaria is rife, having a small dose of sickle cell haemoglobin (the trait but not the full-blown disease) in your blood means that you are better able to cope with the infection because your red blood cells are more fragile. As a result, the malarial parasites are less able to survive.

If you carry the sickle cell trait, it is important that your partner's sickle cell status is established early on, since there is a chance that your baby could inherit a double dose of the trait and develop the full-blown sickle cell disease (see p.418 and p.425). Similarly, if you carry the A or B thalassaemia trait, you will need to arrange for your partner to be tested, too. A baby with full-blown thalassaemia (see p.425) suffers from very severe anaemia and iron overload, which eventually leads to multiple organ failure.

Hepatitis B and C

These viral infections cause liver disease, but it is unusual for women to be infected for the first time during pregnancy. Both are more common if you have used intravenous drugs, had a promiscuous sex life or have been exposed to infected blood. If you have received a blood transfusion in a country where the screening of blood products is not so rigorous, you may be at risk. The hepatitis B virus does not cross the placenta during pregnancy, but if you carry the virus, your baby will be at risk of infection at the time of delivery. The virus is not transmitted in breast milk, but babies are occasionally infected by blood if the mother's nipples are cracked and bleeding. As many as half of all babies infected with hepatitis B will develop cirrhosis or cancer of the liver in later life. This is why it is so important to know whether you are hepatitis B positive during pregnancy; if you are, your baby can be protected by IgG immunoglobulin treatment at delivery and immunized with hepatitis B vaccine soon afterwards.

Hepatitis C infection is an important cause of liver disease worldwide, but it is only rarely transmitted to the baby during pregnancy or delivery. However, the risk is greatly increased if you are HIV positive (see p.130 and p.414). Screening for hepatitis C is not routine in UK antenatal clinics, but the test may be offered to you if you live in an inner city.

> " …it is essential that your exact blood group is known, included in your maternity notes, and available at any time of the day or night. "

HUMAN IMMUNODEFICIENCY VIRUS (HIV)

Screening for HIV infection is now offered to all pregnant women. If you are found to be positive, you will be offered the best advice and treatment for you and your baby; if you are found to be negative, you will be greatly reassured.

HIV is a retrovirus capable of incorporating itself into the genetic code, especially of white blood cells, which are responsible for fighting infection. HIV infection (see p.415) has now become an epidemic worldwide and, until recently, being HIV positive often led to the development of full-blown Autoimmune Deficiency Syndrome (AIDS). Today the situation has changed dramatically: people who are HIV positive can now receive antiretroviral drugs, which can protect them from the onset of AIDS.

HIV IN PREGNANCY

For pregnant women, knowing that they are HIV positive can improve their personal survival, thanks to the new drugs available. It will also significantly reduce the risk of their babies becoming infected. Delivery by Caesarean section and avoiding breastfeeding reduce the risk. These measures coupled with maternal antiretroviral drug treatment at and around the time of delivery cut the chance of a baby being infected with HIV from 20 per cent

to less than two per cent. However, none of these medical advances can be offered if your antenatal carers do not know that you are HIV positive.

OPPOSITION TO SCREENING

Some years ago I was involved in trying to introduce routine HIV screening at St Mary's Hospital, London. Patients, midwives, and doctors were concerned that being found to be HIV positive would be so devastating that it should not be revealed as part of antenatal screening. The Royal College of Midwives actually advised members that routine screening was an invasion of a pregnant woman's privacy.

A CHANGE IN ATTITUDE

Several events helped attitudes change. First was the publication of European studies showing that the measures described above could reduce the transmission of HIV from mother to baby. Next came the introduction of the antiretroviral drugs used singly and in combination, which appeared to offer a greatly improved chance of halting the progression of HIV to full-blown AIDS.

The tragedy in our hospital was that it was only after two six-month-old babies were admitted with life-threatening infection caused by AIDS that the real importance of antenatal screening for this disease began to be fully understood by all parties concerned.

The mothers of these two babies had not been offered testing for HIV during pregnancy by their local hospital. Having witnessed the horror of their children's suffering they wanted to support the introduction of routine screening.

POSITIVE APPROACH

During the months that followed, the uptake of HIV screening in our antenatal clinic rose from 30 per cent to over 95 per cent.

Much of the credit for this change in practice must go to the two specialist midwives who introduced the service. Their positive and supportive approach towards HIV screening was crucial in changing the attitudes of patients and their medical and midwifery colleagues. Today HIV screening is a routine part of antenatal care.

Your blood test results

The results of your blood tests will be available in about two weeks and will be filed in your hand-held booking notes. The date of your next antenatal visit should follow the antenatal care pathway (see p.161). If your care is hospital-based, the date of your next visit may vary between different hospitals. In my own unit we usually see women at about 16–17 weeks – after their serum screening blood test result is available – in order to discuss the results of these tests and ensure that any necessary action is taken. Any important abnormal test results may be duplicated and filed in a separate set of hospital-based notes for the few women who have been identified as having high-risk pregnancies.

Common concerns

You may not have many concerns at this point. The risk of miscarriage is diminishing; you have survived the early pregnancy complaints; and you are not yet pregnant enough for the later ones.

Although your risk of miscarriage is now considerably reduced, any bleeding in early pregnancy invariably raises the fear of miscarriage occurring, especially if you have suffered one in the past, or experienced problems earlier in this pregnancy. So if you do experience some vaginal bleeding, see your doctor and have an ultrasound scan at the earliest possibility – in the majority of cases it will reassure you that nothing is wrong and that the bleeding is insignificant. If this is the case, it is a good idea to make sure that your doctor examines you internally and looks carefully at your cervix. In early pregnancy, the flood of hormones can make its surface very fragile and prone to bleeding, particularly if you develop a mild infection, such as thrush. If there is any concern about the appearance of your cervix, your doctor will probably take a cervical smear.

Varicose veins

Although varicose veins tend to be much more common in later pregnancy (see p.235) some women, particularly those who had varicose veins in a previous pregnancy, will have symptoms of aching and discomfort much earlier. If this applies to you, do make sure that you start wearing good support tights every day. Prompt attention to varicose veins in pregnancy can greatly reduce the problems that tend to develop at a later stage.

> " In early pregnancy, the flood of hormones can make the surface of your cervix very fragile and prone to bleeding… "

Your sex life

Some women find pregnancy brings added sexual fulfillment. The marked increase in vaginal secretions, together with the greater blood flow to all of the genital organs may mean that sex is more pleasurable than before. For many couples, there is the added thrill of being able to have unprotected sex, which can be a highly erotic sensation after years of using contraception. Added to this is the wonderful closeness that arises from the knowledge that you and your partner have created a life together. For many couples, this is a very powerful emotion, which enhances their lovemaking.

However, for many women, sex suffers. In spite of the many "sexy" images of famous women in late pregnancy that we are subjected to in newspapers and magazines, the fact remains that many mothers-to-be do not consider themselves to be very sexually appealing during their pregnancy and may start to feel this way as early as the third month when their shape starts to change. Being pregnant may change your perception of yourself and your partner's perception of you as a sexual partner and there are also physical and emotional reasons why your sex life may be different or diminished during pregnancy. During the first three months a woman may experience a lower libido because she feels sick or exhausted; her breasts might be too tender to touch; she might have had some bleeding or have reason to worry about the risk of miscarriage; or she might simply not feel like having sex. Later on, heartburn, indigestion, tiredness, sheer size, and inability to get comfortable mean that women may have sex less often and find it less enjoyable. Even though loss of libido is an extremely common occurrence, it can still come as a shock to both partners.

If you are feeling insecure about these issues, it is vital that you talk to your partner. You need to reassure each other that your feelings for each other have not changed just because one or both of you is not very interested in making love.

Clothes and hair

Most likely your clothes are starting to feel tighter round the waist now, but it is sensible to resist the temptation to rush out and buy a completely new wardrobe of clothes at this early stage. If this is your first pregnancy you

66 In spite of the many 'sexy' images of famous women in late pregnancy, the fact remains that many mothers-to-be do not consider themselves to be sexually appealing… 99

ENROLLING FOR ANTENATAL CLASSES

▶ **You will not start your antenatal classes** until your sixth or seventh month but many get booked up months in advance, so start researching now what is available in your area. Some are termed parent education rather than antenatal classes, but most aim to cover similar ground.

A good antenatal class should explain the physiology of pregnancy; describe the best breathing techniques for labour; and advise you how to remain as active as possible. Your class tutor should discuss labour fully and honestly, giving a full description of pain-relief options. She should also give advice on basic baby care, including feeding, for the days and weeks following the birth. Some classes have follow-up groups after the birth.

▶ **All antenatal classes encourage fathers-to-be to attend**, although your partner should not feel pressurized to attend every session. Some courses arrange one-off classes for men so they can discuss their feelings in a more open way and learn how they can prepare to be supportive during labour.

▶ **All hospital maternity units run antenatal courses**, as do midwife teams. These can be very useful if you are planning a hospital birth. You will have ample opportunity to put questions to the midwives and other obstetric personnel and this will make you all the more familiar with the way the labour ward works. Some units now offer online antenatal classes. By the time you arrive for the birth, you will be even more relaxed about your surroundings.

▶ **There are many independent courses** available including Active Birth Centre and National Childbirth Trust classes (see p.437 and p.438). In some areas Active Birth sessions and Birth and Beyond workshops are now offered by the NHS.

▶ **Even if this is not your first baby**, enrolling in an antenatal class is still a good idea. You may be a little rusty when it comes to remembering the details of labour or the correct breathing techniques.

▶ **One of the best spin-offs from attending an antenatal class** is the chance to meet women who are having babies at around the same time as you and who live in your area. Many women find that they make wonderful, enduring friendships in their antenatal classes.

can usually get by with some looser tops from your existing wardrobe perhaps with one or two pairs of trousers or skirts with an elasticated waist. Wearing your partner's jeans for a few weeks may be an option. If you have been pregnant before, you may well find that you need to change into roomier garments earlier than you did in your first pregnancy. Once the muscles of the abdominal wall have been stretched by pregnancy, they are never quite as tight as they used to be.

Trips to the hairdresser are a good way to boost morale, but many women tell me they are concerned that the chemicals in hair dyes might be potentially dangerous. There is no evidence that this is so; most permanent and non-permanent dyes contain chemicals that have been in use for many years and are unlikely to be toxic in the kind of doses used to colour hair every few months. However if you are worried, you could stick to highlights, which only colour the hair shaft rather than expose the whole scalp to dye, and if you colour your own hair, wear gloves and do it in a well-ventilated space.

ANTENATAL TESTS

Screening and diagnostic tests for fetal abnormalities make up one of the most complex areas of antenatal care. I can appreciate that if you have been sailing through pregnancy so far, these may be topics you feel reluctant to engage with – but I would urge you to read on. I hope the information here will help steer you through the options available and enable you to base your choices on the most up-to-date evidence and information. This will give you confidence in any decisions that you may need to make.

All screening tests are optional and you and your partner have the choice of whether or not you wish to have them. There is no right or wrong answer; each couple will have to decide what is right for them after considering all the available information. Although the vast majority of babies are born healthy, when problems do occur they tend to do so during fetal development because of an inherited genetic condition, an acquired problem due to, for example, an infection or drug or for no known reason. If an abnormality is detected through screening, it gives you and your partner the chance to prepare yourselves emotionally and practically for the prospect of caring for a child with a disability or for the possibility of terminating the pregnancy. (For a fuller discussion on congenital abnormalities see pp.144–7.)

Do I need to have tests?

All women have a chance of delivering a baby with an abnormality, but a number of factors increase the risk and these should be taken into account when you decide which, if any, tests to have. You are at increased risk if:

- you have had a previous pregnancy that was affected by an abnormality
- you or your partner has a family history of genetic disorders or abnormalities
- you are over 35 years of age
- you take or have taken drugs that are known to harm a developing baby
- you have a pre-existing medical problem such as epilepsy or diabetes.

What is available?

First trimester screening is expensive to provide because it requires scanning and counselling expertise to achieve high detection rates and ensure good follow-up care. Although provision varies from one health authority to the next, many more hospitals are now exploring the possibility of introducing first trimester screening to high-risk groups of women even if they are unable to provide this facility for everyone. The two main categories are screening tests and diagnostic tests and the difference between them is important.

Screening tests are usually offered initially and these will identify most, but not all, of those at risk of carrying a baby with an abnormality. They cannot diagnose a problem; they simply establish a risk figure on which women then have to base their decision whether to go on to have further investigations. Screening tests include a variety of serum (blood) tests and ultrasound scans (see p.124 and p.174), which include a specialized scan called a Nuchal Fold Transluclency Scan (NTS). With every test you need to consider the detection rate and the false positive rate (see chart below). A false positive means that a test result that is positive is later shown to be negative. A positive screening test prompts antenatal carers to offer an invasive test to confirm the diagnosis, so if the false positive rate is high, many women with pregnancies that are actually free of problems are exposed to further tests that they do not need.

Diagnostic tests give a clear answer as to whether or not a fetus has an abnormality, but these invasive tests are not routine, since they all require samples of the amniotic fluid, placenta or fetal blood to be taken from inside the uterus and these procedures carry a small additional risk of miscarriage. The only definitive tests for Down's syndrome (see p.147) are chorionic villus sampling (CVS), amniocentesis, and cordocentesis. Whether or not you choose to have one of these tests will depend on your views on abnormalities and how you would want to act if you knew for certain that your baby was affected by one.

How accurate are the tests?

The detection rate of Down's syndrome has effectively trebled over the last 15–20 years in specialist centres thanks to the work of committed obstetricians and scientists in the field of more effective first trimester screening.

The most important practical problem in antenatal screening is that it is difficult to achieve

SCREENING TEST COMPARISONS

The development of new tests over time has raised detection rates for abnormalities such as Down's syndrome from 30 per cent to 85 per cent. The most recent advance in screening – the integrated test – has the lowest false positive rate at just 1 per cent, resulting in fewer invasive tests.

Method of screening	Timing (weeks)	False positive rate	Detection rate	Number of babies found to be affected after test result is positive
Maternal age		5%	30%	1:130
Double test (p.137)	14–22	5%	66%	1:66
Triple test (p.137)	15–20	5%	77%	1:56
Quadruple test (p.137)	16–20	5%	81%	1:50
NT scan (p.137)	11–14	5%	80%	1:47
Combined NT and serum test (p.137)	11–14	5%	85%	1:45
Integrated test (p.138)	10–13/15–22	1%	95%	1:9

TIMING OF TESTS

Date	Test
11–14 weeks	Nuchal Fold Translucency Test (NTS) (screening)
16–18 weeks	Double, triple or Bart's serum test (screening)
18–22 weeks	Fetal anomaly scan (see p.174) (diagnostic)
11–14 weeks	OSCAR – NTS with B-hcg and PAPP-A serum tests (screening)
10–13 weeks and 15–22 weeks	Integrated test (screening)
11–14 weeks	Chorionic villus sampling (CVS) (diagnostic)
14–16 weeks	Amniocentesis (diagnostic)
20–40 weeks	Cordocentesis (diagnostic)

a high detection rate of affected babies and at the same time maintain a low false positive rate. In the past, we had only maternal age of 35 years or more to identify those women who are at greater risk and most maternity units routinely offer these women amniocentesis. However, if the mother's age alone is used to decide whether an invasive test such as amniocentesis or CVS is performed, only 30 per cent of babies affected by Down's syndrome will be identified. If maternal age is combined with serum screening, the detection rate rises to 65 per cent, but that is still only two-thirds of affected babies. However, when Nuchal Fold Translucency Scanning (NTS) is performed at 11–14 weeks the detection rate rises to 80 per cent, and when the NTS is combined with a blood test that measures free B-hcg and PAPP-A hormone levels, the detection rate is as high as 85 per cent.

A further advance in screening is the integrated test (see p.138), which has a detection rate of 95 per cent and a false positive rate of just 1 per cent. In

effect, this means that almost 9 out of 10 babies with Down's syndrome can be detected, and only 1 in 100 women will be wrongly identified as at risk and offered further tests that prove to be unnecessary.

Nuchal Fold Translucency Scanning (NTS)

This screening test was developed at King's College Hospital, London, in the 1990s to improve the detection of Down's syndrome as early as possible in pregnancy. The scan is performed between 11 and 14 weeks by hospital-based specialists and is based on an ultrasound measurement of the depth of fluid present under the skin behind the neck of the fetus (see box, right). Although an NTS is not offered to every pregnant woman in the UK, it is usually available on request, and you may have to pay for the test.

An increasing number of physical markers for Down's syndrome are being identified. For example, Professor Kypros Nicolaides at the Fetal Medicine Centre in London has shown that these babies often lack a nasal bone, have protruding tongues, a single hand palmar skin crease or have abnormal flow patterns in their heart valves or blood vessels. By examining the baby's profile during the NT scan, he believes that the detection of Down's syndrome can increase to over 95 per cent, and the false positive rate be reduced to less than 1 per cent.

Serum screening tests

The various different serum screening tests that are available measure two, three or more substances in your blood to predict whether your baby is at risk of Down's syndrome, certain other chromosomal (genetic) abnormalities or an open neural tube defect such as spina bifida (see p.146 and p.419). Serum screening tests are probabilities, or estimates of risk, and they do not provide you with a definite answer. When you undergo a test, it is important that you remember the following:

• An abnormal serum screening test (screen positive) does not mean that your baby has one of these abnormalities, but it does identify that you are at greater risk, and as a result your carers will discuss whether you want to undergo further tests.

• If the baby is found to have a chromosomal disorder, you will be faced with the choice of whether or not to continue with your pregnancy.

Carrying out the test

Serum tests are usually performed at about 15–16 weeks at your local maternity unit, at your GP practice, or in your home by your midwife. The best known test, which is often referred to as the double test or alpha-fetoprotein test, measures two substances in the blood, alpha-fetoprotein (AFP) and free Beta-hcg. In babies with Down's syndrome, the AFP level tends to be lower and the HCG higher. The double test detects two out of three cases of Down's and four out of five cases of neural tube defect. The triple test adds

HAVING AN NTS

During an ultrasound scan at 11–14 weeks, the technician measures the fetus and the depth of the fluid under the skin behind the neck of the fetus (the nuchal translucency).

This screening test can only give you an indication of risk and is not a conclusive answer as to whether or not your baby has Down's syndrome.

▶ **If the fluid measurement is below 3mm**, your baby is unlikely to have a problem. This will be the result for 95 per cent of women.

▶ **If the measurement is between 3 and 7mm**, there is a probability that your baby has Down's syndrome – the higher the measurement, the higher the chance.

▶ **If your NTS measurements are high or borderline**, you will be counselled about the implications and offered the option of undergoing an invasive antenatal test, such as a chorionic villus sampling or amniocentesis.

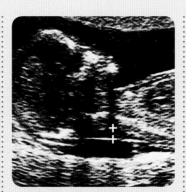

LOW RISK This fetus has only a small depth of fluid behind its neck and is at low risk of Down's syndrome.

Only 5 per cent of pregnant women will find themselves in this situation.

▶ **If you decide not to have an invasive test** following an NTS measurement that was high or borderline, I strongly advise you to ensure that you have a detailed anomaly scan at 20 weeks. This is because babies with a thicker nuchal translucency have an

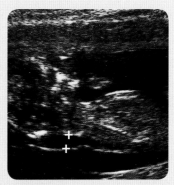

HIGH RISK The larger depth of fluid marked here puts this fetus at a higher risk of Down's syndrome.

increased chance of heart, gut, and other structural abnormalities that will be visible on an ultrasound scan. If some or any of these are identified, your antenatal carers will be able to arrange for appropriate paediatric help and advice before, during, and after the delivery should you decide to continue with the pregnancy.

> ❝ There are no right or wrong answers to these dilemmas, which is why you need to think and discuss how you would want to act upon an abnormal test result. ❞

another hormone, oestriol, to the calculation and the quadruple, or Bart's, test includes both inhibin A and pregnancy associated protein A (PAPP-A, low levels of which are also predictive of pre-eclampsia and poor fetal growth). The blood sample is sent to a specialist laboratory and analyzed for the different substances. The results are then fed into a computer programme along with your age and the exact gestational age of your baby. The results are usually available within five working days and, depending on the type of antenatal care you have chosen, you either have to phone for the result or will be contacted by your doctor or midwife. In the vast majority of cases, the test results will be low risk, but for the few results that show a high risk, it is very important that you receive the news as early as possible in order to provide you with the maximum amount of time to arrange further investigations should you wish to have them.

Your risk assessment

Out of the computer comes a risk assessment, such as 1 in 45 or 1 in 450. Translated into simple terms these numbers mean that for every 45 or 450 pregnancies, one baby is likely to be affected by the abnormality and either 44 or 449 babies are unlikely to be at risk of the abnormality. Hence, large numbers are good news and lower numbers will raise the alarm that a baby may have a problem.

It sounds simple, but the reality is quite complicated. Some couples will consider that a risk of 1 in 45 is worrying, while others will interpret that 1 in 45 is a risk that they are prepared to accept. At the other end of the scale, most couples and their doctors will consider a serum screening result of 1 in 450 as very reassuring while for others, the possibility that their baby may be affected by a small but finite chance of an abnormality, prompts them to undergo further tests. Of course, what the numbers cannot possibly take into account is your past experience and your personal views about having a baby affected by an abnormality, or alternatively, electing to terminate a pregnancy with a proven abnormality. There are no right or wrong answers to these dilemmas, which is why you need to discuss openly and honestly how you would want to act upon an abnormal test result.

Integrated screening

This antenatal screening test was developed in the private sector and has now been introduced in some specialist maternity units. This combination of tests provides a high detection rate for Down's syndrome, Edward's syndrome (see p.416), and neural tube defects such as spina bifida. It also has a much lower false positive rate when compared to other screening tests. The integrated test is performed in two stages:

• **Stage 1** The first part of the test is best performed at the end of the first trimester between 10 and 13 weeks. The date on which you should have stage 1 of the integrated test is decided by menstrual dating, or by the results of any earlier ultrasound scans. A detailed ultrasound scan is then performed to confirm the exact gestational age of your pregnancy and measure the nuchal translucency. A blood sample is taken at the same time to measure your levels of PAPP-A, and you will be advised when to have the second blood sample performed.

• **Stage 2** The second stage of the test ideally takes place in the second trimester at 15–16 completed weeks of pregnancy, but can be undertaken up until 22 weeks. Your midwife will take a second blood sample, which will be analysed for alpha-fetoprotein (AFP); unconjugated oestriol (uE2); free beta human chorionic gonadotrophin (free B-hcg); and inhibin-A (inhibin).

Calculating the risk

The measurements of the five blood tests and the NT result are fed into the computer, along with the mother's age, to estimate her risk of having a baby with Down's syndrome or an open neural tube

NEW DEVELOPMENTS

OSCAR stands for One Stop Clinics for Assessment of Risk. These tests take place in specialist clinics between 11 and 14 weeks of pregnancy. An NT scan and blood test for free B-hcg and PAPP-A are performed and the results are available within a few hours and combined with the mother's age and past obstetric history to provide an immediate computerised risk assessment. If the risk is shown to be high, the couple can opt for an invasive test immediately and receive a provisional result within 48 hours.

NIPD stands for Non Invasive Prenatal Diagnosis. This new screening test analyzes the cell free DNA (genetic code) in maternal blood that originates from the fetus. It offers a strong indication of whether the fetus is at high or low risk of Down's syndrome but avoids the risk of miscarriage from invasive tests.

defect. The results of the integrated test are usually ready within 3–5 working days of the second blood sample being taken. Normal (negative) results are sent to the GP or antenatal clinic, and a letter is sent to the woman advising her that the results are available. Screen positive results are telephoned or faxed to the GP or antenatal carer. The integrated test result depends on both blood samples being analyzed. You can have your risk of Down's syndrome estimated on the basis of the first-stage information alone, but this is not nearly so accurate as the combined results from the two-stage integrated test.

Test results

If the risk calculated from the integrated test is 1 in 150 or greater (which means 1 in a lower number than 150), the integrated test result is reported as screen positive for Down's syndrome and the woman will be offered a diagnostic test, usually an amniocentesis. Approximately 1 in 100 of all women screened will be in the screen positive group and after amniocentesis about 1 in 10 of these women will be shown to have a baby with Down's syndrome. This means that 10 invasive procedures will be performed to identify one baby affected by Down's syndrome. These figures are a great improvement when compared to the double serum screening test alone, in which over 60 invasive tests are performed to detect a single case of Down's syndrome (see table p.135). The integrated test also identifies 6 out of 10 women carrying a baby with Edward's syndrome (see p.416) – a detection rate of 60 per cent.

Neural tube detection

The level of AFP alone is used to determine whether there is an increased risk of having a pregnancy with an open neural tube defect, such as spina bifida. Women with a raised AFP level (2.5 times the normal average or greater) are reported as screen positive and are then offered further tests such as a detailed ultrasound scan. Most babies with anencephaly (see p.419) and some 86 per cent of babies with an open spina bifida can be detected in this way. Approximately 1 in 100 of all women screened will fall into the screen positive group for an open neural tube defect, and about 1 in 20 women with screen positive results have an affected pregnancy.

Factors that alter results
A variety of factors that can affect the various blood levels may need to be taken into account when calculating your integrated test result:
• Blood levels for some markers tend to be lower in overweight women and those with insulin-dependent diabetes.
• Levels for some markers may be higher in slender women and those of Afro-Caribbean origin.
• Levels may differ in women who are pregnant following IVF treatment.
• All blood markers are raised in twin pregnancies and are therefore unreliable.
• Vaginal bleeding just before the second blood test can raise AFP levels, as can amniocentesis testing.

If you have had a previous pregnancy affected by fetal abnormality, the result will always be reported as screen positive. Amniocentesis is usually offered, even if the integrated test result records a risk that is smaller than 1 in 150.

Chorionic villus sampling (CVS)
This antenatal diagnostic test is usually performed at 11–13 weeks (although it can also be performed later in pregnancy) and involves obtaining a small tissue sample (a biopsy) from the placenta (see box, right). Since the baby and the placenta

develop from the same cells, the chromosomes in placental cells are the same as in the cells from the baby. The majority of women who undergo a CVS test do so to exclude Down's syndrome. However, CVS is also used when a specific gene disorder is suspected, such as sickle cell anaemia or thalassaemia major (see p.418). Using CVS, fresh tissue can be collected and tested before 12 weeks, which means that a pregnancy with a severe chromosomal abnormality can be diagnosed in time for a suction termination of pregnancy to be performed, if this is what the parents choose.

Disadvantages of CVS
No invasive antenatal test is completely problem-free and before you decide to undergo CVS, you should consider the following:
• The risk of miscarriage after CVS appears to be slightly higher than for amniocentesis, affecting approximately 1 per cent of women who undergo CVS. This higher risk may be because the test is performed earlier in pregnancy, and the pregnancy may have been going to miscarry anyway, but it is still cause for concern.
• There is also evidence that when the CVS is done very early, the baby may develop an abnormality in the growth of its limbs.
• Occasionally, the placental tissues contain mosaic cells (abnormal cells that suggest that the baby has a chromosomal abnormality) when no significant abnormality is present. In this situation, you will probably be advised to undergo an amniocentesis at a later date to check the results.

Amniocentesis
Amniocentesis is the most commonly performed invasive test. It involves taking a sample of the amniotic fluid around the baby, which is then sent to the laboratory for analysis. The test is usually

HAVING A CVS TEST

If you undergo a chorionic villus sampling test, you will first be given an ultrasound scan to identify exactly where the placenta is lying. The test requires a small sample of tissue from the placenta, and the amniotic sac has to be avoided during the procedure.

▶ A local anaesthetic is injected into your abdominal wall to numb the area before a fine double-barrelled needle is introduced into your uterus at the correct site to access some chorionic villi – the frond-like projections in the placenta.

▶ A syringe containing some special culture fluid is attached to the end of the needle and the placental cells are sucked up into the syringe.
▶ The tissue obtained is fresh living placenta, which means that when it reaches the cytogenetics laboratory, culture and analysis is much quicker than from fetal skin cells cultured from an amniocentesis sample. You will probably receive a provisional test result within 72 hours and a conclusive result in about 10 days.

THE PROCEDURE
A sample of chorionic villi is sucked into a syringe attached to the needle.

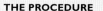

needle and syringe

ultrasound transducer

placenta

uterus

area being sampled   cervix   vagina

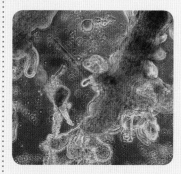

CVS SAMPLE A magnified image shows a tissue sample taken from the budding chorionic villi.

performed at 14–16 weeks of pregnancy, but can be performed at any gestational age. You will be offered an amniocentesis test if:

• you are more than 35 years of age
• you have a personal or family history of a baby with Down's or another chromosomal abnormality
• you have had an abnormal nuchal translucency scan result or a high-risk serum screening result in your current pregnancy.

When the amniocentesis sample reaches the cytogenetics laboratory, the fluid is spun hard to collect cells from the baby's skin together in a pellet. These cells have floated off the surface of the skin into the amniotic fluid in much the same way that our skin cells float off into bath water. These fetal skin cells then have to be encouraged to grow in tissue culture, which takes time (usually three to four weeks) and much expertise. They then have to be brought to a stage where they are actively dividing (called the metaphase stage) to perform the chromosomal analysis. Sometimes the cells cannot be encouraged to grow or are very slow in growing, which can delay your result. Rarely, the cells that are cultured are found to be your own and not your baby's; in these circumstances you would need to undergo a further amniocentesis.

Occasionally, the placental tissues contain mosaic cells (abnormal cells that are not representative of the baby's general chromosomal make-up). In this situation you will probably be advised to undergo a second amniocentesis at a later date to check the results of the first test. Amniocentesis is not usually performed until 14–16 weeks of pregnancy because before this time, the number of fetal skin cells may be insufficient to set up a culture and obtain a result. Removing fluid from the amniotic pool at too early a stage may also cause problems with the development of the baby's lungs.

Pros and cons of amniocentesis

A positive aspect of amniocentesis is that it is extremely rare for the results to be wrong and the risk of miscarriage is low. Although generally quoted as 1 per cent, in units that are performing

HAVING AMNIOCENTESIS

This procedure takes about 20 minutes and is performed using ultrasound guidance to find the best point to insert the amniocentesis needle. The optimal spot is where the needle can enter through the uterine wall and reach a pool of amniotic fluid, without touching either the placenta or the baby.

▶ The operator may inject some local anaesthetic into your skin at this spot to reduce any discomfort, but the amnio needle is so thin that you will find this procedure is less troublesome than a blood sample being taken from your arm.

▶ Once positioned in the right place, a syringe is attached to the outer sheath of the needle and the sample of amniotic fluid (about 10–20ml, the equivalent of 4 teaspoonfuls) is sucked into the syringe.

▶ The needle is then removed and the baby is scanned carefully to ensure that all is well.

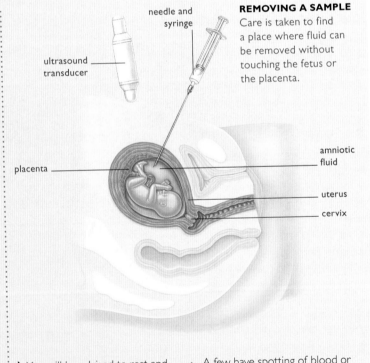

needle and syringe

ultrasound transducer

REMOVING A SAMPLE
Care is taken to find a place where fluid can be removed without touching the fetus or the placenta.

placenta

amniotic fluid

uterus

cervix

▶ You will be advised to rest and avoid strenuous activity for 24 hours. Some women feel slightly sore for an hour or two afterwards.

A few have spotting of blood or leaking of amniotic fluid from the vagina. This usually stops within a short time.

many of these procedures the risk is much lower – in the order of 1 in 300 or 0.3 per cent. The risk of miscarriage is highest within two weeks of having the amniocentesis performed. It is relevant that only pregnancies with potential problems are going to undergo this test, so later complications may not be directly related to the procedure and may have been going to happen anyway.

The downside to amniocentesis is that you will not have the results before about 17–18 weeks of pregnancy. This means that if the result shows an abnormality and you choose to terminate the pregnancy, you would have to undergo an induced labour to deliver the baby vaginally (see pp.294–7).

New developments in chromosomal analysis

If you are particularly distressed by the thought of a three-week wait for your results, you should ask about a new technique that has become available in some specialist centres called amnio PCR. Using a powerful molecular biology technique – the polymerase chain reaction (PCR) – the DNA in the fetal skin cells can be multiplied massively to provide sufficient quantities to allow the diagnosis to be made within a couple of days.

Fluorescent in-situ hybridization, or FISH, is another new form of sample testing that is becoming more widely available. This method tags pieces of DNA from a specific chromosome with fluorescent coloured markers. These are then placed on the cells that are being tested where they glow (fluoresce) with a specific colour that is easily seen under the laboratory microscope. The beauty of this technique is that the cells being examined do not have to be nurtured to the point where they are actively dividing

to see whether or not the correct number of chromosomes are present.

Cordocentesis

This procedure involves taking a sample of the baby's blood from the umbilical cord and is only performed after 18 weeks when the blood vessels in the umbilical cord are large enough to be clearly visualized. Under ultrasound control, a needle is inserted through the mother's abdominal wall into the uterus and guided into a blood vessel in the cord close to where it emerges from the placenta. The risk of miscarriage is between 1 and 2 per cent and the test is only undertaken by experienced operators in specialist units.

Cordocentesis is the quickest way to diagnose a chromosomal abnormality because the fetal blood can be directly and rapidly analyzed. Less commonly, cordocentesis may be used to measure the fetal haemoglobin in a pregnancy affected by rhesus incompatibility (see p.128 and p.425). Fetal blood transfusions are also performed by cordocentesis.

Occasionally, the possibility that a fetus has been infected with rubella or toxoplasmosis needs to be confirmed in later pregnancy with a blood sample taken from the umbilical cord.

Fetoscopy

In this procedure, a thin, illuminated telescope is inserted through the cervix and into the uterus to look at the baby, particularly the limbs, genitals, spine, and skin, together with the colour of the amniotic fluid. Some rare liver and skin disorders in the fetus can be diagnosed by fetoscopy and tissue samples obtained for laboratory confirmation. It is a high-risk intervention, which may lead to late miscarriage or preterm delivery and is only performed in exceptional circumstances.

CONGENITAL DISORDERS

Congenital means "born with". The term includes all genetic disorders and any physical or structural abnormality that may be present in a baby. This section will help you to understand how and why many congenital disorders arise and give a context to many of the antenatal tests that have been described already. An increasing number of abnormalities can now be diagnosed antenatally, enabling parents and carers to plan treatment, although some become apparent only after a baby is born.

Genetic disorders are caused by abnormalities in our genetic material that are either inherited or arise when a previously normal gene mutates (undergoes a change that makes it function abnormally). Some genetic disorders in the fetus are known to be due to the presence of a single or several abnormal genes. Others result because the number, shape or arrangement of one of the chromosomes is abnormal. Still more are due to a complex interaction between environmental factors and genes, which is not fully understood. Spina bifida and cleft lip/palate are two examples. Only a few, mainly Down's syndrome and spina bifida, are screened for regularly in pregnancy, although diagnostic tests and genetic counselling are available to couples who have particular risk factors or a family history of genetic diseases or other congenital abnormalities.

Chromosome abnormalities

Before, during, and after fertilization the two sets of chromosomes (one from your egg and one from your partner's sperm) that make up your baby's complement of 23 pairs undergo a complex series of divisions and rearrangements. If one of the chromosomes is abnormal, or too many or too few chromosomes are left in the fertilized egg, an abnormal embryo or fetus may develop. Most are miscarried early, but sometimes the pregnancy continues and an abnormal baby is born.

About 6 babies in every 1,000 are born with a chromosomal abnormality. In stillborn babies the figure rises to 6 in every 100. The most common abnormalities are disorders in the number of chromosomes (either too many or too few) with their names reflecting the number of the pair of chromosomes they affect.

Trisomies occur when three copies of one chromosome are present. Most trisomies are due to abnormal cell division (meiosis) in the egg, which occurs before fertilization. They are much more common in older women, because older eggs are more likely to be abnormal. The most common trisomies are Down's syndrome/Trisomy 21 (see p.147); Patau's syndrome/Trisomy 13 (see p.416) and Edward's syndrome/ Trisomy 18 (see p.416).

Monosomies arise when one chromosome is completely missing. The commonest type of monosomy, Turner's syndrome (see p.416), is the loss of an X chromosome in girls.

Triploidy is when the embryo has an extra set of 23 chromosomes (see p.416).

Extra sex chromosomes occur in disorders such as Klinefelter's syndrome (see p.417), in which boys have an extra X chromosome.

Translocations (see p.416) are abnormal arrangements of the correct number of chromosomes. When the transfer of genetic material occurs between two chromosomes, genetic material can be lost, augmented or simply exchanged.

Dominant genetic diseases

In these inherited diseases, only one abnormal gene is necessary for the disease to develop. Males and females are equally affected and have a 50 per cent chance of passing the gene and the disease on to their children. Unaffected individuals cannot pass on the gene or the disease. Dominant diseases are rarely fatal in early life because affected individuals would die before passing on the genes.

There is invariably a family history of the disease, but because dominant diseases are expressed to a greater or lesser degree in different individuals this may be difficult to establish without the help of a specialist geneticist. In familial hypercholesterolaemia (see p.417), for example, babies of affected parents can be tested at or after birth for high blood levels of cholesterol. Some of the dominant neurological disorders, such as Huntington's Disease (see p.417) and myotonic dystrophy, can now be diagnosed antenatally, thanks to advances in gene mapping

INCIDENCE AND CAUSES

▶ Major congenital abnormalities (such as heart or neural tube defects) are present in 4 per cent of newborn babies and cause 1 in 4 perinatal deaths.
▶ Minor congenital abnormalities, such as an extra toe or finger, are present in at least 6 per cent of newborns.
▶ About 40 per cent of congenital problems are inherited as a result of genetic factors.
▶ Around 10 per cent are acquired due to damage during development by infection (5 per cent), and exposure to drugs (2 per cent), chemicals, X-rays or metabolic disorders, such as uncontrolled diabetes.
▶ About 50 per cent of congenital disorders are unexplained, although it is likely that the majority of these will be found to have a genetic origin or result from a mixture of environmental and genetic factors.

technology, which can pinpoint the abnormality in DNA samples obtained by amniocentesis or CVS.

Recessive genetic diseases

In these diseases, two copies of the abnormal gene (one from each parent) are needed for the disease to develop. The recessive gene is usually masked by a normal dominant gene, and hence there may be no family history of affected individuals. However, when both parents are carriers, all of their male and female children have a 1 in 4 chance of inheriting two recessive genes and developing the disease, and a 2 in 4 chance of becoming a symptomless carrier of the disease.

Many recessive disorders can be diagnosed prenatally. Cystic fibrosis, sickle cell anaemia, and

❝ The most common congenital abnormalities are caused by disorders in the number of chromosomes – there can be either too many present or too few. ❞

thalassaemia (see p.418) are detected by DNA analysis from amniocentesis or CVS samples, whereas biochemical disorders such as Tay-Sachs disease (see p.418) and phenylketonuria (see p.418) are diagnosed from blood samples.

Sex-linked genetic diseases

Diseases such as haemophilia, Duchenne's muscular dystrophy (see p.418), and Fragile X syndrome (see p.419) are caused by a recessive gene located on the X (female sex) chromosome. The disease only affects men, because women have a second X chromosome to mask the effect of the recessive gene. Women are carriers of the disease, which means that their children have a 50 per cent chance of inheriting the abnormal gene. A daughter may not inherit the gene at all, or she may become a symptomless carrier because the second X chromosome will prevent her from

developing the disease. A son has a 50 per cent chance of developing the disease, because the Y chromosome inherited from his father will be unable to mask the disease. There is no male-to-male transmission of X-linked disorders, but occasionally an X-linked disorder may arise from a new random gene mutation.

Neural tube defects

Neural tube defects (see also p.419) are one of the most common serious congenital abnormalities. In the absence of antenatal screening, about 1 in every 400 babies is affected. Although the exact gene or genes have not been identified, these disorders tend to run in families. Incidence varies widely from one region to the next and has a strong connection with diet. Babies born with neural tube defects such as spina bifida are often severely handicapped and require frequent surgical procedures and hospitalization. Disability typically consists of weakness or paralysis of the legs and urinary and faecal incontinence.

Genetic counselling

Couples who know they have a family history of genetic disease or have already had a child with an inherited disorder are strongly encouraged to undergo genetic counselling when they are planning to get pregnant. They may wish to undergo antenatal diagnostic procedures such as chorionic villus sampling, amniocentesis or specialist ultrasound scans during pregnancy. Furthermore, for certain conditions it is now possible to offer them preimplantation genetic diagnosis (PGD). PGD is a technique in which eggs are fertilized in vitro and one of the cells of the tiny embryos are analyzed to ensure that it is free of the genetic disorder before being implanted into the mother's uterus.

PRENATAL DIAGNOSIS

You may need genetic counselling and/or prenatal diagnosis if you have or have had:
▶ A child with a birth defect, chromosome abnormality or genetic disorder
▶ A family history of any of the above
▶ A child with undiagnosed mental retardation
▶ An abnormal antenatal serum screen result
▶ A fetus with suspected abnormal ultrasound findings
▶ A maternal medical disorder that predisposes your baby to congenital abnormalities
▶ Exposure to an environmental hazard (teratogen) in your current pregnancy
▶ A parent known to be a carrier of a genetic disorder
▶ A history of recurrent miscarriage or fetal loss
▶ A previous neonatal death

DOWN'S SYNDROME

Although Down's syndrome (trisomy 21) is the most common chromosomal abnormality seen in live-born babies, numbers have fallen from 1 in every 600 births to 1 in 1,000 in recent years, thanks to improved accuracy in antenatal testing.

In 95 per cent of cases of Down's syndrome there is no family history. In three per cent of cases, the extra chromosome 21 is attached to another chromosome (a translocation) and is inherited from one parent, who usually shows no signs of the problem. In the remaining 2 per cent of cases, mosaicism is present, which means that some cells in the body contain a third chromosome 21, whereas others have the normal two.

The risk of Down's syndrome increases sharply with age (see below), but since older pregnant mothers are routinely offered screening, most Down's babies are now born to women under 35. As a result, screening for all pregnant women is becoming routine.

Although about 50 per cent of Down's syndrome babies miscarry, 9 out of 10 full-term Down's babies survive the first year of life. These babies are, however, at high risk of abnormalities of the heart or intestine and problems with hearing and eyesight, and usually have reduced muscular tone and are floppy. Physical features include slanting eyes, a single skin crease on the hands and feet, and a protruding tongue. The bridge of the nose is shallow or absent, which often means that the child is snuffly and susceptible to colds and chest infections.

All Down's children are mentally handicapped, but the severity of the handicap is variable and difficult to predict before birth. Recent advances in the way Down's children are educated has led to many leading relatively independent lives as adults. The average life expectancy is about 60 years of age, although leukaemia is common in childhood, and thyroid disease and a form of Alzheimer's disease are common in adults.

The Nuchal Fold Translucency Scan is an early screening test for Down's (see p.137). Routine ultrasound scans may detect other markers such as the absence of a nasal bone, or heart, kidney, and gut abnormalities. The skin creases on the baby's hands and the eyelids are also indications that a baby may be affected. Nevertheless, some babies with Down's syndrome have no obvious structural signs, and are not detected until after birth.

RISK OF DOWN'S SYNDROME

Maternal age at EDD Risk of Down's syndrome

Under 25	25	26	27	28	29	30
1:1500	1:1350	1:1300	1:1300	1:1100	1:1000	1:900
31	32	33	34	35	36	37
1:800	1:680	1:570	1:470	1:380	1:310	1:240
38	39	40	41	42	43	44
1:190	1:150	1:110	1:85	1:65	1:50	1:35
45	46	47	48	49	50	
1:30	1:20	1:15	1:11	1:8	1:6	

*EDD= expected delivery date

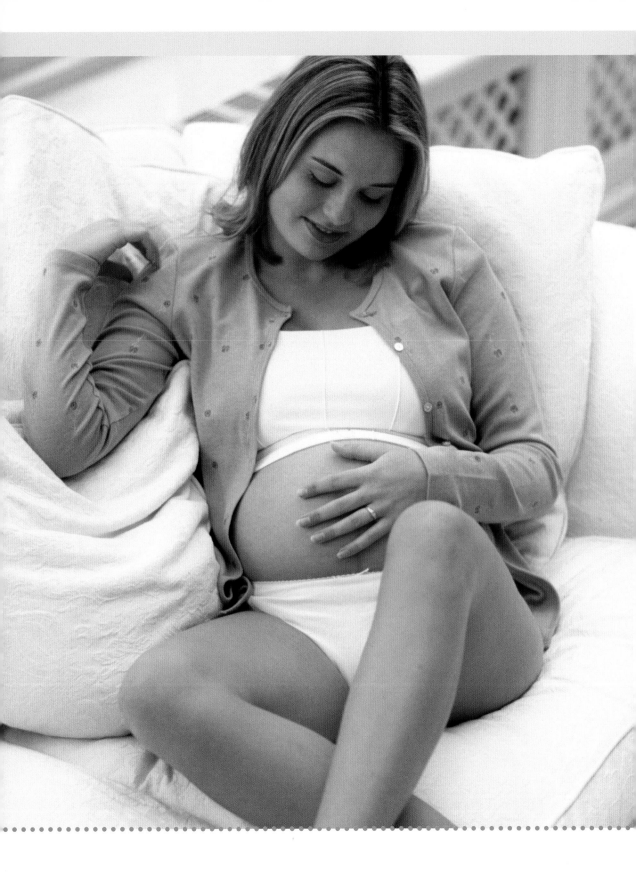

▶ **WEEKS 13–26**

The second trimester

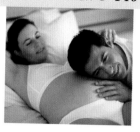

In the second trimester, your baby will grow steadily and the basic structures and organ systems that were established in the early weeks will be further developed and consolidated. The overall size of the fetus will increase three- to four-fold, and its weight a dramatic 30-fold. Although over the coming weeks you will begin to look noticeably pregnant, this is often a time of renewed energy, good health, and a sense of wellbeing.

CONTENTS

Your baby

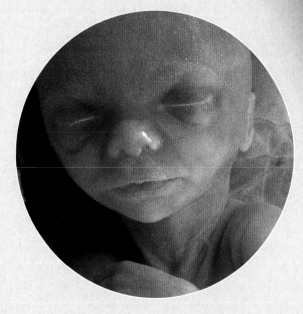

WEEK 14

The eyes are now positioned at the front of the face with the eyelids tightly closed.

WEEK 16

The difference between the male and female genitalia is increasingly obvious. This male fetus now has a solid scrotum and a rudimentary penis.

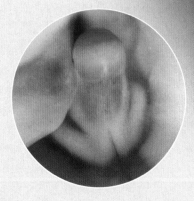

66 Your fully formed baby grows rapidly during the second trimester and can soon be felt kicking in the uterus. 99

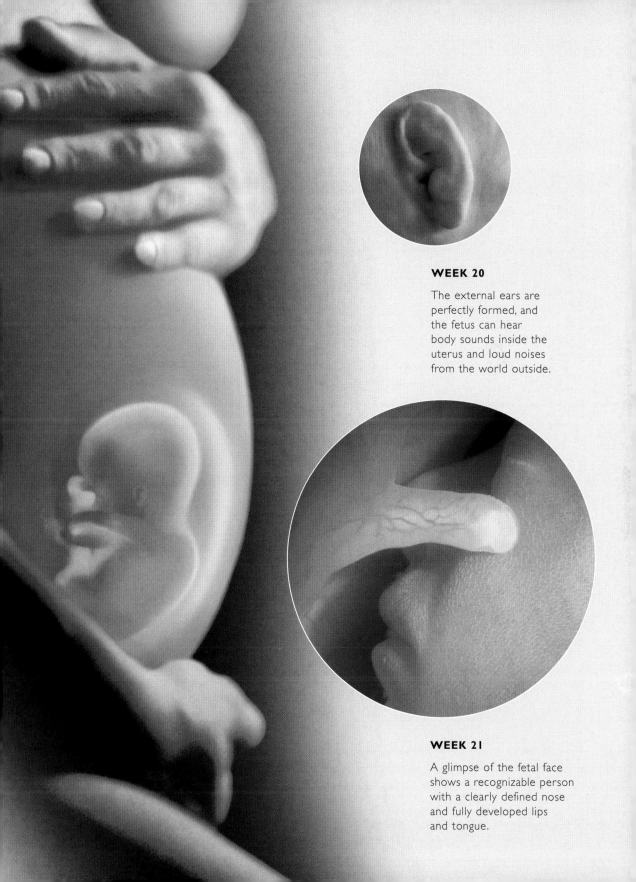

WEEK 20

The external ears are perfectly formed, and the fetus can hear body sounds inside the uterus and loud noises from the world outside.

WEEK 21

A glimpse of the fetal face shows a recognizable person with a clearly defined nose and fully developed lips and tongue.

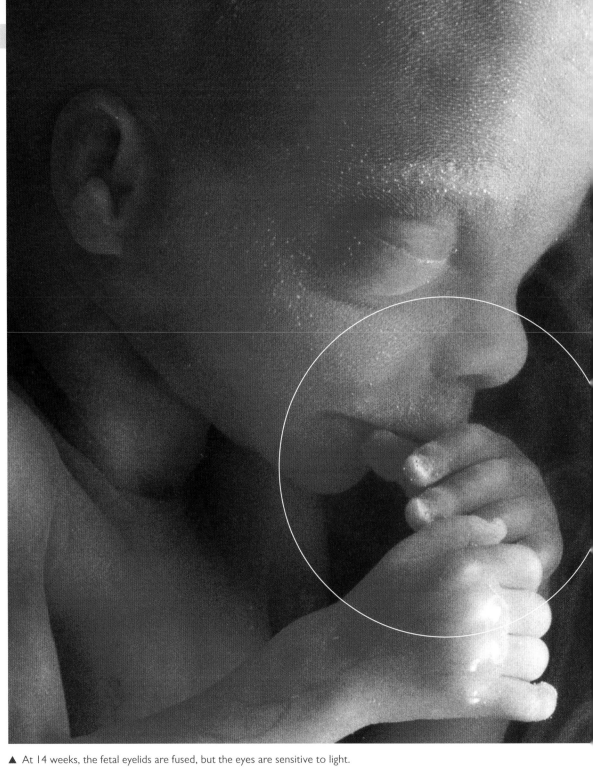

▲ At 14 weeks, the fetal eyelids are fused, but the eyes are sensitive to light.

1	2	3	4	5	6	7	8	9	10	11	12	13	14	15	16	17	18	19	20

▶ WEEKS 0–6   ▶ WEEKS 6–10   ▶ WEEKS 10–13   ▶ WEEKS 13–17   ▶ WEEKS 17–21

▶ FIRST TRIMESTER   ▶ SECOND TRIMESTER

▶ **WEEKS 13-17**
The developing baby

YOUR BABY IS LOOKING more and more like a human being. **Although the head is still relatively large, the length of the body is increasing rapidly. The development of the legs is catching up with the arms and very quickly overtakes them in length. The limbs now appear to be in better proportion with the rest of the body.**

Fingernails can be visualized and toenails will start to develop in a few weeks. The trunk has straightened out, but the body still looks thin and is only covered by a layer of fine translucent skin through which the underlying blood vessels and bones can be seen clearly. Very soon, a protective layer of brown fat will start to form, which will help to keep the baby warm.

The facial bones are complete, and the facial features are more delicate and much easier to recognize. The nose appears more pronounced, and the external ears now stand proud of the sides of the head. The tiny bones in the inner ear have hardened, which allows the fetus to hear sounds for the first time. The eyes are looking forwards, although they are still quite widely spaced, and the retina at the back of the eye has become sensitive to light. Although the eyelids are fully formed, they will continue to remain closed for most of the second trimester. However, your baby has already started to be aware of bright light beyond your abdominal wall. The recent development of facial muscles means that your baby can now make – but not yet control – facial expressions. If you happen to have an ultrasound scan at this stage, you may well see your baby frowning, grimacing or even squinting at you. Eyebrows and eyelashes start to develop, and the downy hair on the head becomes coarser and now contains some pigment. Inside the mouth, taste buds are appearing on the tongue.

Intricate movements
Perhaps the most important step forward in your baby's development is that all the connections between the brain, nerves, and muscles have been made.

life size

At 13 weeks, the fetus is about 8cm (3in) long and weighs 25g (about 1oz). By the start of the 17th week, its size has increased dramatically to 13cm (about 5in). Its weight now averages about 150g (5oz).

21	22	23	24	25	26	27	28	29	30	31	32	33	34	35	36	37	38	39	40

▶ **WEEKS 21–26**   ▶ **WEEKS 26–30**   ▶ **WEEKS 30–35**   ▶ **WEEKS 35–40**

▶ **THIRD TRIMESTER**

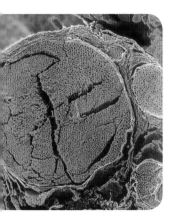

NERVE FIBRES
Signals pass quickly from the fetal brain to the muscles and limbs now that the nerve fibres are coated with fatty myelin sheaths.

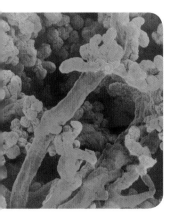

CHORIONIC VILLI
The frond-like villi (coloured green) in the placenta allow the exchange of gases and nutrients with the mother's blood.

The nerves linking the muscles to the brain begin to develop a fatty coating of a substance called myelin, which helps to transfer messages to and from the brain. This means that the fetus is now capable of a wide range of quite intricate movements. The limbs can now move around their joints because the muscles that control this movement are now able to contract and relax. The arms are now long enough for the hands to meet together over the fetal body. When the hands touch they grasp each other and anything else they encounter – such as the umbilical cord. The fingers now curl and the arms and legs flex and extend. The fetus can make a fist or suck its thumb.

Despite all this activity, most first-time mothers are not aware of these fetal movements because the amniotic fluid acts as a cushion and the baby is still not large enough to stimulate directly the nerve endings in the wall of the uterus. Some second-time mothers who know what to expect report that they can feel "quickening" – fluttering sensations in their abdomen, but definite fetal movements are not usually recognized until about 18 or 20 weeks.

The placenta

The placenta continues to grow in size and produce essential hormones (see pp.158–9), which are needed throughout pregnancy to ensure that the baby's growth is on target and the mother's uterus and breasts continue their growth and development. As well as providing all the oxygen and nutrients that your baby needs until the time of delivery, the placenta has now formed a very sophisticated barrier that will help to combat the risk of many infections for the rest of your pregnancy. In addition, the placenta will dilute the effect on the baby of any medical drugs, nicotine, and alcohol taken by the mother. By the end of the 16th week of pregnancy, the placenta has thickened to a depth of 1cm (less than ½ inch) and now spans around 7–8cm (3in).

The amniotic fluid

The amniotic fluid, which fills the sac surrounding the fetus, plays a very important role in fetal development at this stage. It allows freedom of movement and the development of essential muscular tone, while protecting your baby from knocks and bumps. During the first trimester, the amniotic fluid was absorbed through the fetal skin, but in the early weeks of the second trimester the fetal kidneys start to function. From now on your baby will swallow amniotic fluid and excrete the fluid back into the amniotic cavity. Although the amount of amniotic fluid remains relatively constant, it is being absorbed and replaced continuously. The presence of the right amount of amniotic fluid is particularly important for the development of the fetal lungs. Although your baby will continue to obtain all its oxygen and nutrient supplies from the placenta until birth, the lungs must be able to float in a full bath of amniotic fluid in order to expand and develop optimally in preparation for breathing in the outside world. At this stage, the bath contains about 180–200ml (6–7fl oz) of amniotic fluid, which is equivalent to the contents of an average paper drinking cup. During this period the fetus starts to shed some of its own skin cells into the amniotic fluid. This is an important milestone because these cells can be used to determine the chromosomal status of your baby if you decide or are advised to have an amniocentesis test (see pp.140–2). Until now the skin cells available were too few to be a reliable source of information about your baby, which is why amniocentesis is usually not recommended until 15–16 weeks of gestation.

17 WEEKS OLD On a 3-D ultrasound the fetus is seen wriggling and floating, but its movements are cushioned by the amniotic fluid and may not yet be felt.

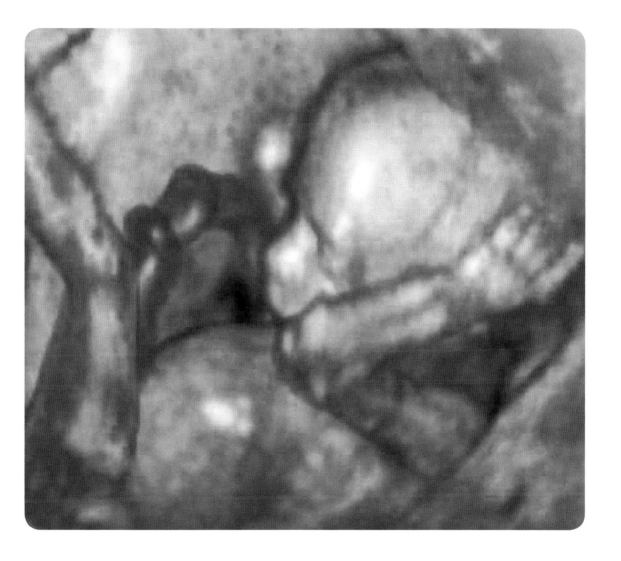

Your changing body

You will probably have noticed that your waist has become a little thicker by now and your tummy has become rounder, but the exact time in weeks at which you become noticeably pregnant to other people depends very much on your pre-pregnancy weight and shape.

Nevertheless, during the next few weeks you will be conscious of the fact that you are starting to "show" and that work colleagues and friends who are not in the know are starting to look quizzically at your abdomen. At the beginning of the second trimester, your uterus has grown to the size of a small melon and as a result can now be felt rising out of your pelvic cavity. From now on, its size can be easily assessed by gentle abdominal palpation.

> ...work colleagues and friends who are not in the know may now be looking quizzically at your abdomen.

Skin pigmentation

Increased skin pigmentation is very common in pregnancy and usually starts to be noticeable at the end of the first or the beginning of the second trimester. The extra oestrogen being secreted by your body stimulates cells in your skin called melanocytes to produce pigment that darkens the skin. The areola around your nipples may be the first noticeable change; as well as becoming darker, the areola usually increases in size as well. Moles, birthmarks, and freckles are also likely to enlarge in size and darken in colour, as will any areas of scar tissue. Most women develop a linea nigra or "black line" of pigmentation, which stretches down the centre of their enlarging abdomen. The linea nigra can be prominent in some women from early in the second trimester, whereas in others it does not appear until a little later in pregnancy. All these changes in colour are entirely normal and usually fade away after the baby is born.

Increased blood flow

None of these changes to your body would be possible without an increase in your circulating blood volume and important adaptations in the way that your heart and blood vessels work. The water content of your blood increased early in your pregnancy, but now the volume of red blood cells is becoming measurably larger. Your cardiac output (the amount of blood that is pumped through your heart per minute) continues to increase. Your stroke volume (the volume of blood pumped by your heart at every beat) and heart rate will also increase, but thanks to the action of progesterone hormone, your blood vessels will cope with these dynamic changes by becoming more dilated and relaxed.

At the beginning of the second trimester, 25 per cent of your blood is being directed to the uterus in order to support your growing baby and placenta, which is an enormous increase compared to the 2 per cent that your uterus used to receive before you became pregnant.

The blood flow to your kidneys will continue to rise until the 16th week, after which it levels off. The filtering capacity of your kidneys, which started to increase in the first trimester, is now 60 per cent higher than it was before you were pregnant and will stay at this level until the last four weeks of your pregnancy, when it will fall again. However, the tiny tubules in your kidneys, which are responsible for reabsorbing all the substances that pass through them, are now working overtime. Hence, it is not uncommon for your urine to contain small amounts of sugar and protein.

How you may feel physically

Now that your pregnancy has entered its second trimester, you will be much more confident that this baby is going to become a reality. On a physical level, you will most probably be feeling less nauseous and be regaining some of your usual vitality.

You have probably started to tell people that you are pregnant and find you have become the focus of much attention, congratulations, and advice about what you should and should not be doing as a pregnant woman. Advice is usually offered freely, not just by close family members and friends but also by people you hardly know, and although it is almost always well meaning, there are times when it may be confusing and even distressing. There is no need for you to be elated one moment and desperately worried the next, so be careful who you discuss your pregnancy with at this stage. You also need to ensure that you treat unsolicited advice and cautionary tales with a large pinch of salt.

Minor irritations

There are some minor problems that may become noticeable in the early weeks of the second trimester. For example, some of you will notice that your nose is permanently stuffy, although you are not suffering from a cold. You might even be experiencing nosebleeds, blocked ears, and bleeding gums.

> ...ensure that you treat unsolicited advice and cautionary tales with a large pinch of salt.

THE MAJOR PREGNANCY HORMONES

From the first day of your pregnancy, most of the subtle and more dramatic changes in your body and the way it is functioning are under the control of key hormones. These are produced from existing sources and glands within your body but also, increasingly as the pregnancy progresses, by the placenta and the developing baby.

HORMONE	WHAT IT DOES	WHERE PRODUCED
HUMAN CHORIONIC GONADOTROPHIN (HCG)	Maintains secretion of pregnancy hormones oestrogen and progesterone by the corpus luteum in the ovary until the placenta takes over.	Produced in large quantities by the young placenta, peaking at 10–12 weeks, then declining rapidly.
OESTROGEN	Increasingly high levels in pregnancy boost the blood flow to body organs and promote the dramatic growth and development of the uterus and breasts. Softens collagen fibres in connective tissue to allow ligaments to become more flexible.	Over 90 per cent is a type called oestriol, which is produced by the placenta; fetus is also involved in the oestrogen production process.
PROGESTERONE	Relaxes blood vessels to cope with increased blood flow. Has similar relaxing effects on digestive and urinary tracts. Hypnotic effect may induce placid feelings in pregnancy. Relaxes muscles and helps ligaments and tendons to loosen to accommodate the growing uterus and prepare the birth canal for delivery. Prevents contractions until birth is due. Prepares the breasts for lactation.	Until weeks 6–8, corpus luteum produces progesterone to maintain the pregnancy. By the end of the first trimester, progesterone is produced entirely by the placenta.
HUMAN PLACENTAL LACTOGEN (HPL)	Similar to growth hormone, HPL accounts for 10 per cent of the placenta's protein production. Diverts mother's glucose stores to the fetus; also has effects on maternal insulin production and uptake to help the transfer of nutrients to the fetus. Has a role in breast development and in milk secretion after delivery.	Produced by the placenta from five weeks onwards; levels rise throughout pregnancy.

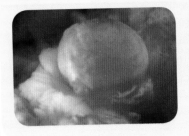
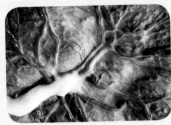

Hormone factories The key site of hormone production in early pregnancy is the maternal ovary (far left), but by 12 weeks the placenta and fetus take control. The placenta both produces hormones and martials all the fetal and maternal resources to produce oestrogen.

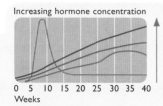

Increasing hormone concentration

KEY

― Human chorionic gonadotrophin
― Oestrogen
― Progesterone
― Human placental lactogen

0 5 10 15 20 25 30 35 40
Weeks

Key hormones A graph illustrates the surge in HCG hormone early in pregnancy and the steady rise in levels of oestrogen, progesterone, and HPL throughout pregnancy.

HORMONE	WHAT IT DOES	WHERE PRODUCED
PROLACTIN	Stimulates breasts to produce milk. Prolactin levels increase during pregnancy, but their effect is blocked until after the birth.	Produced in the anterior lobe of the pituitary gland in the brain.
RELAXIN	An insulin-like substance in the blood that helps soften the pelvic ligaments for delivery and also aids cervical ripening (softening and thinning) ready for dilatation and childbirth.	The ovaries produce relaxin.
OXYTOCIN	Causes the muscles of the uterus to contract. Levels rise in the first stage of labour and are further stimulated by the widening of the birth canal. Oxytocin helps the uterus to contract after childbirth and is stimulated by the baby sucking on the nipple during breastfeeding.	Produced by the posterior lobe of the pituitary gland. Receptors in the uterus increase in late pregnancy, enabling oxytocic drugs to be used to induce and augment labour.
CORTISOL AND ADRENOCORTICO-TROPHIC HORMONE (ACTH)	Production increases from the end of the first trimester onwards. Effects contribute to stretch marks and high blood glucose levels. Cortisol has an important role in helping to mature the fetal lungs.	Cortisol secreted by the maternal adrenal glands and the placenta. ACTH from the pituitary gland prompts release of cortisol.
ANDROGENS (TESTOSTERONE AND SIMILAR HORMONES)	Vital building blocks for the production of oestrogen during pregnancy. Some testosterone is needed for the development of the male external genitalia.	Produced largely by the fetal adrenal gland. Fetal testes also produce testosterone.

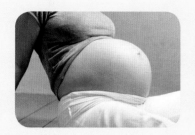
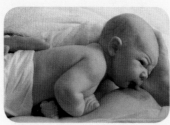

Hormone effects The expansion of your uterus is made possible by a boost in blood flow due to oestrogen, and the softening effect of progesterone on your ligaments and muscles. After birth, prolactin and oxytocin stimulate your breasts to produce milk.

> You may find that you are increasingly forgetful – a symptom that is referred to jokingly as maternal amnesia.

These symptoms are nothing to worry about, but because they are due to the increased blood flow to the mucous membranes of your nose, mouth, ears, and sinuses, they are likely to remain with you for the rest of the pregnancy. So it makes sense to think about ways to alleviate these symptoms, even though it is unlikely that you will be able to get rid of them altogether until the baby is born.

Try to avoid spending too much time in hot, dry environments at work and home, especially those with central heating and air conditioning, both of which dry out the atmosphere. You can improve the atmosphere by using cheap, portable humidifiers in the rooms you use most frequently. Placing a saucer of water on the radiators in your home or office or hanging a wet towel close to a radiator has a similar effect. If you are troubled by repeated nosebleeds, then discuss this with your doctor who may suggest that you visit a specialist.

You may find that you are increasingly forgetful – a symptom that is often referred to jokingly as maternal amnesia. I think it is simply a reflection of the fact that women are so preoccupied with the excitement of pregnancy during this period that other things seem less important and fail to register. Even if you find yourself forgetting things and unable to multi-task in your usual way, rest assured that this vagueness often abates later in pregnancy and you will almost certainly be back to your normal self after the birth.

Your antenatal care

Even though, like most women, you will remain physically fit and well throughout pregnancy, it is usual to see your antenatal carers every four to six weeks during the second trimester.

The exact timing of your visits depends upon when you booked, the results of your blood and urine tests, the type of care you have chosen, and whether you have any particular problems that need attention, but the procedure at each routine check-up is usually much the same.

• Your urine will be tested for protein. It is important to exclude any infection if protein is persistently present by sending a sample for laboratory culture.

• Your blood pressure will be measured with the correct size of cuff to make sure that you are not at risk from some of the common complications of pregnancy.

• Your doctor or midwife will most likely examine your hands and feet to ensure that you have no swelling or oedema.

• Your abdomen will be examined and the distance between your symphysis pubis (pubic bone) and the fundus (the dome-shaped top of your uterus) will be measured in centimetres to ensure that the uterus is growing steadily by about 1cm (½in) per week. This measurement is known as the symphyseal-fundal height (SFH in your antenatal notes): at 14 weeks it will be about 14cm (5½in) and by 16 weeks it will be about 16cm (6in). Of course, measurements vary depending on a woman's height and build, together with the number of babies she is carrying and the quantity of amniotic fluid. If you are carrying twins or more, your fundal height will be much higher than would normally be expected for the number of weeks of your pregnancy.

• Your carers will also listen to your baby's heartbeat by placing a special monitor called a sonicaid over your uterus. This uses Doppler sound waves (which are completely safe for use in pregnancy) to record your baby's heart rate, which at this stage in pregnancy will be about 140 beats per minute – approximately double your own.

• Nowadays, most antenatal carers do not weigh pregnant women at every clinic visit but they may want to keep a check on your weight if you started your pregnancy overweight or if you suffer from diabetes (see p.408).

Notes and blood tests

The results of all your scans and blood tests will be entered into your hand-held notes. These provide you with clear documentation of what has happened to you in the past and during your current pregnancy, which you can immediately share with any doctor or midwife that you may

YOUR ANTENATAL VISITS

In the shared-care system that operates in my own maternity unit, most mothers are cared for jointly by a team of midwives and doctors both in the community and in the hospital. Your antenatal visits should follow the same general pattern as the pathway below, based on the NICE guidelines (see p.87).

6–8 weeks	First contact visit; receive hand-held notes
10–13 weeks	Booking visit; dating scan; NTS scan
16 weeks	See midwife
20 weeks	Detailed fetal ultrasound scan; Mat B1 forms available now
24 weeks	See midwife/GP
28 weeks	Hospital visit: blood tests for anaemia, glucose tolerance test if appropriate; birth plan advice; arrange parent education visit; receive anti-D injection if blood group is Rhesus negative
32 weeks	See midwife/GP
34 weeks	Discuss results of screening tests; discuss labour and birth preparations, pain relief, birth plan; receive anti-D injection if appropriate
36, 38, 40 weeks	See midwife/GP
41 weeks	Hospital visit with doctor. Discuss possible membrane sweep and induction of labour
42 weeks	Attend the maternity day-care unit at hospital – CTG (baby's heart rate tracing). Ultrasound scan to assess volume of amniotic fluid and fetal wellbeing

need to consult. Having your own notes close at hand also means that you can review your progress in the journey through pregnancy any time you want to. Most pregnant women are very good at remembering to bring their notes to antenatal appointments, which means that lost records are rarely a problem.

Things to consider

At this stage of pregnancy your immediate concern is probably finding something suitable to wear to work. You may also be wondering if some of the side effects of pregnancy can be prevented – for example, by taking extra care of your skin.

Stretch marks

The vast majority of pregnant women will develop some stretch marks during pregnancy. These are caused by the collagen beneath the skin tearing as it stretches to accommodate your enlarging body. Stretch marks can make an appearance at an early stage in pregnancy and tend to occur initially on the breasts, as these are the first parts of the body to start expanding, and then on the abdomen, hips, and thighs. The number and extent of stretch marks varies greatly from one woman to the next and is determined mainly by your genes and your age. As you get older your skin loses its elasticity, making stretch marks more likely. There is some evidence that if you are physically fit and well toned before pregnancy and ensure that your weight gain during pregnancy is gradual, you can limit their appearance.

If you do develop lurid stretch marks – and remember, few women do not – rest assured that, with time, their pink appearance (together with any itching) will fade. They will not disappear altogether but will become a lighter silvery shade that makes them less visible. There are numerous anti-stretch mark creams on the market, but despite what the manufacturers would have us believe, I'm afraid that no cream applied to the surface of your skin can have much effect on what is happening to the deeper layers of collagen that lie well below the surface. That said, massaging creams into your skin to keep it smooth and supple is very pleasurable – and any good moisturizing cream will do.

What to wear

You will find that some of your favourite clothes no longer fit, but try to resist the temptation to go out and buy a whole new wardrobe. You are well advised to wait and buy clothes for the last trimester, by which time

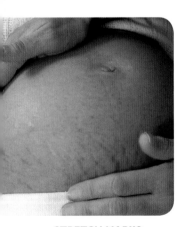

STRETCH MARKS
If you are prone to stretch marks there is nothing you can do to prevent them. However, their livid appearance will fade with time and they will be much less noticeable.

there will be very little in your current wardrobe that you will be able to wear. You also need to consider the change in season between now and the final months of pregnancy. So look carefully at your current wardrobe, put away anything that has become out of the question or feels even slightly uncomfortable and concentrate on what still fits and can be worn for the next few weeks.

It is very tedious to have only a limited selection of clothes so this is a good time to review some of your partner's T-shirts, sweatshirts, and jeans to see if any are suitable. Borrowing larger sizes from your partner or friends is a great way to see you through this transition period. You will then be able to save your clothes budget for the later stages of pregnancy when you are likely to be desperate for a few new things to wear.

Cosmetic effects

If you feel that having tanned legs and arms and a brown bump are essential to your self-esteem, be aware that, in general, you will tan more quickly during pregnancy because the amount of pigment in your skin has increased. It is a good idea to avoid long periods in the sun to minimize the risk of burning, as well as the risk of prematurely ageing your skin. Sunbeds should be avoided for much the same reason. When you are in the sun, make sure that you use a high-factor sunblock on your face, neck, and shoulders. Alternatively, try self-tanning products, which are all safe to use in pregnancy.

If you want to get rid of unwanted hair, depilatories are safe to use, but shaving or waxing may be your preferred option if you want to minimize contact with chemicals. Avoid waxing over any heavily pigmented moles or varicose veins.

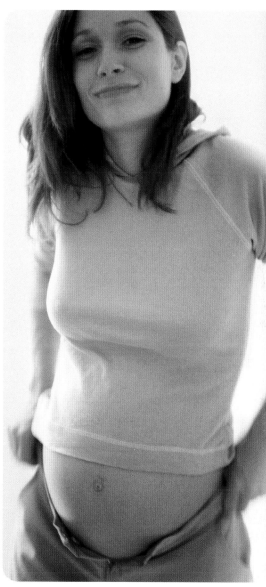

TIGHT FIT Put away anything that no longer fits and see if you can borrow a bigger size.

Those of you with tattoos and piercings may have a few questions now that you are pregnant. A belly ring or bar will become uncomfortable as your abdomen grows and is unlikely to stay in place when your navel begins to protrude in late pregnancy, so have it removed sooner rather than later. Nipple rings can be left in place for now, but will need to be taken out if you want to breastfeed. Tattoos on any area of your body that expands may change beyond all recognition. It goes without saying that you should not have new piercings or tattoos in pregnancy because of the risk of infections such as hepatitis B and C (see p.129) and HIV (see p.415).

DIET AND EXERCISE

During the second trimester, you will probably find that
you have regained your appetite and are able to resume
normal eating habits. You are also likely to feel more
energetic – ready to pick up your old exercise routine
or start a new one.

EATING WELL

Make the most of this trimester
by eating well because by the next,
you may well find that your appetite
and digestion go awry again, this
time because your growing baby is
compressing your digestive system.
For most women, lack of time rather
than inclination leads to a less than
ideal diet during pregnancy. One
solution is to stop worrying about
producing elaborate nutrient-
balanced meals and concentrate
instead on regular snacks chosen
from a range of healthy foods. You
can supply yourself and your baby
with everything you need by ensuring
that you keep some of the following
foods available:

▶ wholemeal bread and pitta
bread and fillings such as grated
cheese, lean ham, well-boiled
eggs, mashed sardines, salmon,
tuna fish, hummus, baked
beans, Marmite, salad, tomatoes,
and vegetables
▶ chopped fresh vegetable sticks –
carrots, peppers, cucumber,
and celery
▶ fresh fruit – washed and prepared
▶ fruit juices, semi-skimmed
milk, mineral water, herbal and
fruit teas or decaffeinated tea
and coffee
▶ unsweetened wholegrain breakfast
cereals, porridge
▶ low-fat yogurt and fromage frais
▶ dried fruits – apricots, prunes,
raisins, and figs
▶ nuts and seeds (sunflower and
sesame seeds)
▶ wholemeal crackers
▶ cereal snack bars

GOOD POSTURE

Posture becomes increasingly important now that your shape is
changing fast. Try to stand tall, as if your head is being stretched
upwards by a thread, aligning yourself in a straight line from the top
of your head, down through your pelvis and perineum to your feet.

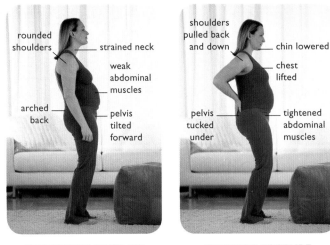

rounded shoulders — strained neck — weak abdominal muscles — arched back — pelvis tilted forward

shoulders pulled back and down — chin lowered — chest lifted — pelvis tucked under — tightened abdominal muscles

INCORRECT POSTURE   **CORRECT POSTURE**

Keep some of the more portable items in a fridge at work and carry crackers, fresh and dried fruit, nuts, and a small bottle of mineral water or fruit juice in your handbag.

PREGNANCY PROBLEMS

One of the fears that women have during pregnancy is that bad diet will give rise to a range of complications. Conditions that are affected by diet include pre-eclampsia (see p.426), gestational diabetes (see p.427), and intrauterine growth restriction, IUGR (see p.429). However, I must stress that many women who develop complications have perfectly good diets – certainly no worse than others who remain untouched by these problems. Women are quick to blame themselves – and their diets in particular – as being responsible for other problems such as premature labour and high blood pressure. Let me reassure you straight away that these conditions are not diet-related.

EXERCISING SAFELY

High-impact sports, such as jogging, skiing, and horse riding, will become progressively inadvisable over the second trimester. Jogging is not dangerous for your baby, but it puts pressure on your joints, tendons, and ligaments and can lead to lasting damage. During skiing and horse riding, your growing bump alters your centre of balance, making a fall more likely. If any of the above is your preferred method of keeping fit, consider switching to other forms of exercise – cycling, walking, and swimming are among the best.

PELVIC FLOOR EXERCISES

This is one set of exercises that you should do on a regular basis – I cannot emphasize enough how important they are. Your pelvic floor resembles a hammock of muscles, which support the bladder, uterus, and bowel and surround the urethra, vagina, and rectum. Loss of tone in these muscles and/or damage from a prolonged vaginal delivery can lead to stress incontinence – small leakages of urine when you cough, laugh or sneeze. This often continues after the birth and later in life, especially after the menopause, when lack of oestrogen compounds the problem.

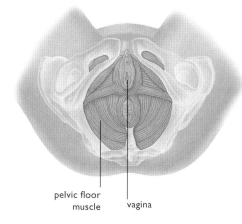

Your pelvic floor During pregnancy, your pelvic floor muscles soften and relax and become stretched under the pressure of the enlarging uterus.

pelvic floor muscle   vagina

Practise pelvic floor exercises every day throughout pregnancy, and continue them after the birth. One way to remember to do them is to practise them at particular times, for example, when you brush your teeth or wait for a bus or train – after a while they will become automatic.

▶ **Empty your bladder** before starting the exercises. (It is no longer recommended to try to stop urine flow midstream.)

▶ **Tighten and release the muscles** around your urethra, vagina, and anus. You should feel a lifting sensation in your pelvic floor muscles. Hold for a few seconds, then relax slowly. Build up to 10 squeezes, taking 10 seconds for each and resting briefly between squeezes.

▶ **Now squeeze and relax the muscles more quickly** holding for about a second at a time. Repeat 10 times.

▶ **Now squeeze and relax each set of muscles** around your urethra, vagina, and anus in turn from the front to the back and from the back to the front. You can perform these regularly during the day.

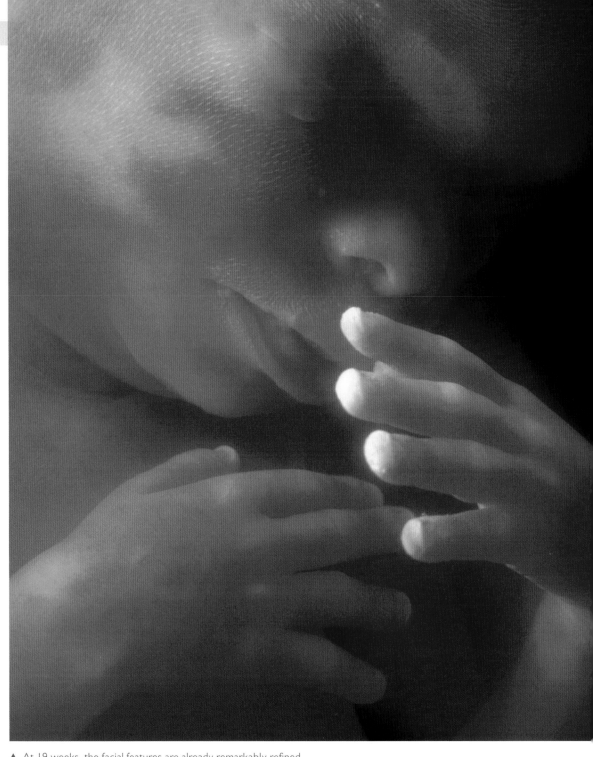

▲ At 19 weeks, the facial features are already remarkably refined.

| 1 | 2 | 3 | 4 | 5 | 6 | 7 | 8 | 9 | 10 | 11 | 12 | 13 | 14 | 15 | 16 | **17** | **18** | **19** | **20** |

▶ WEEKS 0–6   ▶ WEEKS 6–10   ▶ WEEKS 10–13   ▶ WEEKS 13–17   ▶ WEEKS 17–21

▶ **FIRST TRIMESTER**   ▶ **SECOND TRIMESTER**

▶ **WEEKS 17–21**

The developing baby

THE GROWTH OF YOUR BABY'S TRUNK AND LIMBS continues very rapidly during this time and, as a result, the head now appears in better proportion with the rest of the body. By the end of week 20, the head makes up less than one third of the total length of the fetus.

Your baby's legs in particular have undergone an amazing growth spurt and are now longer than the arms. From this point onwards, the rate of growth of the trunk and limbs will start to slow down, although the fetus will continue to gain weight at a steady pace until the time of delivery. This relative slowing in physical size is an important milestone because it marks the fact that the baby is now developing in different ways. The lungs, digestive tract, nervous, and immune systems are all starting to mature in preparation for life in the outside world. The skeleton can now be seen clearly on an X-ray because further calcium has been deposited in the bones to harden them.

Your baby's sexual organs are now well developed and the differences between the male and female external genitalia are increasingly obvious. Inside the body of a baby girl, the ovaries contain the three million eggs that she will be born with; the uterus is fully formed and the vagina is starting to become hollow. A baby boy's testicles have not descended from the abdominal cavity into the scrotum, but a solid scrotal swelling alongside a rudimentary penis can often be seen between the boy's legs on an ultrasound scan. An ultrasound scan at 20 weeks should be able to determine the sex of your baby, provided she or he is facing the right way. On the chest wall of both boys and girls, early breast tissue (mammary glands) has developed and nipples can be seen on the skin surface.

Improving senses

Although your baby's eyelids are still generally closed, the eyeballs can roll from side to side, and at the back of the eye, the retina is light-sensitive because nerve connections to the brain have been established. Your baby's taste buds are so

life size

At 19 weeks, the fetus now measures about 15cm (6in) from crown to rump. Its weight now averages about 225g (8oz). By the end of 21 weeks, its length is around 17cm (7in) and the weight averages 350g (12oz).

| 21 | 22 | 23 | 24 | 25 | 26 | 27 | 28 | 29 | 30 | 31 | 32 | 33 | 34 | 35 | 36 | 37 | 38 | 39 | 40 |

▶ **WEEKS 21–26** ▶ **WEEKS 26–30** ▶ **WEEKS 30–35** ▶ **WEEKS 35–40**

▶ **THIRD TRIMESTER**

> " The fetus may move around vigorously if exposed to loud noises such as music at a pop concert. "

well developed that they can now distinguish between sweet and bitter flavours (although these are unavailable in utero) and many of the first "milk" teeth have developed inside the gums. The mouth opens and closes regularly, and an ultrasound scan may capture your baby sticking its tongue out at you. Although it still has no conscious thoughts, it now hears sounds very clearly such as those of your heart beating, blood pulsing through the vessels in your lower body, and your digestive system churning around. It is often suggested that one reason why newborn babies usually stop crying when they are placed over their mother's left shoulder is that they recognize the comforting memory of her heartbeat.

The fetus can also hear sounds from outside your body and may jump or move around vigorously if exposed to loud noises such as music at a pop concert. The pattern of the fetal heartbeat, now clearly audible if an electronic monitor or sonicaid is placed on your abdomen wall in the correct place, also changes in response to loud external sound. The skin has also become responsive to touch and when firm pressure is placed on your tummy, your baby will move away from the intruding stimulus.

New nerve networks

All of these sophisticated developments in your baby's senses are due to the fact that the nervous system is developing rapidly and maturing steadily. New nerve networks are being formed continuously and acquiring fatty, insulating myelin sheaths, which enables them to transmit messages to and from the brain at great speed. A fibrous sheath starts to grow around the nerve bundles in the spinal cord to help protect them from mechanical damage. These adjustments to the nervous system help your baby to become much more

FETUS AT 19 WEEKS ···

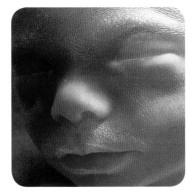

A fine covering of downy hair forms on the eyebrows and upper lip.

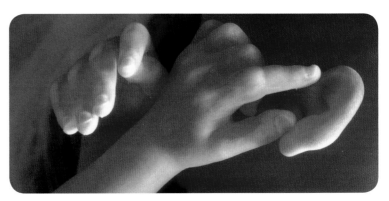

Your baby now hears sounds very clearly – your heart beating and the rumblings of your stomach.

active. Even though you may not be able to feel all the movements yet, your baby is constantly on the move, twisting, turning, stretching, grasping, and doing somersaults. This increase in muscular activity allows movements to become more refined and purposeful, improving motor skills and co-ordination and helping stronger bones to develop.

Skin and hair

The fetus starts to look a little plumper and less wrinkly during this stage of pregnancy as thin layers of body fat begin to form. Some of this fat is insulating brown fat, which starts to be deposited in pockets at the nape of the neck, behind the breastbone, around the kidneys, and in the groin areas. Babies that are born prematurely or are underweight have very little brown fat, which is why they have such difficulties trying to maintain their body temperature and become cold very quickly.

There is still very little fat beneath the skin, so the blood vessels, particularly those around the head, are clearly visible and the skin continues to look red and translucent. However, your baby's entire body is now covered with a fine downy layer of lanugo hair, which was first seen around the fetal eyebrows and upper lip at about 14 weeks. Lanugo hair is thought to be one of the mechanisms that help the fetus to keep warm until it has sufficient fat stores. This is probably why babies born before 36 weeks are usually still covered in lanugo, while those born at term have shed most of the hair during the last few weeks in the uterus. This fine covering of skin hair also helps to ensure that the baby remains covered in the thick white waxy coating, called vernix caseosa, which starts to be secreted from the sebaceous glands in the skin during this second trimester. The vernix protects the fetal skin from fingernail scratches and prevents it from becoming waterlogged during the many weeks that it is immersed in amniotic fluid.

Support systems

The placenta continues to be the fetal life-support system and is now fully developed functionally. However, it will continue to grow, trebling in size by the end of a normal pregnancy. Up until now, it weighed more than the fetus, but from this point onwards the fetal weight overtakes that of the placenta.

It is quite common to find the placenta lying low in the uterus during the 20-week ultrasound scan, but this is not a cause for concern at this stage. Although the placenta is firmly attached to the uterine wall, the uterus surrounding it will grow considerably both upwards and downwards during pregnancy. The lower segment of the uterus starts to form in preparation for delivery at around 32 weeks, with the effect that the majority of placentae are no longer low lying when visualized on an ultrasound scan. Of course, the placenta does not change its position; rather the uterus grows around the placenta at a different rate and at different times in the pregnancy. In fact, the uterus continues to grow until about 37 weeks, and at term less than 1 per cent of women have a low-lying placenta (see p.240 and p.428).

The pool of amniotic fluid around the fetus continues to increase: by the end of the 20th week it contains about 320ml (11fl oz). This is a dramatic increase when compared to the 30ml (1fl oz) of amniotic fluid that was present in the uterus at 12 weeks. The temperature of the fluid is carefully maintained at 37.5°C, which is slightly higher than the mother's body temperature. This is another method by which the fetus manages to keep warm.

Your changing body

For some women, weight increases gradually, while others notice a big spurt one week and no apparent increase during the next. Overall, you will gain, on average, 0.5–1kg (1–2lb) per week during this period, and by week 21 you will definitely look pregnant.

> ...your blood pressure has not shot through the roof because most of your blood vessels have become more dilated and flexible...

At 18 weeks, the fundus of your uterus can be felt midway between your pubic bone and navel (umbilicus) when your midwife or doctor gently palpates your tummy; by week 21, it will probably be at or just below your navel. The symphyseal fundal height (the distance between the top of your uterus and your pubic bone) will be 21cm (8¼in). Although this measurement is not as accurate as a scan, it is a quick way to establish that your baby is growing satisfactorily.

Feeling the heat

The volume of blood in your circulation continues to increase steadily and by 21 weeks it will measure nearly 5 litres (8¾ pints). This increase is needed to supply the many organs in your body that are now working much harder than usual. The uterus is receiving the biggest share of this extra blood flow, which is vital to perfuse the placenta and provide sufficient oxygen and nutrients for your baby; an extra half litre of blood (16fl oz) will continue to be pumped to your kidneys every minute for the rest of your pregnancy. A higher than normal proportion of your blood flow is also going to your skin and mucous membranes and their blood vessels have become dilated to accommodate it. This is one of the reasons why pregnant women have blocked and stuffy noses, feel the heat, sweat more profusely, and feel faint during pregnancy.

Extra blood volume

To deliver all this extra blood to your organs, your cardiac output must continue to increase gradually and by 20 weeks, your heart is pumping about 7 litres (12 pints) of blood per minute. However, your heart rate (the number of times your heart beats every minute) cannot be allowed to rise too much or you would start to experience palpitations. The extra blood volume and the stronger pumping activity of your heart should logically result in your blood pressure rising dramatically, but important changes in the blood vessels throughout your body are taking place, which usually prevents these problems from developing.

One of the major reasons why your blood pressure has not shot through the roof is because most of the blood vessels in your body have become more dilated and flexible (known medically as a fall in their peripheral resistance). They contain much more blood then they used to, thanks to the action of progesterone and other hormones, and this extra blood volume and your dilated blood vessels can lead to unwelcome physical symptoms such as varicose veins (see p.235) and haemorrhoids (see p.217). This fall in peripheral resistance ensures that, in most cases, blood pressure alters very minimally during the first 30 weeks of pregnancy, unless complications such as pregnancy-induced hypertension develop (see p.426). After 30 weeks there is a normal tendency for the blood pressure to rise, but this increase should never be fast or excessive.

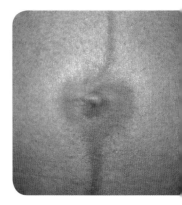

LINEA NIGRA This line of pigmentation down the abdomen is usually more noticeable in women with dark or olive skin.

Changes to your skin

Because of the dilated blood vessels in your skin and the high levels of oestrogen in your body, you are likely to notice tiny red marks called spider naevi appearing on your face, neck, shoulders, and chest.

The pigmentation in the skin around your nipples, genitalia, and the linea nigra down your tummy will continue to be more noticeable. This line, which is more prominent in some women than in others, marks the point where the right and left abdominal muscles meet in the midline. These strap muscles will start to separate from now on to accommodate your growing uterus, but why this should be accompanied by increasing pigmentation on the surface of your abdominal skin is a bit of a mystery.

Some women develop chloasma – also called the mask of pregnancy – on their face. In fair-skinned women the chloasma appears as darker, brownish patches mainly on the bridge of the nose and cheekbones and sometimes around the mouth. On darker skin, the patches appear lighter than the normal

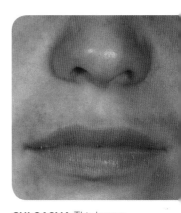

CHLOASMA This brown pigmentation usually develops symmetrically on the cheeks and other areas of the face.

skin tone. Since all of these skin pigmentation changes are due to pregnancy hormones, they usually disappear or fade quite quickly after the baby is born.

How you may feel physically

By now, you are probably rediscovering your pre-pregnancy energy levels. Indeed, many women find that, although they now look pregnant, they don't feel very different physically from the way they did before their pregnancy began.

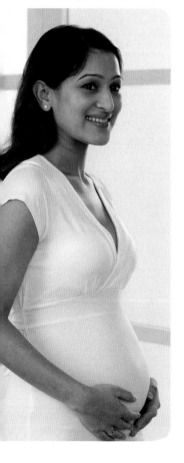

FIRST FLUTTERS It may take a while before you are certain that you are feeling your baby move.

Your appetite will return, indeed it may well increase, and you will find that you can once again enjoy normal meals. Make the best of this time in pregnancy and ensure that you follow a well-balanced nutritious diet (see pp.43–9). It will not be very long before your appetite is upset again, this time because of heartburn, indigestion, reduced stomach capacity, constipation, and all of the other gastrointestinal problems that develop in later pregnancy as the baby grows inside your abdominal cavity and your digestive system becomes sluggish.

Your libido may also have returned and for many couples this is a reassuring sign that pregnancy has not permanently changed their physical relationship. Indeed, some find that their sex life becomes particularly enjoyable during this trimester. A variety of factors contribute to this. Physically you are generally feeling better, which is important since nausea and tiredness are real passion killers, and your hormone levels are less likely to be swinging all over the place. In addition, both you and your partner may be feeling more relaxed in this trimester, having had time to get used to the idea of you being pregnant.

The first time you become aware of your baby's movements is a physical experience that is almost inseparable from the emotional response that follows it. If you have not had a baby before, you may dismiss these first fluttery sensations as wind, but after a while you realize they are unrelated to your digestion; they feel quite different. No one can predict the exact date when you will feel your baby moving around, but it is likely to happen now or very soon.

Your emotions

By now you have probably told most of the people with whom you have regular contact that you are expecting a baby, but even if you have been keeping the news to yourself, your changing shape will have given others a few hints that you are pregnant. Whether you are at home or at work, you are likely to find that everyone around you wants to talk about your pregnancy. Like many women, you may enjoy this new-found closeness with relative strangers and welcome the chance to share your excitement about the pregnancy. There are very few occasions in life when we embark on a deeply personal conversation with a complete stranger and then allow them to pat our tummy or place a paternalistic arm around our shoulders. This happened all the time when I was pregnant and I confess that, after some initial feelings of surprise, this generous display of warmth and goodwill confirmed for me that I was going through a very special time, and that everyone around me recognized this fact. Having said that, I do appreciate that some women view this outside interest in their pregnant state as an unwanted invasion of their privacy. If you find yourself in the latter group you will need to find ways to protect yourself from becoming resentful and angry, since there is little doubt that society tends to view pregnant women as some sort of public property.

Overall this is one of the most enjoyable stages in pregnancy and you are probably feeling more serene and calm than usual. Try to enjoy the relative peace of the second trimester because the third trimester will probably bring with it some emotional highs and lows, not to mention some physical discomfort.

> " ...you may enjoy this new-found closeness with relative strangers and welcome the chance to share your excitement about the pregnancy. "

Your antenatal care

You will see your antenatal carers every four to six weeks during the second trimester for checks on your urine, blood pressure, and the height of your fundus. Your baby's heartbeat will be listened to using a sonicaid monitor or a pinard's stethoscope (see page 161).

If you have not already been given the results of your booking blood tests and serum screening tests and received your hand-held notes, this will all be arranged at one of your antenatal appointments during this stage of pregnancy.

The fetal anatomy or anomaly scan

All maternity units in the UK offer women an ultrasound scan at about 20 weeks (see pp.174–5), although the exact timing varies from one unit to another to complement additional antenatal tests such as serum screening blood tests. However, it is usually performed between 18 and 22 weeks and is frequently referred to as the fetal anomaly scan because at this stage of pregnancy, your baby's organs and major body systems are sufficiently

YOUR 20-WEEK SCAN

By around 20 weeks, your baby is sufficiently developed
for most of the major organs and body systems to
be viewed on ultrasound and checked for signs of
a problem. For most women this scan will reassure
them that all is progressing well.

Below is a summary of the most common checks during this scan, but they will not necessarily occur in this order because your baby will be moving around constantly and may not always be in the right position. Measurements and observations of your baby will be taken as the opportunity allows. The sonographer will only tick off the boxes on the checklist when everything has been seen clearly. So if the position of your baby makes this impossible at first,

you may be asked to walk around and then return for further measurements or even come back in a week or so for a further attempt.

▶ **The fetal heartbeat** is usually the first item to be checked. The sonographer will also look for the four chambers of the heart. If a specialist heart scan is needed, this usually takes place at 22–24 weeks.

▶ **In the abdominal cavity**, the shape and size of the stomach, intestines, liver, kidneys, and bladder

will be examined and the sonographer will check that your baby's intestines are now completely enclosed behind the abdominal wall. The diaphragm, the muscular shelf that separates the chest from the abdominal cavity, should be complete and your baby's lungs should be developing. Although abnormalities in any of these organs are uncommon, you will find information about some of the problems that may be identified on pages 416–22.

▶ **Your baby's head and the spine** will be examined, starting with the covering bones of the skull, to check that they are complete. The fetal spine has straightened, which means that the sonographer can move the scanning probe up and down, checking each bone, or vertebra, to make sure that there is no evidence of spina bifida (see p.419).

▶ **The brain** contains two ventricles, or fluid-filled cavities, positioned on the left and right side of the midline, which are lined with a special system of blood vessels called the choroid plexus. Rarely, the ventricles are enlarged (see cardiac abnormalities, p.421) or the choroid plexus contains

HOW YOUR BABY MEASURES UP

The measurements taken during the scan help to establish whether your baby is the right size for your dates. They are recorded as abbreviations in your notes, with measurements in millimetres, which are checked against charts of normal values. This provides an estimate of the size of your baby in terms of weeks out of 40.

BPD	Biparietal diameter (the distance between the side bones of your baby's head)	45mm = 19+/40
HC	Head circumference	171mm = 19+/40
AC	Abdominal circumference	140mm = 19+/40
FL	Femoral length (length of the thigh bone)	29mm = 19+/40

These measurements suggest that this fetus is appropriately grown for 19 plus weeks of gestation. Assuming that the scan was performed at 19–20 weeks, the baby is the right size for dates.

DETAILS FROM A 20-WEEK SCAN

chin   lung   liver   bowel

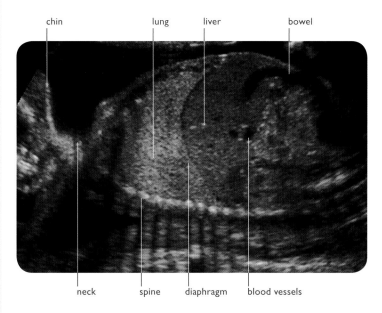

neck   spine   diaphragm   blood vessels

UNDERSTANDING YOUR BABY'S SCAN This right-side image of the fetus shows the chin and neck (far left in the image) and the lung is visible as a pale area above the diaphragm, the dome-shaped sheet of muscle that separates the chest from the abdomen. The liver appears as a large shadow below the diaphragm, punctuated by two blood vessels, which appear as black circles. The dark M shape (top right in the image) is the fetal bowel.

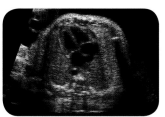

FETAL HEART The four chambers of the heart and blood vessels are visualize.

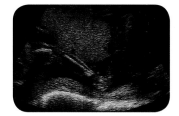

LEG AND FOOT The length of the femur (thigh bone) is a good growth indicator.

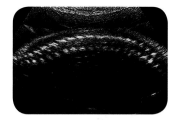

SPINE Each individual vertebra in the spine is counted and checked.

cysts (see p.419). In the unlikely event that these problems are identified, you will be offered further scans.

▶ **The position of the placenta** will be recorded as lying on the anterior or posterior wall, or at the fundus (top) of the uterus. It is quite common for the placenta to be low-lying at this stage and you may be advised to have another scan at about 32 weeks to check that it is positioned higher.

The umbilical cord will be checked and the place where it inserts into the placenta may be noted. Most of the time it is in the centre, but if it is at the very edge of the placenta (known as velamentous cord insertion, see p.430) there may be concern.

▶ **The volume of amniotic fluid** will be assessed to ensure that there is neither too much, a condition known as polyhydramnios (see p.427), nor too

little (oligohydramnios, see p.427). In either case you will need to have further investigations that include a scan in a few weeks' time.

▶ **The sex of your baby** can sometimes be determined if the scan reveals a penis between the fetal legs. But it is not always possible to conclude that you are carrying a girl because the penis can be hidden. For this reason, some hospitals are unwilling to disclose these findings.

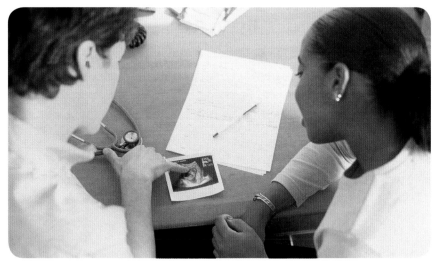

UNDERSTANDING YOUR SCAN Your doctor will be able to help you interpret exactly what you are seeing.

developed for it to be possible to detect the vast majority of potential structural abnormalities. The vast majority of anomaly scans will demonstrate that your baby appears to be developing normally. Far from being a cause for concern, it will offer you and your partner great reassurance, not to mention the thrill of seeing your baby in great detail. For many couples, this is the magical moment when they realize that their pregnancy is going to result in a real human being. Most maternity units will offer you a printed picture for your family album; my twin girls are still entranced by the photo of themselves at the 20-week scan.

Confirming results

For some women, the scan result may show one or more causes for concern. Many abnormalities are accompanied by physical signs that are described as markers for a disorder or syndrome. For example, about 70 per cent of babies with Down's syndrome have structural abnormalities in their heart or gut, a single skin crease in the palm of their hands, and slanting eyes with epicanthic folds that can often be visualized on an ultrasound scan. When a scan picks up a physical sign that suggests Down's syndrome, I almost always advise the parents to have an amniocentesis test (see pp.140–3). They then have a diagnosis they can be certain of and can be given full counselling and advice on their next step.

Although the 20-week scan provides vital information, I should make it clear that a normal scan cannot guarantee that a baby does not suffer from an abnormality. About 30 per cent of babies with Down's do not have an obvious structural marker. It is also impossible to diagnose antenatal problems such as mental retardation, autism or cerebral palsy. Scans do have limitations, even when the sonographer is expert and the machinery is state-of-the-art.

Common concerns

Most of the complaints that crop up in the second trimester are minor, and many of them are due to your blood vessels dilating to cope with the extra volume of blood circulating in your body.

Feeling dizzy or faint is a very common symptom during the second and third trimesters of pregnancy, and is rarely a serious problem. As I explained earlier, the blood vessels around your body, and particularly in the veins of your pelvis and legs, now contain a much larger volume of blood. When you stand up quickly, you may feel momentarily dizzy because all that extra blood in your leg veins needs a bit of extra time to be redistributed to your head and other organs. Headaches are another common complaint. Most of the time they are due to tension and anxiety or the fact that you are suffering from nasal congestion. However, always seek advice promptly if you find that you are suffering repeated headaches because occasionally they are a first sign that you are developing high blood pressure (see blood pressure problems, p.426).

Skin rashes

Pregnant women are very susceptible to a wide range of skin rashes, which are usually due to the massive hormonal changes occurring in your body. However, always check with your doctor or midwife if you experience persistent problems.

It is not unusual to develop dry patches of flaky and highly itchy skin, most commonly on your legs, arms, and abdomen. Applying simple emollient (moisturizing) creams such as E45 or Diprobase usually helps, but occasionally an antihistamine or even a low-dose steroid cream may be needed to relieve the irritation. The dilated blood vessels in your skin may mean it looks pinker, or even blotchy, which can sometimes be mistaken for a rash.

Since your skin needs to get rid of the extra heat from these dilated blood vessels, it is normal for you to sweat more. As a result, you may develop a sweat rash under your arms or breasts and in the groin areas, where sweat accumulates and does not have much chance to evaporate quickly. Wearing looser clothes, preferably cotton, and avoiding synthetic fabrics close to your skin will reduce the problem as will careful hygiene and using unscented soaps and deodorants. Occasionally, a sweat rash can become infected with yeast or other fungal organisms (for example, thrush see p.216). These are not serious, but can make you itchy and uncomfortable and you may need to be prescribed a topical antifungal cream to help clear the infection.

APPLYING CREAM Using moisturizing cream will help improve itchy, flaky skin on your legs, arms, and abdomen.

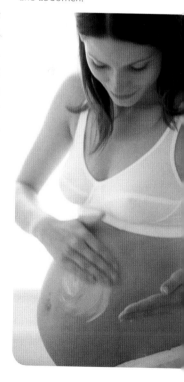

Things to consider

The chances are that the clothes that you need to wear now are quite different from those that you imagined you would be wearing at this stage. Feel pleased with yourself if you resisted the temptation to buy new outfits at the first sign of a bump.

> ...many women feel the urge to go on holiday – a sort of 'make hay while the sun shines' type of break.

Now is the time to give some thought to what clothes you really need to be comfortable at work and at home. Think of this exercise as being similar to packing to go on holiday when your baggage allowance is restricted. There is no shortage of sources for maternity clothes – they can be found in the big department stores, in certain high street chains, and in specific specialist shops and mail order catalogues – but careful selection is the key.

Mix and match separates are usually the best solution, since they offer the greatest flexibility and you can accommodate repeated changes in your size relatively easily. The main difference between special pregnancy tops and normal jackets or shirts is that the front is longer than the back so that, once your bump has been taken into account, both are the same length. However, the back of some jackets have a way of expanding to fit your enlarging shape, so if you need to wear suits or jackets to work, you could well find that buying yourself one good jacket and changing the skirt or trousers as and when your growing abdomen demands it, is the best way to deal with your changing size.

When it comes to skirts and trousers, the priority is to find clothes with a comfortable, expanding waistline. In the short term, buying leggings a couple of sizes larger than usual works well, but you will soon find that this is not the long-term answer, since the elastic waist starts to dig into you as the weeks go on. Proper maternity skirts and trousers have clever button elastics or panelling at the top, both of which allow for your expanding waist and provide comfort for the later stages of your pregnancy. You might also want to invest in some drawstring trousers or a dress with no waist to see you through a good part, if not all, of the remaining months.

Maternity tights provide more support than ordinary tights and even though you will probably have to buy different sizes as your pregnancy continues they are a good investment. I can remember how much more comfortable I felt when I was wearing them and how conscious I was of my tired and aching legs when I did not. Avoid knee-high socks, as these can block circulation at the top of your calf and encourage the formation of varicose veins. Cotton-rich ankle socks allow your skin to breathe and do not impede circulation.

If swimming is part of your exercise routine, buy a swimming costume that will see you through the whole nine months. You will feel a lot more comfortable in a proper maternity swimming costume, many of which can be bought for around the same price as an average swimming costume.

A 40-week pregnancy spans several seasons and most of your major clothing purchases need to be for the season when your body shape has altered most significantly. If your first and second trimesters fall in the summer months, you may have several items of loose clothing in your wardrobe to tide you over until your shape demands a formal shopping expedition. If your third trimester is in the winter months, resist the temptation to buy an expensive winter coat in a larger size, since you are unlikely to want to wear it next winter after your baby has been delivered. In the meantime you could borrow a coat from a friend, or buy an A-line design with no front fastenings, which can be used indefinitely.

A change of scenery

During the second trimester many women feel the urge to go on a holiday or weekend away – a sort of "make hay while the sun shines" type of break. Now that cheap flights are available to all corners of the globe, I find the question of travelling in pregnancy and how safe it is crops up continually. Most of the answers are to be found in the Staying Safe in Pregnancy section, which includes a full discussion about travel in pregnancy, safety of immunizations, and the various precautions you should take (see pp.36–7).

As far as advice specific to this stage of pregnancy goes, if you have had previous pregnancy complications, think carefully about travelling abroad at this time; the last thing you need is to find yourself a long way from home, should something unpredictable happen. Coping with an unforeseen problem is distressing enough without having to deal with a foreign language, a different healthcare system, and the uncertainty of whether your health insurance will cover the situation. However, if you have no history of problems and your doctor has passed you fit to travel, then it is highly unlikely that you will encounter any pregnancy-related problems during your holiday.

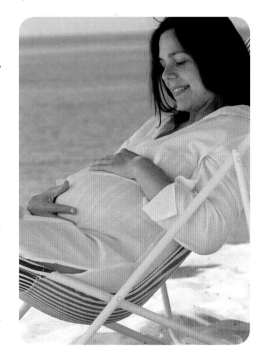

TAKING A BREAK This stage of pregnancy can be a good time for travel as long as you have no pregnancy problems.

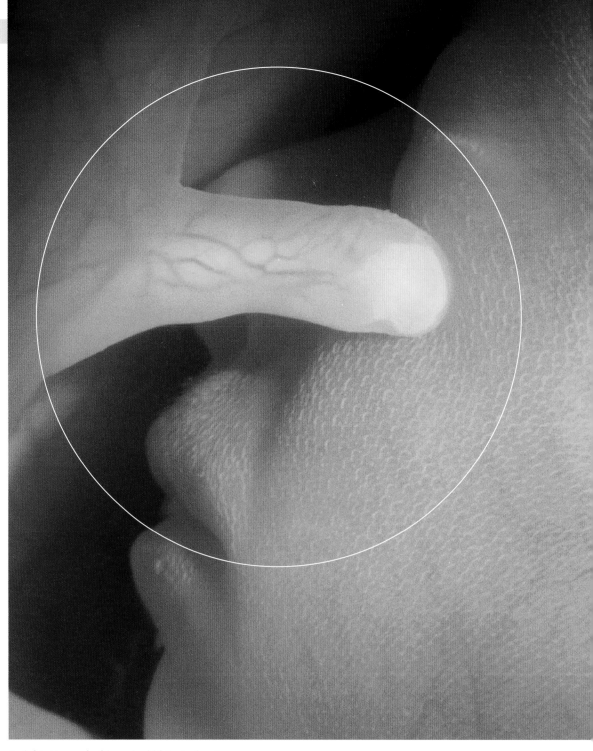

▲ A fetoscope of a 21-week-old fetus in the uterus.

1	2	3	4	5	6	7	8	9	10	11	12	13	14	15	16	17	18	19	20

▶ WEEKS 0–6   ▶ WEEKS 6–10   ▶ WEEKS 10–13   ▶ WEEKS 13–17   **WEEKS 17–21**

▶ **FIRST TRIMESTER**   ▶ **SECOND TRIMESTER**

▶ WEEKS 21–26
The developing baby

YOUR BABY IS CONTINUING TO GROW in length and to put on weight steadily, although it will be some time before it develops a plump, chubby appearance. The facial features are now very well developed and eyebrows, eyelashes, and head hair are clearly visible.

The skin still looks pink and wrinkly, but no longer appears completely translucent, because some subcutaneous fat is being laid down. Two distinct layers of skin have developed: the surface layer or epidermis and a deeper layer called the dermis. The epidermal skin layer now carries a surface pattern on the fingertips, palms, toes, and soles of the feet, which is genetically determined and gives rise to a unique set of finger- and toe prints for this future human being. The underlying dermis grows little projections containing blood vessels and nerves. The surface of the skin remains covered with a fine layer of lanugo hair and a thick coating of white vernix caseosa. This waxy protective coat will remain until just before birth: babies that are born prematurely are often still covered with a thick layer of vernix, whereas babies born late or post mature, have lost all their vernix, and as a result, their skin is dry and flaky.

Inside the body

Several important developments are occurring inside your baby's body. The nervous and skeletal systems continue to mature, which means that, instead of just wriggling or floating, movements become more deliberate and sophisticated, including kicks and somersaults. The fetus practises thumb-sucking and starts to hiccough. Any object that the hands encounter is firmly grasped and, amazingly, this grip is strong enough to support the whole of the baby's body weight.

The brain is developing and its activity can be monitored electronically on an EEG (electroencephalogram). By 24 weeks, the fetal brainwave patterns are similar to those of a newborn infant. The brain cells that have been programmed to control conscious thought are beginning to mature and

life size

The 21-week-old fetus measures around 17cm (7in) and weighs about 350g (12oz). By the end of the second trimester, it will have increased in size to 25cm (about 10in) from crown to rump and weighs just under 1kg (about 2lb).

| 21 | 22 | 23 | 24 | 25 | 26 | 27 | 28 | 29 | 30 | 31 | 32 | 33 | 34 | 35 | 36 | 37 | 38 | 39 | 40 |

▶ **WEEKS 21–26**   ▶ **WEEKS 26–30**   ▶ **WEEKS 30–35**   ▶ **WEEKS 35–40**

▶ **THIRD TRIMESTER**

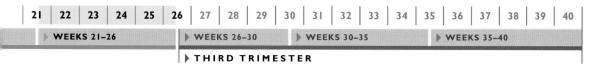

research suggests that, from this time onwards, the fetus starts to develop a primitive memory. Certainly, your baby can now respond to noises in your body and also to loud outside sounds and your physical movements. It is thought that a baby can now distinguish between his mother's and father's voices, and is able to recognize them after birth. Studies have shown that babies are able to recognize a particular piece of music that they have "heard" repeatedly in utero. This theory might explain why my young daughters always seem to feel comfortable and relaxed when they hear Italian opera or Nina Simone – both are acquired tastes, but the twins were exposed to them repeatedly while I was pregnant.

The eyelids will be open towards the end of this period. Although most babies have blue eyes at birth, the final colour of their eyes is not known until many weeks after delivery.

A cycle of sleeping and waking has started to develop. Unfortunately, this is not always synchronized with your daily pattern and you may find yourself worrying about the lack of movements during the day, only to find that you are kept awake for most of the night because the baby is buzzing around.

The fetal heart rate has slowed considerably from 180 to 140–150 beats per minute by the end of the second trimester. From this point onwards, monitoring the heart rate pattern on a cardiotocograph (CTG) machine becomes one of the most useful methods of assessing your baby's wellbeing.

The fetus is opening and closing its mouth regularly as large quantities of amniotic fluid are ingested. The fluid is digested and waste products from the metabolic processes in the fetal body are passed across the placenta, via the umbilical cord, to be disposed of in the mother's blood. The remainder, which is effectively excess water, is then excreted back as urine into the pool. At 26 weeks, the volume of amniotic fluid has risen to about 500ml (16fl oz or almost 1 pint) and the entire pool is changed or recirculated every three hours.

The fetal lungs are still relatively immature and it will be several weeks before they can breathe unaided. Nevertheless, your baby has started to make breathing movements and will practise them until the time of delivery. The lungs are full of amniotic fluid, which helps the fetus to develop more air sacs (alveoli), which need to be buoyant in the amniotic fluid in order to multiply properly and later to expand. A network of tiny blood vessels around the sacs is forming; this will be essential for the transfer of oxygen to the rest of the baby's body after birth. If the waters

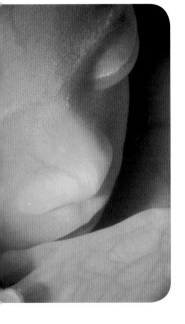

TOUCHING The hands move towards the face and touch and grasp anything they encounter.

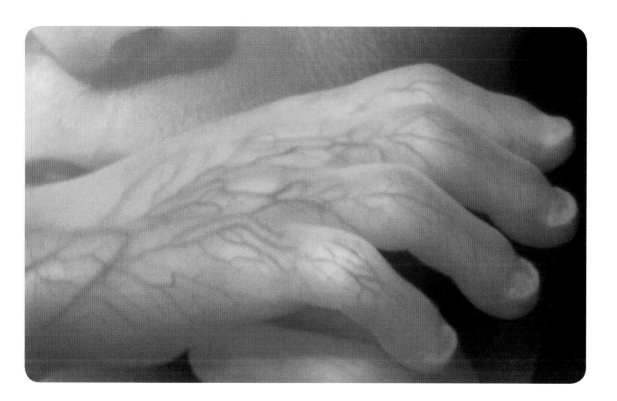

break before the end of the second trimester, the baby's lung development is almost always compromised and breathing difficulties after birth are invariably a problem.

A viable baby

Even though the lungs are still relatively immature, the fetus has now reached a stage of potential viability, which means that it may be able to survive outside the womb, albeit with the help of neonatal medical expertise and a ventilator to assist with breathing. The legal definition of fetal viability in the UK is now set at 24 weeks and every baby born after this time is registered as a birth. This is because babies born before this date are very unlikely to survive and will be classified as a miscarriage (see p.431) or a stillbirth if the baby shows any sign of life at delivery (see p.432). After 24 weeks, the chances of survival begin to increase, although until about 30 weeks, there is still a high chance of the baby suffering from a physical or mental disability (see p.339). Nevertheless each day that passes after 26 weeks is accompanied by an increase in lung maturity and a reduced risk of other problems as well. As I will explain in the next section, the first few weeks of the third trimester of pregnancy are crucially important in terms of potential fetal survival.

SKIN AND NAILS
A layer of underlying fat has been laid down, but blood vessels are still visible. Fingernails have developed and also a unique surface pattern on the fingertips.

Your changing body

During the next few weeks, most women will gain about half a kilogram (about 1lb) in weight every week, although the exact amount varies between women and between weeks. Ideally, you should gain 6–6.5kg (13–14lb) during this second trimester.

> ...you may notice that your skin is looking particularly rosy and healthy and your hair is thick and glossy.

If you find you are putting on quite a bit more weight than is recommended during this last part of the second trimester, remind yourself that only about one kilogram of this weight will have gone to your developing baby. The rest can be attributed to your growing uterus and breasts and the increased blood and fluid volume that your body now contains, but also to your maternal fat stores (see p.42). Lots of extra pounds gained now will be difficult to shed after the birth. If your weight gain continues to be excessive as you move into the third trimester, you will be at greater risk of developing gestational diabetes (see p.427) and pre-eclampsia (see p.426), not to mention feeling unnecessarily tired and being troubled more than usual by backache. So do try to eat a sensible balanced diet and restrict your sugar and carbohydrate intake. If you do need to control your weight, reducing your calorie intake gradually will not harm your baby's growth. Some women put on very little weight in pregnancy, but as long as their diet contains all the necessary nutrients, this is nothing to worry about.

The expanding uterus

Your uterus continues to expand, and between 21 and 26 weeks will rise above your belly button (umbilicus). This growth has been achieved by an increase in the size of the muscles of the uterus, which are still attached to the same supporting ligaments. It is not surprising that many women experience stitch-like pains down the sides of their abdomen as the uterus expands and stretches these ligaments to their limits. The height of the fundus measures approximately 22cm (7½in) at 22 weeks; 24cm (9½in) at 24 weeks; and 26cm (10in) at 26 weeks.

To accommodate the increasing size of your uterus and baby, several other changes occur. As the uterus moves upwards in your abdominal cavity, your rib cage will move upwards too, by as much as 5cm (2in) and the lowest ribs begin to spread sideways. This frequently causes discomfort or pain around the ribcage and may mean that you start to feel breathless. The stomach and other digestive organs become compressed and progesterone continues to relax the muscles in the gut. As a result, it is common to experience heartburn, indigestion, and constipation at this stage in pregnancy (see p.187).

A pregnancy bloom

Between 21 and 26 weeks, the increase in your cardiac output continues to rise slowly but steadily, along with the volume of blood in your circulation, but your stroke volume and heart rate are levelling off and will not increase further. To deal with these cardiovascular changes, your peripheral resistance must reduce even further to ensure that your blood pressure does not alter significantly.

The up side to all of this extra blood flow and the enormous quantities of pregnancy hormones, is that you will probably notice that your skin is looking particularly rosy and healthy and your hair thick and glossy. This is because women shed less hair during pregnancy and the increase in their metabolic rate means that hair also grows faster than usual. After the birth, you will start to lose hair in much greater quantities than usual – but to a large extent you are simply losing post-birth what you would normally have lost during the nine months.

Changing centre of gravity

Your posture will have changed by this stage in your pregnancy. The enlarging uterus and baby are slung forwards in the middle of the body, which means that a pregnant woman is forced to find ways of restoring her altered centre of gravity. Added to this mechanical load, the ligaments of the pelvis have been softened by the pregnancy hormones contained in the vastly increased blood flow to the pelvis. This is an essential change since the pelvis needs to relax sufficiently in order to be able to accommodate the passage of a 3kg (6½lb-plus) baby through its previously rigid walls. However, this means that your pelvis can no longer function as the stable girdle that it once was and your pregnant body must find a way of compensating for these changes to their stability. The simplest way to deal with this mechanical challenge is to lean backwards, arch your back, and ensure that your legs take on a wider gait than normal, but this change in posture is frequently accompanied by backache, since the ligaments of your abdomen, back, and pelvis are placed under strain.

Your fast-growing tummy is beginning to affect the way you move, sit, and lie. You will start to notice that you feel unstable wearing high-heeled shoes and that certain chairs are less comfortable than others. You may need to support the small of your back when you are sitting, and when you are lying down, there will be certain positions that are much more comfortable than others. These changes and effects are especially noticeable if you are expecting twins. You will find some practical advice on adopting a good posture and preventing back pain later in this section (see p.193) and more specific advice on backache later in this trimester (see p.218 and pp.243–4).

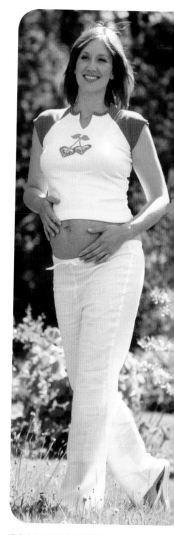

GOOD HEALTH Through the second trimester of pregnancy, many women appear to be glowing with good health.

How you may feel physically

Even first-time mothers will now be very aware of their baby's movements every day and left in no doubt that these sensations are the work of a lively, growing baby. I think this is one of the most exciting milestones reached by women in their journey through pregnancy.

You will also find your baby's movement very reassuring, because you will now be able to monitor the welfare of your baby yourself, instead of having to rely solely on the information you receive from your doctor, midwife or the latest scan report. I remember vividly my own astonishment and overwhelming joy, when during a meal one evening, a commotion in my tummy occurred, which resulted in my plate being bounced across the table in front of me.

Unwanted advice

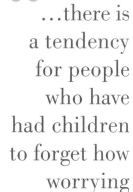

...there is a tendency for people who have had children to forget how worrying scare stories can be...

Every woman carries her pregnancy differently, and however you are carrying yours, it is more than likely that your baby is exactly the right size. Yet it can be difficult to remember this advice when everyone seems to have an opinion as to whether your pregnancy is too big or too small for your dates. Throwaway lines such as "Goodness you have put on a lot of weight" or "You're getting as big as a house" can be truly upsetting, particularly if you are already feeling self-conscious about the extra pounds you have put on. Conversely, "Are you sure that you are eating properly?" and "You do look small. Is everything all right?" may be well intended, but are guaranteed to alarm you at a vulnerable moment. If this constant analysis of your size in pregnancy begins to bother you, I suggest that you explain as calmly and as tactfully as you can, that you find it distressing and you would prefer family, friends, and colleagues to stop. After all, people do not usually pass judgement on your body shape when you are not pregnant.

Another problem may arise if you are so engrossed in the subject of pregnancy you find yourself inadvertently encouraging people to open up and recall all sorts of things about their own pregnancies that might be better left unsaid. Some of their anecdotes will be encouraging and useful (particularly if you have a specific problem that you are worried about), but others can be downright frightening. I think there is a tendency for people who have had children to forget how worrying scare stories can be for those who are currently going through a pregnancy. Again, my advice is to be honest. Gently but firmly explain that you would rather not hear another tale of a premature birth or an

PROBLEMS WITH DIGESTION

At this stage of pregnancy, problems with your digestion become much more common. You may well have started to experience mild or even severe symptoms of heartburn and indigestion and suffer episodes of constipation, too.

INDIGESTION

As your enlarging uterus begins to compress your abdominal organs, the capacity of your stomach is reduced and your whole digestive system begins to slow down. Food remains in your stomach and intestines for longer, making you prone to indigestion – a sensation of a heavy lump at the bottom of your stomach. At times you may have a constant dull or stabbing pain around your abdomen, sometimes with back pain.

HEARTBURN

You may also have heartburn due to the fact that the valve between your oesophagus and stomach has become relaxed and is no longer very efficient at preventing food mixed with acid gastric juices from regurgitating back. This irritates the lining of your oesophagus causing a searing or burning sensation behind the front of your ribcage.

As long as the symptoms pass within a couple of hours, they are not a cause for alarm. In the meantime, there are several ways to minimize your digestive problems:

▶ **Eat little and often**, avoiding heavy, fatty, highly spiced or pickled foods, which make symptoms worse.

▶ **Drink a glass of milk** or eat a pot of natural yogurt before meals and before bedtime. This can help to relieve heartburn by neutralizing stomach acid.

▶ **Sit bolt upright** when you are eating to reduce the compression to your stomach.

▶ **Avoid lying down** for at least an hour after you have eaten and keep your head well propped up at night on several pillows to reduce the problem of heartburn.

▶ **If your symptoms** are severe, ask your doctor to prescribe you an antacid such as Gaviscon or Maalox.

CONSTIPATION

Your sluggish digestion can also make you constipated, leaving you feeling heavy and irritable. Try some of the following remedies:

▶ **Boost the fibre** in your diet by eating more fresh fruit and vegetables and wholegrain bread and cereals.

▶ **Increase your fluid intake** by making sure you drink at least 2 litres (4 pints) of water per day.

▶ **Take regular exercise**. As little as a 20-minute walk each day can help to relieve constipation.

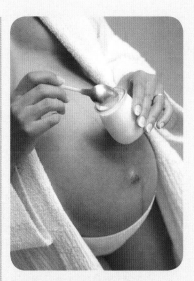

EASING HEARTBURN Natural yogurt may help to relieve symptoms.

▶ **Bulking laxatives** such as Fybogel or Lactulose are effective because they contain complex sugar compounds, which the human gut cannot digest. They absorb water, helping to produce a bulkier, softer stool that can be passed without straining and discomfort.

▶ **Laxatives** containing senna are not recommended in pregnancy because they irritate the gut, which has the potential to trigger uterine contractions.

excruciating labour. Far from being offended, most people will understand and some will also realize (and most probably deeply regret) that they have caused you unnecessary anxiety.

Your antenatal care

You will continue to have antenatal appointments with your midwife or GP (see page 161), and by now will know what to expect in terms of the various checks. For the majority of women, this period of their antenatal care is a quiet and enjoyable time.

Although I feel it is important to cover the further investigations that may form part of antenatal care here, I want to add that it is very unusual to encounter any of these serious complications during this stage of pregnancy, either with your health or with that of your baby.

It is unlikely that you will undergo a further routine ultrasound scan during this period unless problems that need further investigation were identified at the 20-week scan. If the scan suggested anything abnormal in the development of your baby's organs, for example, an intestinal blockage or problems with the kidneys or urinary tract, you will have additional scans between 21 and 26 weeks, possibly at a specialist centre. If the abnormality is confirmed, you may be advised to undergo a late amniocentesis (see pp.140–3) or fetal blood

PREDICTING PREMATURE BIRTH

Nowadays, the majority of babies that are born prematurely survive and develop normally, but those that are born very prematurely (before 30 weeks) still have a significant risk of handicap if they survive (see p.339). So any test that may help to predict which babies are at risk needs to be carefully considered.

Some 2 per cent of women have a very short cervix and it is thought that half of these may give

birth very prematurely as a result. Some units are now using vaginal ultrasound scans throughout the second trimester to help identify these pregnancies and offer preventive treatments. If your hospital is participating in this research, you will have the length of your cervix checked using a vaginal ultrasound probe. If your cervix is found to be shorter than average, you will be closely monitored.

Some researchers believe

that inserting a stitch in the cervix to lengthen and close it may be of help, although this procedure is not without risk. Some hospitals offer progesterone treatment to prevent contractions and/or steroid treatment to reduce the risk of breathing complications if the baby is born prematurely. It is too soon to know whether this type of antenatal screening will become routine practice, but the provisional results look promising.

sample test (see cordocentesis, p.143) to see whether or not the baby is affected by a chromosomal or genetic problem. The results from the amniocentesis usually take three weeks because the skin cells in the amniotic fluid have to be cultured before they can be examined for chromosomal abnormalities. This will seem like an eternity for worried parents-to-be, but new molecular biology techniques at some specialist centres can greatly speed up the time taken to establish the baby's genetic make-up (see p.143). The results from a fetal blood sample are also available more quickly because it is possible to analyze the white blood cells immediately.

If you have had a previous baby with a heart abnormality or if there is a family history of cardiac problems, early referral to a fetal cardiologist is advised, as at times early cardiac scans at 12 or 16 weeks can offer great reassurance to the expectant mother. This is followed by a detailed cardiac scan at 22 weeks. The other type of ultrasound scan you may be offered is a Doppler blood flow scan (see p.257), which examines the way blood is flowing in the vessels of the uterus, placenta, and umbilical cord. Research has suggested that reduced blood flow through the uterine arteries at this stage in pregnancy may be a way of identifying women at high risk of developing high blood pressure (see blood pressure problems, p.426) or problems with the growth of their baby (see p.214 and intra-uterine growth restriction, p.429). As a result, some specialist units now screen women with Doppler scans at 24 weeks. The small minority of women (5 per cent) in whom the blood flow is reduced can then be carefully monitored for changes in their blood pressure. The Doppler blood flow scan can also be used to look at the flow of blood in many of the baby's arteries and veins, which is a good indicator of the baby's general wellbeing.

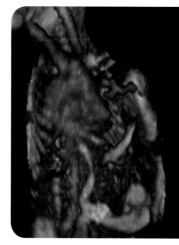

BLOOD FLOW
A Doppler scan shows blood flowing through the major fetal vessels. The heart is seen as a large red structure centre left, and the yellow-coloured blood vessels, bottom right, lead to the umbilical cord.

Common concerns

Concerns in pregnancy are usually a mixture of niggling complaints and anxieties about things you may have heard or the way your pregnancy is progressing. I hope the advice here sets your mind at rest on a few issues, but remember that your doctor or midwife will also be happy to talk through any worries that you may have.

It is quite common to feel dizzy or light-headed when you change your position suddenly at this stage of pregnancy because of the massive changes in the way your increased blood volume is distributed in your body. A significant proportion is being directed to the uterus to support the placenta and baby and large quantities of blood are being stored in your pelvic and leg veins because of the reduction in peripheral resistance. When you stand up quickly it takes a few minutes for the blood in your pelvic and leg veins to redistribute; meanwhile, there is a shortage of blood to the brain, leaving you light-headed and even inclined to faint. Similarly, if you have been standing for long periods, the extra pooling of blood in your legs may leave your brain short of blood, especially when it is hot and your blood vessels dilate even more to cool you down.

There are steps you can take to reduce these dizzy spells or, worse, fainting fits, both of which can be quite frightening and unpleasant.

• Make sure that you do not get up too quickly from a sitting or lying position. Aim to let the blood flow adjust gradually.

• Try to avoid becoming overheated, particularly in hot weather. One of the commonest times for feeling dizzy or faint is when you try to get out of a hot bath too quickly because this leaves your circulation completely unable to deal with the shifts in blood volume needed to prevent you feeling light-headed.

• Take care to eat regularly and choose foods such as complex carbohydrates (see p.44) that release energy gradually, so that your blood sugar levels are prevented from rising and then falling too quickly.

• If you feel faint or dizzy, sit down and put your head between your knees or lie down and raise your feet above your head or at least above your pelvis, so that the blood in your leg veins returns to your brain as quickly as possible.

Even if you suffer from regular dizziness, your baby is not in any danger because the blood supply to the uterus and placenta is being maintained at your expense. However, when you lie flat on your back, the weight of the uterus can end up pressing against blood vessels in the pelvic area, depriving your placenta (and hence your baby) of oxygen, so avoid this position.

The main danger of dizziness is if you suddenly start to see stars while driving up the motorway or getting on a train. For this reason, interrupt travel regularly. If you have to stand for long periods, make sure that you keep shifting your weight from one leg to the other. Better still, walk around if you can.

Checking fetal movements

Many women I meet in the antenatal clinic are worried about how many fetal movements they should be feeling each day or night – anxieties that can be made worse by the doctor or midwife asking at each visit "Is the baby moving well?" If this is your first baby it is obviously difficult for you to know, so I owe a big debt to the distressed pregnant woman who pointed this out

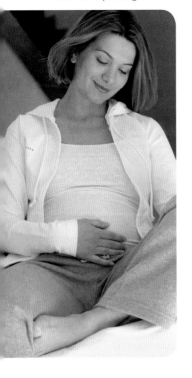

PATTERNS OF MOVEMENT You will begin to recognize your baby's patterns of movement and become alert to any changes.

to me many years ago when I was at the start of my training. As a result of this lesson, I changed my methods of finding out about fetal movements.

The issue of fetal movements is important in pregnancy for the simple reason that they are one of the best ways for you and your antenatal carers to assess the wellbeing of your baby. Having said that, I don't intend to offer rigid rules about how many movements you should be feeling per day or night, at any stage during your pregnancy journey. This is because every pregnancy is different and every baby develops its own pattern of movements, which can change as the pregnancy progresses. Some babies are more active than others generally and all babies go through periods in the day when they are quieter or are engaged in more vigorous pursuits. Over the weeks, you will get a feel for your baby's own pattern of activity, perhaps noticing that your baby responds with a kick when you are in a certain position or becomes still at certain times of the day. So, instead of advising that you should feel 5, 10, 20 or 50 movements every 12 or 24 hours, you should look out for any dramatic changes to your baby's pattern of movements and should one occur, consult your midwife or doctor as a matter of urgency. In particular, if you do not feel your baby move during a 24-hour period, then seek advice immediately.

> ❝ ...every pregnancy is different and every baby develops its own pattern of movements... ❞

Abdominal aches and pains

Abdominal pain is always worrying and, for pregnant women, it invariably raises concerns that the baby is at risk. During the second trimester, the most likely explanation for the twinges and aches in the lower abdominal area that virtually every woman experiences at this stage in pregnancy is that the ligaments supporting your enlarging uterus are being put under enormous strain. However, if you develop regular abdominal pain, or notice that you have become tender to touch anywhere in your abdomen, tell your carers about it immediately so that it can be investigated promptly. There are several possible causes and, although these are not common, they can have potentially serious consequences. The most serious is pain in the uterus itself, which may be the first signs that you have had some bleeding behind the placenta from a placental abruption (see p.428) or are at risk of premature labour (see p.340). The pain may be sharp and stabbing or a dull, constant ache and may or may not be accompanied by vaginal bleeding. Whichever, your midwife or doctor will want to examine your uterus.

A uterine fibroid (see p.423) is a benign mass of muscle in the uterine wall, which may begin to cause problems in the second trimester because the

> You should always try to avoid lifting heavy weights in pregnancy, but if you have young children, this is likely to be impossible at times.

high levels of oestrogen and progesterone hormone present will encourage the fibroid to grow along with the rest of the uterus. Occasionally, this rapid growth means that the centre starts to degenerate, which results in severe pain in the uterus and abdomen, localized to a particular spot. Pain from fibroid degeneration is very unpleasant, but usually resolves itself with bed rest and painkillers without causing any problems to the baby. Occasionally, large fibroids that are positioned in the lower part of the uterus or beside the cervix will lead to problems near the time of labour if the baby's head does not have sufficient room to descend into the pelvis.

Nausea, vomiting, and/or diarrhoea accompanied by abdominal pain is uncommon in pregnancy, but is almost always due to food poisoning or viral gastroenteritis. It is usually self-limiting and although very unpleasant, it resolves quickly with no harm to you or your baby. There is no need for any medical treatment apart from ensuring that you drink plenty of fluids to replace those you have lost. Very occasionally, symptoms may be due to listeria infection (see p.50 and p.413), which is a potential cause of late miscarriage and intrauterine death and is best treated with penicillin antibiotics.

Appendicitis is another rare, but important, cause of persistent abdominal pain in the second trimester of pregnancy. However, it can be very difficult to make the diagnosis in pregnant women, since the appendix is no longer lying in its usual position in the lower right corner of the abdomen but has been displaced by the growing uterus.

Urine infections are another important and common cause of abdominal pain in the second trimester. It is usually felt in the lower part of your abdomen, above the pubic bone and is likely to be accompanied by discomfort when passing urine. Remember that you may not notice the early symptoms of a urine infection, such as cystitis, before organisms have travelled up the dilated urinary tract to the kidneys and developed into pyelonephritis. In mid and late pregnancy, urine infections can lead to irritability of the uterus and premature contractions, not to mention long-term damage to your kidneys if they go untreated. For this reason, if you have abdominal pain in pregnancy, your urine will be tested and you will probably be started on a course of antibiotics while you wait for the results. These drugs will not affect or damage your baby. If you do have a urine infection, it is essential that you finish the course, even if your symptoms disappear quickly, and also that you have a further urine sample examined to make sure the infection has cleared. Urinary infections that are inadequately treated will recur and, worse still, may then become resistant to the more usual antibiotic treatments.

PREVENTING BACK PAIN

Back pain is so common in pregnancy it is unusual for a woman not to suffer from it. You are likely to begin to notice it around the end of this trimester, so here are some tips that may help to reduce its severity and prevent it becoming worse.

▶ **When you are upright**, adopt a good posture: stand tall, and hold your shoulders back (your back should always be in a straight line). Remember that if you slouch over your expanding tummy, your back will arch and this will aggravate your lower back pain. Try not to stand for long periods of time.

▶ **Invest in some good flat or low-heeled shoes**, preferably with support for the arches of your feet and sturdy soles. Wearing high heels from this point onwards will make you feel more unstable, and increase the strain on your back.

▶ **Sit well: this is particularly important** if you spend long periods working at a desk. Make sure that both shoulder blades and the small of your back are against the chair back and that the seat supports your thighs. The chair should be at the right height for you to keep your feet flat on the floor and the computer screen should be at eye level.

▶ **When you are driving** check that the car seat supports the small of your back and that you can reach the hand and foot controls easily. Your seatbelt may feel uncomfortable but you must wear it for every trip.

▶ **When you are resting, raise your feet** and legs to take the pressure off your back and pelvis. Later on in pregnancy you may need a firmer mattress to help support your back. You will also find that sleeping on your side will help to reduce the strain in the ligaments of your back.

▶ **When you get out of bed**, first turn on your side and, keeping your back straight, swing your legs over the side of the bed. In this position you will be able to push yourself upright using the strength of your arms without placing any strain on your back.

▶ **Regular gentle back exercises will help** the muscles and ligaments of your back to stretch and become more supple. Pelvic tilt exercises are especially helpful as are exercises that help to strengthen the muscles of your back (see p.219).

▶ **Try not to gain too much weight** – every extra pound places further strain on your back.

LIFTING HEAVY WEIGHTS

You should always try to avoid lifting heavy weights in pregnancy, but if you have young children, this is likely to be impossible at times. When your toddler needs to be carried use this method: squat down and hold him close to you; keep your back straight and use the muscles in your legs to push yourself upwards as you stand. Use the same technique to lift any heavy weight.

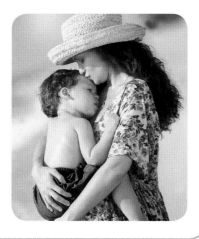

Dental health

As well as visiting the dentist regularly, it is often a good idea to see a dental hygienist for some general advice on gum care. Sore gums that bleed when you brush or floss your teeth are very common; they become soft and spongy thanks to the increased blood supply and hormones of pregnancy. To help firm your gums and prevent bacteria infecting the broken skin, increase the number of times you brush your teeth. Recent research has suggested that gum disease in pregnant women may contribute to the development of problems such as late miscarriage and premature labour. Although the mechanisms are not completely understood, it is possible that a constant focus of inflammation or infection in the mouth can result in complications in other areas of a pregnant body.

Things to consider

I hope that you have already enrolled in an antenatal or parent education class because the best ones tend to book up well in advance. If you haven't found a place yet, make it a priority to do so.

The more knowledgeable and prepared you are for your labour, the more relaxed and confident you will feel; added to which, you will find that the opportunity of sharing worries, feelings, and experiences with other parents-to-be is a source of comfort and relief. Even if this is not your first baby, do sign up for a refresher course – you will be surprised how quickly you have forgotten the details of labour and breathing techniques. Also, there is a constant evolution in how a hospital deals with labour and what sort of pain relief it can offer, so even if you had your first baby in the same hospital, there may have been changes that you are unaware of.

Parents and in-laws

If you are one of those lucky individuals who usually enjoys an uncomplicated relationship with their parents and in-laws, or step-parents for that matter, you may be surprised to find that things are not quite as straightforward as

❝ Your mother may be offering all sorts of advice about pregnancy and child-rearing already and may be put out if you plan to deal with your pregnancy and newborn differently. ❞

they were before you became pregnant. There are so many different permutations of a family unit nowadays that I could not begin to cover them all, but I think it is useful to reflect on the fact that, although pregnancy invariably brings joy to a family, or extended family, it can also give rise to conflicting emotions that can reverberate upwards through the generations as well as downwards.

Your mother may be offering all sorts of advice about pregnancy and child-rearing already and may be a bit put out if you are taking the view that life has moved on in the intervening years and that you plan to deal with your pregnancy and newborn baby differently. Similarly, your mother-in-law will have her own views, too, that don't always chime exactly with those of your own mother. Both are capable of loaded questions such as, "Why are you working so hard?" or, "Are you planning to give up work after the baby is born?". If these are beginning to trouble you, ask your partner for help. Presenting a united front and demonstrating clearly that you are making decisions together about issues such as childcare and work may help to silence the critics in the family.

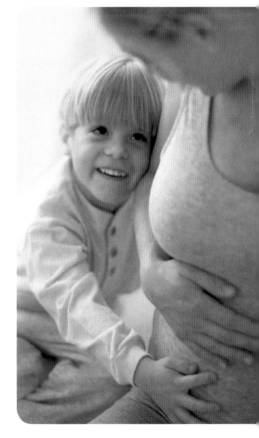

NEW ADDITION An older child may want to ask exactly how his new brother or sister will arrive in the outside world.

Telling children about the baby

If you already have a child or children, the other delicate issue you will shortly have to address, if you have not already done so, is when to tell them that they will soon have a baby brother or sister. Of course the timing depends, to a large extent, on the age of the child. A two year old may not have noticed your changing shape and will certainly not have linked it to the fact that there is a growing baby inside you. However, older children will certainly be aware of your altered appearance, so it is much better that they hear the news from you instead of accidentally from someone else.

If you have not told them already, reflect for a moment on why you have not. I suspect that this will be because you are worried that any existing children may fear they are going to lose some of your love and attention by having this new person in the family. This is a logical concern for a small child who cannot yet know that parents have limitless love when it comes to their children. So you need to tell them this important fact repeatedly.

The other thing to remember about young children is that they have little perspective of time and have no way of understanding that your pregnancy is going to continue for another six months or so before they see the end product. Children absorb most information they are given but often choose to process it in their own time, usually at a later date. So, when you are trying to have a sensitive conversation about the future baby, do not worry that your toddler appears to have no interest in the subject and suddenly interrupts to ask if he can have a biscuit. Equally, do not be surprised when the next day, or the next week, he returns to the subject of the future baby without any warning. Just pick up the threads of the conversation and continue to reassure him.

Your girlfriends

During the second trimester of pregnancy, your relationship with girlfriends who don't have children or are not planning to have them in the near future can become strained. Now that your attention is focused on visits to the antenatal clinic, how many times a day you can feel your baby kick, and which parentcraft class you want to join, your friends may well find your new topics of conversation rather limited. They may be wondering what happened to the pre-pregnant you and whether that person will ever re-emerge.

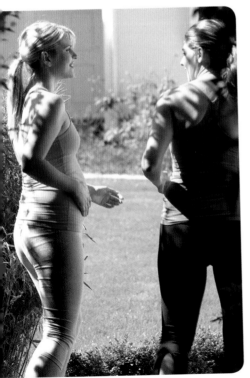

GIRLFRIENDS Your relationship may change but you don't need to lose touch with your non-pregnant friends.

The reality is that you are moving on to a different phase of life, and this change in your relationship will be even more noticeable after your baby is born. But there is no reason why a close friend cannot be equally important to you, just because your lifestyle has taken on a new direction. If you rate your friendships, there is every good reason to continue them.

As far as nights out are concerned, whiling away an evening in a crowded pub or club may no longer be an attractive option in pregnancy, but you can make the most of meals out and get-togethers at friends' homes while you still have the freedom to do so. Reassure them that there will be nights out after the birth even if they end a little earlier, either because you need to get as much sleep as possible or because your babysitter will want to go home. Having a baby does not mean that you do not want to see your friends, or that you have to become such a baby bore that you are no longer able to involve yourself in friends' lives and concerns or listen to their current news.

What's in a name?

Before pregnancy, you might have assumed that the only possible difficulty in choosing a name would be to whittle down a long list of names to a few contenders. Now that you are pregnant, you may be surprised to find that the whole exercise is more complex than you had imagined.

Part of the problem may be that you find it difficult to relate to your baby at this stage. Some mothers-to-be start chatting away happily to their baby when it is only a few inches long, but believe me, there is no need to feel disturbed if it is taking you a little longer to develop the relationship. Knowing the sex of the baby at the earliest possible opportunity helps some parents to think about their unborn baby as a real person and this may also help when it comes to choosing a name; others feel this takes away some of the excitement of the birth. For the latter group, choosing two sets of possible names for their baby boy or girl can be one of the magical parts of the pregnancy.

The next problem is that you may soon be feeling pressurized by suggestions from family and friends. Some women deal with the issue by inventing a completely absurd name, which shocks their relatives into silence; others opt for a vague, non-committal approach. Having said all that, it is also common for parents to make their final choice during the birth, or days, or even weeks, afterwards when the legal requirement to register the child's name forces them to make a decision. There are only two outcomes I can guarantee: the first is that you will look at your child as she grows up and will not be able to imagine her being called anything other than the name you gave her. Secondly, when your child grows up, she will tell you repeatedly how she wished you had given her a different name.

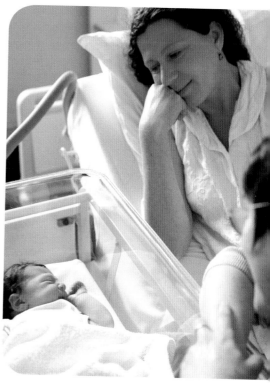

CHOOSING A NAME
Sometimes the perfect name does not become apparent until you meet your baby face to face.

The surname dilemma

If you are married or in a long-term relationship, the issue of which surname your baby uses may be open for debate. Although the assumption is that the child will take the father's surname, there is no legal reason why this should be so and you may have strong feelings that your own surname should be used. One increasingly favoured option is either to double-barrel the surnames or to use the mother's name as an additional first name.

My personal view is that life is quite complex enough for young children today without adding unnecessary speculation from outside parties about the identity of the parents. Call me old-fashioned, but I have always found that being known as Mrs Summerfield at home and at the girls' school and Professor Regan at work has had some very positive advantages and has never given rise to any uncertainty for my children.

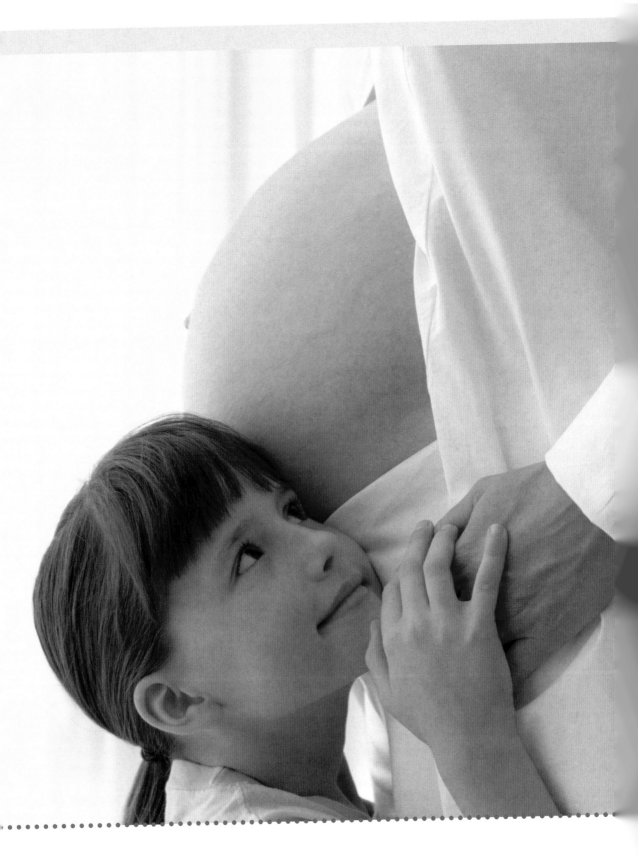

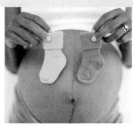

▶ **WEEKS 26–40**

The third trimester

Your baby is capable of surviving if delivered now, albeit with medical assistance, but the remaining weeks in the uterus are vitally important. All your baby's development is now focused on maturing the lungs, digestive system and brain so they can function in the outside world. As your abdomen expands hugely to accommodate your growing uterus and baby, your thoughts turn increasingly towards the birth.

CONTENTS

Your baby

IN THE THIRD TRIMESTER

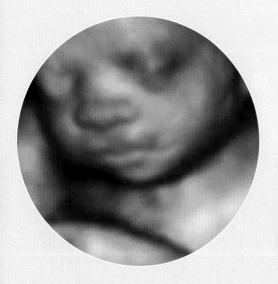

WEEK 27

The baby begins to develop a pattern of rest and sleep alternating with active periods.

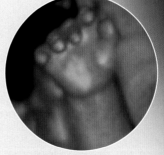

WEEK 28

Skin creases are visible on a chubby hand with perfectly formed fingernails.

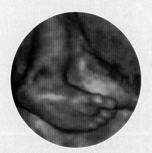

WEEK 29

Movements are strong and purposeful and include hefty kicks, punches, and rapid changes in position.

66 During the weeks between now and delivery all the baby's body systems are maturing ready for life outside the uterus. 99

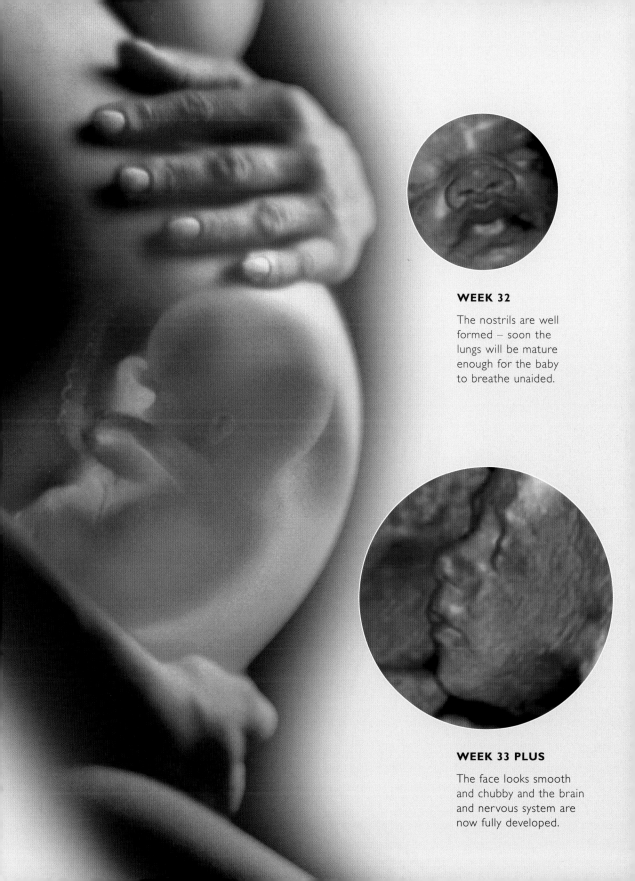

WEEK 32

The nostrils are well
formed – soon the
lungs will be mature
enough for the baby
to breathe unaided.

WEEK 33 PLUS

The face looks smooth
and chubby and the brain
and nervous system are
now fully developed.

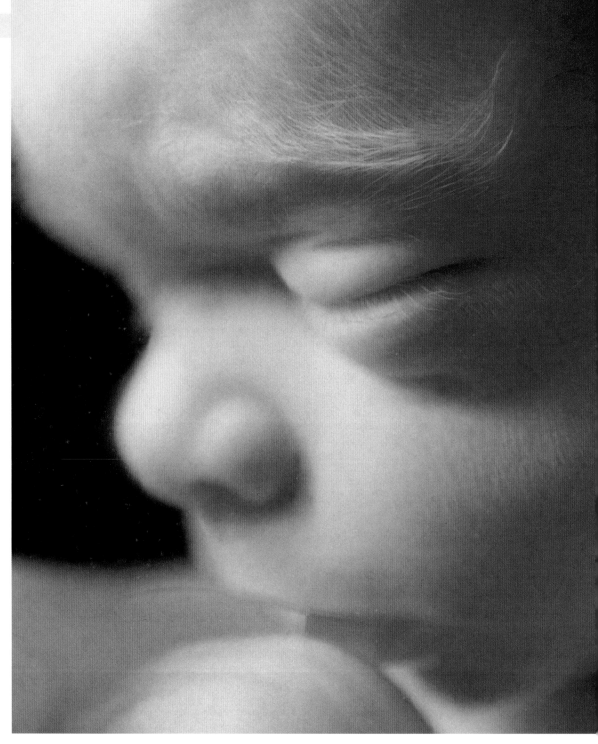

▲ By 27 weeks, the eyelashes and eyebrows are fuller and the fetus can blink.

| 1 | 2 | 3 | 4 | 5 | 6 | 7 | 8 | 9 | 10 | 11 | 12 | 13 | 14 | 15 | 16 | 17 | 18 | 19 | 20 |

▶ WEEKS 0–6   ▶ WEEKS 6–10   ▶ WEEKS 10–13   ▶ WEEKS 13–17   ▶ WEEKS 17–21

▶ FIRST TRIMESTER   ▶ SECOND TRIMESTER

▶ **WEEKS 26–30**

The developing baby

DURING THE NEXT FEW WEEKS, your baby continues to grow in length, while the body weight increases quite significantly because white fat is being deposited under the skin. The baby now looks plumper as the abdomen and limbs fill out and the skin starts to lose its wrinkly appearance.

Subcutaneous fat helps your baby to regulate its own body temperature, an essential development for life after delivery, although this ability is only partially acquired in the uterus, and newborn babies still lose heat very quickly. As the fat is laid down, the lanugo hair becomes sparser and soon only a few patches over the back and shoulders will remain, although the coating of white vernix will stay until about 36 weeks. The hair on the scalp will lengthen and the eyebrows and eyelashes will become fuller. Skin creases can be seen on the hands and feet, and little fingernails and toenails are also clearly visible. The testes of male babies start to descend into the scrotum.

Now that the eyelids are open, your baby will start to blink and will become much more aware of differences in light. This new sense allows the baby to be more responsive to external stimuli; many mothers notice their baby has developed a distinct pattern of rest alternating with activity. The baby is also able to start focusing at this stage, although the distance is limited to about 15–20cm (6–8in) until after the birth.

Getting ready to breathe

From now until the end of the pregnancy the further development of the lungs is vitally important. By about 29 weeks, most of the smaller airways (bronchioles) are in place and the number of alveoli (little air sacs), which lie at the end of the bronchioles, are increasing. The formation of alveoli continues throughout pregnancy and after birth. In fact, the lungs do not become fully matured until a child is eight years old, which is why many childhood respiratory problems resolve or improve as children get older.

not life size

At the start of the third trimester, an average fetus measures 25cm (approx 10in) from crown to rump and weighs just under 1kg (about 2lb). By 30 weeks, its length is about 28cm (11in) and it weighs about 1–1.5kg (2–3lb).

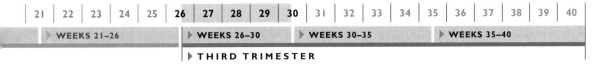

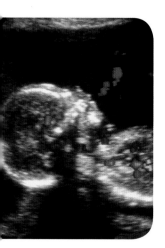

PRACTICE BREATHING
The flow of amniotic fluid in and out of the baby's mouth as it practises breathing movements is seen as red patches on this colour Doppler scan.

The next step in lung maturity is the production of a lipid called surfactant, made by the lining cells of the lung, which coats the air sacs in a very thin film. The surfactant works by reducing the surface tension inside the alveolar air sacs, in rather the same way that washing-up liquid disperses grease on dishes. This process is important because when the baby takes a first breath of real air, the air sacs need to be as elastic as possible to be able to expand successfully. When the first breath is exhaled, the air sacs must be prevented from collapsing in readiness for the next lungful of air. A baby born before 35 weeks cannot yet produce sufficient quantities of surfactant and this, coupled with the inadequate development of the bronchioles and alveoli, means that the newborn baby's lungs are too rigid to deal with the constant flow of air entering and leaving them. Should you be unlucky enough to have a premature birth, you will probably be given an injection of steroids before the baby is born; this helps to stimulate the lungs to produce surfactant (see p.342). The neonatal doctors may also decide to spray artificial surfactant into your baby's lungs after he or she is born in order to make them more elastic.

Of course, your baby is not breathing air at present because the placenta is still supplying all its oxygen requirements. Nonetheless, your baby will have started to make rhythmic breathing movements as it continues to develop its lungs, in preparation for the birth. These movements of the chest wall can be seen on an ultrasound scan and explain the "hiccoughs" you sometimes feel – short jerky movements that are quite different from other activity you can feel going on inside you.

Your active baby

You will be very aware of fetal activity between 26 and 30 weeks. Although conditions inside the uterine cavity are becoming cramped, there is still enough room for the odd somersault and complete change of position. The amniotic fluid is not being produced at the same rate as a few weeks ago so movements are no longer so well cushioned and hence more noticeable than previously. It is very common to see dramatic changes in the shape of your abdomen when the baby heaves itself into a different position. Some women worry that they will be damaged or that their baby will suffer an injury as a result of all this vigorous activity. Neither will occur. There is still enough amniotic fluid to protect the baby and the thick muscular wall of your uterus is more than enough to prevent damage to your internal organs. Before leaving the subject of movements, I want to remind you that there is no correct number of movements or kicks that you should experience every day (see pp.190–1), but any sudden changes in your baby's regular pattern of movement needs to be reported to your doctor or midwife immediately, just in case your baby is in trouble.

There is no correct position for the baby to be in at present, but many babies at this stage are still lying with their head uppermost. This often results in the mother feeling the head butting against her ribcage, which can be quite unpleasant and can sometimes be the cause of quite sharp pain. Like every other problem in pregnancy, it will not last forever. Most babies turn round to embark on their journey into the outside world head first.

Maturing systems

Your baby's nervous system continues to become more intricate and sophisticated. Constant movements of the muscles help to make movements and reflexes more finely co-ordinated. Your baby will practise the sucking reflex on a thumb or fingers whenever the opportunity presents itself, but the ability to suck from the breast will not be fully developed until 35–36 weeks.

The fetal bone marrow has now taken over as the main producer of the baby's red blood cells. This will help your baby become more independent after delivery because these cells will transport oxygen around the blood stream. A simple immune response to infection is now in place.

As your baby reaches 30 weeks, its ability to survive in the outside world has improved dramatically and, as a result, the vast majority of babies that are born at this gestation will cope extremely well, with a bit of help from the special-care baby doctors. From now onwards, every day spent in utero reduces the time that your baby would need to spend in a neonatal unit. Even though the baby's physical size is not changing dramatically, its functional maturity is taking a considerable leap forwards.

By 30 weeks, the placenta will weigh about 450g (just under 1lb), which is a massive increase compared to the 170g (6oz) it weighed at 20 weeks. Every minute, it receives about 500ml (16fl oz) of blood from your circulation.

YOUR BABY'S BRAIN

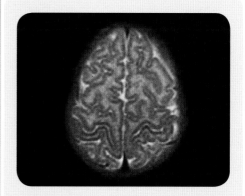

The brain grows in size and now starts to fold over to fit inside the bony skull. An anatomical slice through the upper part (cortex) of the fetal brain now looks like a walnut or a map of the Scandinavian fjords, with lots of little inlets and inwards projections. The protective myelin sheath that began to form around the nerves of the spinal cord many weeks ago now extends to the nerve fibres entering and leaving the brain. As a result, nerve impulses can travel much faster from the brain to the rest of the body. This ensures that, in addition to more intricate movements, the baby is able to learn new skills.

Your changing body

Your uterus is continuing to expand at a steady pace. By 26 weeks it has reached above your umbilicus or belly button and during the next few weeks you will notice that your abdomen is enlarging both upwards and sideways.

By the 30th week, the height of the uterine fundus measures approximately 30cm (12in) from your pubic bone. I say approximately because there is much individual variation and it is important not to become worried if your fundal height is a few centimetres lower or higher than the standard textbook measurements. Your doctor and midwife will measure your uterus at each visit and if there is any serious discrepancy in size, they will arrange for you to undergo a series of growth scans (see p.214) together with some other investigations to ensure that all is well with your developing baby (see pp.256–9).

INSIDE YOUR ABDOMEN Your uterus grows both upwards and outwards, reducing the available space for your stomach and intestines.

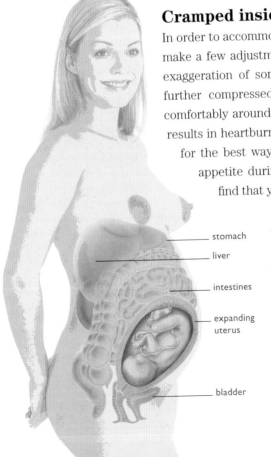

stomach
liver
intestines
expanding uterus
bladder

Cramped inside

In order to accommodate this enlarging mass, your other body organs need to make a few adjustments so you may experience some new symptoms or an exaggeration of some previous ones. The intestines and stomach become further compressed upwards because they can no longer fit themselves comfortably around the sides of the uterus. This upward displacement often results in heartburn and/or indigestion; look back to the feature on page 187 for the best ways to deal with this. Similarly, even if you had a healthy appetite during the second trimester of pregnancy, you will probably find that you can no longer manage to eat a large meal at one sitting.

Your bladder is also unused to this extra pressure in the abdominal cavity and can no longer hold the quantities of urine it used to be able to cope with; this causes its own set of irritations (see p.215).

You may also experience some rib pain or discomfort, since your ribcage is now pushed outwards to make more room for the increasing contents of your abdominal cavity. Some women are lucky and go through the whole of their pregnancy without any rib pain. However, if your body frame is smaller than average or you are carrying twins or triplets then you are very likely to notice rib discomfort. It will be made worse if your baby is an especially strong

SHORT OF BREATH

You will notice a definite change in your breathing pattern during the third trimester. There are several reasons for this:
▶ First of all, the high levels of progesterone hormone increase your body temperature and breathing rate.
▶ In addition, as your ribs flare outwards, your diaphragm has to stretch further and in the process becomes less flexible. This reduced movement of the diaphragm forces you to try to breathe more deeply.
▶ Lastly, the expanding uterus pushes the abdominal contents up against the diaphragm, leaving the lungs with less room to expand when you try to take a deep breath.

With all these conflicting pressures it is hardly surprising that pregnant women frequently experience episodes of breathlessness, dizziness, and light-headedness towards the end of their pregnancy. If you look back to page 190 you will find practical advice on ways to reduce some of these symptoms.

kicker or spends a lot of time in the breech position (see p.269) because the fetal head will bump up against your diaphragm and ribcage. You may be particularly uncomfortable when you are sitting down, as this compresses everything even more. If you have a desk-bound job, it is sensible to make a few adjustments to your routine. Try to ensure that you get up and walk about regularly. When you are feeling particularly uncomfortable, keep changing your sitting position until you find a better one. Make a determined effort to keep a good posture.

A surge in circulation

From 26 weeks onwards, your circulatory system embarks on another surge. The total blood volume is now about 5 litres (8¾ pints) – a 25 per cent increase over normal, although the maximum blood volume will not be reached until about 35 weeks. This increased blood volume means that your cardiac output (the quantity of blood pumped by the heart at each beat) continues to increase during the next few weeks. However, further relaxation of the blood vessels around your body is no longer an option because all your blood vessels are now at maximum capacity. In fact, from this point onwards, your peripheral resistance will have to increase slightly and your blood pressure will start to rise, although this should be a small and very gradual change.

Your body tissues also become thicker because there is so much fluid on board that it has to be accommodated somewhere – so it is very common and perfectly normal for your fingers and legs to become slightly swollen. Having said that, if you notice that your face, fingers or legs have suddenly become much puffier or swollen, these may be early signs of pre-eclampsia (see p.426) and you need to be seen and checked over as a matter of urgency.

CIRCULATION CHANGES

The graph shows a steep rise in cardiac output and blood volume from mid-pregnancy onwards and a corresponding dip in the peripheral resistance of the body's blood vessels.

KEY

— Cardiac output

— Stroke volume

— Heart rate

— Blood volume

— Peripheral resistance

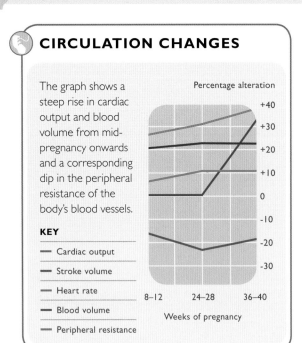

Percentage alteration

+40
+30
+20
+10
0
-10
-20
-30

8–12   24–28   36–40

Weeks of pregnancy

Pre-eclampsia usually develops after 30 weeks, and then only in a minority of women. Rarely, it develops earlier and, when it does, it is likely to become severe.

The continuing changes in your circulatory system means that the blood flow to your skin and mucous membranes is increased. In response, the peripheral blood vessels dilate and this is why pregnant women in the third trimester notice that they "feel the heat" and sweat more easily, sometimes profusely. Many women also find that the palms of their hands and the soles of their feet are red in colour and feel as if they are on fire. This is called palmar erythema. All of these skin changes are entirely normal and will disappear after you have delivered. They merely reflect the fact that you need to get rid of the extra heat that your increased metabolism and your baby's metabolism is generating. If the blood vessels in your skin did not dilate, you would not be able to maintain your body temperature or your baby's at a constant level and you would literally overheat – just like a car with a broken radiator.

Breasts and colostrum

Your breasts will feel a lot fuller by now, due to the combined and continued action of the hormones that are responsible for breast growth in pregnancy. The veins on the surface of your breasts become more prominent and more visible during this last trimester and the nipples and areolae continue to darken.

Under the influence of pregnancy hormones, the internal structure of your breasts has been changing and developing ready for lactation and breastfeeding (see p.396). While the placenta is still in the uterus, high levels of oestrogen and progesterone block the action of the key hormones that trigger milk secretion, but you may notice from this stage onwards that you are producing some clear liquid, which leaks from the nipple at all sorts of strange times, for example, when you are in the bath or making love. This liquid is called colostrum and it is the fluid that your baby will suckle for the first few days of life, before your real milk comes through. Colostrum contains sugar, protein ,and antibodies – in fact, all your baby's nutritional needs – and doubtless the reason why it has started to be produced now is to cater for those babies that decide to make an early appearance into this world. Having said that, please do not worry if you do not see any colostrum throughout your entire pregnancy. I can assure you it is there, it is just that you are one of the fortunate women from whom it has not actually leaked out.

How you may feel physically

You are likely to be actually enjoying your enlarged size by now, even if at times you feel rather compromised by it. Remember to walk tall and keep your back straight, since bad posture will put a lot of pressure on your lower back during these last three months.

I think it is useful to make a few suggestions here about how you can address the predictable tiredness and loss of energy that may have started by now. Many pregnant women tell me that, however much they rest, they are still tired and lacking in energy. The usual advice is to spend time with your feet up, but this is more difficult to do when you have a job and/or other children, not to mention the rest of your life to run. So the message needs to be – think realistic not idealistic. Try to find ways to reduce your commitments at work and at home.

Delegation is often the answer and I suspect that you will be pleasantly surprised by how receptive your colleagues and your family are if you just give them the opportunity to help you. So instead of trying to be superwoman, identify someone else to go to the extra committee meetings at work. Ask your partner to go to the school parents' evening, or send your apologies. Look at the household chores with a fresh eye. Do they really need to be done or could they be left to a later date when you are feeling more energetic? If the answer is yes, as may be the case with basic shopping and housework, then think about ways to employ someone to do them. If this is not possible, then you will need to ask your partner, another family member or a supportive friend for help.

As any mother of more than one child will tell you, there can be real problems dealing with your first child or other children when you are heavily pregnant. When your two-year-old toddler is having a tantrum and refuses to have a bath, you need to step back a few paces and give yourself a break. Ask yourself – is this bath really necessary? If the answer is no, then skip the bath. If the answer is yes, go for a compromise of waving a sponge around the face and grubbiest parts of your child. Remember that becoming fraught about daily domestic issues will help no one and you need to make sure that you conserve your physical and emotional energy for things that really do matter.

> 66 When your two-year-old toddler is having a tantrum and refuses to have a bath, you need to step back a few paces and give yourself a break. 99

Your emotional response

You are definitely in the home straight now – well past the halfway mark in this pregnancy journey. This is a real transition period in emotional terms, because the birth of your baby, which used to be a rather abstract notion, suddenly becomes very real.

Your baby has a very good chance of survival now, so you may be starting to become impatient, wishing away the next few months. At the same time you may be experiencing contradictory feelings of panic at the thought of having a baby to look after in the near future. If this is your first baby, you are probably starting to worry about how qualified you are to be let loose on a newborn infant. After all, many women nowadays have never changed a nappy, let alone held a very young baby, before they are handed their own in the delivery room. If this is not your first child, you will understandably be concerned about how your other children will adapt to the challenge of another little person who will have demands on your time and attention. You may also worry about how this new baby will fit into your already hectic life.

Since the possibility of birth now exists for real, you are doubtless also starting to think about how you will cope with labour and delivery. If this is your first birth, you will be conscious that you are about to sail into uncharted waters. If you are reading this book stage by stage, I would suggest that now is the time to jump ahead and read the sections on pain relief, labour and birth, and life after birth to familiarize yourself with the practical and emotional aspects of childbirth and beyond. Like most other important events in our lives, the better informed you are, the more capable you will be of dealing with the challenge positively and confidently. Do make sure that you start your antenatal or parentcraft classes now, if you have not already done so.

A positive body image

If you are normally a fit, healthy woman, the physical downsides of pregnancy can come as something of an emotional shock. You may become increasingly frustrated by your growing bulk, which is preventing you from leading your life as you used to. On the other hand, you may be loving every minute of your new-found voluptuousness. Some women who are usually very slender and weight-conscious tell me that they feel suddenly liberated by, and enormously proud of, their large, rounded belly. They view their body as an

> 66
> Some women who are normally slender and weight-conscious feel suddenly liberated by their large, rounded belly.
> 99

affirmation of their sexuality, especially as it might be the first time that they have ever had a generous cleavage! Similarly, women who have previously been worried about their body size, may for once be reconciled with their larger shape and positively enjoying it. The truth is that the way we feel about our heavily pregnant bodies has a lot to do with how well we feel on a day-to-day basis during the latter stages of pregnancy and the way in which our partners react to our distended bellies and swollen breasts (not to mention extra all-round weight). Some women become deeply attached to their growing bump and a little sad at the prospect of losing it, while others feel that the day when it disappears cannot come quickly enough.

Involving your partner

Some men are closely involved in their partner's pregnancy from the beginning, but many more do not show much interest in the details of pregnancy, labour, and life after birth until rather late in the day. If this is the case with your partner, you may be starting to feel concerned that he is still not as involved in your pregnancy as you might have wished. Indeed, some men are reluctant to become demonstrably involved at all. They are not necessarily being unsupportive, it is just that men and women tend to be on different wavelengths during this unique time.

Women tend to immerse themselves totally in their pregnancy, because it is both physically and psychologically part of them. It is not really surprising that men are less able to do the same, since they are, by definition, physically detached. Many tend to carry on with their lives as if nothing has changed. Although they may recognize that life will change dramatically after the baby arrives, it may be difficult for them to translate this somewhat abstract notion into the day-to-day reality.

If you are first-time parents, pregnancy provides you with the opportunity to start shifting your relationship from the couple that you currently are, to the family that you will shortly be. However, I do think it is important to remember that trying to mould your partner into your ideal of what he should be during your pregnancy is unlikely to be successful. He is going to need to adapt in his own way and in his own time – albeit with a few prompts from you. He is undoubtedly just as keen as you are that everything goes smoothly during labour itself and afterwards, so perhaps the most important thing that you can do now is to ensure that he is sufficiently well informed to offer you some practical and emotional help throughout. Then he will be able to look back on the event and feel he was as involved in thebirth of his child as he wanted to be.

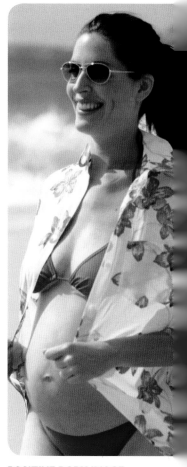

POSITIVE BODY IMAGE
How you feel about your heavily pregnant body is usually a reflection of your overall health and wellbeing at this stage of pregnancy.

Your antenatal care

As long as there are no complications in your pregnancy, you will need to see your antenatal carers only once during the next few weeks. This appointment with your midwife is an ideal opportunity to reassure yourself that all is going well.

Antenatal schedules vary but it is usual to have a routine appointment at 28 weeks. A blood count and antibody test will be performed (see below) and your urine and blood pressure will be checked. Your doctor or midwife will examine your hands and legs and any sudden swelling will be investigated with blood tests to ensure that you are not developing pre-eclampsia.

You may already be experiencing mild practice contractions called Braxton Hicks' contractions (see pp.237–8) that travel down your uterus and cause it to harden momentarily, although these become more common after 30 weeks. However, if you are experiencing any prolonged or painful uterine activity, especially if it is accompanied by lower back pain, do report it straight away.

THE GLUCOSE TOLERANCE TEST

Gestational diabetes (see p.427) is a common complication in pregnancy, largely because of the strain that pregnancy puts on a woman's kidneys and metabolic system. In severe cases, the symptoms are similar to those of diabetes itself and these include extreme thirst, a need to urinate frequently, and tiredness. However, many pregnant women who develop gestational diabetes have no symptoms, which is why the routine screening test has been introduced in all UK maternity units. NICE recommend an oral glucose tolerance test (OGTT) performed at 28 weeks, although if you have a past history of gestational diabetes, a BMI of 30 or more, or if glucose was found in your urine at a previous antenatal visit, you may have the test earlier, at 16–18 weeks. The test is very simple:

▶ You will be asked to provide a urine sample first thing in the morning on an empty stomach.

▶ Still starved, you will have a base-line blood sample taken at the maternity unit and then be asked to drink a glucose (sugary) solution, such as an energy drink or lemonade.

▶ A further blood sample will be taken after an hour and then after two hours. The results, which are usually available within 24 hours, provide a valuable assessment of how well you metabolize sugar.

If you are found to have gestational diabetes you will need to follow a low-sugar, low-carbohydrate diet for the rest of your pregnancy. If this does not control the problem effectively, you may need to take tablets to reduce your high blood sugar levels or possibly have regular insulin injections.

Although only a small percentage of women continue to have the problem after the delivery, having gestational diabetes increases your risk of developing Type 2 or late onset diabetes later in life by 50 per cent.

Blood tests at 28 weeks

Your haemoglobin (blood count) will be tested between 26 and 30 weeks to ensure that you have not developed anaemia (see p.424). If your haemoglobin is less than 10.5g, you will probably be advised to take some iron tablets. It is important to build up your red blood cell count now, since your haemoglobin is likely to drop further towards the end of pregnancy, thanks to the increased fluid content in your blood stream. However, gastrointestinal upsets, constipation problems, and sometimes diarrhoea are common side effects of iron tablets so if you have problems, ask for a different brand. The liquid preparations available in your local chemists may be kinder on your digestive system. Above all, aim to eat iron-rich foods, particularly those that contain lots of fibre, such as dried apricots and raisins.

The antibody screen uses a portion of the same blood sample to check your blood group again and make sure that you have not developed any red cell antibodies. This is particularly important if you are Rhesus negative (see p.128 and p.425). Although the time of greatest risk is at delivery when a Rhesus-negative mother may become sensitized to blood from her Rhesus-positive baby, these women are all offered an injection of anti–D at 28 weeks, even if this is their first pregnancy.

Your baby's position

As well as measuring the height of your fundus and listening to the fetal heartbeat, your antenatal carers will palpate your abdomen and at this stage may be able to determine the position in which your baby is lying. From now on, your antenatal notes will carry a record of the baby's position at each check-up. (For a full description of these different positions and the abbreviations in your notes see pp.268–70).

The lie of your baby at this stage is most likely to be longitudinal (vertical), but it could also be transverse (lying horizontally from side to side in your uterus) or oblique (at an angle). The presentation refers to the part of your baby that is nearest to the pelvis. It can be a cephalic presentation (head down) or a breech presentation (head up). If the lie of your baby is transverse, there is no presenting part at the present time. This is nothing to worry about, since the lie and presentation of the baby can change many times between now and the onset of labour. Similarly, do not be concerned if your doctor or midwife cannot determine which way up your baby is lying between 26 and 30 weeks. Even the most skilled clinicians may find it impossible to decide whether your baby is head down or head up at this stage.

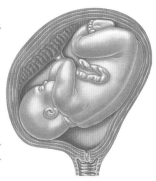

OBLIQUE LIE The baby is lying at an angle across the uterus.

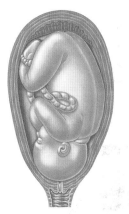

LONGITUDINAL LIE In this lie the baby is vertical with its head or bottom down.

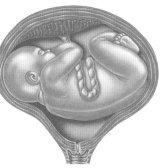

TRANSVERSE LIE The baby is lying horizontally across the uterus.

CHECKING YOUR BABY'S GROWTH

At each antenatal visit, your carers monitor the growth of your baby by palpating your abdomen and measuring the fundal height of your uterus. If a more detailed check is needed, this is usually done with a series of ultrasound scans.

GROWTH SCANS

Fetal growth scans are revealing because most problems at this stage in pregnancy are likely to affect the rate at which your baby is growing. The size of the baby's head, limbs, and abdominal girth will be recorded, and the relationship between the various measurements examined carefully because late pregnancy problems may not affect all aspects of growth equally.

IDENTIFYING THE PROBLEM

Intrauterine growth restriction (IUGR) manifests itself in different ways depending on the cause (see pp.256–7 and p.429). For example, if the placenta is not working well (as can be the case if the mother has high blood pressure or pre-eclampsia) the growth of the baby's head will be maintained but usually at the expense of the growth of the baby's abdomen.

This is because the blood supply carrying oxygen and nutrients from the placenta will be diverted to the baby's brain, and the abdominal organs receive less. To compensate, the baby's liver will start using fat stores with the result that the liver (and abdominal girth) become smaller. This growth pattern is known as "head sparing growth retardation" – a rather frightening term, but one that sums up a clever survival mechanism that ensures that the fetal brain is protected in a potentially difficult situation.

COMPARING MEASUREMENTS

Your baby's measurements will be compared with previous and future measurements because the rate of growth over time is what determines whether it is safe to leave the baby in utero or whether the baby needs to be delivered immediately.

If your baby is not growing very well but is not in distress, you will be asked to return for another scan in 7–10 days. This may seem a long time to wait, but it is difficult to interpret changes in measurements within a shorter interval of time.

INTERPRETING GROWTH CHARTS

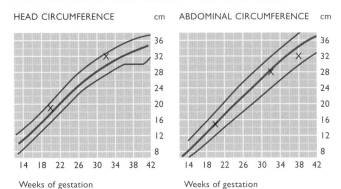

HEAD CIRCUMFERENCE   cm

ABDOMINAL CIRCUMFERENCE   cm

Weeks of gestation

Weeks of gestation

ON EACH GRAPH the 50th percentile (red line) is the average and the 90th percentile line (above) and the 10th percentile line (below) represent the upper and lower ranges of normal growth. On the head circumference graph, the baby's head is growing steadily. On the abdominal circumference graph, the velocity of growth of the abdomen is showing a decline, possibly because blood and nutrients are being directed to the heart and brain at the expense of organs in the abdomen.

Common concerns

This is a weightier section now, reflecting the fact that pregnancy-related problems and irritations are more numerous in the third trimester. Fortunately, there are remedies and strategies that will help to reduce some of their effects.

Urinary frequency during the day is common – the usual reflex signals that start when the bladder is full cut in much earlier when there is an increasingly heavy baby pushing down on it from above. Although there is nothing that can be done about this further mechanical design fault of pregnancy, do remember that if you need to pass urine very frequently and can only expel a tiny amount on each occasion, you may have developed a urinary infection and need to make sure that your urine is properly tested (see p.192).

You may have started to leak small quantities of urine when you sneeze, cough or laugh; this is called stress incontinence and is common towards the end of pregnancy. Renewed attention to pelvic floor exercises can reduce the problem, as can cutting out tea, coffee, and alcohol, which have a diuretic effect.

Sleep patterns in the third trimester are often disturbed and your bladder will make a significant contribution to this by ensuring that you have to get up several times a night to visit the toilet. Several of my patients have suggested that these night-time interruptions are designed to help you adjust to the inevitable lack of sleep after the baby is born. They may be right, but when I was pregnant I would have preferred to sleep undisturbed at night between 26 and 40 weeks and find out about night-time vigils at a later stage.

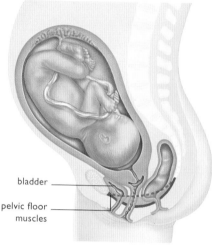

bladder

pelvic floor
muscles

BLADDER PROBLEMS
During a cough or sneeze you may leak urine. The problem is due to the weight of the baby pressing on your bladder and also weak pelvic floor muscles, shown above as a solid line (with a dotted line indicating their pre-pregnancy position).

Vaginal infections

It is normal for vaginal discharge to increase from the second trimester of pregnancy onwards. However, it should always remain clear and mucus-like, odourless or just mildly smelling – similar to the discharge you may have experienced before the start of your period. You may find that you need to use a thin panty liner. If the discharge becomes yellow-green coloured, develops a stronger smell, or your vulva, vagina, and anal region become reddened and painful, particularly when you pass urine, tell your antenatal carers. They will take some swabs to check for vaginal infection, which if left untreated may increase your risk of going into premature labour.

DEALING WITH THRUSH

Many pregnant women are troubled by thrush (candidiasis) in pregnancy. The following remedies may help to relieve symptoms:
▶ Cream and pessary remedies can be bought over the counter or prescribed by your doctor. Pessaries, inserted into your vagina, are the most effective because they tackle the root cause of the infection by increasing the acidity of your vaginal secretions. They will not harm your pregnancy, and a single pessary may resolve the problem. Creams applied to the vulva may reduce the discomfort temporarily, but they won't resolve the underlying problem.
▶ Personal hygiene is important. Make sure that you always wipe your anal region from front to back (rather than back to front) after passing a stool. Bathe regularly and keep your vulva clean and dry. Avoid highly fragranced soaps and bubble baths, particularly if the vulval skin is reddened and sore.
▶ Adding a few drops of vinegar to your bath or bathing the vulval area with a weak solution of cider vinegar may relieve symptoms. Alternatively, you could try live yogurt to balance the body's natural bacteria and fight fungal infections. You could try smearing the yogurt into the vaginal entrance to relieve the itching.
▶ Wearing cotton underwear, and avoiding wearing tights or close-fitting trousers and jeans will give the skin around your genital area more air to breathe.
▶ Reducing your intake of sugar and yeast may prove useful if you have recurrent episodes of thrush infection, since they can both aggravate the problem.

Most itchy vaginal infections are due to thrush (candida infection), which is an innocent, albeit uncomfortable, side effect of pregnancy (it is not sexually transmitted). You will notice an itchy, curd-like discharge (which looks a bit like cottage cheese) around your vagina. Thrush is not a cause of premature delivery and most women experience at least one episode of it during pregnancy. It is largely due to the vaginal environment becoming less acidic during pregnancy thanks to the effects of pregnancy hormones, and this encourages the growth of the yeast-like fungus (*Candida albicans*), which is normally present in small numbers in the vagina and gut. Another common cause of thrush is antibiotic treatment because the antibiotics kill off some of the normal house-keeping bacteria in the gut and vagina, allowing the candida organisms to gain a hold. Some women suffer recurrent episodes of thrush during pregnancy.

Headaches

Headaches are common in pregnancy and are usually nothing to worry about. However, some women suffer from migraine attacks that can leave them quite debilitated. If you are suddenly experiencing severe headaches, report them to your doctor or midwife promptly. Please do not be tempted to wait until your next antenatal appointment, because severe headaches at this stage in pregnancy can be a sign that your blood pressure is too high (see p.426). Even if your headaches prove to be nothing serious, your doctors will be able to suggest some safe remedies.

Itching skin

By the end of pregnancy, your skin will have stretched by an extra 77–155 square cm (1–2 square feet) and can become dry and itchy as it becomes increasingly taut over your enlarging tummy. Stretchmarks – which often make their appearance around now – can make the problem worse. Expensive creams marketed specially for pregnant women, to prevent or reduce stretchmarks, are unlikely to do more than relieve dry itchy skin temporarily. I can promise you that cheaper remedies – simple, non-perfumed emollient creams or oil such as baby oil or olive oil – are just as effective at keeping your skin supple and well hydrated. The other practical step you can take to reduce the itchiness is to start wearing cotton clothes, as these help keep the skin cool. If the itching persists or becomes severe you may need a blood test (see p.242 and p.424), so please tell your midwife.

Haemorrhoids

Many women become troubled by piles (haemorrhoids) by this stage in pregnancy. These are dilated veins around the inside and outside of the anus, or back passage, which are caused by the pressure of the baby's weight in your pelvis. Piles frequently cause throbbing pain and itching around the anal area and they may also bleed. You may find that you can feel a swollen tender vein protruding out of your anus or notice some light red bleeding on the toilet paper after you have passed a stool. If you are constipated, you are more likely to strain in an attempt to empty your bowels and this can cause the haemorrhoids to swell further, so make sure you drink plenty of water each day, increase your intake of dietary fibre and take regular exercise. Lifting heavy weights can aggravate the problem. Over-the-counter creams that contain a lubricant and a light local anaesthetic will help to relive the discomfort, as can cold packs, particularly when you have had a long and tiring day.

Leg cramps

Many pregnant women suffer from leg cramps, particularly at night. You may find that you wake up suddenly, gripped by painful, violent spasms in one of your legs or feet. Some doctors think that the pressure of the uterus on certain nerves in the pelvis may be the trigger while others suggest they may be due to low calcium or salt levels, or an excess of phosphorus. However, none of these theories has been proven so don't even consider trying to adjust your levels of these minerals with supplements or dietary changes. When you get a cramp attack, simply flex the leg, calf or foot in the opposite direction. So if your calf gets cramp, for example, stretch it out by straightening your leg and flexing your foot towards you as you simultaneously massage the calf area until the

> **If you are suddenly experiencing severe headaches, report them to your doctor or midwife promptly.**

RELIEVING BACK PAIN

Women used to be told that they had to put up with backache in pregnancy because nothing could be done about it. In fact there are several practical measures that help relieve symptoms – you don't have to put up with debilitating pain.

The kind of back strain that tends to occur at this stage of pregnancy is generalized back pain. Later in the trimester you may develop more specific back problems, such as sciatica, pubic symphysis dysfunction, and sacroiliac joint pain – these are covered in detail on pages 243–4.

First of all, make sure your doctor identifies exactly what the problem is: the back is such a complex area that the pain could be due to any number of causes. Without a correct diagnosis, treatments could be inappropriate or dangerous.

By all means consider consulting an osteopath, but do make sure that you choose a trained practitioner (see pp.437–8). A skilled osteopath will relieve symptoms of back ache (or joint pain) by gentle manipulation and massage, but you should never agree to undergo any realigning of vertebra – especially in the lower spine – by "clicking" them back into place or using short, sharp manipulations.

Once your doctor has made a diagnosis, back exercises designed for pregnancy may be useful (some are shown here). Referral to a physiotherapist may also be helpful.

PROTECTING YOUR BACK

Because your bump now weighs heavily, you may find that walking even short distances can pull on your abdominal ligaments or give you lower backache. Your pelvic ligaments are now under more strain than ever and, as they are more elastic than usual, it is inevitable that they complain when made to work harder. Turn back to the tips on page 193 to remind yourself how to protect your back when lifting and how to support your back while you sleep.

STRENGTHENING MUSCLES

Regular exercise will help build stronger back muscles and improve your posture and, as a result, support your spine and lumbar region and help reduce – if not prevent – back pain. Physical activity will also enable you to sleep better, as you will feel calmer in yourself, thanks to endorphins released during exercise, which have a slight pain-killing and mood-enhancing effect.

AN ORTHOPAEDIC BELT

Another practical way to reduce back strain is to buy an orthopaedic belt (these are usually advertised as

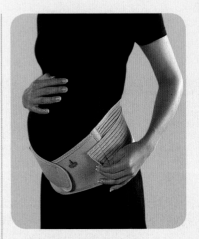

SUPPORT A belt may bring instant relief.

maternity belts in magazines and online). The belt is positioned just below your enlarging bump and straps around your pelvis with velcro fastenings. Wear it through the day and take it off at night. I remember how important my belt was to me at this stage in pregnancy. I was carrying twins, and am short (about 1.5m or 5ft 2in), which meant that by 26 weeks, I was feeling extremely unsteady on my feet and the backache was awful. As soon as I put on my belt, the relief was immediate. Why they are not recommended regularly to pregnant women is a mystery to me.

BACK EXERCISES

If your back is giving you problems, try some of the exercises below. They will help to strengthen the muscles that give support to your spine and pelvis and will keep you supple, which will be of great benefit during labour. As always, stop exercising if you feel any discomfort, and if you are unsure about any specific exercise, ask the advice of an obstetric physiotherapist (contact him/her through your midwife or doctor).

▶ **Knee hug** Lie on your back with your arms hugging your knees (make space for your bump) and gently roll a little from side to side to release tension in your lower spine and pelvis. This is very soothing for your lower back.

▶ **Spinal twist** Lie on your back with your knees bent and feet together, arms out at shoulder height. Slowly drop your knees to one side, while turning your head to look in the opposite direction. Feel your spine twisting gently. Raise your knees back up and repeat on the other side.

▶ **Spinal relaxation** Lie on your back, with your knees bent, shoulder-width apart, with your arms by your side. Push up on your legs so that your thighs, pelvis, and back as far as the shoulder blades are lifted off the floor. Lower your back down slowly, exhaling at same time. Repeat five times.

▶ **Pelvic tilts** Lying on your back with your knees bent, pull in your lower abdominal muscles, squeeze buttocks, and press the curve of your back into the floor. Hold for 10 seconds (don't hold your breath) and release slowly. Repeat five times, building up to 10.

▶ **Knee squeezes** Lie on your back, with your knees bent and your feet together. Squeeze any object roughly the size of your clenched fist between the knees (such as a can of baked beans). Hold the contraction for 10 seconds and repeat 10 times, twice a day. Progress on to an object the length of your forearm (such as a roll of kitchen paper) only when the previous exercise is absolutely pain-free throughout the contraction. This exercise is particularly good if you are suffering from pubic symphysis dysfunction.

▶ **Birth ball** Sitting upright on an inflated birth ball will help to promote good posture.

KEY BACK STRETCHES

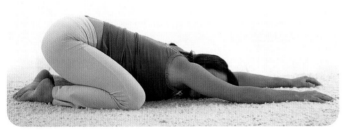

SPINAL STRETCH Sitting down on bent knees, legs slightly apart to make way for your bump, stretch your arms out in front of you along the floor. Feel the stretch right along your spine.

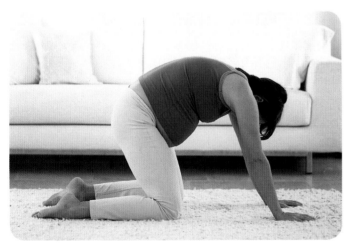

CAT HUMPS Kneeling on all fours, knees and arms shoulder-width apart, arch your back into a hump, clenching your buttock muscles and tucking your pelvis in. Hold, then release slowly until your back is flat again. Repeat five times.

> *You may be anxious to ensure that you are not regarded simply as a mother-to-be but also as a working woman and colleague.*

pain fades away. Although leg cramps are uncomfortable, they are nothing to worry about, since they are temporary ailments that will disappear after your baby is born. However, constant leg pain should always be investigated because of an increased risk of deep vein thrombosis (DVT) in pregnancy (see p.424).

Carpal tunnel syndrome

Some of my patients become alarmed because their fingers sometimes feel tingly, as if they had pins and needles in them. Occasionally, they might even feel a little numb or weak, as if they have lost sensation. This common ailment is caused by fluid retention, which swells the band of tissue (carpal tunnel) at your wrist and puts pressure on the nerves and ligaments that lie in this tunnel, before they enter your hand. The symptoms will disappear after the birth of your baby, as you get rid of all the excess water that you have accumulated. In the meantime, if you become seriously uncomfortable, your doctor will refer you to a physiotherapist, who will prescribe a splint to support your wrist. You could also try sleeping with the affected arm propped up on a pillow, to help drain the excess fluid from your arm. Remember that diuretic drugs to get rid of excess body fluid should not be used in pregnancy (see p.35).

Things to consider

You can tell your employer when you plan to start maternity leave. You should also have filled in a Mat B1 form (available from your midwife from week 20). This enables you to qualify for maternity pay or allowance and leave (see pp.58–63). Your partner should tell his employer now in order to qualify for paternity leave (see p.61).

You can start your maternity leave 11 weeks before your expected delivery date but you may be hoping to carry on working for as long as you can to maximize your paid maternity leave after your baby is born. However, if you need to stop work for medical reasons within four weeks of your EDD, even for one day, you are obliged to start your maternity leave from that point onwards.

If you work in an office where certain styles of clothes are not permitted or are frowned upon, clothes can be a major issue now. Although anyone who sees you will probably instantly realize you are pregnant, you may be anxious to ensure that you look professional. If slipping into comfy leggings and baggy T-shirts is not an option, then you will have to struggle on with wearing a jacket or similarly business-like attire for as long as you can bear it. So do make sure that you borrow or buy a few outfits that will fit the bill.

If you are heavily pregnant during the summer, it may be quite difficult to find clothes that can keep you both cool and decent. You feel like a furnace for much of the time and if it is high summer or you are living in a hot climate, you may feel unbearably hot, puffy, and sweaty. Heat rashes form in all sorts of recesses of your body (under your arms, under your breasts, between your legs). Added to which, if your feet and hands have swollen, shoes start to pinch, and finger rings may become so tight and uncomfortable that they are impossible to wear. There is not much you can do about this, other than avoiding situations where you will feel particularly hot, such as overcrowded restaurants or stuffy cinemas, and wearing loose, light clothes made of natural fibres such as cotton.

Starting antenatal classes

You will probably be starting your antenatal classes now – most hospital-run classes have start dates every four weeks and recommend women start their course between 30 and 32 weeks. Monthly start dates are also the norm for most other forms of antenatal classes. If you do have a choice of when to start, always opt for the earlier date since you never know what might happen. You need to make sure that you will have the chance to attend the all-important sessions on labour and pain relief, before you are forced to find out all about it at first hand in the delivery room. For exactly the same reason, you want to avoid missing the formal visit to the labour ward, if you have not already been shown around it. This is especially important if this is your first birth; if you are expecting twins (50 per cent of twins are delivered before 35 weeks); or if you have had a previous premature delivery.

Your partner may not want to attend all of the classes, but make sure that he at least knows when the special session for fathers is and encourage him to attend this one. It is far better that he has prior warning about the role you would like him to play, rather than leaving him to find out for himself during your labour.

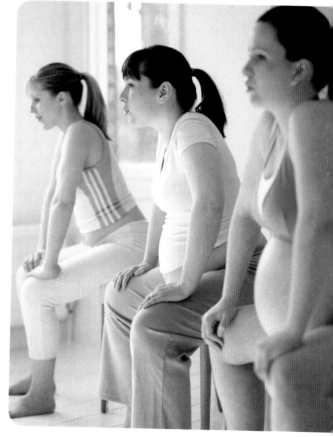

PREPARING FOR BIRTH Breathing and relaxation classes will help to focus your attention on and prepare you for the next stage – your baby's birth.

Your sex life

A couple's sex life is often revitalized in this period of pregnancy since most women are feeling well both physically and emotionally. You may be conscious of the fact that time is running out before the birth of your baby, with the inevitable disruption that this will bring to your night's sleep and, as a result, to your sex life. Tiny babies are not very considerate about their parents' need for intimate times together alone. The only thing that may hinder your sex life at this stage is niggling doubts, so let me deal with a few of them.

• Although rarely discussed, the fact that you may feel the baby moving inside you while you are making love can make you feel inhibited, or it can make you laugh. Although the sensation may be disturbing, it is certainly not a sign that your baby is in any way upset by your lovemaking.

• You may both be worried that you will harm your baby by having penetrative sex or concerned that sex could trigger labour inadvertently since your partner's semen contains prostaglandin (a hormone that is given to women to induce labour). In addition, orgasm causes the uterus to contract.

The reality is that no amount of sexual activity will harm your unborn child or trigger labour in a normal pregnancy, so you can continue an active sex life unless you have been told to stop because of a potential problem or pregnancy complication. Examples include a previous premature delivery or a risk factor for premature labour such as a short or slightly dilated cervix (see p.188); threatened premature labour (see p.340); recent bleeding and/or a very low-lying placenta (see placenta praevia, p.240 and p.428); and ruptured membranes.

Disturbing dreams

On a totally different note, many women report that they experience strange dreams during late pregnancy. They may be sexually explicit dreams or disturbing dreams involving death or illness of babies and children. Both types are common and can cause great anxiety, since you will undoubtedly start to wonder about their meaning. So I think it is important for me to reassure you here that they are not an omen of awful things to come. Like all our good and bad dreams (most of which we do not remember because we do not wake through the dream phase of our sleep) they are a method of coping with our day-to-day concerns and fears. Think of them as a way of sifting through any negative emotions without having to experience them in reality. One of the reasons why these dreams seem more common during the last trimester is that you wake much more often (either because you need to go to the lavatory or because you are uncomfortable) and so are more likely to recall them.

Disturbing dreams are a way of sifting through any negative emotions without having to experience them in reality.

DIET AND EXERCISE

In the third trimester, eating nourishing food and maintaining your fitness has a dual purpose. Both will help reduce fatigue and boost your wellbeing as you enter the last stretch of pregnancy and begin to build your strength for the birth.

GOOD EATING

Your diet is less crucial to your baby's wellbeing than in the first trimester, and unless you are surviving on a diet of chips and canned drinks, your baby is likely to be getting everything it needs.

▶ **Your weight gain should be** around 0.5–1kg (1–2lb) per week during the final three months (see p.42) although it may be minimal in the final weeks.

▶ **Your daily calorie intake** in the third trimester should increase by only 200 calories, which is not very much at all. An extra healthy snack, such as an apple or an orange, each day will supply all you need.

▶ **You may need to eat more frequently** during the last few weeks simply because you feel the need to stoke up regularly. Your body is most likely laying down some final, extra stores in preparation for labour, so choose foods that are nutritious and which will give you vital energy. Since you never know when you will go into labour, the better your diet in the weeks ahead, the better your ability to cope physically with the demands on the day.

▶ **Keep up your fluid intake** (at least eight glasses a day) to ensure that your body is fully hydrated; this will give you more energy.

▶ **Avoid drinking alcohol** as there is no known safe level of alcohol use in pregnancy. An excessive intake can cause fetal alcohol syndrome (see p.435). Smoking starves the placenta – and consequently your baby – of oxygen.

FIT FOR LABOUR

There is no reason why you should not continue to exercise until the day you deliver, unless your doctor has specifically told you to stop.

▶ **Certain activities will now be difficult or uncomfortable** so the chances are that you will have given up white-water rafting, horse riding, and energetic runs.

▶ **If you are used to a particular sport**, you may be able to continue for a little longer, albeit at a gentler pace, provided you feel well and your doctor gives you the all clear (although I'm sure you will know yourself when things are becoming more than you can manage).

▶ **If you haven't tried swimming, pregnancy yoga or exercise classes yet**, try to find time to do so soon. You will be surprised by how good they make you feel.

▶ **Whatever your chosen method of exercise**, make sure that you are doing your pelvic floor exercises regularly (see p.165) and paying attention to your posture.

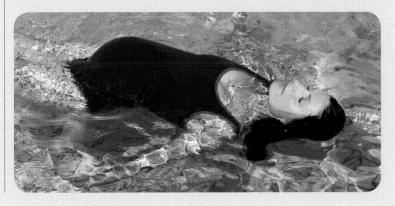

SHOPPING FOR YOUR BABY

There are no fixed rules about what to buy for your baby, but from my own experience and that of the many pregnant women I have talked to over the years, there are certain items that are more essential than others. Broadly speaking, there are two main areas to think about when choosing what you need for your baby's first few months: clothes and equipment.

Choosing baby clothes

Young babies cannot regulate their temperature very well, so they need to be kept well covered during the early weeks, but not so much that they start to overheat. The general rule of thumb is that, for the first two months, babies need one more layer than you yourself would wear on any given day (although this varies depending on the time of year and on the baby, as some feel the cold more than others). Remember also, babies have little or no hair, so on cooler days they will need to wear a bonnet or hat outdoors (never indoors), and if it is sunny, they must have a hat that protects their head, neck, and face.

Comfort, practicality, and ease of washing are the main criteria when choosing baby clothes. Look for clothes that do not restrict your baby's movements; that can be put on and taken off easily without causing your baby distress; that do not have fiddly bows, ribbons, and lace for him catch his fingers in; and that allow his skin to breathe. Babies grow so fast that clothes for newborns may only last a couple of weeks and, if you and your partner are taller than average, you may even have a baby who at birth is already wearing clothes for older infants. So, apart from two or three all-in-one stretch suits for newborns, I would advise you to go straight for the next size up when choosing your baby's clothes. Don't shy away from borrowing newborn clothes if they are offered – they get very little use and can be handed back within a month of the birth.

Make sure that the clothes you buy are made of a breathable fabric that can be machine washed at

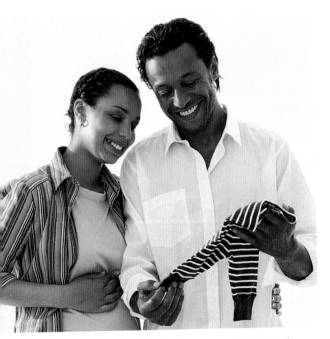

THE RIGHT SIZE Most babies grow so fast they only wear newborn-sized clothes for a matter of weeks.

a reasonable temperature (minimum 40°C/104°F) and tumble-dried if you want to dry them that way. Cotton is the best fabric for breathability, comfort, and ease of washing; synthetic-only fabrics are less suitable, particularly in the early weeks. Wool is good in winter, but it can be irritating worn next to a baby's delicate skin. Make sure all-in-one suits are quick and easy to undo – in the early months, you will be changing at least 10 nappies in a 24-hour period. Go for the styles that have popper fastenings around the bottom to ensure that your baby is not put through the unnecessary contortions of taking the whole garment off every time he needs a new nappy. All-in-one suits without feet have the advantage that they will not cramp your baby's toes as he grows.

If you are having an autumn or winter baby, he will need some warm outerwear, too. All-in-one suits, with integral hoods and booties are ideal. Pay attention to the outer fabric and inner lining, as some suits are warmer than others. Your baby will also need a warm hat (babies can lose most of their body heat very quickly from an uncovered head), and several pairs of mittens and booties to keep his hands and feet warm. Young babies can be relied upon to lose these items regularly by pulling or kicking them off. You will find countless varieties of shoes for babies in shops – all of them unnecessary and potentially harmful if they cramp your baby's toes. Your baby will only need shoes (properly fitted in a children's shoe department) when he begins to walk outside.

Most importantly, remember that you will be given many clothes as presents so try not to buy too much now. Your newborn can only use a few outfits per day, even if he is the sort who throws up after every feed. Before you can blink, they will no longer fit, which is why it is much better to top up on missing items at leisure later on.

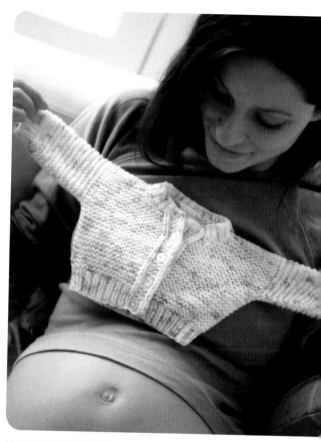

NATURAL FIBRES Clothes made of cotton and wool allow your baby's skin to breathe.

ESSENTIAL BABY CLOTHES

▶ Six cotton vests with wide (envelope) necks
▶ Six all-in-one suits
▶ Two cardigans (fleece-backed cotton or wool for winter, lighter cotton for warmer days)
▶ Two pairs of socks or soft cotton booties
▶ One shawl or cotton blanket
▶ One bonnet or sunhat, which shades eyes and neck
▶ One outdoor coat, including hood and booties, or one all-in-one outdoor suit, depending on season
▶ One pair of mittens, depending on season

CHOOSING A PRAM

I cannot recommend a particular pram or buggy (it would be out of date before you had finished reading this section), but I can offer a few points to keep in mind when you are choosing transport for your newborn:

▶ For the first few months, your baby's spine needs proper support and he will need to be able to lie totally flat. Any pram or pushchair that does not have a flat position should be rejected. If you buy a travel system, you can use the car seat clipped onto the pushchair, but only for short trips.

▶ Think about where you live. Some of the raciest pushchairs have a very long chassis and big wheels – ideal for cross-country jogging but hard to manoeuvre up and down steps and in shops and on busy streets.

▶ For winter babies, look for a pram that is well insulated and offers protection from the elements.

▶ Whatever time of year you give birth, you will need to have a rain hood, and if you are having your baby in spring or summer, you will also need a sunshade.

▶ Do make sure that the folded-down pram or pushchair fits inside your car boot and the car seat fits in your car. Most baby shops and departments will let you try them out before you buy them.

Buying baby equipment

When you become pregnant for the first time, you discover a whole new world of products aimed at mothers, parents, and children. If you have had little contact with babies up until now, you might be astonished at the variety of what is on offer and even if this is not your first child, you may be surprised to see items in the shops this time round that were not around as little as 18 months ago. Be in no doubt, many of these so-called essential products are conceived by the fertile imaginations of those who work in the baby and childcare industries, aided and abetted by all kinds of marketing wizardry.

Go to any babycare section in a department store or leaf through any mother and baby mail-order catalogue and you are suddenly confronted with everything from endless varieties of prams and buggies – with horrifying price tags to match – to a plethora of little gadgets, which may or not be of any use. After all, you ask yourself, how important is an in-car bottle and jar warmer? While there is no denying that many products are genuinely helpful and make our lives easier, it can be very difficult if you are a first-time parent to distinguish between what is a true must-have and what is a nice but entirely optional extra.

Prams and pushchairs

The choice of pram or pushchair is probably the most important and costly item. Technically, a pram is a carrycot on a chassis that can then be taken off and used for the baby to sleep in at night because it has sufficient depth to accommodate a mattress. A pushchair may allow the baby to lie completely flat but it cannot be used for him to sleep in at night because it cannot be taken off the chassis and, crucially, it lacks the depth to accommodate a mattress.

Whether you go to a specialist baby shop or a department store, the sales assistant is likely to blind you with science as he or she demonstrates how all the various models work. Before you know it, like a child's transformer toy, travel systems, prams, and pushchairs are being clicked up and down, folded or taken apart to become forward and back facing pushchairs, carrycots, car seats ,and more besides. Some of the new generation of prams and pushchairs now have four-wheel drive and larger wheels allowing you to jog with your baby across the most rugged terrain.

As with all aspects of buying equipment, speak to as many people as you can who have recently had babies, as their advice will be unbiased and they can explain the pros and cons before you even begin to look round the shops. You will then have a clearer idea of what you are looking for and what your main criteria are.

If the price tags of prams is alarming (and they often are) grandparents-to-be might like to contribute; alternatively, consider borrowing one from a friend or relative, or buying second-hand. Because of the high price and high turnover of nursery equipment, there is a thriving second-hand market in all these goods.

A baby sling is a useful and inexpensive addition to having a pram or pushchair. It allows you to keep your baby close to you (with the bonus that he may well sleep very peacefully through any trips) and to have both hands free. It also saves the bother of hauling your pram around in and out of shops and people's houses. Slings range from traditional hammocks that lie across the body to high-tech sporty models with adjustable straps and back supports. Whichever one you choose make sure it supports your newborn baby's head. Try the sling on before you buy it to make sure that you can put the baby in it and fasten it by yourself.

Car seats

The other essential item you will need is a car seat: in fact, if you give birth in hospital, you will not be allowed to leave unless you have one properly installed in your car. Some are part of a travel system – a suite of items that attach to a pushchair base; or can be lifted out of the car and used as a babyseat. Many car seats for newborns are designed to last only around six months, so this is an item that you could

consider borrowing from a friend if you know its history. If you buy a second-hand seat, check that it has not been involved in a serious accident, because there is a risk that it may no longer be safe as a result.

BABY SLING The most comfortable slings have wide straps that support your back and shoulders and a well-placed head support for your baby.

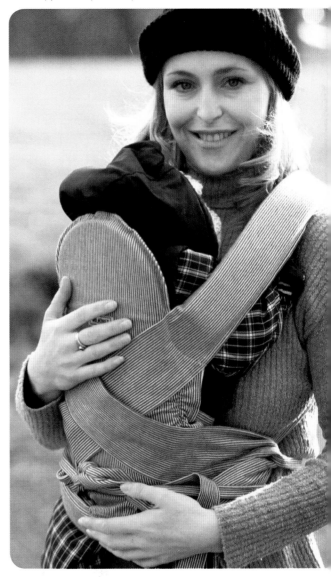

Cribs and cots

What will your baby sleep in at home? There are various options, from carrycots, Moses baskets and cribs to proper cots. Essentially, all options are fine from the start and, to be honest, many babies spend their first few weeks in rather less customized beds and are none the worse for it. The important thing is to buy a new mattress. A few years ago, there was a cot death scare that suggested a link between old mattresses and an increased risk of Sudden Infant Death Syndrome (cot death). This theory has now been discredited, but there is still a good reason for buying a new mattress: a second-hand one will have an indentation from the previous baby and will not give your newborn good support for his spine. Some parents keep their babies in carrycots and Moses baskets during the day, then transfer them to a cot at night, with the idea that the baby will gradually recognize that the latter is specifically for a long sleep at night. This is certainly worth a try, although it may make little difference before the baby is around three months old, by which time, he will have outgrown carrycots and Moses baskets anyway. Babies move more freely and sleep better in a proper cot from the start, so there is really no need to invest heavily in the other options as you will soon be dispensing with them.

As far as bedding is concerned, cotton is best, especially as it is important not to let your baby overheat by piling on layers of woollen blankets. You can check if your baby feels cold by feeling the nape of his neck: if it feels warm, then he is fine. For each type of bed, you will need a minimum of two cellular blankets, two fitted sheets and two top sheets. Babies should not have pillows, because their heads need to lie flat on the mattress. Even though cot bumpers, quilts, and duvets are widely available in shops they are not recommended for small babies because they may move over the baby's head and hinder breathing.

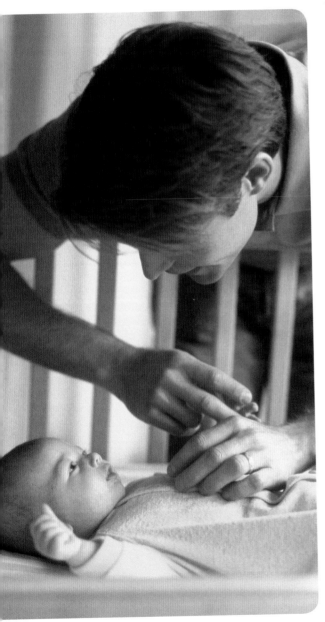

COT SAFETY Your baby is safest with his feet near the base of the cot so he cannot slip down under the blankets.

Nappy-changing and feeding equipment

Regarding smaller items of baby equipment, you will need a plastic-covered changing mat and a plastic bucket or bin (with a lid) in which to put disposable or terry towelling nappies. Nappy disposal units store used disposable nappies in a sealed, fragranced container until you are ready to empty them. This is hardly an essential item but it reduces the amount of times you have to empty your bin and avoids unpleasant smells. A baby bath can make bath time easier on your back and nerves as you struggle with a small, slippery baby.

If you plan to use terry towelling squares, which are more environmentally friendly, you will need to buy at least 30 of them to cater for as many as 10 nappy changes a day, together with plastic pants, pins, and nappy liners. They may appear to cost less than disposables but you need to take into account the fact that they need laundering either by you (make sure you have a good washing machine and dryer) or by a nappy laundering service (this latter option works out at roughly the same cost as using disposables). The more modern-shaped re-usable nappies are fully washable and tend to fit better than terry nappies, because they come in different sizes, although all types require a nappy liner (and plastic pants to protect clothes from soiling). You will find more information about the baby products you may want to buy closer to your delivery date on pages 224–7.

Feeding equipment

If you plan to bottle-feed from the start, you will need at least six bottles, as you will be feeding your baby up to seven or eight feeds per day (or at least making up that many feeds).

If you plan to breastfeed, you should still buy two or three bottles so you will be prepared if or whenever you decide to start using bottles. Remember that babies can take your expressed milk, as well as formula milk, from a bottle so it is as well to be organized. Buy slow-flowing teats, otherwise your baby will struggle to swallow fast enough.

You will need to sterilize bottles until your baby is six months old using one of the following:
• A sterilizing tank uses water and sterilizing agent in tablet or liquid form. Bottles and teats have to be submerged for several hours.
• The newer electric or microwave steamers use steam to sterilize bottles and teats within a matter of minutes. Most kits are sold with bottles.

These are the essential items to have ready before your baby's birth, but by all means go out and buy whatever seems useful afterwards. The early weeks and months are all about making life easier and, within reason, you should look for anything that helps you to do just that.

ESSENTIAL EQUIPMENT

▶ Pram or pushchair that allows baby to lie flat
▶ Rain hood
▶ Carrycot or Moses basket, or a cot (or both options) with new mattresses
▶ Cotton bed-clothes, including, for each size of bed:
  Two fitted sheets
  Two top sheets
  Two cellular blankets
▶ Rear-facing car seat
▶ Plastic changing mat and plastic bucket (with lid)
▶ Bottles (six if bottle-feeding, two if breastfeeding) plus slow-flow teats.
▶ Sterilizing equipment
▶ Baby sling with good head support

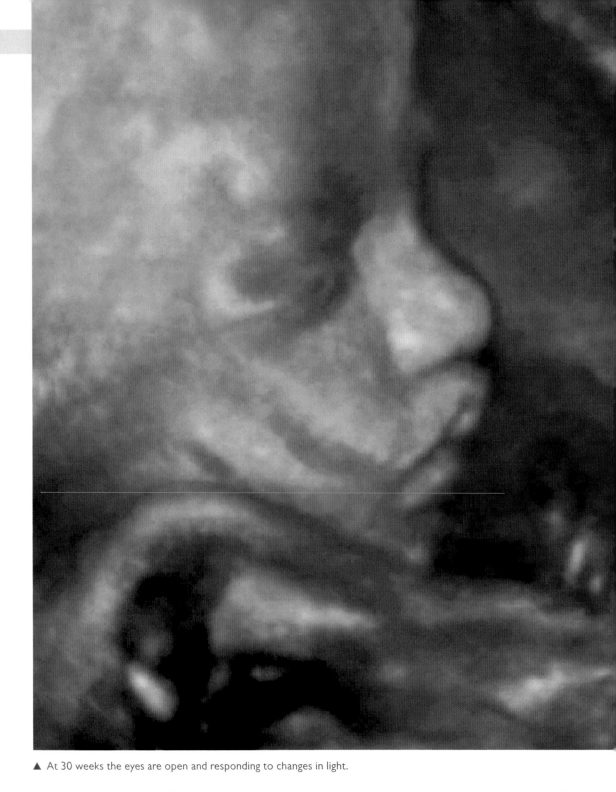

▲ At 30 weeks the eyes are open and responding to changes in light.

▶ **WEEKS 30–35**
The developing baby

YOUR BABY IS CONTINUING TO GROW IN LENGTH, but the really noticeable difference is in your baby's weight. The layer of subcutaneous fat is increasing and the skin now looks pink and less wrinkled, especially in the face, which now looks smooth and chubby.

From 28 to 32 weeks, the weekly weight gain is as much as 500g (17oz) and continues at a rate of about 250g (9oz) per week between 32 and 35 weeks, which means that the average baby weighs 2.5kg (or 5½lb) at 35 weeks. A baby born around this time will still look a little on the lean side but will no longer have the wrinkly, red, emaciated look of a few weeks ago. The surface coating of white waxy vernix will be very thick, but the lanugo hair is fast disappearing and will probably be present only in patches on the shoulders and back. If delivered now, your baby will be less in need of these protective mechanisms to combat the cold since its control of body temperature is becoming much more reliable.

Your baby's eyes are opening and closing now, blinking and learning to focus, since the pupils are able to contract and dilate in response to differences in light filtering through the wall of the uterus. The brain and nervous system are also fully developed, although some of the reflexes and limb movements will still be poorly co-ordinated if the baby is born now. The fingernails extend to the end of the fingertips, but the toenails will need a few more weeks to reach the end of the toes.

The sucking reflex becomes properly established at this stage and the baby will be repeatedly sucking on his thumbs and fingers. However, most babies born before 35 or 36 weeks still need a little more practice, which can mean that breastfeeding is more difficult to establish. This is one of the reasons why the definition of a premature baby is still, strictly speaking, a baby born before 37 weeks. Although most babies born after 28 weeks have an excellent chance of survival, thanks to the special care they receive after the birth, there is no technical advance that can make a premature baby suck as effectively as a full-term baby. So if your baby is born at or before 35 weeks, you will probably need some specialist help from midwives and breastfeeding counsellors.

not life size

By 30 weeks, the fetus is about 28cm (11in) long and weighs about 1–1.5kg (2¼–3⅓lb). At 35 weeks, its weight has increased to about 2.5kg (5½lb) and the fetus now measures 32cm (13in) from crown to rump and as much as 45cm (18in) from head to toe.

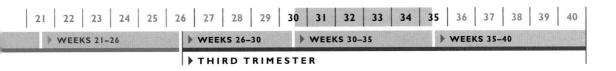

| 21 | 22 | 23 | 24 | 25 | 26 | 27 | 28 | 29 | **30** | **31** | **32** | **33** | **34** | **35** | 36 | 37 | 38 | 39 | 40 |

▶ **WEEKS 21–26**   ▶ **WEEKS 26–30**   ▶ **WEEKS 30–35**   ▶ **WEEKS 35–40**

▶ **THIRD TRIMESTER**

The lungs are maturing so fast between 30 and 35 weeks that every day that passes reduces the time that your baby is likely to need assistance to breathe. In practical terms, a baby born at 34 weeks may need some help in breathing, for days or even weeks, whereas one born at 36 weeks is almost always able to breathe unaided. In these next few weeks, your baby crosses the divide; its lungs undergo the final steps of maturation that allow them to function independently.

The fetal adrenal glands, on the top of the kidneys, are pumping out cortisol to help stimulate the production of surfactant in the fetal lungs. They are working so hard that they are the same size as the adrenal glands of an adolescent and are producing 10 times the quantity of cortisol as those of an adult. Soon after your baby is born they will shrink back down and only become active again at puberty.

Sex hormones

In boys and girls, the fetal adrenal glands continue to produce large quantities of an androgen-like hormone (DHEAS), which has to be processed by enzymes in the fetal liver before it can be passed on to the placenta for final conversion to oestrogen. In boys, the fetal testes are producing testosterone and some of this is converted by special target cells in the genitals to another male hormone that is essential for the development of the external genitals. It is quite common for these high levels of hormones to result in the external genitals of both boys and girls appearing large and swollen at birth. In the case of boys, the scrotal skin that surrounds the testes can be darkly pigmented. All of these changes disappear in the next few weeks as hormone production settles down.

3-D ULTRASOUND AT 30–35 WEEKS ··

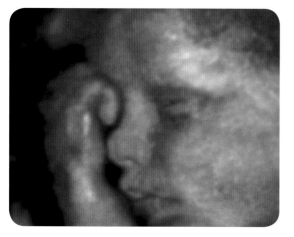

REFLECTIVE Images of a perfectly formed face begin to reveal a suggestion of the personality within.

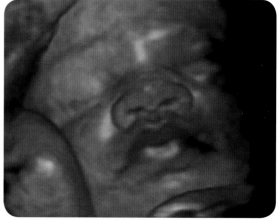

SLEEP PERIODS Movement is now restricted by space and, during quiet periods, the baby sleeps.

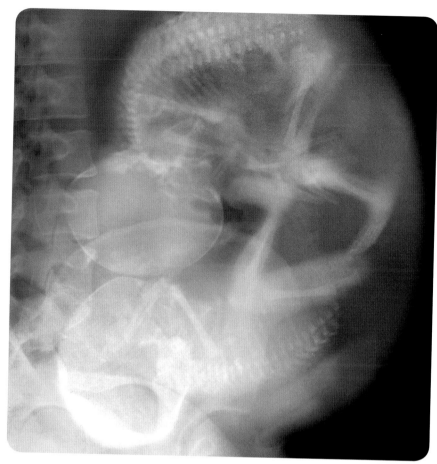

TWIN PREGNANCY An X-ray of a twin pregnancy reveals both babies lying transversely across the abdomen with both heads close to the mother's spine. Unless they change position, this will cause problems in normal labour and vaginal delivery. A Caesarean section is the most likely option to deliver the babies safely.

Movements and lie

Your baby's movements will be strong but most probably slower than before for the simple reason that your baby can no longer move around so freely because space inside the uterus is now at a premium. However, if your baby's movement pattern changes from being very active to very quiet, or vice versa, seek advice urgently. Mothers-to-be are usually the best judge of whether problems in utero are brewing and you should never be worried that you are bothering people unnecessarily. It really does not matter how many false alarms there are.

Most babies are lying longitudinally (vertically) by week 35, but there are situations in which the baby may be transverse (horizontal) or oblique (diagonal). The risk of an abnormal lie is increased when the amniotic fluid level is high (see polyhydramnios, p.427); when the placenta is in the lower segment of the uterus (see placenta praevia, p.240 and p.428); or when there is more than one baby.

Your baby's presentation is determined by which part of the baby is closest to your pelvis: head down is described as a cephalic presentation while bottom down (and head up) is called a breech presentation (see p.269). Cephalic is the most common presentation and by term, 95 per cent babies are in this position. At 32 weeks, as many as 25 per cent of babies are breech, but this percentage has dropped to just 4 per cent by 38 weeks. After 35–36 weeks the baby is much less likely to change presentation because the lack of space prevents major movements.

The amniotic fluid

Your baby excretes about half a litre (16fl oz) of urine daily and at 35 weeks the amniotic fluid reaches a peak volume of 1 litre (1¾ pints). After this time the volume starts to decline and can be as little as 100–200ml (3½–7fl oz) in a pregnancy that is post mature (overdue). Low levels of amniotic fluid (see oligohydramnios, p.427) can be a sign of a growth-restricted baby or a baby with kidney problems, while excessive amniotic fluid, or polyhydramnios (see p.427), may be seen in twin pregnancies and is sometimes associated with physical abnormalities in the baby or diabetes in the mother.

FLUID LEVELS

Levels of amniotic fluid increase rapidly from mid-pregnancy onwards reaching a peak at 40 weeks. After 40 weeks the fluid level needs to be checked regularly to ensure that the post-mature baby is not put at risk due to a decline in fluid.

Your changing body

Now and for the next few weeks, the height of the fundus measured in centimetres will be about the same as the stage of your pregnancy in weeks. This changes slightly when the baby's head descends and causes the height of the fundus to drop slightly in most pregnancies.

Whatever the exact measurements at this stage, your uterus has expanded your abdomen so much that your belly button may have become inverted, giving it quite a prominent appearance. If this coincides with summertime and light clothing, it is often clearly visible through your clothes. Its change in appearance is not permanent; it will pop back into place once your baby is born.

Your blood volume will probably reach a peak of 5 litres (8¾ pints), although some women will have a further increase between 35 and 40 weeks. Most of the increase is due to the plasma or fluid content in your bloodstream, but the number of oxygen-carrying red cells does not increase at the same rate. This dilution of red cells by the increasing plasma fluid is a common cause of anaemia in late pregnancy (known as dilutional anaemia). Certainly, your blood count will be checked during this stage of pregnancy. However, only rarely is there a serious problem as a result of lack of red blood cells, because the amount of haemoglobin (oxygen-carrying pigment) is now much higher than before you became pregnant. Rest assured that your baby is happily creaming off all the oxygen and nutrients it needs.

Varicose veins

If you are going to be troubled by varicose veins, this is the stage in pregnancy when you are most likely to notice them. Varicose veins are dilated veins just under the surface of the skin, most of which occur in the legs and anal region (see haemorrhoids, p.217). Wherever they pop up in pregnancy, they are caused by an unavoidable mechanical problem – the weight of your enlarging uterus pressing down on the main veins in your pelvis. These veins feed blood back to your heart and lungs, but they are now very dilated by your increased blood volume. When they meet a large obstacle in their path, such as your expanded uterus, the back pressure that develops forces your blood to pool in the dependent (smaller) veins in your legs, vulva, and anal margin. Since your baby is going to get bigger over the next few weeks the discomfort from varicose veins is likely to get worse. Symptoms usually improve after the delivery of your baby, but for some women varicose veins become a long-term problem.

Varicose veins in the vulval area are not as common, but they are often a cause of concern because they look unsightly and can become tender and uncomfortable. The symptoms are best treated in the same way as haemorrhoids. Although there is the potential for vulval varices to bleed heavily if damaged at the time of a vaginal delivery, this is only very rarely a problem. Furthermore, they usually disappear completely after the birth.

TIPS FOR DEALING WITH VARICOSE VEINS

▶ **Buy some good support tights.** For maximum relief, put them on in the morning before you get out of bed.

▶ **Rest with your feet up** as high as possible whenever you can. This will help blood to drain from the veins in your legs.

▶ **Walk briskly.** This will keep the muscle pumps in your legs working and help return the blood to your heart.

▶ **If you have to stand** for any period of time, keep shifting your body weight from one leg to another, instead of distributing it equally between both.

▶ **Keep a check on your weight gain.** Carrying extra pounds puts even more pressure on your legs.

How you may feel physically

It is very common for women to feel uncomfortably large and unwieldy at this stage of pregnancy, particularly if it happens to coincide with the summer months when heat increases the risk of developing swollen hands, feet, and legs.

Even if you do not feel like the proverbial beached whale, you may well be moving around more slowly and laboriously than you normally do. Day-to-day tasks such as getting out of the car or putting on a pair of socks or tights require a radical alteration of your usual technique. Although none of us likes to feel physically compromised and dependent on others for help, the best way to deal with these situations is to see the funny side and keep reminding yourself that this is temporary. If you are philosophical about your restricted movement now, it will also help to prepare you for the fact that young children will inevitably slow you down. After the birth, you will no longer be able to shoot out of the house in three seconds flat, grabbing your car keys and bag as you go. You will just have to take things a step slower. Do try, though, to stay as active as possible during this last stage of your pregnancy – it will help you to feel physically and mentally prepared for the challenges ahead of you, particularly labour.

FINDING A POSITION
You may be most comfortable lying on your side with cushions supporting your bump and upper leg.

Hard to sleep

By now, you may not be sleeping well and this will affect how you are feeling physically during the day. It becomes increasingly difficult to find a comfortable position at night. Lying on your back needs to be avoided, because the weight of your uterus will press on the major veins returning blood to your heart, making you feel very faint and reducing the blood supply to your baby. The possibility of lying on your front disappeared some weeks ago, and it is likely that your only practical option now is to lie on your side, with your upper leg bent forwards at the knee and, if necessary, supported by a pillow. However, you cannot stay in the same position all night,

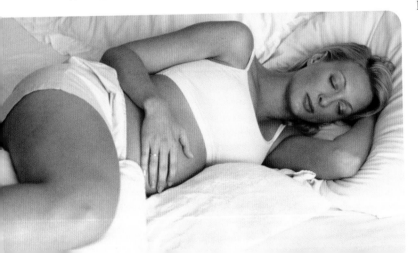

MOVING SAFELY

Getting up from the floor or bed after relaxation or exercise can put strain on your abdominal muscles, which are already stretched to full capacity. Your altered centre of gravity will also be making large-scale movements difficult.

The following technique has been devised by yoga teachers to help you get to your feet safely. As with any strenuous manoeuvres at this stage of pregnancy, move slowly and remember to breathe throughout.

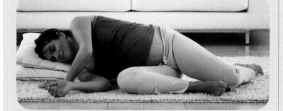

Step one With your knees bent, roll on to your right side bringing your the knee beneath you up to waist level. Keep your left hand aligned with your bent knee.

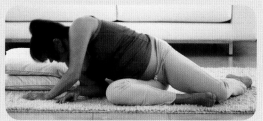

Step two Shift your weight on to your left hand and knee. Position your right knee under your right hip and your right hand under your shoulder and come up slowly on all fours.

and as you near term, turning over in bed becomes a major operation, involving shifting your increasing bulk, not to mention all the supportive pillows around the bed. Added to which, your bladder is giving you regular wake-up calls and your baby may be continually kicking and wriggling.

This poor-quality sleep can make you extremely tired and irritable, which is why it is so important to try to find time to rest during the day. Even if you are still working full time, ensure that you reserve half an hour per day to sit down with your feet up. If you are at home, an hour's nap on your bed after lunch will really help to make up for poor sleep at night. If you establish a routine in which you break off from your tasks to rest during this antenatal period, it will be easier to continue after the birth when tiredness and lack of sleep are inevitable. You are going to need to train yourself to take advantage of the times when your newborn is sleeping to catch up on some rest or sleep for yourself and restore your energy and sanity.

Braxton Hicks' contractions

From now until the end of your pregnancy the uterus starts to practise contracting mildly in preparation for labour. These painless tightenings, called Braxton Hicks' contractions, start at the top of the fundus and travel down the uterus causing it to harden for about 30 seconds. The 19th-century obstetrician John Braxton Hicks, from St Mary's Hospital, London, was the first to describe

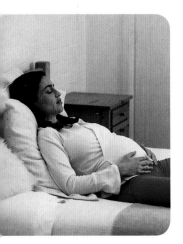

BREATHING Practising deep, slow breathing can help you get rid of tension and regain control between contractions.

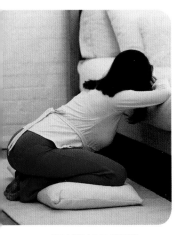

BEARING DOWN Exhaling with your knees wide apart and your head and elbows supported can help you to prepare for second-stage contractions.

them. He realized that this painless activity towards the end of pregnancy was because the uterus needed practice to contract strongly enough to expel a baby through the birth canal and into the outside world. The contractions also help to direct more blood into the placenta during the last few weeks of pregnancy.

Although some women are completely unaware of having Braxton Hicks' contractions, for others they can become quite strong and uncomfortable towards the end of pregnancy. If this is the case for you, try changing your position, getting up and walking around, or having a warm bath, since all these simple remedies can help to relax the uterine muscles. Practising some of the relaxation and breathing techniques you are learning for labour is also likely to be of benefit, as may be getting your partner to give you a back massage.

If this is your first pregnancy, it may be difficult for you to know whether you are having strong Braxton Hicks' contractions or early labour pains so the rule here is that if you are not sure, go straight to your midwife or nearest labour ward and ask for help. Similarly, it is essential to report any prolonged or painful uterine activity immediately, particularly if it is accompanied by lower backache, since you may be threatening to go into premature labour. As a mother of premature twins who spent a month in special care after delivery, I can assure you that this is a frightening and distressing experience for every parent, so do make sure that you take every precaution to avoid delivering prematurely. Another possible cause of uterine pain and low backache is a placental abruption (see p.428), which needs urgent investigation.

Your emotional response

Top of the list of anxieties that patients share with me at this stage is the fear that their labour will be difficult, that it may go disastrously wrong, or that they will disgrace themselves during the delivery (see Q&A opposite).

As always, the fear of the unknown is far more difficult to deal with than the reality. So once again, try to discard any horror stories that you have been party to and hold on to the fact that most pregnant women are extremely healthy and their babies have a trouble-free entrance into this world.

Another common feature of late pregnancy is that women often find it hard to concentrate on specific tasks. Many of my patients tell me that their minds repeatedly wander off to baby-related issues and for those of you who are still at work, this can be quite a problem. It may come as a bit of a shock to find yourself dreaming the days away and unable to focus on the job in hand. Tasks that used to demand high priority may no longer seem very important and pressing. I think the best way to manage this situation is to try to identify the key tasks and ensure that they are finished, sideline non-essential jobs and make sure that you do not take on anything new that is challenging or unlikely to be accomplished within a short time span. You should then be able to leave work comfortable in the knowledge that you have left things in a reasonable state.

Another feature of this last trimester is that sad or bad news tends to affect you more than usual. There is no doubt that pregnancy triggers intense emotional responses in many of us and makes us much more vulnerable to sad situations, particularly those involving children. Watching a programme about any form of child deprivation or the loss of a child, for example, is likely to reduce you to floods of tears, even if in the past you were able to take such things in your stride. The only practical advice that I can offer here is to try to limit your exposure to situations that are likely to make you feel very distressed.

 EMBARRASSING SITUATIONS

Q&A

▶ **I hate feeling out of control. How can I avoid disgracing myself during labour?**
Nothing you do during your labour and delivery will be considered disgraceful. This will be one of the few times in your life when you cannot be totally in control of your own body so instead of feeling embarrassed and agitated, just accept it. As for anyone in the delivery room being horrified or disgusted by anything that happens, or upset by you groaning, swearing or shouting at them – forget it; the midwives and doctors have seen and heard it all before. They would not be doing the job that they have chosen to do if they did

not understand the practicalities of what happens when a 3.5-kg (7½-lb) baby is pushed through a woman's birth canal.

▶ **What if my waters break when I am in a public place?**
It is unlikely that your waters will break in the middle of the supermarket or other public place but even if they do – so what? I have never heard anyone complain about having to help a pregnant woman whose membranes ruptured unexpectedly. But I have heard lots of people talk about how pleased they were to be able to help when this entirely natural event occurred. The reality is that it is very rare for the amniotic fluid to gush out –

it is usually a trickle because most babies are head down, pressing on your cervix and preventing too much liquid from escaping.

▶ **I am worried that I might have a bowel movement during labour. Should I have an enema?**
Having a bowel movement in labour can happen because of the baby's descending head placing pressure on the rectum. However, it is unlikely that there will be much stool in front of your baby's descending head, so any problem is likely to be minimal. Compulsory enemas in early labour were routine practice years ago but are vanishingly rare in modern-day maternity units.

Your antenatal care

Your doctor or midwife will want to monitor you more closely towards the end of your pregnancy. Take advantage of their expertise to ask questions about any procedures or symptoms that worry you.

All the usual routine checks will be performed, but your carers will be especially alert to signs of late pregnancy complications such as gestational diabetes (see p.427) or slow growth of your baby (see intrauterine growth restriction, p.427). Pre-eclampsia (see p.426) becomes increasingly common after week 30. Although it may develop without symptoms there are usually some indicators. Any of the following should prompt you to see your doctor or midwife urgently to check for protein in your urine:

• Your finger rings are suddenly too tight and your feet too swollen for your shoes.

• Your face becomes puffy and swollen.

• Headaches have become constant or unbearable and you have flashes of light at the edge of your vision.

The height of your uterine fundus will be measured and if it is higher or lower than your dates suggest, you may be advised to have an ultrasound scan to check the size and wellbeing of your baby. If this shows that the baby is too small or too large for your dates, or that the liquor volume is increased or reduced, further investigations (see pp.256–9) will be arranged. It may even be necessary to make plans to induce early delivery of your baby.

 PLACENTA PRAEVIA

A placenta that remains low in the uterus causes problems if all or part of it is in front of the baby's head, overlapping or covering the internal part of the cervix (the cervical os). The first sign is often one or more episodes of painless bleeding, sometimes as early as 30 weeks, which needs to be assessed immediately in hospital. If only the lower edge of the placenta covers the cervix (minor placenta praevia), the baby's head may be able to pass through the dilated cervix, so a vaginal delivery may be possible. If the placenta is lying centrally over the cervix (major placenta praevia), there is a high risk of haemorrhage before or during labour. A Caesarean section is the only safe option (see p.428).

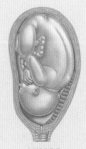

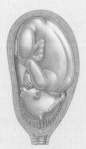

MINOR **MAJOR**

Palpating your abdomen will enable your carers to determine the position in which your baby is lying. If your baby is breech (bottom down) it still has time to turn around and adopt the cephalic (head down) position, which is the best position for a normal vaginal delivery. However, if the baby's position persists as breech, you may be advised to undergo external cephalic version (ECV), a manual procedure to turn the baby round in the uterus, which is usually performed after 37 weeks (see p.271). Do remember that even the most skilled doctors and midwives can get the position of your baby wrong. Any obstetrician who says that he or she has never missed a breech presentation is either untruthful or has not been doing the job for long enough to have it happen!

A full blood count is usually performed at either 28 or 32 weeks to check for anaemia (see p.424). The same blood sample will be used to check that you have not developed any unusual red blood cell antibodies that might cause problems at a later stage, should you require a blood transfusion, for example, if you bleed severely during the delivery (see p.425). If you are Rhesus negative (see p.128 and p.425) you will be given an anti-D injection and your blood will be checked to ensure that no rhesus antibodies have been produced.

A further ultrasound scan will be carried out at about 32–34 weeks if you were found to have a low-lying placenta earlier in your pregnancy. This is done to determine whether its position has changed. Even if the scan shows that your placenta is low, there are still several more weeks during which the lower segment of the uterus will continue to develop, so the chances of a low placenta causing problems at the time of delivery are reduced as the pregnancy becomes more advanced. The incidence of placenta praevia (see left) is only 1 in 200 at term, whereas before 32 weeks it can be as high as 20 per cent.

Diabetic pregnancies

All diabetic pregnancies will be under close surveillance from 35 weeks for late pregnancy problems (see p.408 and p.427). Poorly controlled glucose levels result in the baby being overweight (macrosomia), which increases the risk of shoulder dystocia (see p.430), birth injuries, and stillbirth. If your diabetes is well controlled and your baby's growth is normal, you may be able to wait for labour to begin and have a normal vaginal delivery. In uncomplicated diabetic pregnancies, there is no indication that an elective Caesarean section improves the outcome.

However, many maternity units have a policy of induction (see pp.294–7) for diabetic mothers at 38–39 weeks, using continuous fetal monitoring and regular checks on the mother's blood sugar levels throughout labour and delivery. This is because after 38 weeks, diabetic pregnancies are at increased risk of birth trauma, stillbirth, and neonatal complications. If fetal distress develops or

> Remember that even the most skilled doctors and midwives can get the position of your baby wrong.

there is poor progress in labour, an emergency Caesarean section is sometimes required. After birth, babies born to diabetic mothers are thoroughly assessed because they can develop hypoglycaemia (low blood sugar levels) during the first hours of life. They are also at increased risk of respiratory distress syndrome (see p.375), particularly if they are delivered prematurely.

Common concerns

Most of the physical ailments that you are likely to experience in late pregnancy are related to your increasing size and will probably persist until your baby is delivered. That said, if your baby's head engages in the pelvis during the last few weeks, you may have some relief from them.

If you have been troubled by backache, this may well get worse over the next few weeks.

If you are seriously troubled by breathlessness, try to cut down on unnecessary exertion while remaining reasonably active. Lying down flat often makes breathlessness worse, so you may find that you need to rest and sleep in a semi-propped-up position during the last trimester of pregnancy.

Palpitations

Missed heartbeats, a short run of fast heartbeats or just being acutely aware of your heartbeat (often loosely referred to as palpitations) are common in late pregnancy. Normally they are nothing to worry about and are simply the result of changes in your blood circulation coupled with the mechanical disadvantages of having a large mass in your abdominal cavity. However, if you develop chest pain or severe breathlessness with palpitations or if they are occurring more and more frequently, you should consult your midwife or doctor.

Severe itching

It is very common to develop patches of dry, flaky skin in late pregnancy, but some women suffer from a severe form of itching on their abdomen and especially on the palms of their hands and soles of their feet, which does not respond to the usual moisturizers. Occasionally this is the first sign that you are developing obstetric cholestasis (see p.425), which is a rare condition in pregnancy caused by bile salts being deposited under the skin. If it is severe, it can lead to maternal jaundice, liver failure, premature delivery, and even stillbirth so it is important to report severe, persistent itching to your antenatal carers, quickly.

Losing fluid

If you experience small gushes of fluid from your vagina when you make a sudden movement, it is most likely due to stress incontinence. However, at this stage of pregnancy, you should also consider the possibility that your membranes have ruptured (your waters have broken) and you are leaking amniotic fluid. If you are unsure, save a sample in a clean container and seek advice from your midwife or doctor. They may perform a speculum examination, by asking you to cough and testing any fluid that is visible in the vagina to determine whether it is amniotic fluid or urine. If your membranes have ruptured, both you and your baby are at risk of developing an infection so if there are no signs of uterine contractions developing within 24 hours of this occurring, most antenatal carers will suggest that you are induced (see pp.294–7) as long as you are at least 34 weeks pregnant.

Localized backache

If you have been troubled by backache, this may well get worse over the next few weeks. In addition to the generalized discomfort you have probably experienced up until now, you may well find that mild, generalized lower backache has been replaced by specific and clearly localized pain because specific disorders such as sciatica frequently develop towards the end of pregnancy (see below). Although back pain is common during pregnancy, it is important to take severe lower back pain seriously and seek advice from your midwife or doctor.

Sciatica is characterized by a sharp, constant or intermittent pain in the lower back or buttocks, which sometimes shoots down the back of one or both legs. The sciatic nerve is the largest nerve in the body and runs from the spinal cord, through the buttock and into the back of the leg. When it is crushed or compressed by your baby's head anywhere along its route, the sharp pain is frequently accompanied by numbness, tingling, weakness, and occasionally a burning sensation. If the pain or weakness becomes severe, you will need to see your doctor to rule out the possibility of a slipped disc.

Gentle manoeuvres to encourage the baby's head to change position and relieve the pressure on the sciatic nerve can be helpful, but this is sometimes easier said than done. Improving your general posture and performing regular pelvic tilt exercises will bring relief (see p.219) as will yoga and stretching exercises, such as lying down flat on a firm mattress and trying to lengthen your spine by raising your head on pillows or books.

Coccygeal pain is pain in the very lowest part of your spine and tenderness when you press into the natal cleft of your buttocks. The coccyx is a sort of hinged appendage made up of four tiny bones at the end of your sacrum (the

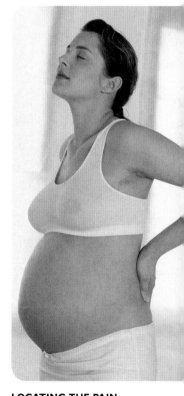

LOCATING THE PAIN
A severe pain in your lower back is likely to have a specific cause and needs appropriate treatment.

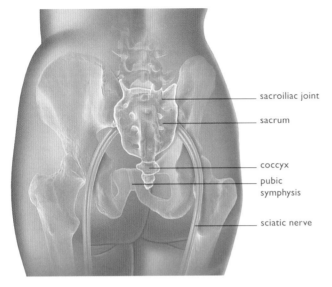

sacroiliac joint

sacrum

coccyx

pubic
symphysis

sciatic nerve

TROUBLE SPOTS
Localized back problems
are usually due to the
softening of ligaments
supporting the sacroiliac
joint, the pubic symphysis
joint between your pubic
bones or the coccyx. Pain
that radiates down one
leg may be due to the
baby's head pressing on
a sciatic nerve.

large triangular bone at the base of the spine).
Lax supporting ligaments can cause the coccyx
to become displaced from the sacrum during
late pregnancy and during delivery. A previous
bruising impact injury to the area, such as a
fall, often contributes to the problem. The pain
can be excruciating, particularly when sitting,
and if this is the case, try applying local heat
such as compresses and hot water bottles, or
taking a hot bath. You can also take paracetamol,
but try to limit it to times when nothing else
brings relief.

Sacroiliac pain is usually experienced as
a steady pain in the middle or lower back. At
the lower end of the spine your sacrum inter-
connects with the left and right iliac bones at the sacroiliac joints (see picture),
to help provide you with a stable pelvic girdle with which to walk and maintain
an upright posture. Towards the end of pregnancy, hormones relax the
ligaments to prepare for the passage of your baby through the pelvic canal and
this, together with the increasing weight of your uterus, can make the sacroiliac
joints unstable. This can result in severe pain, especially when walking, standing
or bending. You may need to see your doctor, physiotherapist or osteopath.
Meanwhile, wear comfortable low-heeled shoes and try to ensure you maintain
good posture – keep your shoulders back, walk tall, and don't lean backwards.

Pubic symphysis dysfunction is pain affecting the symphysis pubis, the
narrowest point of your bony pelvic girdle lying just in front of your bladder. As
the ligaments around the joint loosen in late pregnancy, the two pubic bones
(pubic rami) may rub against each other uncomfortably when you walk and
particularly when your legs rotate outwards or your knees move wide apart. If you
are suffering from this type of pain, avoid straddling movements by keeping your
knees together and swinging your legs around from the hips when you get out of
the car, bed or bath. Putting cold packs over the painful area under your underwear
for 10 minutes every three hours may reduce the swelling and pain. Knee squeezing
and pelvic tilts (see p.219) or sitting on a birth ball can help ease the discomfort.

If the two pubic bones actually separate from each other (a condition called
diastasis of the symphysis pubis) the pain can be very severe. Although bed
rest and local heat treatment can help, most women who develop this rare
complication in late pregnancy are forced to limit their weight-bearing
activities and often need to use elbow crutches to move around.

Things to consider

By this time you will probably have started to develop your own views about how you would like your ideal labour and delivery to be conducted. You can talk to your midwife about your birth preferences or consider writing a birth preference plan.

To make the process simpler, I have included a brief summary of the major childbirth philosophies as well as some advice on compiling your own list of birth preferences, which can be incorporated in your hand-held notes. However, before you make any decisions about the way you would like your labour and delivery handled, I suggest that you read the sections on pain relief, monitoring, and labour and birth to form a clear idea of what might be generally available and what to expect.

The change of title from the more usual "birth plan" is deliberate because I think that it is more useful to think of this document as a list of preferences. To me, a birth plan implies a rigidity of approach – as if it is a set of rules and

---

TOPICS FOR YOUR BIRTH PREFERENCE PLAN

Nowadays most maternity units make great efforts to help women fulfil their wishes during labour and delivery. Good communication with your carers will help them to work towards your requests wherever possible and prevent disappointments and unrealistic expectations.

Things to consider
▶ Who would you like to be with you during labour and birth – your partner, mother, friend?
▶ What are your views on being cared for by student midwives and doctors?
▶ Are you prepared to have your

membranes ruptured and to be given drugs to speed up your contractions (see pp.294–7)?
▶ What are your views about fetal monitoring (see pp.291–2)?
▶ How active or mobile do you wish to be during labour?
▶ Would you want your partner to be with you during a Caesarean delivery (see pp.360–9)?
▶ Do you have views on episiotomies or perineal tears (see p.330–1)?
▶ Do you want to hold your baby immediately following the birth or after first checks have been made?
▶ Who do you wish to cut the umbilical cord?

▶ Do you wish to receive an oxytocin injection to speed the delivery of placenta (see p.333)?

Questions to ask
▶ Will you be allowed to eat and drink normally in early labour?
▶ Is it OK to wear your own clothes?
▶ Will you have access to a bath, shower or birthing pool?
▶ What types of pain relief are available and is there a 24-hour epidural service (see pp.311–5)?
▶ Are different positions encouraged during delivery?
▶ Is there a time limit for the second stage of labour, even if progress is being made?

commandments to which you and your medical and midwifery carers must comply. As we all know, the most carefully laid plans can go awry and labour can take an unpredictable turn, so the best way to avoid distress and disappointment about the final outcome is to be as flexible as possible.

At my own hospital, we offer women a double-sided sheet of A4 paper with a selection of issues that they may find helpful to consider. The points are arranged in boxes with space provided for women to make notes after they have considered the issues. We then encourage them to discuss their ideas with their midwife before drawing up a list of preferences that can be included in their notes. There are some distinct advantages to this method:

• Your list sends a message to the team delivering your baby that you have thought about your labour and want to participate in the decision-making.

• Drawing up your list of preferences will help you to feel more composed, because you will spend time thinking about your views on labour and delivery. If you find that you need more information about the many eventualities that could occur there is still time to seek out the missing facts.

• Forward planning also gives your partner the chance to understand your preferences and know what you expect of him during labour.

UMBILICAL STEM CELL COLLECTION

Stem cell collection is a new service available to parents which I mention here for information rather than as an advocate. At a cost of around £1,000 it offers parents the opportunity to have stem cells harvested from their baby's umbilical cord and stored as an insurance against potential illness in later life. Stem cells, which are found in embryonic tissue as well as umbilical cord blood, have the potential to develop into different types of body cells. Although stem cell treatment is still in its infancy, its most promising uses are in diabetes, degenerative disorders, such as juvenile arthritis and Alzheimer's disease, and as a substitute for bone marrow in diseases such as leukaemia.

You can find leaflets advertising umbilical cord sampling in some maternity units and on the internet. You will need to join a scheme at least eight weeks before the birth. When your baby is born, a phlebotomist from the company will come to the hospital to harvest your baby's cord blood. After the birth the sample will be couriered to a laboratory to be frozen and stored for possible future use.

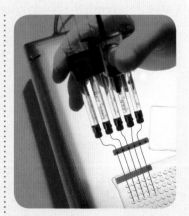

Testing cells Stem cells found in umbilical cord blood can develop into white and red blood cells and platelets. White blood cells from a sample are being tested here.

Disadvantages of birth plans

The sheer length of the document can be a problem, so do bear in mind that three closely-typed pages will be harder for your carers to take on board than a page of succinct bullet points. When you are compiling your wish list, try to take a positive approach and focus on what you would like to happen rather than making a negative list of things that you do not want to happen. Some midwives will be put off by a lengthy list of "Don't do this and don't do that." However, there are other important reasons why birth plans can end up being counter-productive:

• There are so many different ways of experiencing labour that no birth plan can possibly anticipate them all. Indeed, I think that the more detailed the birth plan, the more likely it is for events to fall short of expectations.

• Some women who have spent a lot of time and effort constructing a "natural" birth plan feel desperately distressed and disappointed if their labour takes an unexpected turn and requires sudden medical intervention. I understand their disappointment, but when they tell me that they now feel a failure as a woman because they were unable to deliver their baby naturally, it is my turn to feel distressed. No one who nurtures a baby in their womb for the best part of a year and then delivers it safely into the outside world, by whatever route, can be considered anything other than extraordinarily successful. Similarly, when I hear comments such as, "control was wrested away from me by the doctors as if I did not matter", I do not feel defensive or cross. My immediate worry is that this woman is at greater risk of developing postnatal depression because she feels so negative about her birth experience and considers that she has been let down by her carers and by herself.

• Every person involved in the delivery of your baby (including you) has a common goal: the safe delivery of a healthy baby to a healthy mother. Your antenatal carers will want to help you experience the delivery of your dreams, but there may be occasions when your wishes are just not compatible with protecting your safety and that of your baby. In this situation, it is really important that you listen to the advice that is offered by the experts and understand why it may be necessary to override your birth plan.

My personal view is that ensuring your antenatal team understand that you would like to be closely involved in any decision-making is far more important and valuable than any written statement that you make about your labour and delivery. Women give birth every minute of the day with no birth plan whatsoever – they simply use their voice to express their preferences, to ask questions, and to ensure that the medical team communicate with them.

> Women give birth every minute of the day with no birth plan whatsoever – they simply use their voice to express their preferences…

APPROACHES TO CHILDBIRTH

A number of childbirth philosophers have had a significant influence on the way that pregnant women and their maternity carers approach labour and childbirth. Below is a brief summary of their ideas and how they have been put into effect.

In the 1950s and 1960s, birth became highly medicalized in the Western world and the obstetrician's word was gospel. Hardly surprising, therefore, that in the decades that followed, advocates of a more natural approach to childbirth sprang up to question what had become the accepted way of giving birth. Collectively their teaching and ideas have altered many aspects of antenatal and postnatal care, some of which we now take for granted because they have become such an integral part of obstetric care.

▶ **Dr Grantley Dick-Read**, a UK physician, recognized in the 1930s that fear of childbirth was one of the major contributors to pain during labour. He introduced the idea of teaching breathing and relaxation techniques to help reduce fear and tension. He was also the first person to include fathers in the antenatal education process and to encourage them to be present in the delivery room. Antenatal preparation is now considered essential to help women cope with the physical and emotional demands of labour.

▶ **Dr Ferdinand Lamaze** developed a similar approach in France, using teaching about childbirth and relaxation techniques to counteract labour pains. Lamaze argued that women could be conditioned to deal positively with labour pains in the same way that the Russian scientist, Dr Pavlov, had trained his dogs to respond to a learned stimulus. Both Dick-Read's and Lamaze's methods have had an enormous influence on the way women now prepare for and manage their labours. Indeed, the National Childbirth Trust (NCT) uses Lamaze breathing and relaxation techniques alongside preparation and education in their antenatal classes. It seems strange to us now to think that 50 years ago women frequently went into labour in terror, ill informed and reliant on anecdotal evidence!

▶ **Frederick Leboyer's** method of delivering babies is based on the theory that many problems in later life stem from trauma experienced at the time

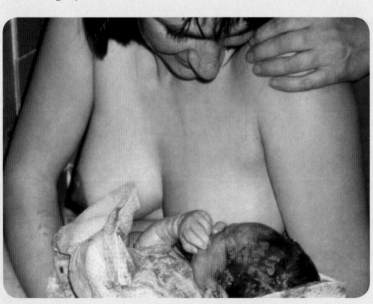

LEBOYER BIRTH The baby is delivered and put immediately into her mother's arms.

of birth. In his book *Birth without Violence*, Leboyer argued that babies needed to be born into calm, gentle surroundings where noise and sudden movements are kept to a minimum. In a gentle Leboyer birth, the baby is placed immediately on the mother's skin and the umbilical cord is not cut until it has finished pulsating. He also advocates placing the baby in a warm bath immediately after delivery – a soothing replica of the watery world it has just left behind.

Soft lighting in the delivery room and facilities for water births are Leboyer influences, which are becoming commonplace in many maternity units. Although it may not always be appropriate to give birth in semi-obscurity with only one midwife in attendance, thanks to Leboyer, newborn babies are no longer held head down by their feet and welcomed into the world with a slap on the bottom.

▶ **Sheila Kitzinger** emerged during the 1960s as one of the key figures in the natural childbirth movement. A founder member of the National Childbirth Trust (although she is no longer involved with them), Kitzinger argues that women should be allowed to reclaim some control over the way in which they give birth and participate actively in the process of birth. Having said that, she does not advocate natural birth techniques where they may endanger the mother or baby's welfare, but does campaign for the avoidance of unnecessary obstetric intervention. She believes that birth can be made a powerful, positive, and personal experience for mothers even

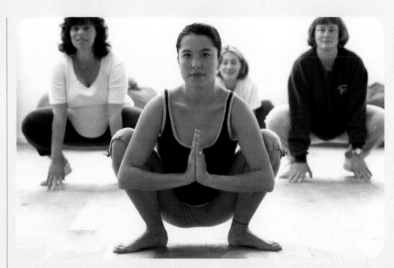

ACTIVE BIRTH CLASS Exercises strengthen the hips, pelvis, and thighs for delivery.

when the labour becomes complicated, involves medicalized pain relief or ends in delivery by Caesarean section. As a result of her work, women are no longer shaved routinely or subjected to enemas when they go into labour, and episiotomies (see pp.330–1) are no longer routinely performed at delivery – at least not in the UK.

▶ **Michel Odent** is a French surgeon who uses active childbirth techniques at his specialist unit in Pithiviers, which boasts the lowest rate of episiotomies, forceps, and Caesarean deliveries in France. His belief is that women confined to bed with their legs in stirrups, labour slowly and painfully because they face an uphill struggle to deliver their baby. His view is that women should be allowed to return to a primitive state (either upright or on all fours) in labour. Their instincts and loss of inhibitions help to produce natural painkilling chemicals in the brain called endorphins, often eliminating the need for drugs to relieve pain.

▶ **Janet Balaskas** founded the Active Birth Movement in 1981 and from her Active Birth Centre in North London organizes a network of private classes teaching women yoga, massage, breathing techniques, and relaxation to help them prepare for labour. The Active Birth Movement and also the National Childbirth Trust (see Useful Contacts, pp.437–8) emphasize the importance of postnatal support, focusing particularly on practical help with breastfeeding.

Of course, the reality is that many women dip into some, or all, of the above childbirth philosophies and extract the bits that they find helpful, but do not follow them down to the last letter. There is nothing to prevent you, for example, learning about yoga and massage or breathing and relaxation techniques, and then choosing to have an epidural, should the pain become too difficult to bear.

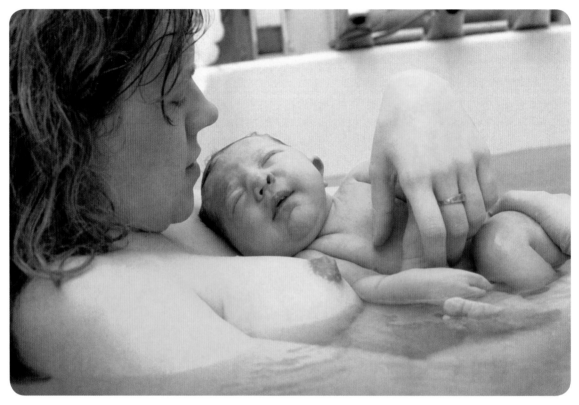

BIRTH POOLS Spending your labour in water is now an option in some maternity units although there may be only one birthing pool available.

Water births

Birthing pools and water-assisted births have become increasingly fashionable over the last 10 to 15 years, largely out of enthusiasm for the gentle birth ideas of French obstetrician Dr Leboyer, but also because they can be effective as a method of pain relief (see pp.319–20); so much so, that many maternity units have installed birthing pools in which you can spend some or all of your labour. My own hospital overcame the plumbing problems of an old Victorian building and installed one in the midwifery-led area of our labour ward, and it has proved to be very popular.

If you think that you might like this option, check in advance whether your hospital provides this facility and how likely it is that you will be able to use it. Remember that a single pool will probably be allocated on a first-come-first-served basis, and it is very difficult to predict exactly when you might go into labour. If a birthing pool is not available, you may be able to hire one to take into the maternity unit with you.

If you are hoping to hire a pool for a home birth, the first thing to establish is whether the floor of the room that you are going to use will sustain the weight of a full birthing pool. You will need to set it up close to where you wish to give birth and ensure that you have facilities to both fill it and, most importantly, empty it after the delivery. There are several companies that specialize in hiring out birthing pools in various sizes and at different prices (see Useful Contacts, pp.437–8). When you are calculating the cost of hiring a birthing pool, remember that you will have to finance time on either side of your expected delivery date, since you cannot be sure exactly when you will go into labour. Your midwife should be able to advise you about good local companies, or you could contact the Active Birthing Centre for information.

The nesting instinct

With D- (delivery) day approaching, you may develop an urge to sort out and tidy up everything around the house, in preparation for the birth of your new baby. Although aiming to conserve your energy in preparation for the birth would seem the best plan, many of you will be rushing around, trying to get the house ship shape. This strange compulsion, known as the nesting instinct, grips many women as the end of their pregnancy approaches. So don't be surprised if you find yourself steam-cleaning the carpets, clearing out the kitchen cupboards, attempting to dust the highest of your bookshelves, or suddenly taking it into your head to repaint the living room.

I suspect that this nesting instinct is one of the means we use to help ourselves prepare psychologically for the birth. Many women tell me that they are only able to relax properly when they know that the house is completely ready for the new baby's arrival. Such is the enormous emotional relief and mental release from knowing that things are well prepared that some find they go into labour as soon as they feel their home is ready. Interestingly, women who deliver prematurely sometimes find the adjustment to the practicalities of motherhood more difficult and this may be because they have not had sufficient time to prepare for their baby.

Air travel in late pregnancy

If you are planning a trip abroad at this stage of your pregnancy, you may have some concerns about the safety of air travel and at what point an airline may refuse to carry you. Generally speaking, most airlines do not accept pregnant women after the 34th week of pregnancy, but individual airlines vary. Although many people assume this is because the reduced cabin pressure in an aircraft can induce labour or harm the baby, there is no hard, scientific evidence to support this view. It is my belief that the ruling is based on the fact that some 10 per cent of pregnancies are going to deliver prematurely, and airlines want to reduce the likelihood of having to deal with a labouring woman during their

> This strange compulsion, known as the nesting instinct, grips many women as the end of their pregnancy approaches.

flight. Indeed, this is an ordeal that you probably do not want to willingly inflict on yourself either. Should labour start, there is a small chance you might give birth on the plane (on a long-haul flight) and an even greater risk that you would be faced with the prospect of seeking help from doctors and midwives in a strange place.

If you do decide to fly in your last trimester, make sure that you have taken the precaution of finding out where the maternity units are located at your destination. You should also make sure that the airline is prepared to fly you not only on the outward journey, but on the return one as well.

Planning childcare

Without a doubt, one of the biggest financial outlays for working parents is that of childcare. Sadly, the UK lags behind some of its European neighbours in terms of the cost and availability of high-quality childcare. Nurseries and crèches are not available in every area of the UK, and good ones can be heavily over-subscribed. As a result, many women have to find a childminder or nanny to look after their children, particularly if their working life involves anything other than a strict nine-to-five day. Not surprisingly, many women are forced to conclude, after calculating the full costs of childcare, that it is financially not worth their while to work. This situation needs to change!

Although it may seem premature to be discussing childcare before the baby has arrived, I can assure you that it is never too early to give thought to this crucial issue. If you are planning to go back to work, it is particularly important that you give thought to the sort of childcare that you would both prefer now, so that you have time to inform yourself fully while you are on your maternity leave. You will most likely be considering one of the following options:

Maternity nurses are usually employed to live in your home for about 4–6 weeks after the baby is born. Some independent midwives or doulas will also live with you to offer postnatal care for this period. They will help you with the 24-hour demands of your new baby, including feeding, nappy changing, doing the baby's laundry, and ensuring that you have regular rest periods and a good night's sleep. However, their most important role is to help you work out a future routine for caring for your baby. Some women will welcome the organization and routine they provide, whereas others may find them intrusive, preferring to muddle through in the first few weeks, learning the ropes by themselves. There are plenty of private agencies offering maternity nurses or doulas, but a personal recommendation is the best route to follow. If you decide to employ one, you will need to work out exactly what you want her to do for you. They are invariably expensive.

> Without a doubt, one of the biggest financial outlays for working parents is that of childcare.

Nurseries or crèches are run either privately or by the state, and their hours and flexibility vary considerably. As mentioned above, they are hard to come by, especially good ones, and you will need to make enquiries about what is available locally at the earliest opportunity. All nurseries and crèches adhere to strict legal requirements concerning safety, the ratio of carers to children, the suitability of the location, the space available, and the equipment they provide. All the above points need to be considered carefully, but friends' recommendations are also invaluable.

Registered childminders will look after your child in their own home and are paid per child and per hour, so although a childminder is usually cheaper than a nanny for just one child, if you are asking them to care for two or more children, they can become as expensive as a full-time nanny. Childminders tend to be less flexible, as they often have other children to look after, including, though not always, their own. So if your child falls ill, they may well not be able to look after him – a situation that also applies to nurseries and crèches. In addition, if you work irregular hours or sometimes have to stay late unexpectedly, the childminder may not be able to accommodate your individual needs, in which case you will have to pay for additional childcare to fill in the gaps. Your local council can provide you with a list of childminders in your area, all of whom will have undergone a thorough vetting process before being accepted on the books.

A nanny will look after your child in your own home. Nannies can either live in or live out, they can work for you alone or you can share them with another family. You will need to determine clearly the hours that they work during the day and whether you wish them to undertake other duties, which may include one or two evenings a week babysitting. Speaking from practical experience, the most important thing about employing a nanny is to make sure that you are completely up front about what you expect her to do for you. As with all employee/employer relationships, trust and good communication are crucial. No one can completely protect their family from the proverbial nanny from hell, but you can take some careful steps to ensure that this is unlikely to happen to you.

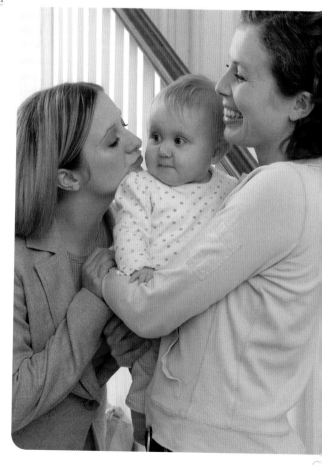

BACK TO WORK Leaving your baby for the first time is a little easier when you are totally confident about her care.

In general terms, live-in nannies earn less money than live-out nannies because you also provide them with board and lodging. However, when you add up the additional costs of having another adult living in your house, not to mention the telephone bills, you will probably conclude that the overall outlay for a live-in nanny is higher than you originally thought. For some couples, the advantage of a live-in nanny is that they have someone in the house to call on in an emergency, whereas others find that another person in their home is an intrusion. Whatever the case, it is important to remember that if you are repeatedly late home from work, frequently expect them to help out on their weekend off or fail to pay them for the extra hours they work, you will soon find that your nanny has become disgruntled and is looking for an alternative job.

A live-out nanny is generally the most expensive childcare option in terms of the salary you pay, but she goes home at the end of the day and you have your home to yourselves. When you are considering the financial implications of employing a nanny, it is important to remember that most nannies will expect you to pay all of their national insurance and tax contributions, in addition to their salary. Setting up a nanny-share arrangement with another family is one way of reducing the expenditure, but this requires a good deal of flexibility.

Start by buying yourself a good book or researching online and follow this up by taking advice from as many friends and acquaintances as possible, even those who are not currently using any childcare. Above all, aim to have clear ideas about what you are looking for before you start to advertise. Even if you decide to pay an agency to find a suitable nanny for you, you must ensure that you interview them and contact their referees personally before you agree to employ them. Advertising and interviewing for a nanny is a time-consuming business, so plan ahead to make sure that she can start work on your preferred date. Resist the temptation to ask the new nanny to shorten the notice that she gives to her current employer and start more quickly. If she does this for you, then she can just as easily leave you at short notice in the future.

Au pair girls/boys are another possible source of childcare and are usually much less expensive. In exchange for a room, board, and some pocket money they will help you to look after your baby or children and undertake light housework duties. However, since they are usually young people from abroad with limited English and, quite possibly, no experience of caring for babies or

66 …the most important thing about employing a nanny is to make sure that you are completely up front about what you expect her to do for you. 99

young children, I think this option is much more suitable for school-age children rather than a newborn baby, particularly since many au pairs want to attend a language school for several hours every day. It is vital that you have total confidence in the person to whom you entrust your child or children and it is unlikely that a young au pair will fulfil your needs in that respect.

Younger grandparents with time on their hands are sometimes more than willing to care for a baby for one or two days a week so this may be an option, especially if you plan to work part-time. There are rich rewards in terms of the close bond that they will develop with their growing grandchild, but you need to be sure that you are not asking more of them than they can manage. Remember, too, that parenting

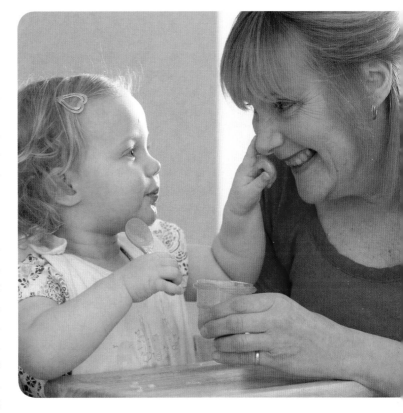

styles differ: their views on, for example, demand feeding, sleep, crying, and treats may conflict with your own, and it is usually more difficult to address a problem with a relative than it would be with a professional carer. Much will have changed over the years since your own parents or in-laws were bringing up a small baby and they may need a refresher course on the complexities of buggies and car seats and on important safety issues, especially if they plan to care for your baby in their own home.

GRANDPARENT CARE
When it works well, grandparent care can be a rewarding experience all round.

If you only need a few hours to yourself for one or two days a week, reciprocal arrangements with a friend with children may be an option, but bear in mind that on your days off you will be caring for two or more children rather than just your own.

Whichever childcare option you choose, you will need to invest a significant amount of time and effort into finding the best solution you can afford for you and your family. Start thinking about the options now, since you need to be very clear about what you require and the timescales involved to find them when you actively start looking. This is usually two to three months before you plan to return to work if you decide on a nanny or childminder, but can be considerably longer if you are looking for a place in a crèche or nursery.

SPECIALIST ANTENATAL MONITORING

Most women and their babies are judged to be fit and well in late pregnancy and are unlikely to need any form of specialist monitoring. However, if your pregnancy goes past its term or you have developed, or are at risk of developing, a late-pregnancy complication, your carers will arrange for you to have some specialist tests.

The kind of problems that are likely to involve specialist monitoring include high blood pressure; a baby that is not growing well; reduced fetal movements; gestational diabetes that is poorly controlled; or a pregnancy that has gone past the due date (to mention just a few). Of course, the exact tests that you are offered will be determined by the particular problem, but on most occasions you will undergo an ultrasound scan to assess your baby's growth together with a general assessment of the baby's wellbeing, called a biophysical profile. This will include a cardiotocograph (CTG) and an electronic trace of the baby's heart rate. Many units will also perform Doppler ultrasound scanning of the blood flow in the uterus, placenta, and in the baby's major blood vessels.

Most maternity units have day-care facilities that are able to provide these detailed monitoring tests. Nowadays, the emphasis is on trying to keep the mother-to-be safe in an outpatient setting, albeit under careful scrutiny.

Fetal growth monitoring

If a problem with your baby's growth is suspected, you may be offered ultrasound scans at intervals of 7–14 days to establish the exact nature and cause. Your baby's head circumference and abdominal circumference will be measured, and also the length of the femur (thigh bone), which is another good indicator of growth.

There are several types of intra-uterine growth restriction (IUGR, see p.429) each with markedly different causes and effects on fetal growth.

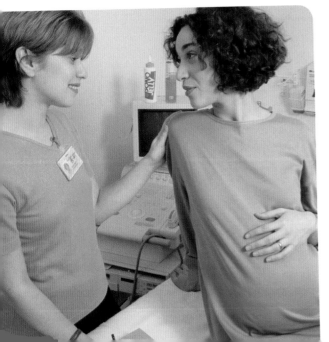

SPECIAL TESTS Usually these are performed in a day-care setting avoiding the need for prolonged stays in hospital before your delivery date.

DOPPLER ULTRASOUND SCANS

This highly sensitive form of scanning is performed like a normal ultrasound scan to assess the amount of blood flowing through the blood vessels in the uterus, placenta, and umbilical cord, and in the baby's head.

▶ **When blood flow is being diverted to the brain and heart** and away from less vital body organs, the main blood vessels in the brain, particularly the middle cerebral artery, dilate (become less resistant) to accommodate the extra volume. This change can be detected by a scanner and gives a clear message that the baby is exposed to stresses such as low oxygen levels (hypoxia), and that action is needed in the near future.

▶ **Reduced blood flow in the umbilical artery** is a useful predictor of risk when a baby is growing slowly. On a normal Doppler scan, blood pressure falls at the end of each heart pumping cycle but the supply to the baby is maintained. However, if the blood flow is interrupted at the end of each cycle, it is a sign that the baby is suffering from a lack of oxygen. If the scan shows blood flowing backwards, immediate intervention is required.

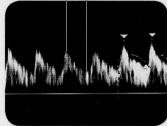

high pressure at start of heart pumping cycle | low pressure at end of heart pumping cycle

NORMAL Although the blood flow to the baby dips at the end of each heart pumping cycle it never stops. The supply is continuous.

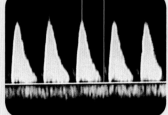

high pressure at start of heart pumping cycle | absent flow at end of heart pumping cycle

ABNORMAL Small gaps between the peaks and troughs show an absence of blood flow to the baby at the end of each pumping cycle.

In symmetrical growth restriction, growth is restricted early in pregnancy and the head and body are equally affected. Many congenital abnormalities, some infections such as rubella cytomegalovirus and syphilis (see p.412 and p.415) and toxins such as alcohol, cigarette smoke, and heroin cause symmetrical growth restriction.

Asymmetrical growth restriction occurs after 20 weeks and is often referred to as placental insufficiency. It develops when a maternal or fetal problem affects placental function, and blood flow becomes insufficient to meet the needs of the growing baby. Examples include pre-eclampsia (see p.426), twin pregnancies, and some fetal abnormalities (see pp.415–21). The baby responds by diverting blood to the brain and heart to protect the growth of these vital organs and the head becomes relatively larger than the abdomen as fat stores in the liver and abdomen are used up. Subcutaneous fat is also absorbed and as a result the fetal limbs may become scrawny.

If your baby is found to be growing too slowly with a head-sparing pattern, you will be offered a Doppler ultrasound scan (see above) to assess the severity of the situation. If there is no immediate danger, you will be asked to return for further growth scans at intervals of 7–14 days. If a subsequent scan confirms that there has been no further growth or that your baby is growing very slowly, you will probably be advised to have an induction of labour (see pp.294–7). In some cases, urgent delivery by Caesarean section is needed.

Fetal heart recordings

Cardiotocographs (CTGs) are pictorial print-outs generated by an electronic machine that assesses your baby's heart rate as well as the activity of the muscles of your uterus. CTGs are most commonly used during labour to assess how the baby is coping with contractions, but they are also used in pregnancy to monitor a baby that is suspected of having a potential problem (see box, below).

Two belts are strapped around your abdomen: one picks up any activity in your uterine muscles, while the other records your baby's heart rate. The combined trace that the machine generates shows whether the baby's heart rate pattern is normal or abnormal and whether your uterus is active (contracting) or quiet (not contracting).

Computerized Oxford CTGs

This type of monitoring is used as a guide to the baby's general state of health and is usually reserved for specialist monitoring in late pregnancy. The Oxford Sonicaid System, for example, sets out a list of criteria that have to be met by the fetal heart rate pattern during a certain time interval. These might include a minimum baseline heart rate, episodes of high and low

 ## INTERPRETING A CTG

Babies in utero normally have a baseline heart rate of 110 to 160 beats per minute. This varies constantly by 5–15 beats, except during periods of sleep lasting around 30 minutes. This variability is an important sign of wellbeing: if there is a lack of variability for more than 30 minutes, it suggests the baby may be experiencing stress.

Healthy babies also have frequent accelerations or increases in their heart rate (defined as an increase of more than 15 beats per minute for more than 15 seconds), which are usually associated with fetal movements, and are sometimes provoked by external stimuli, such as firmly prodding your abdomen, and also uterine contractions.

Decelerations in the heart rate are also very common following fetal movements or uterine contractions. However, repeated decelerations of more than 15 beats per minute for more than 15 seconds are another sign of possible fetal distress, particularly when they have not been provoked by contractions. That said, there are often variations in the way individuals interpret CTGs, which is one of the reasons why computerized analysis of the tracings has been developed.

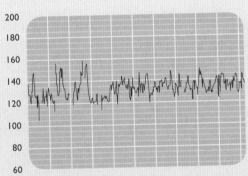

GOOD VARIABILITY The peaks and troughs on this CTG show a healthy pattern of accelerations and decelerations in the fetal heartbeat over a short period of time.

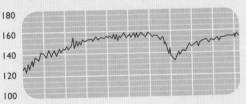

POOR VARIABILITY A CTG showing little variation in the fetal heartbeat over a period of more than 30 minutes suggests that the fetus may be suffering from stress.

variability, presence of accelerations, lack of deep decelerations, and presence of fetal movements. When these criteria are met within a short space of time, this is very reassuring news for everyone involved. The maximum recording time is 60 minutes, but the computer starts analyzing the CTG after 10 minutes. If all the criteria have been met, the analysis stops and it is unlikely that another Oxford CTG will need to be performed.

If the criteria are not met at 10 minutes, the computer will continue to analyze the signals every two minutes, until the criteria are met. If this does not occur within 60 minutes of recording, this will give rise to concern about the baby's wellbeing. Depending on the clinical reasons why you were advised to have this type of CTG in the first place, your antenatal carers will then decide on whether and when to repeat the test.

Very occasionally, a warning signal will be triggered in response to finding a low baseline fetal heart rate (less than 110 beats per minute). In this rare situation, the machine will keep on recording and repeatedly print messages prompting the staff to check that there is no further fall in the fetal heart rate, that there are fetal movements present, and that the heart rate has not developed a sinusoidal pattern (swinging up and down in deep curves), which is invariably a sign that the baby is in imminent danger because of a serious problem such as placental abruption (see p.428).

As with all forms of testing, the computerized analysis may produce a false positive result, suggesting that there may be a problem, when in fact none exists. Although this invariably causes alarm and distress, on balance I think it's much safer to use a test that eliminates the risk of carers failing to identify a baby that is distressed and needs immediate help – even if it does throw up the occasional false positive.

Liquor volume

The volume of your amniotic fluid is usually assessed by measuring the depth of the pools around the baby using ultrasound scanning. When the maximum depth is less than 2–3cm (about 1in) or the sum of the depths of the pools in four separate areas measures less than 7.3cm (3in), intervention and prompt delivery is called for.

Exactly why the volume of liquor surrounding a baby near to term is so important in determining the outcome of pregnancy has been difficult to establish scientifically. The logical explanation is that increased or reduced liquor volume are indications that the fetal kidneys and metabolism are not working optimally, but testing these important functions while the baby is still in utero is nearly impossible. Nonetheless, my personal experience is that evidence of reduced liquor volume should always be taken seriously. When a pregnancy is near to term or past its due date, I almost always make the decision to deliver the baby when told that the liquor volume is very low.

Biophysical profile

This was the first test to recognize the importance of using a combination of factors to estimate fetal wellbeing. It uses a scoring system to assess fetal breathing movements, body movements, muscular tone and posture, as well as the volume of amniotic fluid and the results of a CTG. Nowadays, a reduced volume of amniotic fluid and sub-optimal CTG analysis are considered as the most important indicators that a baby may be compromised and requiring prompt action. Nonetheless, if for example, your liquor volume is low but the CTG is fine, your carers will automatically look at additional parameters to help them to decide whether to watch and wait or whether to intervene.

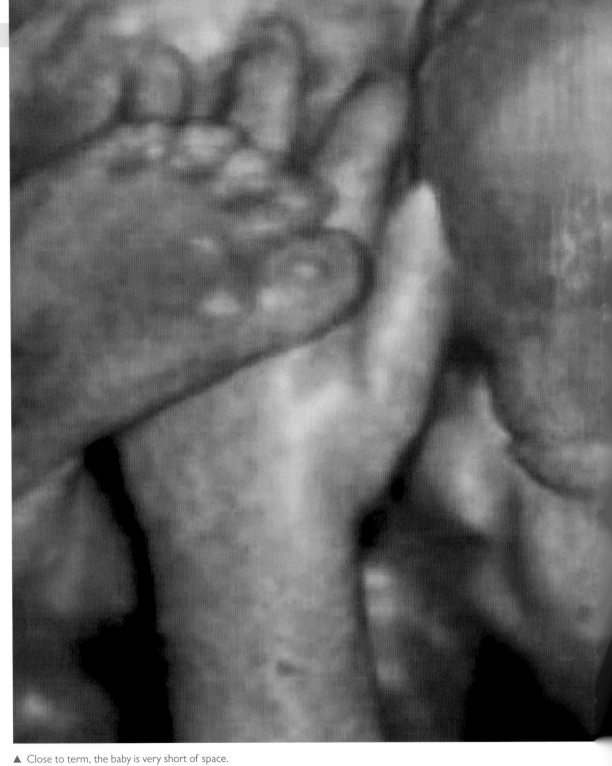

▲ Close to term, the baby is very short of space.

1	2	3	4	5	6	7	8	9	10	11	12	13	14	15	16	17	18	19	20

▶ WEEKS 0–6   ▶ WEEKS 6–10   ▶ WEEKS 10–13   ▶ WEEKS 13–17   ▶ WEEKS 17–21

▶ **FIRST TRIMESTER**   ▶ **SECOND TRIMESTER**

▶ **WEEKS 35–40**

The developing baby

IT IS QUITE A SNUG FIT inside the uterus now. The baby is usually curled up tightly, head pointing downwards, waiting for labour to start. Movements are more limited, but you will probably notice regular changes in the contours of your tummy as the baby shifts position.

Your baby continues to gain weight steadily during this final stage of pregnancy, which is almost entirely due to more fat being laid down under the skin, around the muscles and around some of the abdominal organs. The average term baby will have a plump rounded appearance and will weigh 3–4kg (6½–9lb); it is common for boys to weigh a little more than girls. Although your baby is too cramped to move freely now, you should still be able to feel movement and you may experience the odd sharp twinge as your baby throws a punch and indents the uterine wall. Remember that any sudden change in the pattern of your baby's movements needs to be investigated as a matter of urgency.

Most of the lanugo hair has disappeared, although some slippery vernix is still present to help the passage of the baby through the birth canal. Post-mature babies commonly have cracked and peeling skin because they have been without their protective coating of vernix for longer periods of time; some even have scratch marks on their faces from their long fingernails. The amount of hair babies have at birth is variable, ranging from completely bald, to downy patches to a complete head of hair. Most of it is lost in the first weeks, but this may be hardly noticed because it is replaced simultaneously with proper hair.

Ready for birth

The lungs are now fully mature, and the baby continues to produce large quantities of cortisol to ensure that plenty of surfactant is produced in the lungs and that the transition to breathing air in the outside world goes smoothly. The heart is beating at a rate of 120–160 beats per minute. Dramatic changes will occur in the heart and circulatory system at the time of delivery when the baby takes his first breath (see pp.378–9).

not life size

At 38–40 weeks, your baby will weigh between 3 and 4kg (6½–9lb) and will measure as much as 50cm (20in) from the crown of the head to the tip of the toes.

21	22	23	24	25	26	27	28	29	30	31	32	33	34	**35**	**36**	**37**	**38**	**39**	**40**

▶ **WEEKS 21–26**   ▶ **WEEKS 26–30**   ▶ **WEEKS 30–35**   ▶ **WEEKS 35–40**

▶ **THIRD TRIMESTER**

The digestive system is now ready to accept liquid foods. The intestines become filled with a dark green sticky substance called meconium, which is made up of dead skin cells, remnants of the lanugo, hair and secretions from the baby's bowel, liver, and gall bladder. This meconium plug will normally be passed in the first few days of life, but if your baby becomes distressed or frightened before delivery, he may have a bowel action into the amniotic fluid. If meconium is seen in the amniotic fluid after the waters have broken, it is evidence that the baby has already been put under stress and may need to be closely monitored during labour (see pp.291–2). In boys, the testes descend into the scrotum during this period, which explains why premature babies are often born with undescended testicles.

Your baby's immune system is now capable of protecting against a variety of infections, but this is mainly due to the transfer of antibodies from your own blood. After birth, babies continue to receive antibodies from breast milk. One of the main reasons for trying to establish successful breastfeeding is that you can continue to offer your baby this protection in the first few months of life, before he is capable of producing his own antibodies to infection.

How the head adapts

Your baby's head is relatively much smaller than it was earlier on in the pregnancy, but the circumference is still as big as its abdomen. By full term, the head remains one of the largest parts of the baby's body, so delivering it safely through the birth canal during labour is an important consideration. This is one of the reasons why the fetal skull bones do not fuse together until much later in neonatal life. Although the baby's brain needs to be protected by bone, these are quite soft compared to an adult skull and can slide over each other and overlap. This allows the head to mould to the shape of the mother's pelvis, and greatly eases the passage through the birth canal and vagina.

In a normal pregnancy, the fetal head will move down into the pelvic brim and become engaged in preparation for the start of labour. In first pregnancies, this head descent can start as early as 36 weeks, whereas in second or third pregnancies, the fetal head may not engage in the pelvis until immediately before labour starts.

The placenta at term

Your placenta now looks like a discus and measures about 20–25cm (8–10in) in diameter and is approximately 2–3cm (about 1in) thick. This large surface area enables the transfer of oxygen and nutrients to your baby, and the passage of waste products from baby back to mother. At term, the placenta will weigh around 700g (1½lb), just less than one-sixth of the fetal weight. Although some 45 per cent of pregnancies are undelivered at 40 weeks, most doctors and midwives will advise that the pregnancy not continue after 42 weeks. At this stage, they will probably suggest an induction of labour (see pp.294–7) because the placenta will no longer be functioning as effectively. Its reserves are now pretty well exhausted, which is why the risk of having a stillborn baby is increased in post-mature pregnancies. After 42 weeks, your baby can be more reliably cared for in the outside world.

Your changing body

If your baby's head has started to engage, or settle into the pelvis, your bump will appear to be lying lower in your abdominal cavity. There is sometimes quite a noticeable change in your body shape and you may hear people remarking that you have "started to drop".

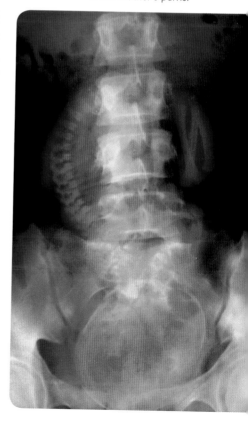

READY FOR BIRTH
A coloured X-ray shows a full-term baby with its head down and engaged in the mother's pelvis.

This does not mean that you are about to go into labour and literally drop your baby; you may still have several weeks to go. It is merely an indication that your uterus and your baby are both getting prepared for the labour ahead. As I mentioned earlier, if this is your first baby, engagement is likely to occur sooner rather than later. This is because the muscles of your uterus are tight because they have not been stretched by a previous labour and so are able to exert more pressure on the baby's head. Also, the arrangement of the pelvic bones is slightly altered after a previous vaginal delivery and this may delay engagement.

If your baby's head has started to engage, your breathing may be easier now and the decrease in pressure under your diaphragm and ribs may make eating a complete meal a possibility. This is why engagement is sometimes referred to as lightening (of the abdominal pressure). The downside to this change is that the baby's head (if head down) is pressing directly on your bladder. You will need to pass small amounts of urine frequently, and at night your increased bulk will make getting in and out of bed to visit the lavatory quite a major undertaking. Further loosening of your pelvic ligaments and joints will occur in preparation for the birth and this can result in a variety of aches and pains in the pelvic area and an increasingly sore lower abdomen. The problem is made worse because your posture changes again as your baby moves into your pelvis. Your own weight gain usually slows up and may even stop during the final few weeks of pregnancy although the baby can put on as much as 1kg (2½lb). But if you suddenly feel swollen and puffy, see your midwife or doctor urgently to check that you are not developing pre-eclampsia (see p.426).

Hormone effects

The pregnancy hormones produced by your placenta will result in further changes to your body. Your breasts will swell even more and may fill up with milk, even squirting small quantities at unexpected times. However, not every woman experiences this symptom and you may never see a drop of milk or colostrum leaking from your breasts until after the baby has been born and you start to breastfeed. Many women notice an increase in their vaginal discharge, which may look slightly brown or pink, particularly if you have had sex recently. This is usually nothing to worry about and is merely a further sign that your cervix has become softer because of the increased blood supply it is receiving. As a result it can become bruised and bleed slightly, even with light contact. However, any bright red vaginal bleeding, particularly if it is accompanied by pain, should be reported as a matter of urgency.

> 66
> ...this is not the time to worry that you cannot bother your midwife again because you have already called her three times this week...
> 99

How you may feel physically

You have now reached your maximum size and find that you bump into things and feel quite clumsy. You need to take care when going up and down stairs because your centre of gravity has altered significantly and you can no longer see your feet.

During these last few weeks of your pregnancy, Braxton Hicks' contractions (see pp.237–8) will be a constant reminder of the fact that labour could start at any time. True labour contractions are much stronger and more painful, but if you are in any doubt about what you are experiencing you should always seek advice. Your doctor or midwife will encourage you to come into the maternity unit and be checked over, rather than stay at home feeling anxious. This is not the time to be ignoring abdominal pain and hoping that it will go away. Nor is it the time to worry that you cannot bother your midwife again, because you have already called her three times this week with the same symptoms. It does not matter how many false alarms there are, it is essential that uterine pain is always investigated promptly and carefully.

However much you are trying to rest at this stage, you will probably still be feeling tired because you are unlikely to be getting enough of the continuous, uninterrupted sleep that you need to restore your mental and physical energy. Good-quality sleep involves cycles of four different stages from light sleep to deep sleep followed by REM (Rapid Eye Movement) sleep, which is when you dream. If you are woken during any of these stages, the sleep cycle goes back to stage one when you fall asleep again. As a result, you miss out on the all-important deep sleep and REM stages and wake feeling poorly refreshed. Even if you manage to doze and sleep for quite long stretches of time, the repeated lack of good-quality sleep will mean that you become progressively more weary and exhausted.

Impatience and frustration

The most common emotions women experience at this late stage of pregnancy are impatience that they are still waiting for D–day to arrive and frustration because there is no way of knowing when it will occur. By now, many women feel quite desperate to reach the end of their pregnancy, however enjoyable it has been.

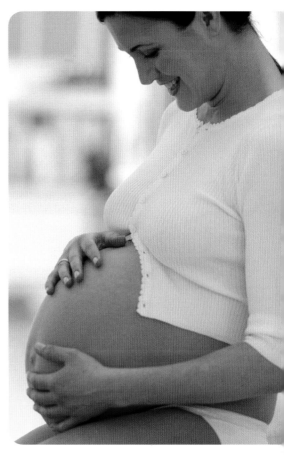

MAGNIFICENT By the end of your pregnancy, your bump can be a source of amusement coupled with sheer amazement.

If you are feeling much like this, remind yourself that the end is in sight. Even if you go overdue, there is only a set number of days left to go. Nevertheless, one of the other pressures you will have to deal with at this point is that, the closer you get to your due date, the more you will have to field enquiries about when you are due, and telephone calls asking if you have had the baby yet. Your friends and family obviously mean well when they show such interest, but many of you will feel even more irritated by being constantly reminded that your long-awaited baby has still not arrived.

Labour represents an enormous emotional and physical challenge and I suspect that many of you will be viewing it with a mixture of excitement and apprehension, since it is almost impossible to predict exactly how it will proceed and how your body will respond. As several women have commented to me recently, it is easier to train for a marathon than for labour. If you still feel seriously apprehensive, have a detailed discussion with your carers so they can understand and address your fears.

Your antenatal care

During the last stages of pregnancy, you will have check-ups at 36, 38, 40, and 41 weeks. Be sure to tell your doctor or midwife about any new or unusual symptom, any issues that are worrying you or anything that does not feel quite right with the baby, even if you cannot put your finger on the exact problem.

All the usual antenatal tests will be performed and you may have another blood count if you have been feeling very tired, or have been taking iron tablets for anaemia that has been previously diagnosed. Your carers will look for obvious signs of severe fluid retention (oedema) and if you have noticed any sudden swelling in your fingers, ankles or face, arrange for blood tests and more frequent checks of your blood pressure if there is any suspicion that you are developing pre-eclampsia. Women with late pregnancy complications are usually asked to come to a day-care centre or a special area in the unit which provides more detailed monitoring (see pp.256–9).

Your doctor or midwife will palpate your abdomen carefully at each of your antenatal visits and record the findings in your hand-held antenatal notes. At this stage of your pregnancy, it becomes important to assess the lie and presentation of your baby and whether the presenting part has started to engage in the pelvis. These findings influence the plans that are made for your labour, may determine the type of delivery that is best for both you and your baby, and will help your antenatal carers to assess your progress when labour is underway.

> " ...a deeply engaged head is usually a good sign that labour will be swift and uncomplicated. "

Is the head engaged?

Pregnant women are often unsure about what is meant by the term engagement, so a brief explanation of engagement and the abbreviations used to describe it in your notes may be useful. Strictly speaking, the baby's head is not properly engaged until more than half of it (three-fifths of the head) has passed through the pelvic brim in the mother's abdomen. The best way to assess engagement is with an abdominal palpation.

• **(High/Fr)** – if your carers can feel all of the head in the mother's abdomen, your notes will record that the baby's head is high or free.

• **(NE/Neng)** – when they can feel more than half (three-fifths or four-fifths) of the head above the pubic bone, they will either write in the notes that the baby is not engaged in the pelvis or state exactly how much of the head is palpable abdominally, for example, ⅗ or ⅘.

• (**E/Eng**) – when they can feel less than half the head (just two-fifths of it) above the pubic bone, the baby's head is engaged. If there is only one-fifth or no fifths left to feel, the notes will record that the head is deeply engaged.

The other way to assess engagement is by performing a vaginal examination. Nowadays these are rarely done in the antenatal clinic, although they are performed regularly during the labour to monitor the progress of your baby's downwards descent through the pelvis. However, there may be occasions when an antenatal vaginal examination is helpful. For example, it can be difficult to assess the height of the head abdominally in very overweight women, near to term. Similarly, when the baby's head is very deeply engaged and the shoulder is positioned just above the pelvic brim, it can be difficult to decide which part of the baby is being palpated. Accuracy is important here because, if you go into labour with your baby's head high and free, there is the potential for all sorts of serious complications such as cord prolapse (see p.430) to occur. On the other hand, a very deeply engaged head before labour is usually a good sign that the labour will be swift and uncomplicated.

If you are a first-time mother and your baby's head is still not engaged, you will probably have an ultrasound scan to check that there is nothing preventing your baby's head from engaging, such as a low-lying placenta or a uterine fibroid or ovarian cyst. If the baby's head cannot travel past the obstruction, delivery usually has to be by Caesarean section. Occasionally, the high head may be because your pelvis is too small to allow the fetal head to engage – the medical term for this problem is cephalopelvic disproportion (CPD). This is

ENGAGEMENT ···

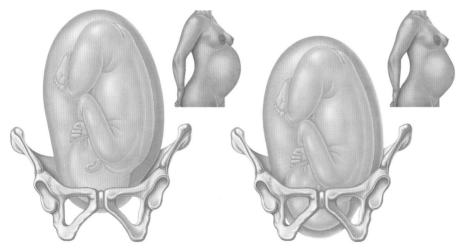

NOT ENGAGED
The baby's head is still at the brim of your pelvis and the uterus is at its maximum height.

ENGAGED The baby has dropped into the pelvis, producing a sudden change in the outline of your bump.

NOT ENGAGED　　　　　**ENGAGED**

always a relative diagnosis: a woman with an average-sized pelvis may develop CPD if her baby is very large, but in her next pregnancy may have a smaller baby and not experience any disproportion. True CPD – where the mother's pelvis is too narrow to allow even the smallest of babies to engage – is rare. However, if it is suspected, you will probably be advised to have an internal examination and an MRI scan to provide accurate information about the size of your pelvis.

Having said all that, high heads can settle down and engage in the pelvis right up until the last minute of pregnancy. Adopting a wait-and-see attitude is usually the best policy when it comes to engagement.

> When I was training I was taught to think of posterior positions as similar to trying to fit a right shoe on to a left foot...

Presentation and lie

Your antenatal notes will probably contain written entries from several different people by the time you reach term, and as they may all include their own abbreviations to describe the lie, presentation, and position of your baby, you may be feeling rather confused at this stage. The following information should help to give you a clearer picture of your baby's position.

• As I have mentioned previously, the lie of your baby is either longitudinal (L/long), which means a vertical position in your uterus, transverse (T/Tr), lying horizontally, or oblique (Obl), in a diagonal position (see p.213).

• The presenting part of your baby is the part that lies closest to the cervix and the one that will therefore present itself to the world first. In a longitudinal lie, this can be either cephalic (C/Ceph), which means head down, or breech (B/Br), which means bottom downwards. When the lie is transverse or oblique, there is no presenting part. By 35–36 weeks most babies are cephalic presentations, and by term 95 per cent will be head down, 4 per cent will be breech presentations, and 1 per cent will be transverse or oblique.

• The position of the baby refers to the relationship between the baby's spine and the back of its head (occiput) and the inner wall of the uterine cavity. Hence the baby's position can be anterior (in front), lateral (to the side), posterior (at the back), and facing either to the right or left. An anterior or lateral position at the onset of labour is considered normal.

• The attitude of the baby describes the relationship between the head and the rest of the baby's body. The normal attitude is fully flexed or curled up with the limbs and head tucked into the body. If the baby's head and neck are extended backwards, this will result in an abnormal brow presentation (see p.430).

Posterior presentation

If the baby takes up a posterior position in the pelvis, meaning that the occiput rotates towards the mother's spine and the baby is effectively facing forwards, the labour is likely to be longer and more difficult. The baby's head simply does not fit so well into the pelvis in a posterior position and the normal mechanics of labour are interfered with. When I was training, I was taught to think of posterior positions as similar to trying to fit a right shoe on to a left foot – possible but clumsy. Fortunately, only about 13 per cent of babies (and they are usually first babies) start labour in the posterior position, and about 65 per cent of these turn during the labour and can be delivered normally. Occasionally a baby is born spontaneously positioned "face to pubes".

A breech presentation

If your baby is breech at 35–36 weeks, it is still possible that it may turn spontaneously. If your baby is breech at term, as occurs in about 4 per cent of pregnancies, a vaginal delivery may be possible (see p.357). However, since breech labours and deliveries are usually more complicated, your antenatal carers may be reluctant to care for you in your own home or non-specialist maternity unit.

During the first stage of labour, a breech baby will not dilate the cervix as effectively as a cephalic presentation and as a result labour is more likely to be prolonged and the baby more prone to develop distress, requiring emergency interventions. If your waters break and your baby is still in a breech position, you are at risk of a cord prolapse and need to go to your maternity unit immediately. This is because a breech baby does not fit the pelvis as snugly as a down baby head would do, so the umbilical cord can slip past the baby's bottom or legs and fall through the cervix, which is a potentially life-threatening situation for your baby. Another major concern is during the second stage of labour, because there is no way of knowing whether your pelvis can accommodate the largest part of the baby's body, the head, before the limbs and trunk have been delivered. There are three main breech positions:

• **In a frank breech**, the legs are flexed at the hip and the knees are extended straight up in front of the baby – this is the best position for a vaginal delivery.
• **In a complete breech**, the legs are flexed and folded tightly in front of the baby – a vaginal delivery is sometimes possible.
• **In a footling breech**, the legs are extended below the baby and one or both feet are presenting first – a vaginal delivery is inadvisable.

In days gone by, women who were carrying a breech baby underwent X-rays and more recently ultrasound scans and MRI scans of their pelvis to assess whether the size of the pelvic outlet was wide enough for them to attempt a vaginal delivery. Nowadays, you are unlikely to have these unless you specifically request a vaginal breech delivery. The main reason for this is that recent research suggests that Caesarean section may be safest mode of delivery for a breech baby, in terms

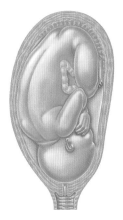

ANTERIOR PRESENTATION

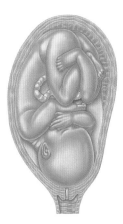

POSTERIOR PRESENTATION

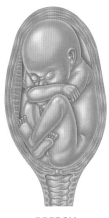

BREECH PRESENTATION

YOUR BABY'S POSITION

Your baby's position is determined by where its occiput and spine are lying in the uterus as the baby passes into the pelvic brim. The six most common positions are shown here along with their abbreviations and percentages indicating how often they occur. Direct anterior (OA) and direct posterior (OP) positions, in which the baby is facing directly towards or away from your spine, are rare. Breech presentations are defined by the position of the baby's bottom (sacrum). The most common is right sacro anterior (RSA) with the baby's spine towards the front of the uterus.

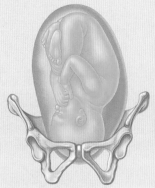

LOL: LEFT OCCIPITO-LATERAL (40%) The baby's back and occiput are positioned on the left side of the uterus at right angles to your spine.

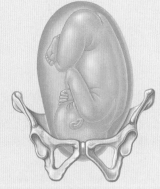

LOA: LEFT OCCIPITO-ANTERIOR (12%) In this position, the baby's back and occiput are nearer to the front of your uterus on the left.

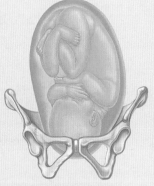

LOP: LEFT OCCIPITO-POSTERIOR (3%) The baby's back and occiput are towards your spine on the left side of your uterus.

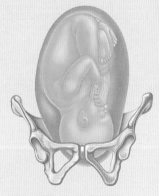

ROL: RIGHT OCCIPITO-LATERAL (25%) The baby's back and occiput are at right angles to your spine on the right-hand side of your uterus.

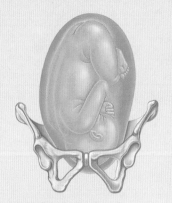

ROA: RIGHT OCCIPITO-ANTERIOR (10%) The baby's back and occiput are towards the front of your uterus on the right-hand side.

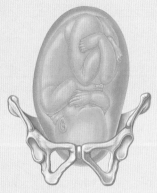

ROP: RIGHT OCCIPITO-POSTERIOR (10%) In this position, the baby's spine and occiput are towards your spine on the right-hand side of the uterus.

of both labour and delivery complications and possibly the long-term neurological development of the baby. If you are keen to have a vaginal delivery, it is worth considering allowing your midwife or obstetrician to try turning the baby around manually, a procedure called external cephalic version (ECV), which has a 50–70 per cent success rate. The procedure is not suitable in every case and is contraindicated if you have had complications in a previous or current pregnancy.

ECV is done in the labour ward or specialist day-care ward at about 37–38 weeks and should only be attempted by an experienced practitioner. There should be immediate access to emergency delivery if complications arise. You will have an ultrasound scan and a CTG of the baby's heart and be asked to empty your bladder before the obstetrician attempts to rotate your baby inside the uterus by gentle sustained pressure, keeping the baby's head well flexed. Raising the end of the bed may help to disengage the breech from the pelvis and you may be asked to inhale some salbutamol or be given a subcutaneous injection of terbutaline to relax the uterine muscles. The scan and CTG are usually repeated after the procedure, and if your blood group is Rhesus negative, you will be given an anti-D injection. About 50–70 per cent of ECVs are successful and the baby remains head down.

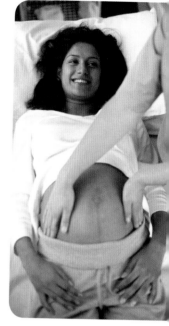

POST-MATURE Your carers will assess the position and engagement of your baby's head.

When your baby is overdue

If your due date arrives and you have not yet gone into labour, your pregnancy is referred to as post-mature or overdue. About 45 per cent of women are still pregnant at 40 weeks, but the majority deliver during the next week and only 15 per cent go beyond 41 weeks.

What happens when your baby is overdue depends on the type of birth you are hoping for and the policy on induction of labour (see pp.294–7) at your maternity unit. The sequence below is what is offered in my own hospital and although timings may vary, the basic procedures will be the same in all antenatal clinics.
• First, your midwife and doctor will check the accuracy of your expected delivery date, using a combination of last menstrual period (LMP) dates and early scan measurements – wherever they are available. Many units advise you to continue until the 41-week check-up, either at home or in the antenatal clinic, after which they will assess the position and engagement of the fetal head and will advise an internal examination to assess how ripe the cervix is.
• If the head is well down and the cervix sufficiently soft and dilated, your carers will usually offer to "sweep" the membranes around the baby at the top of the

cervix to release chemicals called prostaglandins, which may help to start uterine contractions. If this is not an option, your carers will discuss the pros and cons of induction (starting labour artificially) versus waiting for a little longer.

• If you decide to wait, you will probably be asked to attend the maternity day-care unit for a post-maturity assessment (see below) at 41 weeks and 3 days. If the assessment is satisfactory and no problems are found, you may wish to continue your wait, in which case your baby will be assessed again at two-day intervals until 42 weeks, when you will most likely be advised to undergo induction of labour. In my experience, it is unusual for women to choose to continue beyond 42 weeks, but if they do, regular CTGs and biophysical profile scoring will be needed.

• If at any stage, your post-maturity assessment is abnormal in any way, your carers will discuss the need to induce labour and deliver your baby. Although research shows that induction is likely to result in a higher incidence of prolonged labour and instrumental deliveries, there are conclusive studies showing that it does not increase the Caesarean section rate. On the other hand, leaving the pregnancy until the end of 42 weeks may increase the risk of fetal distress or even unexplained stillbirth, if the placenta stops functioning well. Even when the placenta is working well and the baby is continuing to grow after 41 weeks, there is also the risk of a difficult or obstructed labour if the pregnancy is left too long because the baby becomes increasingly large.

It is unusual for the assessment findings to be so dramatic that they prompt an immediate decision to deliver the baby but, if this is the case for you, you may be advised that Caesarean section is the safest course of action. Having said that, everyone involved in looking after you will do his or her very best to achieve an induction of labour and vaginal delivery, if this is what you would prefer.

> " Having sex is another option that, theoretically, should encourage labour to start... "

• If you need to have a post-maturity assessment, your carers will start by checking the exact size of your baby (see pp.256–7) and the amount of amniotic fluid in the uterine sac (see p.259). The results may prompt them to perform a detailed Doppler blood flow assessment (see p.257). The scanners will also perform a biophysical profile of the baby (see p.259) looking carefully at the limb movements, muscular tone, breathing movements and heart-rate pattern in order to help assess the baby's general wellbeing. Most units will also offer a computerized CTG (see pp.258–9), a pictorial print-out generated by an electronic machine that assesses your baby's heart rate to see whether the criteria for a healthy baby are met within a certain period of time. They will also look at the placenta and grade its appearance and texture, which gives a rough indication of how well it is working. All of these tests are prone to error so should be considered as indicators, rather than as definite diagnoses.

COMMON QUESTIONS IN LATE PREGNANCY

▶ How can I prepare for the pain of labour?

If you have been feeling frightened about the imminent labour and delivery, have a detailed discussion about your anxiety with your midwife and doctor so they can understand exactly what your fears are and respond to them individually. I hope that you will have already had plenty of conversations with your midwife and parent education facilitator about the different options for pain relief available to you during early labour (see pp.308–23). In early labour, many women find TENS machines, breathing exercises, massage and having a long soak in a warm bath especially soothing and relaxing.

▶ My baby seems less active than before. How can I be sure that everything is OK?

Many babies change their pattern of movement during the last few weeks of pregnancy, usually because there is no longer sufficient space in your uterus for them to move around and kick as freely as before. If you have not felt the baby moving during the last few hours, try provoking a kick or jolt, by prodding your abdomen, coughing or changing your position. If this does not work, then you need to seek advice immediately. You will most likely be advised to attend the maternity unit for a heart trace (CTG) (see pp.258–9), to ensure that all is well. You may also be given a fetal movement or kick chart to fill in over the next couple of days, but as I have mentioned before I have mixed feelings about these because I firmly believe that babies develop their own individual patterns of movement late in pregnancy, and that it is a change in this pattern that needs to be reported and investigated promptly, not the actual number of movements or kicks.

▶ I have had enough of being pregnant. What can I do to help start my labour?

Although the following ideas are by no means proven, some are worth a try. Eating a hot curry is traditionally thought to help kick-start some action, presumably because it may encourage a bowel movement. Taking castor oil is a much less enjoyable version of the same idea.

If you have not felt like moving around much for the last few weeks, some exercise may help to move the baby down a bit inside your pelvis. The more pressure exerted on your cervix, the more likely that labour will start. Try taking a long walk to see if this helps to start your labour.

Having sex is another option that, theoretically, should encourage labour to start, because semen contains prostaglandins – chemicals similar to those in the pessaries used to induce labour. So if you're not too exhausted, give it a go. Nipple stimulation is often cited as a way of inducing labour because it releases the hormone oxytocin, which stimulates the uterus. That said, you or your partner would need to stimulate your nipples for around one hour, three times a day, to have any significant effect, so I suspect that this is unlikely to be the most helpful option!

▶ How can I distinguish between vaginal bleeding and a show?

The simple answer is that you cannot know until you have been checked out, so speak to your midwife straight away. A typical show includes the loss of a mucus-like plug, mixed with fresh red and old brown blood, but it is always best to ensure that there is no other cause of fresh red bleeding, particularly if it is accompanied by sudden abdominal pain. (See placenta praevia, placental abruption, and antepartum haemorrhage, p.428).

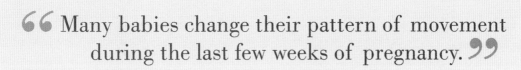

66 Many babies change their pattern of movement during the last few weeks of pregnancy. 99

PREPARING FOR A HOME BIRTH

If you are planning a home birth, make sure that all the practical arrangements are not left to the last minute. You don't want to find yourself hunting for towels from the bottom of the laundry basket in the middle of a contraction.

The midwife who is to attend your delivery will bring all the necessary medical equipment with her (see list, below), but make sure you have discussed with her, several weeks before the expected date, exactly what she expects you to provide. She will also be able to give you some useful tips about additional, non-essential items that you may find helpful during your labour and delivery.

MIDWIFE'S DELIVERY PACK

EQUIPMENT
▶ blood pressure monitor
▶ thermometer
▶ Pinard stethoscope
▶ Doppler sonicaid
▶ gloves
▶ cord clamp
▶ oxygen cylinder
▶ baby resuscitation equipment
▶ antiseptic solutions
▶ urine test sticks
▶ scissors
▶ stitching equipment/ perineal repair kit
▶ intravenous drip set

PAIN RELIEF/DRUGS
▶ gas and air/entonox cylinder
▶ pethidine; co-dydramol
▶ local anaesthetic
▶ syntocinon; misoprostol

PACK A MATERNITY BAG
You might think this is a strange idea as you are not actually going to hospital, but packing a maternity bag (see p.277) is a good way to ensure that all your essential personal items are gathered together in one place, ready for use when the time comes. This will also be useful if things do not go according to plan and you end up in hospital for any reason.

ORGANIZE YOUR BABY EQUIPMENT
Assembling a bag or assigning a drawer or cupboard for all the basic items you will need for the new baby is a sensible idea. You may be planning to deliver at home, but very soon you will be going out and about with your new baby, so don't forget to organize a portable Moses basket or carrycot and a car seat.

PLAN WHERE YOU WANT TO DELIVER THE BABY
The essential requirements are comfort, warmth, and cleanliness. Make sure that you have plenty of plastic sheeting to protect bedding, mattresses, chairs, and the floor and large bin bags to clear up the rubbish. You will also need lots of towels, copious hot water, soap, bowls, and sponges. If you are going to use your bed, it should be easily accessible to your midwife from both sides. Several changes of bed sheets will come in useful, together with extra pillows or cushions.

EXTRA COMFORTS
You may want to have a birthing ball, bean bag or large floor cushions available to you during the labour. There is no reason why you should not use a birthing pool at home, but this will have to be hired well in advance. Although you may prefer to have dim lighting to help you relax during the labour, your midwife will need a good source of light to see what she is doing, especially after the delivery when you may need stitches, so have a portable, directable lamp close at hand.

Things to consider

Most of the considerations at this stage of pregnancy tend to be practical, concerning preparations for the birth and the period afterwards. Having said that, your most pressing concern is likely to be knowing for certain when your labour has really begun.

There are lots of possible indicators but no hard and fast rules, so interpreting exactly what is happening to you when you are in labour, most probably for the first time, is not easy. I've included the key signs and symptoms at the beginning of the Labour and Birth chapter (see pp.283–6) so I suggest you turn to those pages now. As always, seek advice and reassurance whenever you feel unsure – no one will accuse you of wasting time if your symptoms turn out to be a false alarm.

Clothes for comfort

In the last few weeks of the third trimester, you may find it useful to buy some special maternity knickers to accommodate your vastly enlarged abdomen. These garments will never win any fashion prizes, but they can make a world of difference to your comfort, particularly if you have been suffering with underwear that is continually slipping down or riding up into uncomfortable positions. Some women also find that wearing a light girdle, positioned under their bump (not constricting it), helps to support their abdomen and reduce symptoms of backache and weariness. Both of these items can be found in maternity shops and specialist mail-order catalogues.

If you are planning to breastfeed, you will need a couple of good feeding bras so that you are comfortable in hospital and when you return home. These need to be properly fitted in a specialist shop or department store by trained fitters who know how much room to allow for the fact that your breasts will expand when your milk comes in. You will also need to find nightwear with a really low-fronted button opening that will allow you to breastfeed. This may sound overly fussy, but breastfeeding really does become easier if you feel comfortable and at ease. If every feed involves struggling in and out of your clothing, you will become increasingly irritated – especially when you are embarking on your third feed of the night at five in the morning.

This is a good time to choose clothes to wear into hospital – something comfortable that you do not mind becoming soiled – a loose-fitting dress, or

> 66 ...maternity knickers will never win any fashion prizes, but they can make a world of difference to your comfort. 99

a baggy T-shirt with stretchy trousers. You will also need a fresh nightdress for after the delivery and a dressing gown and slippers for the postnatal ward.

Getting ready for your baby

If you are going home from hospital by car, the law requires that you have a special baby car seat in which to take your baby home. Your partner can bring it in when you are ready to leave, together with a bonnet, outside clothes, and shawl or light blanket in which to wrap your new baby. You do not need a Moses basket, carry cot, pram or pushchair until you are safely installed at home.

You may already have arranged a nursery in your home or may choose to have your baby in your bedroom for the first few weeks, when she will need several feeds each night. You will need a Moses basket, or a cot, together with a waterproof mattress, cotton sheets, and warm cotton cellular blankets. Don't use a pillow for your baby, and if you choose to have bumpers around the edges of the cot to prevent your baby hitting the edges, they should be free of ribbons, tassels, and bows so that there is no risk of your baby putting them in her mouth or becoming tangled up in them.

If you plan to breastfeed, you will probably do this in bed during the night, so make sure you have plenty of muslin cloths close at hand, to cope with the inevitable possets of regurgitated milk. You may be planning to move your baby into a separate room after a while, so make sure there is a comfortable chair to sit on for night-time feeds. If you have decided to bottle-feed, then you will need a sterilizing unit and some bottles and teats available when you return home (see p.229). To reduce the risk of gastrointestinal problems it is best to make the bottle feeds up as and when you need them rather than storing them for many hours.

Whichever sort of nappies you have chosen to buy (see p.229), make sure you have a good supply and also cotton wool and baby wipes for cleaning up your baby. Your newborn baby has very sensitive skin and the best way to avoid getting nappy rash is to use cotton wool soaked in ordinary tap water. Wipes are useful when you are travelling or out and about, but opt for the gentlest (hypoallergenic) type for your newborn baby. Some baby products are bulky to carry home and it is worth considering online shopping – many supermarkets and other retailers can supply a wide range of baby products directly to your front door.

❝ Don't forget that grandparents can make an enormously valuable contribution in the first few days after the birth. ❞

Aim to stock your store cupboard and freezer with easy-to-prepare food or ready-prepared meals to get you through the first few days when you return home. This is not the time to feel guilty about the lack of home-made meals. Also make sure that you have enough coffee, tea, milk and biscuits for visitors.

If you have other children, make some plans to entertain them when you first return home with the new baby, so that they do not feel too left out of the limelight. You will find that other mothers of small children are more than happy to rally round and invite yours for tea, a day out or even a sleep-over, depending on their age, given a signal from you that offers of practical help are welcome. Don't forget that grandparents can make an enormously valuable contribution during the first few days after the birth. There is nothing they will like more than having uninterrupted time with your toddler and making her feel special.

YOUR MATERNITY BAG

Try to avoid packing a heavy suitcase suitable for a two-week, long-haul holiday. Remember that your partner, family and friends can always bring in extra or missing items. Unless you find yourself giving birth in an emergency situation and have not had a chance to pack a bag, most maternity units will expect you to supply most of the items that you will need during labour and your stay after the birth.

ESSENTIALS FOR YOUR LABOUR BAG
▶ Nightdress or large T-shirt
▶ Personal toiletries/washing kit
▶ Sanitary towels
▶ Changes of underwear
▶ Camera
▶ Mobile phone with the telephone numbers of people you want to call from hospital. Be sensitive to those around you and to your own needs when using a smart phone. Too much technology may distract you from the task in hand.

OPTIONAL ITEMS
▶ Video camera (check unit policy)
▶ Face spray, sponge, lipsalve, massage oil
▶ Personal stereo, music, magazines, books
▶ Change of clothes for your partner
▶ Food and drink for your partner

THE BABY'S BAG
▶ A pack of newborn-size nappies
▶ Zinc barrier/nappy cream
▶ Cotton wool balls
▶ Two sleepsuits
▶ Two vests

FOR AFTER THE BIRTH
▶ One nightdress (front-opening if breastfeeding)
▶ Disposable knickers or several of your oldest pairs
▶ Extra-absorbent sanitary towels (bulky but a must)
▶ Breast pads
▶ Toiletries
▶ Towel

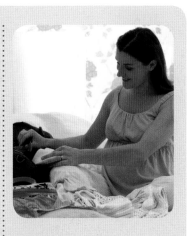

▶ Slippers
▶ Dressing gown
▶ Favourite snacks, high-energy foods, drinks
▶ Ice pack and/or a heated pad

OPTIONAL ITEMS
▶ Ear-plugs and eye mask (to help block out noise and light)
▶ Reading material including a good book about practical childcare
▶ Pillow (many maternity units are unable to provide more than one)

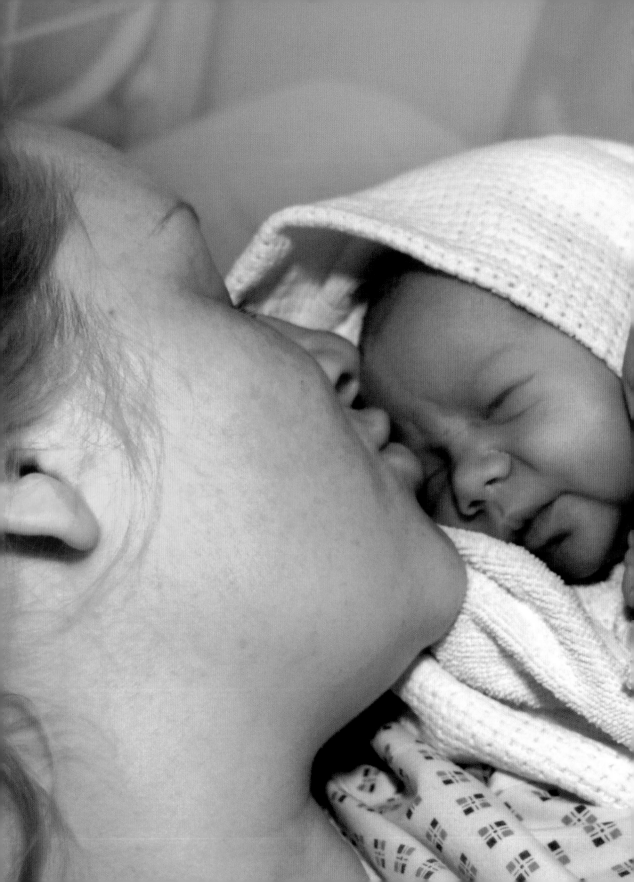

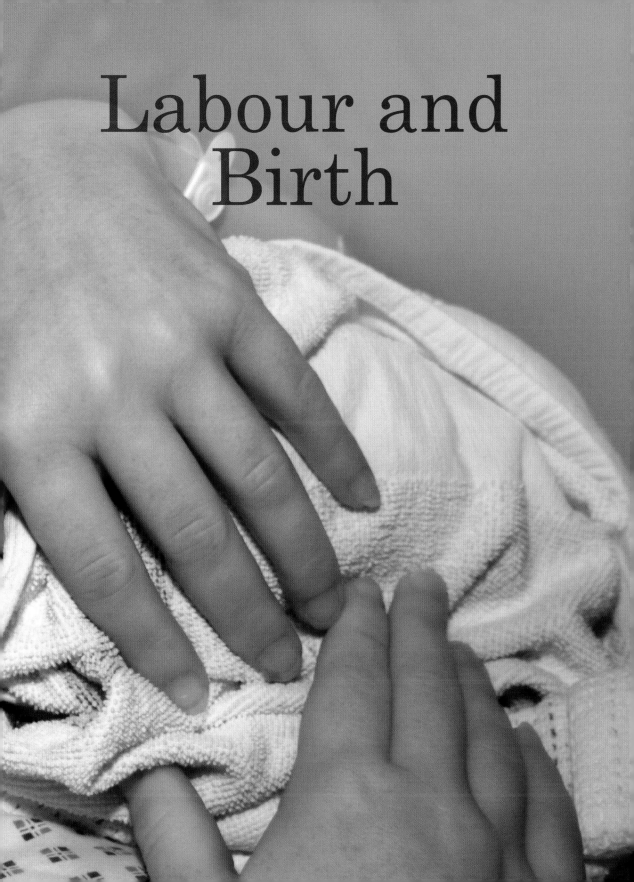

Labour and Birth

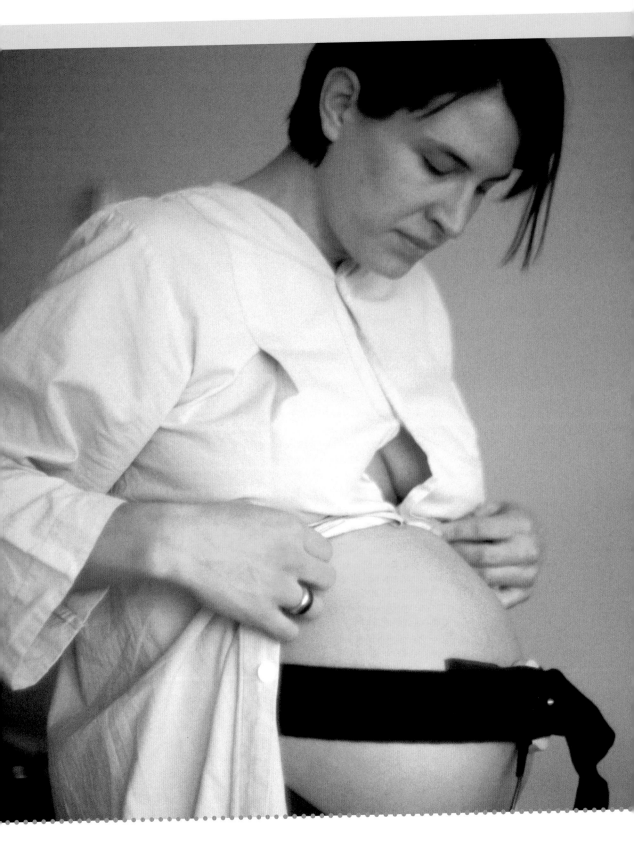

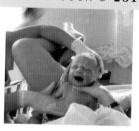

The stages of labour

The only predictable thing about pregnancy is that it always comes to an end – in the vast majority of cases with the delivery of a healthy baby to a healthy mother after a normal labour and vaginal delivery. I regularly reflect on the fact that this is an extraordinary achievement, since decades of research have failed to establish exactly what triggers labour. Indeed, if we better understood this process, we would be able to predict when it was going to happen and take steps to prevent it occurring prematurely.

CONTENTS

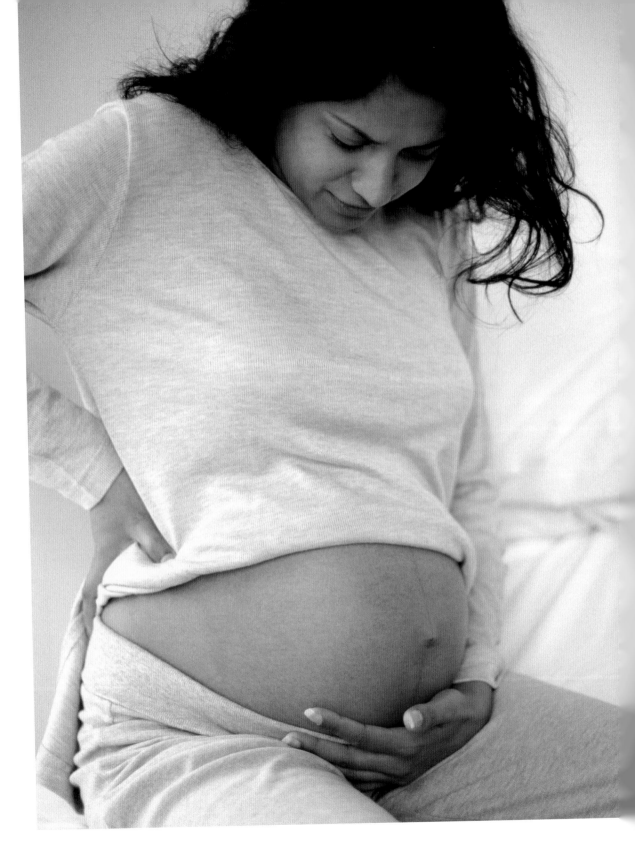

The first stage

GOING INTO LABOUR IS ALWAYS AN EXCITING TIME as your pregnancy nears its end and you embark on the next steps of this amazing journey. During the first stage, your uterus will contract repeatedly causing your cervix to thin, shorten, and dilate. Only when your cervix is fully dilated can your baby's head pass into the birth canal ready for delivery.

There is no right or wrong way to go into labour. Every woman does it differently and no two labours are the same. Interestingly, towards the end of pregnancy, women are often more concerned about the symptoms and signs that they are likely to experience in the pre-labour and early labour phases of giving birth than in the three stages of established labour. The questions they ask are not simple to answer, because the pre-labour stage can last for days or you may skip it completely and be 5cm dilated before you know it.

Symptoms and signs of early labour

There are various signs and symptoms that indicate the end of pregnancy and the start of your labour are not too far away.

Engagement of the baby's head is one of the signs that labour is likely to occur soon for first-time mothers. During the last few weeks of pregnancy your antenatal carers will be assessing the position and descent of your baby's head into the pelvis. When it engages (see p.267 and p.302) you will probably notice that your breathing becomes easier and that your indigestion and heartburn are improved since the pressure in your abdomen has been somewhat relieved. Instead, you will be feeling a new pressure in your pelvis and it is likely that you will need to pass urine more frequently. However, if this is not your first baby, engagement of your baby's head may not occur until shortly before, or even after, labour starts.

Braxton Hicks' practice contractions (see p.237) are likely to become stronger and more frequent in the pre-labour stage. They are usually painless, although some women may find them uncomfortable. It is easy to mistake them for real labour contractions, particularly if they are strong and this is your first baby. However, Braxton Hicks' contractions occur irregularly, rarely more than two per hour, and they fade away, whereas labour pains start slowly but build up gradually in strength and frequency.

> " …every woman goes into labour differently and no two labours are the same. "

Your cervical canal has contained a plug of mucus throughout pregnancy, designed to prevent infection ascending from the vagina into the uterus. As the cervix starts to soften, shorten and dilate, this plug becomes dislodged and the thick discharge that results is referred to as the "show". It is frequently tinged with small quantities of blood, since the mucus plug was attached to your cervical canal by small blood vessels or capillaries. The appearance of the show is often interpreted as a sign that labour is imminent. The reality is that you can have a show and still find yourself pregnant many days later. Nonetheless, loss of the cervical plug is a demonstration that your cervix is changing and is a sign that the end of pregnancy is in sight.

If your vaginal discharge becomes watery or you pass a gush of clear fluid, your waters may have broken (ruptured membranes) or you may have merely leaked some urine. It is important to find out what has occurred so put on a sanitary pad to soak up any further fluid and contact your midwife promptly. She will examine you to decide whether you are leaking liquor or urine (see p.286).

The pre-labour emotional symptoms experienced by pregnant women are varied. Some women find their nesting instinct goes into overdrive and they rush around finishing as many tasks as possible. Others prefer to avoid venturing too far from home in case anything happens. This is undoubtedly a strange and unpredictable period of time, during which you may feel as if you are in limbo. This can give rise to feelings of anticipation, excitement, impatience, anxiety and fear. The fear is usually focused on what might happen in labour and, in particular, on how you will deal with the pain involved. Reading about the available methods of pain relief (see pp.308–23) will help you to feel more relaxed, confident and in control of the exciting developments ahead.

> 66
> Your antenatal carers are there to give you advice and practical help 24 hours a day.
> 99

Recognizing true labour

This is one of the biggest worries for many women. Thinking labour has started in earnest only to be sent home by the hospital is disappointing. But remember that your antenatal carers deal with these uncertainties on a daily basis and it does not matter how many false alarms there are, as long as you and your baby are safe. Most pregnant women do experience symptoms and signs that suggest they have begun to labour (see box opposite) and they now need to seek advice. However, these signs come in no specific order and you may not experience all of them. It is also important to remember that early labour does not always progress in a steady line. You might experience one or several symptoms followed by hours of no activity at all, only for events suddenly to pick up speed again. Overall, there will be a tendency for your uterine contractions to become gradually stronger and more painful, but this increase in strength does not necessarily occur steadily. It is quite common to experience a period of painful contractions followed by a run of contractions that are less intense in strength.

Most first-time mothers are very aware when they are labouring, because the contractions take longer to establish as the uterus has never attempted to expel a baby before. In second and subsequent births, the labour can be quick, and if the contractions have been bearable throughout, there are occasions when the mother will not realize she has reached full dilatation until she experiences an overwhelming urge to push the baby out. However, it is unusual for women not to make it to hospital in time, or to find themselves delivering on their own at home before the midwife arrives (see p.289).

SIGNS OF TRUE LABOUR

▶ Your contractions are occurring regularly every 15 minutes or so (time them).
▶ Your contractions are getting longer, stronger, and closer together.
▶ Walking around or changing positions does not make your contractions go away.
▶ You have pain in your lower back, as opposed to your lower abdomen.
▶ You feel the need to empty your bowels.
▶ You are passing fluid that you don't think is urine (ruptured membranes, see p.286).
▶ Your cervix is undergoing changes (these will be apparent from a midwife's examination).

Contacting your midwife or hospital

Any time you are worried or unsure about what is happening or what you should do, contact your midwife or maternity unit. Your antenatal carers are there to give you advice and practical help and are available 24 hours a day. Whether or not you are advised to go to hospital will depend on many factors:

• whether this is a first, second or subsequent birth
• the strength and frequency of your contractions
• how you are dealing with them at home
• if you have had any vaginal bleeding (more than a show)
• how far away from the hospital you live
• whether your waters have broken
• whether your baby's movements have changed significantly.

Broadly speaking, if you have had no complications during pregnancy and this is your first baby, your midwife will probably advise that you stay at home until your contractions are regular. There are no hard and fast rules but if the contractions are occurring every 15 minutes, lasting for about one minute (time them), and are so uncomfortable that you are forced to stop what you are doing, you should be thinking about going into hospital. If you live some distance away from the maternity unit or are likely to meet difficulties or delays on the journey, you may want to allow plenty of time to get to the hospital.

Another important consideration is how you are coping with the contractions and whether you feel you will need some pain relief in the near future. Many women feel more comfortable, both physically and emotionally, with the knowledge that a variety of pain relief is close at hand once they reach the hospital (see pp.308–23).

Waters breaking

> 66
> ...if your waters break before your contractions start, this invariably kick-starts labour.
> 99

If your waters break (membranes rupture) before the onset of regular or irregular uterine contractions, then it is sensible to seek advice from your midwife or doctor. If you are near to term and you and your midwife know that the baby's head is deeply engaged, you may not need to be checked over straight away and can safely wait at home for several hours to see what happens. However, now that the protective amniotic seal around your baby has been broken, you should not lie in a bath (shower instead) and ensure that you clean yourself carefully after passing a stool to reduce the risk of infection developing in the uterus.

If, on the other hand, your waters break before 37 weeks or if the amniotic fluid is not the colour of clear straw, but tinged green or black, you need to contact the hospital immediately. This sign means that your baby is currently or has been excreting meconium into the amniotic fluid, which invariably means that he has been exposed to stress and that delivery should be sooner rather than later. Meconium is the thick sticky substance present in the baby's digestive system during pregnancy. If the baby is distressed, the response of the nervous system affects the digestive system with the result that some meconium will be expelled from the gut into the amniotic fluid.

In fact, in only 15 per cent of pregnancies do the waters break before contractions have started, and when this does happen it invariably kick-starts labour: 60 per cent of women at term will go into labour within 24 hours of their membranes rupturing. Bear in mind, however, that once the membranes have ruptured, there is a greater chance of an infection developing and affecting the baby in the uterus. As a general rule, most hospitals advise women who have reached 35 weeks or more to undergo an induction of labour if uterine contractions have not started within 24 hours of the waters breaking (see pp.294–7).

Finally, if you see a lot of blood mixed with the fluid that you are passing, or have bright red, fresh bleeding that continues after the waters have broken, you must treat this as a potential emergency. Always call your midwife and make urgent arrangements to attend the labour ward.

Going to hospital

The first thing to do once your midwife or labour ward advises you to come into hospital is to pick up your maternity bag and antenatal notes. I am always impressed by how few women in labour forget to bring their notes with them, despite everything else on their minds.

As for the journey to hospital, if you are planning to travel by car, make sure you and your partner have worked out the route well in advance and also how long the journey will take at any given time of day. I trust that it goes without saying that you should not be driving yourself to the labour ward, except in very unusual circumstances. Strong uterine contractions are distracting and quite incompatible with the concentration needed to be a safe driver.

It is a good idea to have also checked out the parking facilities and to have some loose change in your maternity bag for the car park or street meters. If you arrive at the hospital in a hurry or in an emergency situation, it may not be possible to park the car as you had planned, in which case your driver should leave a note behind the windscreen and inform the hospital security desk that you need to get to the labour ward urgently and that he or she will return to sort out the car as soon as possible. If you don't have access to a car, then you will need to call a taxi or ambulance to transport you to hospital. Make sure that you give clear instructions to find your home and provide a telephone number to avoid unnecessary delays. Ambulance crews are well trained at dealing with the practicalities of labour and ensuring that you and your baby reach hospital safely – indeed they can even be relied on to deliver your baby if the need arises.

Make sure that you know which entrance to the hospital you should use when you get there and exactly how to find the labour ward – many hospitals use a different entrance to the maternity unit at night for security reasons.

> ...it goes without saying that you should not be driving yourself to the labour ward...

Admission to hospital

When you phone the hospital, the labour ward staff may arrange an ambulance to attend you. If you have made your own travel arrangements try to warn the hospital that you are on your way, so they can prepare for your arrival. When you arrive in the labour ward, you will be welcomed by a member of the midwifery team, who will show you around the unit. If you are being cared for by a community midwife (see p.85), your midwife will visit you at home when labour gets underway and will advise when you should go into hospital. She will contact

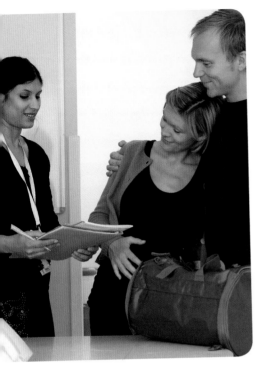

ARRIVING AT HOSPITAL Let the hospital know in advance if you think you are in labour and you are on your way in, so they can prepare for your arrival.

the maternity unit and accompany you into hospital, where she will continue to care for you. After looking through your medical notes, your midwife will check your temperature, pulse, blood pressure, and urine (for protein and glucose) and palpate your abdomen to establish the presentation of your baby and listen to the fetal heart. She will also be assessing your contractions, and will ask you questions about the pattern of activity you have noticed in your uterus so far, whether your waters have broken, and if you need some pain relief. The answers to these questions and the results of the abdominal examination may suggest that you need to have an internal examination to assess the state of your cervix. If you have written a birth plan, this will also be discussed with you.

All the findings will be recorded in your notes and if you have started to dilate (more than 4cm) and are contracting regularly, you will be declared as being "in active labour". Most maternity notes include a partogram – a section with a graphical record of how your labour is progressing with time (see p.303).

What happens next will depend on your midwife's assessment and how your maternity unit is arranged. Some units have early labour rooms in which you will stay until you are transferred to the main delivery unit just before your baby is born. Other units prefer to admit you to a room in which you will be looked after for the duration of your labour and delivery. Whatever happens, your partner will be welcome to stay with you if this is what you want.

If you are not in labour

If your contractions are weak and irregular and your membranes are still intact, an internal examination may not be necessary although you and your midwife will probably conclude that a careful assessment of the cervix will help decide on the next step. If it is decided that you are not in labour and your midwife is happy that both you and your baby are well, she will want to discuss whether you would prefer to stay in hospital for observation, or whether you can safely return home to wait for your labour to become established. The decision will depend on many factors, including how your pregnancy has been so far, your past obstetric history, how anxious or apprehensive you are feeling, and how near you live to the hospital.

There is no need to feel embarrassed if your arrival at hospital proves to be a false alarm – these are very common, particularly with first babies, and you cannot possibly be expected to know when labour has started in earnest.

MANAGING A SUDDEN DELIVERY

It is uncommon for a pregnant woman to have a labour that is so unexpected and speedy that she has to deliver her own baby. However, here is some practical advice in case you do find yourself in this situation.

Try to remain calm. This is always easier said than done, but flying into a panic will only make the situation more difficult to handle. Hopefully, your birth partner will be with you, but if this is not the case, then try to contact a neighbour or friend who is close at hand and can provide you with immediate practical help and support.

Telephone the emergency services and request an ambulance. Explain what is happening to you and also ask them to contact your midwife. Ambulance call centres and crews are well trained in talking women through labour. Make sure you keep your telephone with you at all times.

Wash your hands and your vaginal area with soap and water if at all possible. Put the kettle on to boil and collect together plenty of towels. If you have time, cover a bed or the floor with plastic sheeting, blankets, sheets, newspapers or clean towels and find a washing-up bowl that you can use to catch the amniotic fluid and blood. Then either get on to the bed or lie on the floor.

If you feel an overwhelming urge to bear down, lie down and start panting or blowing in short, controlled breaths. You may have practised this in your antenatal classes and it will help prevent the baby's head delivering suddenly.

If, despite your panting, the baby's head starts to deliver before help arrives, reach down and place your hands on the baby's head at your vulva, applying gentle counter pressure to ensure that the head emerges gradually, instead of popping out. When the baby's head has delivered, check with your fingers that there are no loops of umbilical cord around the neck, and if there are, hook them under your finger and carefully over the baby's head.

Gently stroke the sides of the baby's nose downwards and the neck and chin upwards, to help expel mucus and amniotic fluid from the nose and mouth.

Help has usually arrived by now, and the delivery of the baby's body can be aided by the ambulance crew or midwife. If you have to deal with this on your own, place your hands around the baby's head and apply firm pressure downwards (never pull or jerk) to help deliver the first shoulder. Then gently sweep the head and first shoulder upwards towards your pubic bone. This will allow the second shoulder to deliver and the rest of the body will then slip out easily and can be delivered onto your abdomen. Wrap the baby in towels or blankets immediately to keep him warm.

Do not pull on the umbilical cord, but if the placenta delivers spontaneously, elevate it so that the blood drains into the baby. There is no need to cut the cord.

The most important thing now is to ensure that both you and your baby keep warm until professional help arrives.

❝ Try to remain calm. Flying into a panic will only make the situation more difficult to handle. ❞

The delivery room

It is a good idea to take advantage of the maternity unit tours offered during the antenatal period. These provide an opportunity to see the delivery rooms and to ask questions about the procedures and equipment you are likely to come across during labour and delivery.

The delivery bed will be higher than your own bed for practical reasons. It can be raised and lowered electronically. The end of the bed will be detachable and there will be places for lithotomy poles (see below) to be attached.

The sphygomanometer is an instrument attached to a wide band of inflatable material that is placed around your upper arm to measure your blood pressure. Some are portable hand-held units, others are wall-mounted and the most modern are automatic machines on small trolleys.

Piped gas outlets and tubing in the wall above the bed are something that all hospital delivery rooms are equipped with. These deliver oxygen and pain relieving mixtures of gas and air, via masks or mouth pieces.

The baby resuscitaire is a high, moveable trolley with a platform covered by a mattress for your baby to lie on. The resuscitaire is equipped with an overhead heater to keep the baby warm, a piped oxygen supply, and drawers containing equipment that the paediatrician may need. In addition there will be a simple comfortable cot in the room for the baby to lie in after delivery.

Lithotomy poles or stirrups can be attached to special slots at either side of the delivery bed. These allow your legs to be raised and supported so you can be examined more thoroughly by the doctor or midwife should you need to have a forceps or vacuum delivery or if you require stitching after the birth. They are no longer used routinely for internal examinations during labour.

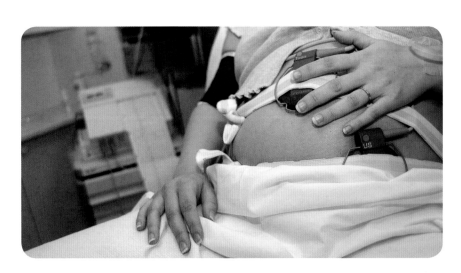

EXTERNAL ELECTRONIC FETAL MONITOR This non-invasive device is used to measure the baby's heart rate and the strength of the uterine contractions.

A drip stand will be attached to the delivery bed or it will be on wheels nearby. There are several situations when it will be essential for you to have an intravenous drip during labour:
• if you decide to have an epidural (see pp.311–5)
• if you are having an induction of labour (see pp.294–7)
• if you require drugs to strengthen your contractions (see p.304)
• if you are bleeding and the doctors need to have immediate access to your veins, to ensure that they can restore your blood pressure if it drops
• if you require IV antibiotics (for Group B streptococcus, for example).

Urinary catheters and bed pans are required in some circumstances during labour when you are unable to travel to a bathroom.

Fetal monitoring equipment

As a medical student I remember an eminent obstetrician telling me that "travelling through the birth canal is the most dangerous journey a human being ever embarks upon." It is not surprising, therefore, that we spend a lot of time trying to monitor the progress of labour and the baby's ability to cope with it.

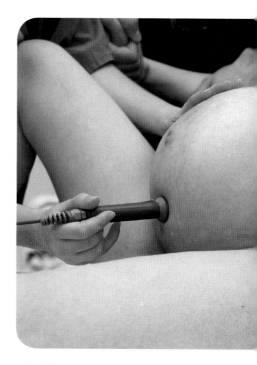

THE HAND-HELD DOPPLER This battery-operated device is used by midwives to listen to the baby's heartbeat during normal hospital labours or home births.

The simplest method of monitoring the fetus during labour and delivery is to listen with a Pinard's stethoscope, placed on the mother's abdomen. This short, hand-held, trumpet-shaped metal instrument used to be the only method of hearing the baby's heartbeat. Alternatively, a hand-held, battery-operated Doppler sonicaid machine can be used at regular intervals.

Electronic fetal monitoring (EFM) measures the baby's heart rate continuously and also the frequency and strength of the uterine contractions and displays the information on a paper printout or tracing, called a cardiotocograph or CTG. A healthy baby has a baseline heart rate of 120–160 beats per minute, which is continuously changing by 5–15 beats – this is described as "good variability". Lack of variability between contractions will alert your midwife to the possibility that the baby is not coping well with the stress of labour. Similarly, a low baseline heart rate of 100 beats per minute or less or a high heart rate of 180 beats per minute are further signs of possible distress. If this occurs, you may be asked to alter your position, which often reduces the problem and the fetal heart returns to normal. However, the most useful information gained from the CTG is how the baby's heart rate responds to the stress of the contracting uterus.

> In most labours... there is no need for the woman to be confined to her bed.

There are two types of EFM: external and internal. External EFM is completely non-invasive. Two small devices are strapped to your abdomen with soft belts – one picks up the fetal heartbeat; the other measures the intensity and duration of each contraction. They are linked by wires to the CTG machine and their findings are also displayed as flashing numbers on the front of the machine. In most labours, intermittent external monitoring (auscultation) is all that is required and there is no need for the woman to be confined to her bed.

Internal EFM is used when the tracing of the baby's heart rate is proving difficult to pick up or when there is clear evidence of fetal distress, or slow progress is being made and the medical team need to know continuously exactly what is happening. The CTG trace obtained is more accurate than the one produced by an external monitor. A small electrode is clipped to the baby's head (or bottom if the baby is breech) and linked up to the CTG machine. This clip can be applied only if the cervix has dilated to 2cm or more and the waters have broken or been ruptured artificially. A belt around your abdomen holds the pressure transducer that measures your uterine contractions. During the first stage of labour, the midwife will listen for one minute after every contraction every 15 minutes; during the second stage, she will listen every five minutes and for one minute after each contraction.

Electronic fetal monitoring was adopted widely and enthusiastically when it was first introduced in the 1970s and was used routinely by some hospitals, either intermittently or continuously, for almost all women. However, recent studies have shown that its routine use in labour increases significantly the incidence of unnecessary interventions for supposed "fetal distress" and does not improve the outcome for the baby during a normal uncomplicated labour.

Fetal blood sampling

If the CTG or EFM print-out shows signs of fetal distress, your doctor or midwife will probably suggest that a fetal blood sample (FBS) is taken. A sample of blood is taken from the baby's scalp and the pH (acidity/alkalinity) is measured in a special machine. The more acidic the reading, the more likely it is that the baby is short of oxygen and that intervention is needed. To obtain the blood sample, you will be examined internally either with your legs raised in lithotomy poles (stirrups) or while lying on your left side (left lateral position).

If the measurements confirm that the baby is distressed, the best course of action will depend on how far advanced you are in labour, together with other considerations. Obviously, if you are only a few centimetres dilated, it will be necessary to deliver you by emergency Caesarean section to avoid delay. However, if you are nearly 10cm dilated or in the second stage of labour, it is often possible to achieve a vaginal delivery more quickly than an abdominal one, albeit with the help of forceps or vacuum extraction in some cases. If the baby is not distressed, it is likely that you will be able to continue labouring safely.

Your birth partner's role

It serves no purpose to be judgmental as to whether or not a father should be present at the birth of his child. Watching someone you care about go through the pain and physical trauma of labour and birth is difficult and some men decide that they don't want to be there, however much they love their partner. That said, it is undoubtedly true that the man who attends the birth of his child will witness an extraordinary event that he will remember for the rest of his life. In addition, he will be able to share it with the mother-to-be and that common experience will often strengthen the bond between them. Encourage your partner to go with what feels right for him.

The most important things a birth partner can do are, first, know what the mother-to-be wants and, second, know what is going on during the labour and delivery. The first can only be achieved if the two of you have had in-depth conversations, and the second is probably best achieved by your partner attending the partners' antenatal preparation session (there is usually at least one class) and reading the labour chapter in this book.

Labouring women have different needs – some want physical reassurance such as massaging, hand holding, and brow mopping. Others need emotional reassurance and verbal encouragement. Your partner will have to be prepared for all eventualities and accept that you might want physical closeness one minute and not want him anywhere near you the next. It is also important for your partner to try not to let his fear or anxiety show.

YOUR PARTNER The most important thing your partner can do is to make sure he is fully informed before the birth so you can rely on him for support as your labour progresses.

Gathering information

A major part of your partner's role will involve liaising with the midwifery and medical staff. There may be instances when something occurs that you do not fully understand. This is where your partner can really help, by asking for clarification to make sure you understand the medical reasons for a particular procedure. He needs to be prepared to ask questions about what is happening in a non-confrontational way and to gather information so you are both kept fully informed and can participate in any medical decisions that need to be taken.

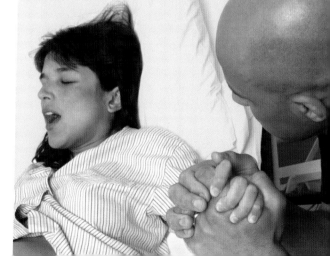

Induction of labour

When labour is induced it is brought forward artificially, before it has started of its own accord. Induction may be necessary if it is decided that the mother or her baby need to be delivered promptly and this is unlikely to happen spontaneously.

> ❝ …there is no such thing as a textbook induction and it is difficult to predict how things will go. ❞

Induction may be used for women who have never shown any signs of going into labour and also a few whose waters have broken but who fail to start contracting within 24 hours. It is important to understand that undergoing an induction of labour does not usually involve a single intervention being performed at a certain time. Induction is a process and it is likely to necessitate a complex set of interventions and interactions, the exact nature of which will be dictated by the events that occur during the labour. Hence there is no such thing as a textbook induction and it is often difficult to predict how things will go. This is why most midwives and doctors are hesitant to recommend induction unless there is a really good reason to do so.

Induction rates vary considerably between different countries, different maternity units, and even between individual obstetricians in the same unit. The rate is influenced by many factors, but particularly by the complexity or otherwise of the pregnancy and the individual obstetrician's perception of what circumstances place the mother or the fetus at risk.

Overall, some 70–80 per cent of inductions result in a vaginal delivery, but the procedure increases the risk of an assisted delivery with either forceps or ventouse extraction (see pp.352–5). The best chances of a successful induction are when the mother has had a previous vaginal delivery, her cervix is ripe, the baby is of average size and the head is engaged in a normally sized pelvis.

Indications for induction

The absolute indications for induction are that the baby would be better cared for in the outside world rather than in the uterus, or that the mother's health demands that the pregnancy ends promptly. All other indications are relative and will frequently include a mixture of fetal and maternal considerations.

There are many reasons why an induction may be considered:
• **Fetal** – when antenatal monitoring suggests that the baby's growth has slowed down or stopped or there are signs that the baby is distressed in utero. This may include a reduction in the fetal movements or volume of amniotic

fluid and is usually because the placenta is no longer functioning properly. Other fetal indications for induction arise if the baby has been affected by maternal Rhesus isoimmunisation (see p.128 and p.425) or the mother has diabetes mellitus which places the baby at increased risk in the last few weeks of pregnancy (see p.408). Similarly, if the baby is known to have an abnormality that will require surgery immediately after delivery, it is often safer for the baby to be delivered at a time when all of the necessary expertise is readily available. The decision to induce will depend on balancing the risks of delivering a baby prematurely with leaving it in utero. However, modern-day neonatal expertise means that most babies delivered at or after 28 weeks will survive without serious problems.

• **Maternal** – severe pre-eclampsia, poorly controlled diabetes, pre-existing kidney, liver or heart disease, and autoimmune disorders may require induction of labour.

• **A combination of fetal and maternal indications** – many of the fetal and maternal indications listed above can lead to the decision that induction is the best way of ensuring the welfare of both mother and baby. However, pre-eclampsia and maternal diabetes are the most frequent combined indications for induction, together with premature rupture of the membranes.

• **Post-maturity** – most units offer induction to women whose pregnancies are prolonged past 41 weeks because it reduces the risks of unexplained stillbirth and other late-pregnancy complications, without increasing the Caesarean section rate.

BISHOP'S SCORES

If an induction is being considered, most maternity units stamp the mother's notes with a Bishop's score table, which helps to make an objective assessment as to whether or not the cervix is favourable for induction. Your midwife or doctor will perform a vaginal examination and cervical dilatation, length, consistency, and position, together with the station that the fetal head has reached in the pelvis (see p.302) are all given a score of 0 to 3. Total scores of 5 or more are considered favourable for induction, because the cervix is ripe.

SCORE	CERVICAL STATE				
	Dilation (cm)	Length (cm)	Consistency	Position	Station of head
0	Closed	3	Firm	Posterior	-3
1	1–2	2	Medium	Middle	-2
2	3–4	1	Soft	Anterior	-1
3	5+	0			0

METHODS OF INDUCTION

When the decision has been made to perform an induction of labour, the method used will depend on whether this is a first or subsequent pregnancy, the presence of a previous uterine scar, whether or not the membranes are intact, and the state of the cervix. It is unlikely that an induction will be planned if the baby is not in a cephalic presentation (see p.268) and the head is not well engaged or nearly so.

You will be admitted to the labour ward and your midwife will examine you and monitor your baby's heart rate with a CTG recording to ensure that there are no signs of fetal distress (see p.291). The examination will start with her palpating your abdomen, confirming the longitudinal lie and cephalic presentation, and assessing the degree of engagement of the head (see p.302). Your midwife will then perform a gentle vaginal examination and use the Bishop's scoring system (see p.295) to assess the state of your cervix. A favourable cervix is critical if the induction is to be successful. Some units offer outpatient induction for low-risk mothers if an ultrasound scan shows normal liquor volumes.

PROSTAGLANDIN GEL OR TABLETS

The hormone prostaglandin occurs naturally in the uterine lining and stimulates the uterus to start contracting. If your cervix is unfavourable, your midwife or doctor will suggest that they put some synthetic prostaglandin tablets or gel into the vagina to help ripen it. A second vaginal dose of prostaglandins may be needed about six hours after the first and some women require further doses to ripen the cervix sufficiently. This is often best done overnight, in the hope that the woman will wake up refreshed the next morning and will either be starting to go into labour or be better prepared to undergo the next part of the induction process. In pregnancies that have been straightforward, this can be carried out on the antenatal ward, but if recognized risk factors are present, the woman will be moved to the main delivery unit for this procedure. After each insertion the baby will be monitored electronically for 30 minutes, but as long as the CTG is normal, intermittent monitoring with the Pinard's stethoscope can then be used (see p.291). As soon as contractions start, another period of electronic monitoring will be advised.

A new preparation of slow-release prostaglandin has been introduced recently, which can be useful for multiparous women (those who have had a previous pregnancy) with an unfavourable cervix.

ARTIFICIAL RUPTURE OF MEMBRANES (ARM)

When the cervix reaches 2–3cm dilatation it is usually possible to

SWEEPING THE MEMBRANES

Before deciding on a date for an induction of labour, it is likely that your midwife or doctor will suggest they sweep the membranes. The doctor or midwife will gently insert one or two fingers through the cervix and literally sweep them around its circumference. This often helps to start the contractions because it releases prostaglandins from the cervix. It can be a little uncomfortable and often results in light bleeding or a "show". However, it is a safe and often effective way of stimulating early labour contractions, which is why you will be offered a sweep at 41 weeks.

artificially rupture the membranes easily by inserting a long, thin plastic hook into the vagina and through the cervix to break the delicate membranes and allow the amniotic fluid to start draining away. This releases further prostaglandins, which help to establish regular uterine contractions. In some inductions, no further interventions are required after an ARM has been performed, because the uterine contractions become well established in a relatively short period of time. However, when this is not the case, you will need to move on to the next part of the induction process – an oxytocin drip.

OXYTOCIN OR SYNTOCINON

Oxytocin is a hormone that is produced by the pituitary gland in the brain and causes the uterine muscle to contract. Syntocinon, a synthetic equivalent of oxytocin, is given via an intravenous drip that is inserted into a vein in your lower arm. The syntocinon drug is injected into a sterile bag of fluid (usually a mixture of salt and sugar solutions), which is then attached to a drip stand. The starting dose is always small and is gradually increased until effective uterine contractions have been established, usually defined as three moderate to strong contractions occurring every 10 minutes. The quantity of syntocinon you receive is carefully measured by a special machine or infusion pump attached to the drip. This allows the dose to be adjusted up or down, depending on the progress of your labour and,

most importantly, how the baby responds to the uterine contractions.

Because uterine contractions that are induced by syntocinon can be strong and start suddenly before the baby has been exposed to more gentle uterine activity, there is a greater risk of the baby becoming distressed. Of course, this potential problem is frequently aggravated by the underlying reasons for which the induction is being performed. For example, if the baby needs to be delivered because of poor growth, then its reserves may already be lower than a baby who is normally grown and going through a spontaneous labour. For this reason, once the syntocinon infusion has started, you will need to be monitored continuously with an electronic monitor (see pp.291–2).

You may find it useful at this point to read the section on the latent phase of labour (see p.298), where I explain the prolonged period of uterine activity usually needed before normal contractions become strong enough and regular enough to dilate the cervix effectively.

Having understood these points, I think it becomes much easier to appreciate why an induction that requires a syntocinon drip often results in an apparently lengthy and more painful labour. Labour is not really longer, but there is quite a lot of catching up to do to reach the

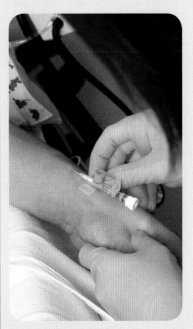

SYNTOCINON The drug is administered via an intravenous drip inserted into a vein in your forearm.

point when the cervix starts to dilate. Furthermore, the induced contractions may appear to be more painful because you have not experienced the gradual increase in uterine activity that occurs in the latent phase of a spontaneous labour. This is one of the reasons why most maternity units suggest you have an epidural anaesthetic if you are induced, and also why the epidural is usually inserted before the syntocinon drip is turned on.

> ❝ A favourable cervix is critical if the induction is to be successful. ❞

Established first stage

Theoretically, the first stage of labour starts when regular painful uterine contractions become established and ends when the cervix is fully (10cm) dilated. This first stage can be further divided into three phases: a latent phase, an established first stage, and a transition phase.

The latent phase

During the latent phase of the first stage of labour, uterine activity starts but the contractions are usually mild and irregular. For many women they feel like period pains or backache and are usually not seriously distressing. This early activity is important because it changes the cervix from being thick and barrel-shaped, measuring about 2cm in length, into a much thinner, softer, shorter structure.

Although you may not be aware of the mild contractions spreading down your uterus, they are thinning the lower part of the uterus and cervix, drawing them up over the baby's head (if that is the presenting part) rather like a glove. This process is called effacement and needs to occur before the cervix can stretch and open up or dilate. The latent phase can last for eight hours (sometimes more for first-time mothers), but if you have had several children it is usually much shorter – indeed you may not even realize that something has started to happen.

The hormones that are secreted during the last few weeks of pregnancy help to soften the cervix in preparation for labour, but the dilatation that occurs in the first stage can only be achieved by the onset of progressively stronger uterine contractions. Hence, in the latent phase, the mild contractions usually occur every 15 to 20 minutes, lasting for no more than 30 to 60 seconds.

FIRST STAGE PHASES ··

As the first stage of labour unfolds, the cervix effaces and dilates. It changes from being a structure that is firmly closed to one that is 10cm dilated and able to allow the baby's head, or other presenting part, to pass through.

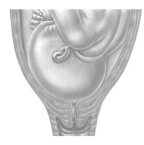

THE LATENT PHASE The cervix thins (effaces) and begins to stretch and open.

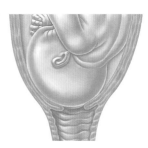

ESTABLISHED FIRST STAGE Contractions are stronger as the cervix dilates.

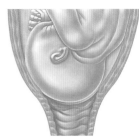

THE TRANSITION PHASE The cervix is fully dilated (10cm) ready for the baby to descend.

Rest assured that if you find the pain you are experiencing in the latent phase distressing, you will be offered pain relief. However, until active labour has started, your midwife and/or doctor will probably advise that this should be entonox gas or an injection of pethidine or diamorphine, rather than an epidural (see pp.308–23). This is because they will want to encourage you to keep upright and active for as long as possible rather than confining you to a bed, in order to allow gravity to play its part in helping you to reach the active phase of labour.

Established first stage

The established first stage is said to have started when the cervix has dilated to about 4cm and the uterine contractions have become more regular and rhythmical. Your midwife will be able to judge if you have reached the established first stage based on what your uterine contractions are like, rather than what has happened to your cervix.

As the first stage progresses and becomes established, the contractions will become more noticeable around the centre of your tummy and will be accompanied by a hardening and tightening of the uterine muscles, which you can feel with your hand. Uterine contractions are painful because the uterus is a massive muscular organ and requires enormous amounts of energy to work efficiently. During a contraction, the blood vessels in the walls of the uterus are compressed and the muscle becomes short of oxygen, resulting in the release of painful chemical substances. These are washed away in the recovery period between contractions.

The other thing to bear in mind about contractions is that they slightly reduce the oxygen supply to your baby, because the blood vessels in the uterus that are supplying the placenta are also compressed. As a result, your baby's heart rate may slow down at the peak of a contraction. This will be carefully monitored as your labour progresses (see pp.291–2) to ensure your baby is not getting too tired or distressed.

Changing contractions

As you enter the established first stage of labour, your contractions will change in nature. First, they become stronger, regular, and more painful. Second, instead of being concentrated in the lower part of the uterus, they now begin at the top and spread downwards through the whole of the uterus. This ensures that the baby's head (or other presenting part) is being pushed against the cervix, since the priority now is to get the cervix opened to a diameter of 10cm. Your contractions will be coming every 10 to 15 minutes,

> 66
> ...the uterus is a massive muscular organ and requires enormous amounts of energy to work efficiently.
> 99

66 …the baby's head and shoulders must descend deep into the pelvic cavity before the second stage of labour starts. 99

then every five minutes, then every two minutes, the timing being calculated from the start of one contraction to the start of the next.

By the end of the established first stage, each contraction will be lasting about 60 to 90 seconds, so there will be little time for rest in between. As they get stronger, you will feel as if you are being gripped round the abdomen by a tight band as the uterine muscles harden and tighten. During each contraction, the pain will usually start slowly, rise to a peak lasting about 30 seconds and then subside.

Between 4 and 9cm the cervix usually goes through the most rapid phase of dilatation, after which there is sometimes a deceleration, or slowing, of dilatation. This is because cervical dilatation is not the only marker of progress in labour. It is also important for the baby's head and shoulders to descend deep into the pelvic cavity before the second stage of labour starts.

The total length of the active phase of the first stage varies because it is determined by whether this is your first baby or not. In a first labour, you are likely to dilate at about 0.5–1cm per hour, whereas if you have already had one or more babies you may dilate considerably faster.

Rupture of the membranes

In 15 per cent of term pregnancies, the membranes rupture spontaneously (SROM) before labour starts and, in the majority of these cases, contractions and progressive cervical dilatation follow within 24 hours. This leaves 85 per cent of pregnancies in which the waters are still intact when labour commences. In most cases, they will rupture spontaneously as labour progresses, but occasionally, and usually in very fast or precipitate labours, the baby will be delivered still surrounded by the amniotic sac.

Some obstetric units still have a policy of artificially rupturing the membranes (ARM) when strong contractions have become established and cervical dilatation has reached 4–5cm. This is because amniotomy or ARM releases prostaglandins, which help speed up uterine contractions. It also removes the fluid cushion surrounding the baby's head, so more effective pressure is exerted on the cervix, further encouraging the progress of labour. However, if your labour is progressing normally, there is no benefit in having an ARM performed routinely, particularly if you feel strongly that you do not want to have any interventions. Also, ARM is associated with an increased need for analgesia.

If your labour has been induced (see pp.294–7) or needs to be augmented because the progress is slow (see p.304) then you may be advised to have an ARM. First, to help the progress of labour, and second because labours that are not completely straightforward need to be watched closely to ensure that the baby does not become distressed. If the CTG shows any worrying features, your midwife will probably suggest that she breaks the waters in order to attach an electronic monitoring clip to the baby's head (see p.292). She will also inspect the amniotic fluid or liquor and ensure that there is no meconium staining present, suggesting that the baby has already been exposed to stress.

ARM is usually a painless procedure (see pp.296–7) when you are already partially dilated. There are a few situations where ARM is not advised, for example, if you labour prematurely. In such a case, it is always best to leave the waters intact for as long as possible, since they protect or cushion the more fragile premature baby during the labour and delivery (see p.341).

The transition phase

This is the name given to the interlude that sometimes, but not always, occurs during the final phase of the first stage of labour, when the cervix has fully dilated and before the intense urge to push that is so characteristic of the second stage of labour really gets under way. The transition phase can last a few minutes or continue for an hour or more. For some women it can be the most difficult part of their labour to deal with because they already feel tired and exhausted by the hours of contractions they have experienced. Some women report that they feel nauseous during this stage. The contractions will be intense, coming every 30 to 90 seconds and lasting for 60 to 90 seconds. Hence there is very little time between them and many women feel frightened that they have completely lost control of what is happening. In some ways this is true, since the labour has developed a momentum of its own and there is no stopping now until the baby is delivered. The good news is that this is not far off, so try to think of the transition phase as a very positive sign that the end of your labour is definitely in sight.

> ...think of the transition phase as a positive sign that the end of your labour is in sight.

Wanting to push

Some women experience an intense urge to push during the transition phase before the cervix is fully dilated. If you start pushing when the cervix is 8 or 9cm dilated, the cervix will develop into a thick, swollen ring around the top of the baby's head, rather than the paper-thin pliable membrane that will allow the head to descend and slip past it. If you do develop the urge to push before you reach full dilatation, your midwife will show you how to pant or take short shallow breaths when you are having contractions, to try to prevent you breathing too deeply and bearing down. She may also suggest that you change to a position that takes the pressure of the baby's head off your cervix (such as on hands and knees with your bottom raised), since an upright position will encourage the urge to bear down. Alternatively, if you have an epidural in place, it may be a good idea to have a small top up at this point so that full dilatation and further head descent can be achieved before you start to do your pushing.

Examinations in labour

The onset of labour depends on the cervix starting to dilate, but progress in labour requires both continued cervical dilatation and also descent of the baby through the pelvic birth canal. There is no absolute size of baby or pelvis that can guarantee good progress in labour, nor is there a magical number of strong contractions that can predict a swift and smooth delivery. This is why it is so important for your midwife to perform an abdominal examination as well as a vaginal/internal examination whenever she is assessing your progress.

How often you are examined during labour will depend on many different factors, not least of which is how long or short your labour lasts. At each

ENGAGEMENT AND STATIONS

Now that you are in labour, it is important to assess how far the baby's head has descended into the pelvis. By definition, engagement means that the largest diameter of the head has entered the pelvic brim, which means that only 0, one-or-two fifths of the head will be palpable in the abdomen. The less head that can be felt on examination, the better the progress of labour is likely to be. You will have a vaginal examination to identify how many centimetres dilated your cervix is and the level that the leading part of the head has descended to within the pelvis. The levels are referred to as stations, which are best thought of as imaginary horizontal lines drawn through the pelvis at centimetre intervals. When the head first enters the pelvic brim it is said to be at −5 station. When the tip of the head reaches the middle of the pelvic cavity it is at zero station. When it reaches the vaginal opening it is at +5 station.

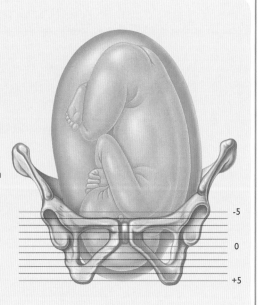

THE DESCENT The position of the head is described according to where it is in cm above (-) and below (+) the ischial spines (the narrow part of the pelvis).

PARTOGRAMS

The best way of monitoring the progress of labour is to use a partogram. This is a large chart consisting of various graphs onto which all of the observations made in labour are entered.

At the top of the partogram all your personal details will be noted, along with any special instructions or reminders to the midwives and doctors. Underneath this are several graphs recording the fetal heart rate, the number of contractions you are having in each 10-minute interval, your temperature, blood pressure and pulse and the results of any urine tests. If you need pain relief or a syntocinon drip, the dosages and the timing of these drugs will also be recorded on the chart.

The most useful part of the partogram is the graph of your cervical dilatation and the station that the fetal head has reached, which the midwife will plot at each assessment. This shows at a glance how the labour is progressing and will quickly identify any delays. Indeed, most partograms have bold black lines already drawn on them showing the anticipated curved pattern of cervical dilatation from 0–10cm. The ideal curve for first-time mothers moves along and up the graph towards the 10cm mark more gradually, whereas the curve for mothers who have already had a baby is shorter and sharper. The ideal curve for head descent will move along and down the graph. Of course, every labour will not follow these guidelines exactly, but if progress is slow (the entries are appearing significantly to the right of the ideal progress line), then interventions are likely to be needed and the earlier this is recognized the better.

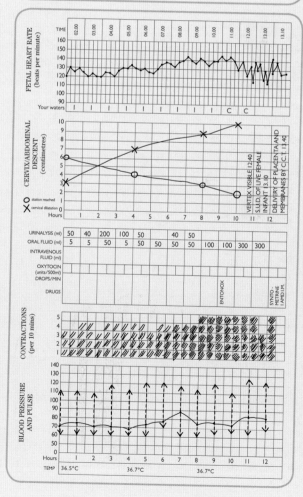

PROGRESS OF THE FIRST STAGE

Good progress is achieved by a combination of three important P factors:

▶ **The powers** – strong uterine contractions that dilate the cervix effectively

▶ **The passenger** – a baby that can fit through the mother's pelvis and is

in a good position for an easy exit

▶ **The passages** – a pelvis that is sufficiently roomy to allow the baby to pass through it.

All three of these P factors are relative to each other, and the progress of your labour will depend on how they interact with each other.

…in the vast majority of pregnancies the lie will be longitudinal and cephalic.

examination, the midwife will palpate your abdomen and confirm the lie and presentation of the baby (see p.268). In the vast majority of pregnancies this will be longitudinal and cephalic, hence the rest of this section on progress in labour assumes that this is the case. If you have a breech presentation or transverse or oblique lie at the onset of labour, you will find details about how these labours are managed on pages 356–9 and page 430.

Augmentation of labour

When the progress of a labour that has started spontaneously slows down it may become necessary to accelerate or augment it. Using a partogram is the best way of deciding when augmentation should be started. If the contractions are satisfactory but the membranes are intact, then an artificial rupturing of the membranes (see p.300) may be all that is needed to speed things up. If the contractions are weak, infrequent or irregular, and the waters have already broken, then a syntocinon infusion will be started to strengthen and regularize the contractions. As with an induction (see pp.294–7) the dose will be small to begin with and then gradually increased, aiming for about three to four moderately strong contractions every 10 minutes.

Continuous monitoring will be needed to ensure that the baby does not become distressed and a further examination will be carried out about two hours after augmentation. Usually this shows that there has been some progress in the cervical dilatation or descent of the baby's head, in which case the syntocinon infusion will be continued until the next examination, in a further two hours' time. All the observations will be added to the partogram (see p.303), and the curve of cervical dilatation should look more normal. Occasionally, however, there is no further progress after four hours, in which case the doctors will be asked to reassess you and may advise that delivery by Caesarean section is necessary.

Prolonged labour

Prolonged labour is usually defined as lasting longer than 12 hours after the mother has been recognized as being in labour. It complicates 5–8 per cent of all labours and is much more common in first-time mothers than those who have had a baby before.

Labour becomes prolonged when the cervix is slow to dilate, or the baby is unable to descend through the birth canal or rotate into the optimal position for a straightforward delivery, or the uterine contractions are suboptimal. In reality, it is often a combination of factors, since dilatation, descent, and rotation are all interdependent. Cephalopelvic disproportion, fetal or maternal obstruction, inefficient uterine activity, and occipito-posterior presentations are the usual causes of prolonged labour, and they are often closely inter-linked.

Cephalopelvic disproportion

Cephalopelvic disproportion (CPD) means that the baby's head is too large for the mother's pelvis. It is a relative term, since a different-sized baby might slip through the same pelvis easily. In first-time mothers, CPD may be suspected if the head has not entered the pelvic brim at term. Further clues may be gained by looking at the mother's height and shoe size – if she is less than 1.5m (5ft) tall and takes size 3 shoes or smaller she may well have a small pelvis that will make a vaginal delivery difficult or impossible.

In cases where there is a strong suspicion of CPD antenatally, doctors will often advise that a Caesarean section should be performed to avoid exposing the fetus to a prolonged and difficult labour. On the other hand, if the head has entered the pelvic brim, and the mother is keen to deliver vaginally, she may choose to have a trial of labour. If this is attempted, progress will be carefully monitored using a partogram (see p.303). If progress is poor, then plans will need to be made for an abdominal delivery.

In second or subsequent pregnancies, the head does not always enter the pelvis until the onset of labour, so predicting CPD may be more difficult. A careful review of the previous labours and the birthweight of the babies may provide useful clues. Some doctors may suggest that an X-ray or CT scan is performed to assess the exact dimension of the mother's pelvis, although this is rarely used nowadays. The reality is that however restricted or capacious the bony measurements may be, the only way of knowing whether or not the baby's head will pass through the pelvis is by monitoring how the labour progresses.

> "The only way of knowing whether or not the baby's head will pass through the pelvis is by monitoring how the labour progresses."

Obstructed labour

This is usually the end result of a poorly managed or neglected labour in which CPD or a malpresentation, such as a shoulder or transverse lie (see p.429), has been missed. Other causes include pelvic masses in the mother, such as a uterine fibroid (see p.422), an ovarian cyst or kidney transplant, or a congenital abnormality in the baby, such as hydrocephalus (see p.419). Happily, I can tell you that obstructed labour is a rare event these days, since most of the causes will be identified before you go into labour.

In a first labour, the uterus contracts strongly to try to overcome the obstruction and then becomes inactive. However, if obstruction occurs in a second labour, the uterus continues to contract strongly leading to the development of a contraction ring in the uterus known as a Bandl's ring. The upper part of the uterus becomes thick and short and the lower part becomes progressively stretched and thinner. In this situation, urgent intervention with delivery by Caesarean section is needed to prevent the uterus from rupturing (see p.428).

Inefficient contractions

Labour will progress normally only if your uterine contractions are efficient and move downwards through the whole of your uterus. When they fail to do so, labour usually becomes prolonged. The inefficient uterine activity can be under- (hypo) or over- (hyper) active and develops in some 5 per cent of first labours and about 1 per cent of all labours. Under-activity – called uterine inertia – often responds to stimulation with syntocinon (see p.297) unless disproportion or another type of obstruction is present. Over-activity – also called incoordinate uterine activity – is when the various parts of the uterus contract independently. These contractions fail to dilate the cervix efficiently and are often very painful. This type of uterine activity may follow the inappropriate use of syntocinon to accelerate labour. Now that epidural analgesia is used so widely the severity and exact location of the mother's pain in labour can be difficult to monitor. For this reason, a partogram is useful in identifying the different types of inefficient uterine activity. If slow cervical dilatation persists and the cervix fails to dilate by more than 2cm over a period of four hours, accompanied by poor head descent, then plans will need to be made for delivery by Caesarean section.

> " Labour progresses normally only when your contractions are efficient, moving down through the whole of the uterus. "

Occipito-posterior presentation

Labour and delivery are more likely to be swift and uncomplicated when the baby is in the occipito-anterior position (OA, see p.270), that is the back of the baby's head (the crown or occiput) is towards the mother's front (anterior). When the baby is in the occipito-posterior (OP) position its face is pointing forwards and the back of its head is pressing against the mother's back (sacrum) with the baby's spine lying on top of the mother's spine. In this position it is more difficult for the baby to flex its neck and chin because the bony crown is pushed up against the bony maternal sacrum, which means that a larger than normal proportion of the head is presenting. This may prolong the labour and it often results in the woman experiencing more pain and discomfort, which she notices most in her lower back. This is why OP positions are sometimes referred to as backache labours.

To take the pressure off your lower back, try getting down on your hands and knees, or sitting with your legs crossed in front of you and leaning forward, or rocking your pelvis. You may find that a vigorous massage of the painful area is helpful. One of the best ways of encouraging rotation of the baby's head is to stay upright and mobile for as long as possible. If you need to lie down, then adopt a position that will encourage internal rotation (your midwife will advise you). Always avoid lying flat on your back, because in this position the complete weight of your baby will be pressing down on your spine and lower back, and this may make you feel faint.

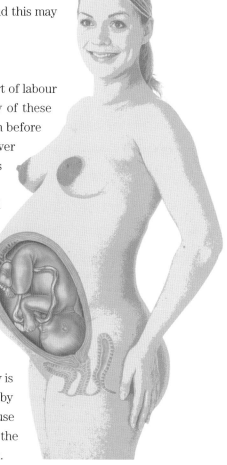

OCCIPITO-POSTERIOR
In this position, the back of your baby's head is towards your back, with its spine pressing against yours.

Rotating the baby

Just over 10 per cent of babies are in a posterior position at the start of labour (see p.270), so this is not an uncommon problem. In the majority of these cases, the babies tend to rotate themselves into an anterior position before the end of the first stage, but the labour invariably gets off to a slower start and the progress is often more painful and protracted, which is very tiring for the mother.

When the baby is in the OP position, both epidural analgesia and augmentation are often required during labour and, not surprisingly, maternal exhaustion and fetal distress are frequent complications of this type of labour. If the baby fails to move into the anterior position by the beginning of the second stage, the midwife will probably suggest topping up your epidural (to prevent any urges to push), changing your position to encourage further rotation, and resting you for an hour or so. If the baby is still OP, a vaginal delivery is still possible but the baby is born facing upwards (face to pubes), which may carry a greater risk of perineal damage. If the baby is in an occipito-lateral position then it may be necessary to rotate the baby into the occipito-anterior position with rotational forceps or the ventouse to achieve a smooth delivery. When this proves to be unsuccessful, the only remaining option for delivery is an emergency Caesarean section.

PAIN RELIEF IN LABOUR

Pain relief is an important issue, since no one wants to be exposed to pain in normal circumstances. However, uterine contractions that are capable of pushing your baby through your birth canal will be painful, although there are effective ways to help alleviate this.

The question of pain relief in labour is a thorny one which has been fiercely debated over the years by pregnant women and healthcare professionals. As with all heated debates, there is a tendency for views to become polarized. Some take the view that childbirth is an entirely natural process, and since they believe that pain is an integral part of this process, will refuse to consider any form of medicalized pain relief. At the other end of the scale are women who will want to have an epidural at the first sign of discomfort, and may even request an elective Caesarean section in order to bypass the process of labour altogether.

I have no real problem with either of these attitudes so long as the woman involved has been given sound advice about all the options available to her before she decides on her approach. There is no way that a first-time mother can know how the pain of labour will affect her, since it is probably the first time in her life that she has been exposed to significant pain. Women who have already experienced labour may have a better idea of their own pain threshold but, since every labour is different, they cannot be expected to anticipate accurately how they will cope with pain this time round. I cannot accept that a woman who is capable of delivering a healthy baby into this world should ever feel that she has failed because she needed pain relief to help her.

My personal opinion is that adopting an open-minded attitude and waiting to see what feels right for you at the time is usually the best approach. I would urge you to be as informed as possible, as there is no doubt that the more you know about the different methods of pain relief available, the better able you will be to make the best choice for you and for your baby on the day.

MEDICALIZED PAIN RELIEF

THERE ARE THREE BROAD GROUPS:
Analgesics, which relieve pain or the perception of pain. These are:
▶ inhalational analgesics such as entonox
▶ systemic analgesics such as pethidine

Regional anaesthesia, which creates a localized block of pain sensation (numbness). These include:
▶ epidurals
▶ spinal blocks
▶ pudendal blocks
▶ cervical blocks

General anaesthesia, which produce a loss of consciousness and therefore no pain is felt.

ANALGESIC DRUGS

Analgesic drugs work on receptors in the brain dulling the pain messages sent to them by the nervous system. Entonox and pethidine are the most common types of analgesic drug used in labour.

Inhalation analgesia

Entonox (nitrous oxide) is an analgesic gas, which, when used as a 50:50 mix with air, numbs the pain centres in the brain and dulls the pain messages being sent to the brain without causing loss of consciousness or significant sedation. However, it is common to feel light-headed and rather as if you are floating or out of touch with your surroundings when using it, which most women in labour look upon as a good thing.

In a recent survey carried out by the National Childbirth Trust, entonox cylinders were readily available in 99 per cent of all maternity and birthing units in the UK and entonox was the main analgesic of choice for some 55 per cent of all women in labour. Its popularity is due to the fact that it acts very quickly and the mother is in control of how much gas she receives. The gas passes out of her system rapidly and has no adverse effects on the baby. It can be used at home births, too.

How to use gas and air

The best way to use entonox is to wait until the start of a contraction, then inhale slowly and deeply through your nose if you are using a face mask and through your mouth if you have been given a mouth piece. Then exhale slowly. After five or six breaths the gas will have reached an analgesic level in your brain and you will notice the pain relief and probably also a floating

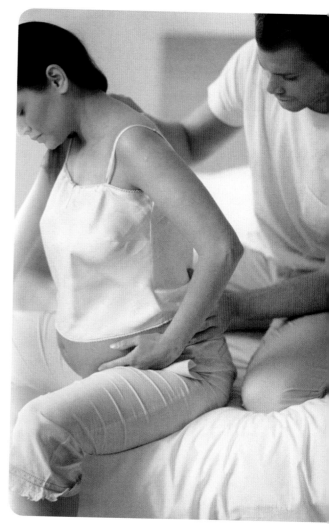

PARTNER PARTICIPATION Partners are taught to recognize the woman's pain and to coach her in abdominal breathing and other methods of deep relaxation.

feeling of wellbeing. You then continue to inhale and exhale until the contraction has subsided.

It is important to stop using the gas between contractions, since continued use does nothing to help reduce the pain of the next contraction, but it will increase your chances of feeling sick and disorientated. Some women used to find that the smell of the rubber face mask made them feel sick, which is why I think the mouth pieces are much better to use. Also, having something in your mouth that you can bite on hard can be very helpful in the middle of a strong contraction.

For many women, entonox is most helpful in the early stages of labour. Some women manage using only entonox throughout, whereas others find they need an additional form of analgesia to cope with strong contractions or during the second stage of labour. I am sure that part of the benefit of using gas and air during the first stage is that it forces you to concentrate on your breathing technique, which helps you to feel more in control of the situation and can also provide a degree of pain relief.

Although entonox readily crosses the placenta, it is eliminated from your body and the baby's body very rapidly, causing no adverse effects, so you do not have to worry that your baby will be delivered laughing or on a high.

Systemic analgesia

Systemic pain relief affects the whole body. Opioids, especially pethidine (a synthetic equivalent of morphine and diamorphine), are widely used in labour. They are members of the family of narcotic (opiate) drugs, which literally means that they induce drowsiness as well as reducing pain. Pethidine relieves pain by stimulating specific receptors in the brain and spinal cord so that the pain messages relayed to the brain by the nervous system are dulled. This is because the same

receptors are used by endorphins – our body's naturally occurring painkillers.

Pethidine is administered quickly and easily by injection, usually into a muscle in your upper thigh or bottom, and you will feel its effects within 15 to 20 minutes. The pain relief will wear off after three to four hours when you will need to have a repeat injection.

Since 1950, midwives in the UK have been allowed to prescribe and administer pethidine injections to women in labour on their own initiative and without needing a prescription from a medical doctor. Pethidine remains the main method of pain relief for some 40 per cent of midwifery deliveries today.

Problems with pethidine

Pethidine has a poor track record as a labour analgesic, since the dosages required for effective pain relief can also result in the mother becoming over-sedated. This can occasionally lead to breathing difficulties and low oxygen levels in the mother between contractions. Pethidine can also be accompanied by additional side effects, such as nausea, vomiting, indigestion, and delayed gastric emptying and many mothers tell me that pethidine makes them feel out of touch with what is happening in their labour.

The other disadvantage of pethidine is that it rapidly crosses the placenta into the baby, where it can cause drowsiness. As the baby becomes sedated, there is often a reduction in the baseline variability on the CTG (see p.291), which makes interpretation of the heart trace more difficult. As a result of respiratory depression, the baby tends to be born with lower Apgar scores (see p.375) and is more likely to require an injection of naloxone, which helps to reverse the effect of the pethidine.

REGIONAL ANAESTHESIA

A variety of regional anaesthetics can be used to block the pain associated with labour, delivery, and the completion of the third stage of labour. All of these depend on blockading nerve fibres by injecting them with local anaesthetic drugs.

The type of regional anaesthetic that is used depends on the procedure. For example, epidurals can be used throughout labour and all types of delivery, whereas spinal blocks are usually reserved for Caesarean sections or manual removal of the placenta. Similarly, a pudendal or cervical block will only provide sufficient analgesia for simple forceps or ventouse deliveries in a woman who has no other form of pain relief available.

Epidural blocks

A good epidural block will numb all sensation in your abdomen and stop you feeling painful uterine contractions. This method of pain relief involves significant medical resources and can be offered routinely only in hospitals which provide 24-hour anaesthetic cover to the labour ward. Do tell your midwife when you are admitted that you might wish to have an epidural, so she can alert the anaesthetists to the fact that they may be needed at a later stage.

How epidurals work

Your spinal cord is covered by a thick membrane or sheath, called the dura, and is further protected by the bony vertebral column that surrounds it (see diagram, p.313). The epidural space lies between the bony vertebral column and spinal cord.

The nerve fibres that control your contraction pains pass out of the spinal cord, pierce the dural sheath and cross through the epidural space before passing between the vertebrae to enter your abdomen. The anaesthetic drugs injected into this epidural space penetrate the nerve fibres and block your pain pathways.

If the dosage of anaesthetic drug is high, some of the motor nerve fibres that control your legs and bladder will also be blocked, which means that

---

WHEN ARE EPIDURALS USEFUL?

▶ At your request: to help with painful uterine contractions in first or second stage of labour
▶ Multiple pregnancy
▶ Premature labour
▶ Prolonged labour: posterior positions; inefficient/irregular uterine

contractions; suspected cephalopelvic disproportion following induction or augmentation of labour (see p.304)
▶ Instrumental delivery: ventouse or forceps
▶ Breech delivery
▶ Elective Caesarean section –

unless there are specific contraindications (see p.362)
▶ Emergency Caesarean section – unless there are contraindications or there is insufficient time
▶ Perineal repairs/episiotomies – where extensive suturing is required

EPIDURALS

▶ Will the procedure be painful?

Since the skin of your back is numbed with local anaesthetic before the epidural needle is inserted, it is unusual for you to feel anything other than mild discomfort.

▶ What happens if the epidural does not work?

If the local anaesthetic solution spreads unevenly in the epidural space, you may find that an area of your abdomen or a patch of your thigh is not effectively blocked. Occasionally, the block is only on one side of your body. However, these problems can be quickly sorted out by the anaesthetist who will adjust the position of the catheter and may ask you to change your position to ensure that the drugs reach all of the nerve fibres evenly. Rarely, the epidural does not "take" and in this situation your anaesthetist will probably decide to completely reinsert it.

▶ I have had a previous back injury. Will I be able to have an epidural?

The answer to this will depend on the nature and severity of the previous back injury. But it is unusual for an existing back injury to make an epidural out of the question. Arrange to meet with one of the obstetric anaesthetists during the antenatal period, so that you can be offered advice as to the best form of analgesia.

▶ Can the epidural catheter damage my spine?

It is extremely rare for the catheter to move inside your spine. If this did happen, your carers would notice it quickly, since the area of numbness would move to a higher or lower level, which they will sort out immediately. It is virtually impossible for an epidural to damage your spinal cord or paralyze you.

▶ Will I be able to push my baby out in the second stage?

The answer to this is yes, you should be able to but it will be more difficult with an epidural. This is because you cannot feel your contractions and will not experience the strong urge to push that accompanies second-stage contractions. This means that you will be less able to judge where you need to direct your pushing efforts. However, your midwife will help by telling you when the contractions are occurring and, between you both, you can find a way of using them effectively. The other way of dealing with the second stage is to let the epidural wear off slightly, so that when you start pushing, you are aware of your contractions and more importantly, you have a better idea of where in your perineum you should be aiming for.

▶ Am I more likely to have an operative delivery?

There is good evidence that epidurals increase the likelihood of an operative vaginal delivery such as a ventouse or forceps, because the woman is less likely to be able to push in the second stage. But epidurals do not increase the Caesarean section rate. My view is that an experienced midwife, working with a motivated mother who really wants to deliver vaginally, can usually manage any uncomplicated delays in labour and achieve a vaginal delivery.

▶ Will my baby be affected?

Some modern epidural solutions contain opioids that cross the placenta and in large doses may cause short-term respiratory depression in the baby. The epidural may cause a fall in your blood pressure, which, if sudden or sustained, could result in fetal distress. This is why CTG monitoring is recommended for at least 30 minutes after insertion of an epidural and after each top up.

> 66 Your midwife will help by telling you when the contractions are occurring. 99

your legs will feel quite heavy and difficult to move and you may no longer be able to tell when your bladder is full.

Preparing for an epidural

If you choose to have an epidural, your midwife will explain the procedure to you and the anaesthetist will answer any questions you may have and will obtain your verbal or written consent to proceed.

You will be asked either to lie on a bed on your left side with your legs bent forwards or alternatively to sit up on the bed and lean forwards, stabilizing yourself by leaning your arms on a table. Lying down is usually more comfortable if you are already contracting strongly, whereas the upright position may be the best choice if you are having the anaesthetic inserted before an elective Caesarean section. Lying on your left side prevents the weight of your uterus pressing on the major veins in your pelvis which could make you feel light-headed and reduce the blood supply to your baby during the 20 to 40 minutes it will take to set up the epidural.

You will need to lie or sit very still during this time, but the anaesthetist will interrupt the procedure every time you have a contraction and wait until it is over. If you have not needed an intravenous fluid drip before now, one will be inserted in your non-writing arm before the procedure starts and an infusion of fluid, usually dextrose-saline, will be started. This ensures that your blood pressure does not drop suddenly when the epidural block starts to work (see p. 315).

Your lower back (lumbar region) will be cleaned with antiseptic; sterile covers will be placed over the rest of your back and legs to reduce the risks of infection; and some local anaesthetic will be injected over the site chosen to insert the epidural,

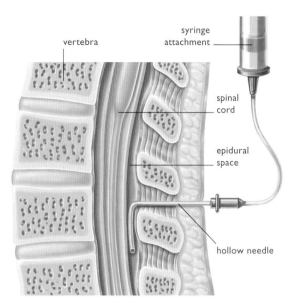

INSERTING AN EPIDURAL A hollow needle is inserted into the epidural space, leaving the spinal cord and its protective dural sheath untouched.

in order to numb your skin and minimize your discomfort. It is unusual for the procedure itself to be painful.

The procedure

The anaesthetist will carefully insert a fine hollow needle between two vertebral bones in the lumbar region of your lower back and from there, into the epidural space (see above). To check that the needle is in the right place, a small quantity of anaesthetic will then be injected. If this numbs your abdomen satisfactorily, then a thin hollow plastic catheter will be threaded through the hollow needle and settled safely into the epidural space. The needle is then removed and a protective bacterial filter is attached to the end of the catheter.

The long length of catheter outside your body will be led up your back and over your shoulder and taped onto your skin. This prevents the catheter becoming dislodged and allows you to receive top-up doses of pain relief throughout your labour. The first proper dose of anaesthetic will then be injected through the catheter and you will experience a sensation like a cold ice cube running down your lower spine as the drugs reach the spot.

The anaesthetist and midwife will check your blood pressure immediately, then every 10 minutes for the next 30 minutes, and at regular intervals afterwards. An electronic trace of the baby's heart (CTG) will also be performed during this period. In most maternity units, continuous fetal monitoring is advised after an epidural has been inserted, but in an otherwise normal labour intermittent CTG monitoring may be possible. Your abdomen will quickly go numb, but epidural anaesthesia that is deep enough to allow a painless

operative delivery, such as Caesarean section or forceps, takes longer to develop – usually 20 to 30 minutes.

Conventional epidurals also block the nerve fibres that control your bladder. As a result, you will not be aware of developing a full bladder and will find it very difficult to pass urine on your own. To overcome this, a urinary catheter will be gently inserted into your urethra to drain your bladder continuously. However, if mobile epidurals are available in your unit (see below) you will probably be able to pass urine without the need of a catheter.

Once your epidural is working effectively, it can be topped up regularly to maintain your pain relief. This is usually needed every three to four hours, but the exact timing will depend on each individual's needs. For women who reach full dilation with an effective epidural, the decision to delay active pushing has been shown to reduce the risk of an instrumental vaginal delivery.

Mobile epidurals

Most hospitals have introduced mobile epidurals, so called because they use lower drug doses to block the pain fibres, but leave the motor fibres controlling your leg movement relatively unaffected. As a result, the woman is usually less numb from her knees down, which means that she can be more mobile and benefit from the fact that gravity may help the progress of her labour. She is also less likely to need a

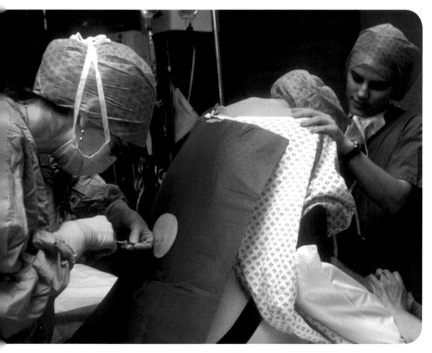

PREPARING FOR AN EPIDURAL Sterile covers are placed over your back and then a local anaesthetic is injected.

urinary catheter to empty her bladder. The other advantage of mobile epidurals is that, since the low-dose top-ups are usually needed every hour, the analgesia can be tailored to suit the stage of labour that the woman has reached.

When an epidural may not be possible

There are few absolute contraindications to having an epidural. They can be summarized as situations where the introduction of the needle could result in a blood clot (haematoma) or abscess (collection of pus) forming and placing pressure on the spinal cord. These are potentially very serious complications, which could lead to paralysis. In reality, they are uncommon, but both inherited and acquired bleeding disorders can place you at risk. Similarly, if you have been taking large doses of anticoagulant drugs (for example, because you have suffered a thrombosis during this pregnancy – see p.424) an epidural may not be recommended.

It is very rare for a pregnant women to have an infection in her lower back, but occasionally it may result from chronic tuberculosis or osteomyelitis

MEDICAL COMPLICATIONS OF EPIDURALS

Hypotension (low blood pressure)
A fall in your blood pressure is a common side effect of epidurals, usually most marked with the first dose. This is because, in addition to blocking pain fibres, the anaesthetic drugs also block some of the nerve fibres that control the size of the blood vessels in your pelvis and legs.
▶ As a result, these blood vessels dilate and the blood will tend to pool in them, reducing the volume of blood returning to your heart and head.
▶ This can cause a reduction in the blood flow through the placenta, which in turn reduces the oxygen supply to your baby.
▶ This is why the anaesthetist will always take the precautions of inserting an intravenous drip before inserting the epidural and checking your blood pressure regularly after the first and subsequent doses of drug are injected. Meanwhile, your midwife will be monitoring your baby on the CTG machine.

Headaches
Headaches are a well-documented side effect of epidurals, but in reality they affect only a small percentage of women.
▶ Severe post-epidural headache is usually the result of accidental puncture of the membrane covering the spinal cord as the needle is being inserted into the epidural space.
▶ The pain is caused by leakage of small quantities of spinal fluid, which results in traction or pulling of the membranes around the brain. It tends to be relieved by lying down.
▶ Similarly, some mothers report a slight tingling or numbness in one of their limbs and some also suffer from back pain.
▶ I do want to emphasize that, although this all sounds frightening, symptoms are only temporary and nothing to worry about.
▶ All these side effects will disappear, most within hours of the birth, some up to a few weeks later.

Backache
Recent studies have concluded that epidurals are not a genuine cause of long-term backache. Postnatal backache is much more likely to be related to pre-existing backache, perhaps caused by poor posture, rather than the use of epidural anaesthetics during labour.
▶ Poor posture and strain on your sacroiliac joints is almost inevitable in the latter stages of pregnancy and during delivery, but many mothers forget the discomfort they experienced antenatally and blame their postnatal backache on the fact that they had an epidural during labour.
▶ Interestingly, recent reports suggest that the use of low-dose mobile epidurals, which allow the mother to remain upright during labour, may reduce the chances of her complaining of postnatal backache.

(a serious infection of the bone pulp). In these situations, the risk of introducing an infection that could cause an abscess in the epidural or dural space will mean that neither epidural nor spinal anaesthesia are an option.

Spinal block

Much of the general information that I have already offered you about epidural blocks also applies to spinal regional anaesthetics. The principles in pain relief are the same – namely to block nerve fibres that conduct pain from the pelvic organs. The difference with a spinal block is that instead of trying to avoid piercing the dural sheath (as is the case with an epidural), the anaesthetist deliberately passes the needle through the epidural space and punctures the dural membrane to inject anaesthetic drugs into the fluid surrounding the spinal cord.

Over recent years, spinal blocks have become increasingly popular for Caesarean sections and emergency obstetric procedures because they are very quick to take effect – the pain relief is almost instantaneous, whereas an epidural will require 20–30 minutes. However, the spinal block is a one-shot technique and lasts for about an hour, possibly two, so it is not a useful method of pain relief throughout labour. Many anaesthetists favour a combined spinal and epidural approach (CSE) for Caesarean sections. The spinal block ensures instant pain relief and the insertion of an additional epidural catheter allows the delivery of top-up

analgesic drugs in the post-operative period. CSE blocks are also useful during labour when rapid analgesia is needed, when there is severe fetal distress in late first stage or second stage of labour.

Pudendal block

This is an injection of local anaesthetic into the vaginal tissues surrounding the left- and right-sided pudendal nerves (these supply sensation to the lower half of the vagina). A good pudendal block will markedly reduce pain in the vagina and perineum during the second stage of labour, but has no effect on the pain of uterine contractions. Hence it is usually reserved for low, uncomplicated lift-out forceps or ventouse deliveries when the mother has been given no other method of pain relief. The pudendal block will last long enough to perform the delivery of the baby and repair the episiotomy or any vaginal or perineal tears that may have occurred.

Since the area that needs to be injected is high up the vagina, the pudendal needle is quite long and thick. However, the doctor will apply a cold anaesthetic spray to the areas that are to be injected. A pudendal anaesthetic will have no effect on the baby and can be used in combination with pethidine or entonox. Although it is usually inserted by a doctor, there is no need for an anaesthetist to be present, and hence pudendal blocks are more commonly used in low-risk delivery units in which there are not 24-hour anaesthetic services available.

> 66 Over recent years, spinal blocks have become increasingly popular for Caesarean sections and emergency obstetric procedures because they are very quick to take effect – the pain relief is almost instantaneous. 99

GENERAL ANAESTHESIA

Although over the past 20 years epidurals have become increasingly popular for deliveries by Caesarean section, to the extent that they have virtually replaced general anaesthesia, a general anaesthetic is still sometimes used for abdominal delivery.

Having a general anaesthetic

All the technical preparations for the operation will be undertaken while you are wide awake in the operating theatre. Your birth partner will then be asked to leave as you are about to become unconscious. You will be asked to breathe deeply from an oxygen mask for several minutes to increase your oxygen levels, and to lie on the operating table on your left side, which further improves the oxygen supply reaching the placenta.

Only when everything is absolutely ready will the anaesthetist ask you to inhale the drugs to make you go to sleep. This will be followed immediately by the insertion of an endotracheal tube (airway) into your mouth and down your throat, to ensure that oxygen can be delivered to your lungs and to prevent you regurgitating food or fluid from your stomach. Further drugs to relax your abdominal muscles will be given intravenously and the surgeon is then able to perform the operation very quickly, delivering the baby in a few minutes, before significant amounts of the anaesthetic drugs have crossed the placenta.

In total, you will be asleep for about 45 to 60 minutes, since it takes a lot longer to stitch all the tissue layers back into place and ensure that the bleeding is under control than it does to open up the uterus and deliver the baby.

REASONS FOR USING A GENERAL ANAESTHETIC

Maternal request
Acute fear of needles, backache, the operative procedure (if a Caesarean section is planned) or a previous traumatic delivery are all valid reasons for a woman to request a general anaesthetic.

Obstetric indications
Extreme emergencies, such as severe placental abruption or cord prolapse, are situations where the baby's life is at risk unless delivery is performed immediately. Severe bleeding may prompt the anaesthetist to perform a general anaesthetic, or even convert your regional block to one, because he will be better able to stabilize your cardiovascular system. Many favour a general for women with an anterior placenta praevia (see p.428).

Maternal indications
Women with heart disease may be best delivered with the help of a general anaesthetic. Similarly, there are a few pregnant women with such severe abnormalities of their spine (such as curvature of the spine or spina bifida) that it is technically too difficult to insert a regional anaesthetic.

Coagulation problems following maternal infection, haemorrhage or pre-eclampsia, can make it unsafe to insert a regional block because of the risk of bleeding into the epidural or subarachnoid space (see diagram, p.313).

NON-PHARMACOLOGICAL PAIN RELIEF

There are various ways in which pain can be reduced without using any drugs, although you should be clear that their effectiveness varies and what might help one woman could prove totally ineffective for another.

Broadly speaking these methods of pain relief can be divided into two main groups:
- methods involving the use of equipment or expert practitioners including TENS, acupuncture, hypnotherapy, reflexology, and water births
- natural methods for use by yourself or with a birth partner including breathing and relaxation, massage, aromatherapy, and homeopathy.

Transcutaneous Electrical Nerve Stimulation (TENS)

The TENS machine is a battery-operated device, connected by wires to small electrodes that are attached to either sides of your lower back by four adhesive pads (see right). It works by conducting a small electrical current through your skin to stimulate the production of endorphins (your body's own natural painkillers) which in turn helps to block the pain impulses carried by your nerves to your brain. Many women choose to try this method of pain relief, particularly in early labour, since they remain free to walk about carrying the hand-held control box with them. The other advantage is that you are in complete control of the frequency and strength of the electrical current. By pressing a small button on the handset at the start of a contraction, you are able to increase or decrease the amount of stimulation, which feels like a tingling sensation in the skin and has an immediate effect in blocking the pain. The TENS will not affect your baby in any way.

The TENS machine cannot be used while you are in water, so you will need to take it off while having a relaxing bath, or if you have chosen to have a water birth.

You can make arrangements to hire a TENS machine from your hospital or through your team of midwives before you go into labour. You will be

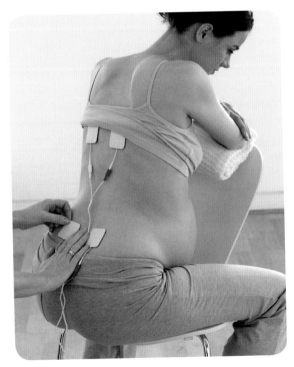

TENS MACHINE This is a popular choice for pain relief in early labour as the mother remains free to walk about and is in complete control of the level of pain relief she receives.

charged for the total length of time you hire it. It is best to plan to collect your machine at about 37 to 38 weeks so you have plenty of time to work out how to use it. TENS is not a good method of pain relief in established labour.

Acupuncture

Acupuncture is another method of stimulating your body to produce endorphins. Instead of electrical currents, firm finger pressure or fine needles are applied to specific points on your body by a trained acupuncturist.

The theory behind acupuncture is based on the age-old Chinese belief that a life force called "chi" flows through the body and that medical disorders occur when there are imbalances in this life force. The balance is restored when the "chi" is unblocked by the insertion of fine needles into key areas of the body. Many women find acupuncture helpful during pregnancy to treat symptoms such as morning sickness, headaches, allergies, indigestion, backache and emotional disturbances including depression. It can be a very effective method of pain relief both before and during labour.

If you want to explore this option, you will need to find an acupuncturist who has experience of treating women in labour and is prepared to attend your labour at home or come into hospital with you.

Hypnotherapy

Hypnotherapy works by suggestion. To relieve the pain of labour this means that you will need to be hypnotized into believing that you can control the pain of your contractions and, as a result, will be less troubled by them. There are several ways to achieve this, but they will all require careful preparation and plenty of practice before you go into labour.

You can hire a hypnotherapist to attend your labour, or you could arrange to have your partner trained to help hypnotize you. Self-hypnosis is a further possibility, but I suspect that for most women, with all that is going on during labour, this may be more difficult to achieve than anticipated. Nonetheless, hypnosis has been shown to be an effective method of pain relief in labour, may reduce the length of labour, and can be a useful tool with which to improve your emotional state both during and post delivery.

Reflexology

In reflexology, gentle pressure or massage is applied to specific points on the feet. This stimulates nerve endings, which helps to relieve problems in other parts of the body. During pregnancy, reflexology can be used to help ease backache, general aches and pains, and in combination with more orthodox medical remedies, to treat problems such as high blood pressure and gestational diabetes. Some therapists believe that attending regular reflexology sessions during pregnancy allows you the option of using this as a method of pain relief during labour. It is also claimed that reflexology can help the progress of labour by making the uterus contract more efficiently and the cervix dilate more speedily. If you decide to explore this option, you will need to spend some time with a therapist during pregnancy and ensure that both you and your partner learn exactly where and how to massage the trigger points on your feet during labour.

Water and water births

There is no doubt that immersion in water can relieve pain, particularly in the early stages of labour. The warmth of the water helps to relax your muscles and the buoyancy of the water also supports your body, thereby relieving some of the pressure of the baby's head pressing down in your pelvis. Provided that your membranes have not ruptured, you can enjoy wallowing in a warm bath either at home or in the maternity unit, for as long as you like during the early stages of labour.

I should mention here that most water-assisted births in the UK do not actually take place under water in the birthing pool. Even if you spend most of the first and second stage of labour in the water, some midwives will still prefer you to be on "dry land" when the baby is actually born. This is quite simply because they will want to ensure that they have maximum access to you and your baby in the final critical stages of the delivery, and also because not all midwives are experienced in supervising water births.

In the past, fears were expressed that delivering a baby under water might lead to problems with him inhaling water into the lungs as the first breath is taken. This is unlikely to happen if the baby is brought to the surface quickly, since the umbilical cord continues to deliver a good supply of oxygen for several minutes after the birth, providing it is not cut.

The other concern is that the mother's body temperature may rise if she remains immersed in warm water for a long period of time. This will result in the baby developing a temperature and increased heart rate, which could lead to hypoxia (lowered oxygen levels). This is why your midwife will be checking your temperature regularly and will advise you to leave the birthing pool if your temperature increases by more than 1°C (33.8°F) during labour or delivery.

Breathing and relaxation

There is no doubt that we all feel pain more acutely when we are tense or frightened. By learning how to relax and breathe properly, you will feel much calmer and, as a result, will be in a much better position to cope with the labour. The breathing and relaxation techniques that you have been taught in your antenatal classes will be put to good use during the last few weeks of pregnancy and particularly when you are in labour. Try to spend a few minutes each day practising breathing in deeply and exhaling slowly. It is a good idea to enlist your partner's help here, so that you can rely on someone else to remind you of these simple but important principles when you need them most.

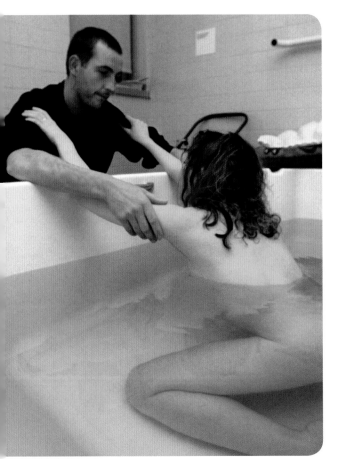

WATER BIRTH Immersion in water is undoubtedly a valuable method of pain relief, particularly in the early stages of labour.

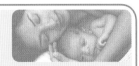

BIRTH STORY

Muriel, 31, has one daughter aged two years eight months
Second baby Killian, born 39 weeks + 5 days, weight 3.1kg (7lb)
Length of labour from first contraction: approximately 12 hours

My first baby, Maela, had been born at home – on dry land. For our second baby, we were planning to have another home birth but this time with the added benefit of a birthing pool. About three days before my due date, I felt a few contractions in the evening. They were quite strong but didn't last very long. The next day, when I took Maela to her nursery, I told the staff that I would have the baby that night. I had a strong feeling that labour would start for good that evening – which it did.

Right from the start, the contractions felt strong, although manageable. As I was still breastfeeding Maela in the evenings, I fed her hoping she would sleep soundly through the night and this increased the strength of the contractions. They were coming every four minutes at that stage and I needed to concentrate on breathing and relaxing. My husband, Steve, started to get the birthing pool organized but we decided not to fill it until Margaret, my midwife, said it was okay to get in.

At about 11pm, I phoned to tell her that my labour had started and she came round to check how I was doing. I was pleased to see her because I wanted to get into the pool, so I asked her to do an internal examination and it turned out that I had not dilated at all but my cervix was fully thinned. Margaret stayed for a little while, then went home. She had told me not to get into the birthing pool, so I had a bath instead and felt it did help a bit. We were taking the contractions one at a time and trying to accept them or even welcome them (not very successfully). At about 3.30am, I did a self-examination as I am an NCT antenatal teacher. I thought I had reached about 4cm dilation, so Steve phoned Margaret again and she arrived at 4am. This time she let me get into the pool and I finally felt I was where I should be to give birth.

The contractions were coming thick and fast and by 7am I wanted to push. I was in a half squatting position in the pool. The contractions had changed and I could feel the baby's head coming down. Margaret told me to look at her and pant. Our little baby was coming.

I grabbed the tiny body, brought it to the surface, and held our little boy's head out of the water. We got out of the pool and I then felt the placenta being delivered. I didn't want the cord to be clamped, so Margaret asked me to cut it myself, which I did. It felt wonderful to at last be holding my newborn baby boy.

> 66 I grabbed the tiny body, brought it to the surface, and held our little boy's head out of the water. 99

In the early stages of labour, you will need to concentrate on breathing in and out slowly as each contraction starts. The secret is to close your eyes and breathe in calmly through your nose, imagining that the breath is filling every part of your body. Concentrate on relaxing all of your muscles as you do so. Then, breathe out slowly through your mouth, this time imagining that you are drawing out and exhaling the pain of your contraction. You may have been shown visualization techniques in your antenatal classes. The principle here is to focus on an image or visit a place in your mind that you find calming and soothing, in order to take your mind off the pain. This is a sort of hypnosis and works better for some women than others.

As the contractions become more intense, you will probably find that you need to take shorter breaths, in groups of two or three, since strong contractions make it difficult to keep up the slow breathing rhythm. At this stage you need to remember that breathing out is the all-important bit, since the breathing in will take care of itself, if you are breathing out properly. My best tip here is to imagine that you are blowing wind through trees and that every breath needs to reach a spot about 30cm (12in) away. I often find that if I sit on the bed beside a woman in strong labour and ask her to ensure that every outward breath hits my nose, that she gets the hang of the new rhythm very quickly. Once achieved, it is easy to get her partner to take up the same position and encourage her to continue breathing out in the same way.

Massage

A good massage is always relaxing and when you are in labour, it can really help to relieve backache. If your baby is lying occipito-posterior with his spine closest to your spine and sacral bones, you will be particularly glad to have someone massage

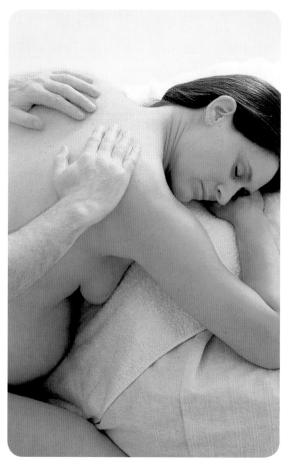

MASSAGE This provides a great opportunity for your partner to become physically involved in helping you to cope with your labour. Encourage him to master the art of giving a good massage while you are pregnant.

your lower back, preferably in slow, firm circular movements just above the cleft of your buttocks.

In addition to the physical comfort this provides, I think that it is also a source of emotional comfort. The fact that someone else is with you and helping you cope with the discomfort or pain helps reduce the feelings of isolation and fear that being in an unknown situation always engenders.

Asking your birth partner to extend the massage to your shoulders, neck, face, forehead, and temples will further help relieve tension and anxiety, enabling you to feel more relaxed during labour. Make sure that the person who is undertaking the massage warms their hands and removes any jewellery. Using scented oils or creams will help the hands slide easily over the skin.

Aromatherapy

In aromatherapy, essential oils are used to soothe and relax the body. It is thought that the scented oils trigger the nervous system to produce natural endorphins and that this helps reduce tension and alleviate some of the pain.

During early labour, the diluted oils can be absorbed through your skin when combined with massaging or by adding them to your bath or birthing pool. Alternatively, you can inhale them from a burner or vaporizer, which gently warms the oils producing a soothing, scented atmosphere.

If you wish to use aromatherapy during labour, you will need to take the oils and the vaporizer with you to the maternity unit. Check beforehand that all of the oils you are planning to use are suitable for use in pregnancy.

Homeopathy and herbs

There is a wide variety of homeopathic and herbal remedies that can be used during labour to help relieve stress and discomfort. However, it is important to ensure that you obtain specialist advice about the types of herbs that are suitable and the doses that should be used. Remember, too, that you need to consult with your midwife or doctors about anything you are taking when you are in labour.

MY PRACTICAL TIPS TO HELP WITH LABOUR PAINS

Here is a selection of practical tips and thoughts that I hope will come in handy on the big day. I was given them by a close friend and have since shared them with many of my patients.
▶ Labour is like walking a tightrope. The aim is to stay balanced and on the rope.
▶ Therefore, one step at a time, one contraction at a time.
▶ Don't think about how much further you have to walk. No one can tell you how much longer it will be before you give birth.
▶ Concentrate on getting through the next contraction with your breathing techniques.
▶ Don't think about how much pain you may be in three

contractions' time, just think about getting through your next "step" on the tightrope.
▶ Levels of pain vary along the tightrope and are unpredictable. What you are going through now could be better or worse in half an hour's time, so there is no point in worrying about it.
▶ Each contraction gets you one step closer to the end of the tightrope – the birth of your baby – so there is a very good reason to keep going.
▶ Try to keep fed and watered wherever possible to keep your energy levels up.
▶ Aim to find ways of distracting yourself to help take your mind off the pain.

▶ Find different positions that help to relieve your pain.
▶ Above all, try your best to stay as relaxed as possible. Tension increases pain.
▶ If you want pain relief, then ask for it sooner rather than later and do not be backwards in coming forwards to request a stronger dose of pethidine or a top up of your epidural, if you need it.

You may find it helpful to write out a list of your own reminders or practical coping tips, which you can then pack in your hospital bag to ensure that they are close by when you need them, or just in case your mind goes totally blank in the middle of your labour.

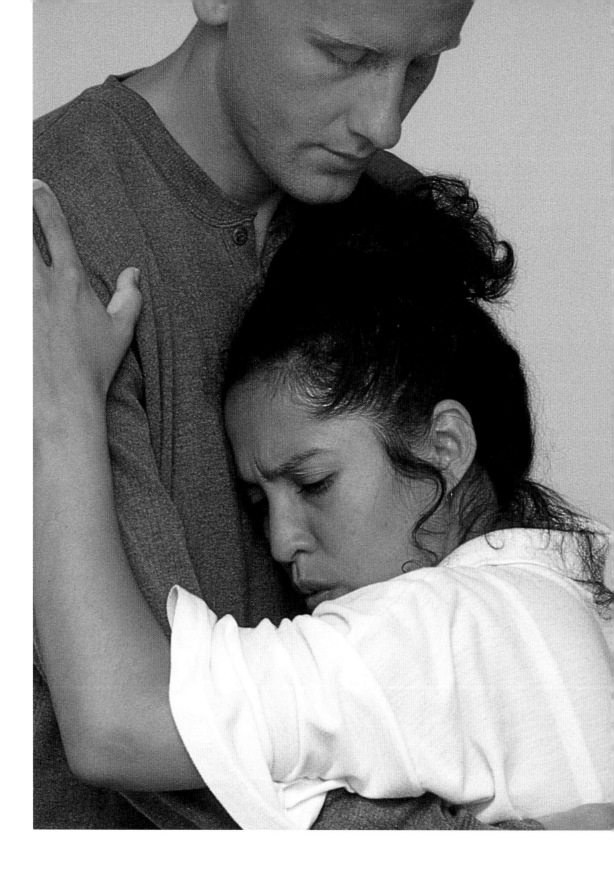

The second & third stages

THE SECOND STAGE OF LABOUR begins when your cervix is fully dilated and ends with the birth of your baby. This is then followed by the third stage when the placenta and membranes are delivered. You will probably be feeling tired as you enter these phases, but the knowledge that the end is in sight will, I hope, spur you on through these final stages.

During the second stage of labour, your baby is forced through your birth canal by the uterine contractions, which are now stronger and more frequent, occurring every two to four minutes, and lasting for 60–90 seconds. At this stage you will probably feel as if you are contracting continuously and that the labour has taken on a momentum of its own, which it has. There is now no stopping a normal labour until the baby has been expelled from the birth canal. In first labours, the second stage may last for two to three hours, although the average length of time is one hour. In second or subsequent labours, the second stage usually lasts for about 15–20 minutes, but can be much quicker and the baby may start to crown before the mother and her midwife recognize that she has entered the second stage of labour.

The third stage of labour – the delivery of the placenta – usually lasts about 10 to 20 minutes, but can be shorter or longer, depending on whether the delivery is actively managed or the placenta is left to expel itself spontaneously (see p.333).

Someone to lean on

Your birth partner has an important role during the second and third stages of labour. He or she will be able to support you physically as you work hard to push your baby out, as well as being able to tell you what can be seen as the baby's head emerges. He or she can also give you invaluable verbal encouragement and reassurance as you both experience the birth of your baby.

66 …during the second stage, you will probably feel as if you are contracting continuously and that the labour has taken on a momentum of its own, which it has. 99

The second stage of labour

For most mothers, the first indication they have completed the transition phase and entered the second stage of labour is that they develop a strong urge to push or bear down. It is important to refrain from pushing until the midwife confirms that you are fully dilated.

> " When it is time to start pushing, it is vital that you work as a team with your midwife. "

Once your midwife confirms that you are fully dilated and that it is time to start pushing, it is vital that you work as a team with her. Remember that the uterine contractions are going to continue involuntarily and what you now need to do is add the force of your voluntary pushing efforts to help expel the baby. Listen carefully to what the midwife tells you to do.

The idea is to push as much as you can as each contraction peaks and to rest in between times. As each uterine contraction starts you need to take a deep breath in, hold it, close your throat, brace your feet, and push downwards to force the baby lower into the pelvis. Aim to contract your diaphragm and abdominal muscles and push down into your pelvis – not into your tummy, which won't help the baby's head to descend. Try to visualize what is actually happening and where you are pushing. The effort needs to be directed specifically into the vagina and rectum, rather than vaguely "somewhere down there". Ideally, try not to hold one long breath, as this can deprive you of oxygen and make you feel light-headed. During a good contraction you should be able to take three separate breaths and achieve three good pushes.

Knowing when to push

If you have an epidural, the top-ups will hopefully be timed so that the effects are beginning to wear off a little by the time you begin the second stage. This means you will be aware of the contractions but will not be in pain. If you are totally numb as a result of the epidural (unlikely with the newer, continuous slow rate of infusion), your midwife will alert you to the start of each contraction, although you may learn quite quickly to recognize them because you will feel your uterus tighten when you place your hand on your abdomen. Furthermore, you and your partner will also be able to see from the CTG monitor print-out when the contractions are beginning and ending. However, I think it is best for you to concentrate on the breathing and pushing and leave your partner and midwife to prompt you when to start and stop pushing. At the end of each contraction try not to relax too quickly because the baby will not continue to progress forwards unless you relax slowly.

COPING WITH THE SECOND STAGE

Try to find a comfortable position that is reasonably upright and always avoid lying flat. By this stage in labour, most women find that they want to be supported on a bed, although some prefer to squat or use a birthing stool. The more upright you are, the more you will be helped by gravity and the quicker your baby will be born.

Many women worry about sounding or looking ridiculous during the second stage of labour. This is not the time to worry about being prim and proper; it is the time to do what feels natural and comfortable for you. If that means grunting and making a lot of noise while you are pushing, that's fine. Similarly, it is pointless feeling worried or embarrassed that you may pass some stool or urine towards the end of the second stage. This is very common and you need to remember that your midwife and doctor have seen it all before.

Interestingly, once they have reached the second stage of labour, most women lose many of their inhibitions and cease being self-conscious. The combination of concentration and instinct take over and there is no time to think about anything other than doing what is necessary to push the baby out.

The other thing that surprises many women in labour is that, compared to some of the late first-stage contractions, the ones in the second stage often seem more bearable. I think this is because you are now actively participating in the labour and this helps to dispel some of the tension caused by painful contractions. Although the pushing is hard work, you will feel a sense of satisfaction as each push brings the birth of your baby closer. Knowing that the finishing line is in sight boosts your energy reserves.

POSITIONS FOR THE SECOND STAGE

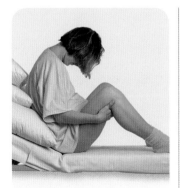

SITTING UPRIGHT Supported by pillows, try to relax your back between contractions.

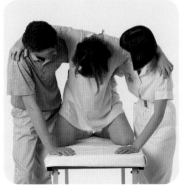

KNEELING A helper on each side supports you, or kneeling on all fours may be more comfortable.

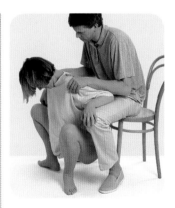

SQUATTING This opens the pelvis wide and uses gravity to help push the baby out.

Descent and delivery

As your baby's head is pushed deeper into the pelvis you will become increasingly aware of pressure in your rectum and may experience pains that radiate down your legs, caused by pressure on the nerves in your sacral area. This stage can be extremely painful as the anus starts to bulge and the vagina and perineum are stretched by the emerging head. At the height of a contraction, the tip of the baby's head will become visible, although, at first, it will slip back up the birth canal when you are not pushing. Gradually, the head stays in place and starts to crown. It is common to experience the sensation of intense stinging or burning because the vagina is stretched to its limit as the head is on the verge of being delivered. It is now very important to follow your midwife's instructions, particularly when she tells you to stop pushing and to pant instead. This helps to avoid the head delivering suddenly, which is dangerous for the baby and may tear your vagina and perineal tissues.

Once the head starts to crown, it usually takes only a couple of contractions for it to be delivered. Your midwife will assess whether you need an episiotomy or whether it is possible to deliver the head safely without one. During the contractions, some midwives will support the perineum, whereas others do not touch it – either method is safe and is the personal choice of the midwife. The midwife will also support the baby's head to help prevent a rapid delivery. Once the head is delivered, the midwife will support it and feel around the neck to make sure the umbilical cord is not wrapped around it. If it is, the cord will be

DELIVERY OF YOUR BABY ·······································

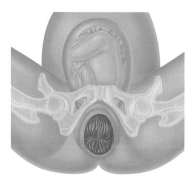 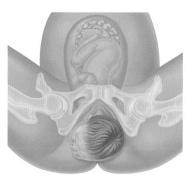 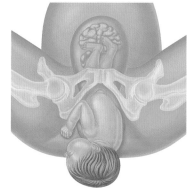

ONCE THE HEAD STARTS TO CROWN it usually takes only a couple of contractions before delivery. Most babies are in an anterior position, so the head will emerge with the nose pointing downwards.

AS SOON AS THE BABY'S HEAD IS FREE of the perineum, the neck will extend and the baby will automatically rotate to face left or right, so that the shoulders are now in the best position to deliver smoothly.

THE FIRST (ANTERIOR) SHOULDER will slip under the pubic bone followed swiftly by the posterior shoulder. The rest of the body slips out and the baby is usually delivered onto the mother's tummy.

gently looped over the baby's head and at the same time the nose and mouth will be wiped free of blood and mucus.

During the next contraction, the first or upper shoulder will be delivered, usually aided by the midwife applying some gentle downwards traction on the sides of the baby's head. As the first shoulder slips free from under the pubic bone, the midwife will gently sweep the baby's head and shoulder upwards, allowing the second or posterior shoulder more room to emerge during the next few contractions. Once both shoulders are delivered, the rest of the baby literally slides out, followed by a further stream of amniotic fluid, which was behind the shoulders. The doctor or midwife will be waiting to catch this slippery bundle, covered with blood, liquor, and vernix. If you request, they will place the baby on your tummy or chest, covered or wrapped in towels to prevent him from getting cold. If you intend to breastfeed, you may want to put your baby to the breast immediately.

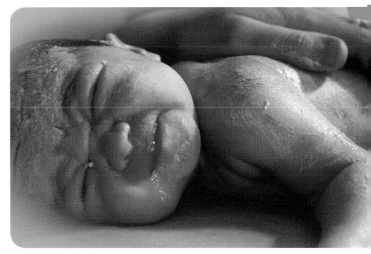

AT BIRTH Your baby will be a slippery bundle, covered in blood, liquor, and vernix.

Managing the second stage

Presuming there are no delays or complications, the second stage will usually be completed within three hours in a first labour and well within two hours for a second or subsequent birth. Throughout the second stage, the midwife will keep a careful watch on the baby's heart rate after each contraction and maternal push, either with a Pinard's stethoscope or an external or internal electronic monitor, depending on what has been happening during the first stage of labour. She will also keep note of the strength and regularity of your uterine contractions. Sometimes they start to fade away during the second stage, in which case you may be advised that a low-dose syntocinon infusion is needed to restore the contractions and enable you to push your baby out promptly.

Every hospital has a policy about how long they will advise a woman to push actively, but because of the risks of fetal distress and maternal fatigue, most units will not encourage you to continue pushing for more than two hours in a first labour or one hour in a subsequent labour before suggesting they assist the delivery with either vacuum extraction (ventouse) or forceps. However, there are no hard and fast rules if you are both coping with the labour, and careful monitoring is important.

EPISIOTOMIES AND TEARS

Ideally you will give birth without needing an episiotomy
or ending up with a perineal tear. However, should the
need arise at the time of delivery, careful consideration
will be given as to which is likely to be the better
option for you. Each has its advantages and disadvantages,
so find out as much as you can about your hospital's
policy on episiotomies and perineal tears during
the antenatal period.

EPISIOTOMIES

An episiotomy is a deliberate incision made in the stretched perineum and vagina to prevent uncontrolled tearing of the mother's tissues as the baby's head is delivered. It used to be thought that an episiotomy not only prevented extensive tears of the perineum but also the development of vaginal prolapse in later life. Since the evidence for the latter is now doubtful, episiotomies are no longer performed routinely.

There are, however, several situations when an episiotomy may be advisable:
▶ tight perineum in a first or subsequent labour
▶ large baby
▶ fetal distress that requires immediate delivery
▶ for a forceps or ventouse delivery
▶ to protect the head of a premature baby
▶ to protect the baby's head in a vaginal breech delivery (however, most breech babies nowadays are delivered by Caesarean section).

If you have strong views about episiotomies – either that you want to avoid one at all costs or that you positively want to have one – then you should make this clear to your midwife early in your labour.

THE PROCEDURE

If your midwife or doctor judge that you need an episiotomy, they will ask your permission before they perform it. They will then swab the area with antiseptic and give you a local anaesthetic in your perineum unless you have an active epidural in place.

The most usual incision is a medio-lateral cut angled away from the vagina and rectum. It is also possible to make a mid-line cut straight down from the bottom of the vagina towards the rectum, but this is rarely performed now. Both types of incision are made with scissors and because the perineum is tightly stretched, almost paper thin, at the time the cut is made, the bleeding is usually minimal. The advantage of a medio-lateral

episiotomy is that it keeps the incision well away from the rectal area. This is particularly relevant if a forceps delivery is anticipated as this may extend the cut. The mid-line episiotomy avoids several blood vessels and is usually easier to repair, but if it extends during the delivery, it is more likely to tear into the rectum.

Once the baby and placenta have been delivered, your midwife or doctor will repair the episiotomy with stitches. They will probably advise that your legs are placed in stirrups to make the repair easier. You will be given a further injection of anaesthetic to ensure you feel no pain during the procedure.

The episiotomy will be sutured in layers, ensuring that all of the tissues are brought together properly to repair the vagina and perineum. The sutures may be interrupted or continuous and either external or buried below the skin. Whatever type is used, they all dissolve and do not need to be taken out.

> ❝ ...make your views on episiotomies clear to your midwife early in your labour ❞

COMMON WORRIES

One of the commonest worries about episiotomies is how much they will hurt afterwards and how long they will take to heal. The reality is that they are painful, particularly on the second or third day after the birth, when the stitches often feel tight and uncomfortable. This is the result of the body's natural healing response, which means that the traumatized tissues inevitably become swollen.

Much relief can be obtained from placing maternity cool packs against the episiotomy area and using an inflated rubber ring to sit on. However, the vagina has an excellent blood supply and most cuts will heal in one to two weeks, so long as the area is kept as clean and dry as possible. Regular bathing with warm water will help relieve discomfort. It is not necessary to add disinfectant solutions and it is important to avoid highly perfumed soaps and oils, which can irritate the healing wound.

In the long term, most women do not have problems with the episiotomy scar, but some experience continuing perineal pain, which can be a source of distress, particularly when it causes problems with sexual intercourse. Massaging the scar tissue with emollient or oestrogen creams can help make the tissues more supple, and pelvic floor exercises will usually help to improve the situation. If the discomfort continues, advice should be sought regarding further surgery.

PERINEAL TEARS

There are four degrees of perineal tear.

▶ **First degree** – these are minor tears to the vaginal skin around the entrance to the vagina. Most will heal well without any sutures.

▶ **Second degree** – the posterior vaginal wall and perineal muscles are torn, but the anal sphincter muscles remain intact. Most will require several sutures to restore the anatomy of the muscles and more superficial tissues.

▶ **Third degree** – the anal sphincter muscles are torn, but the mucous lining of the rectum remains intact. These tears will need careful repair to ensure the muscle layers are realigned.

▶ **Fourth degree** – the anal sphincter muscles are torn to the extent that the rectal mucosa is opened. Considerable skill is required to repair a fourth degree tear because it is essential that the apex of the tear is secured to prevent the development of a rectovaginal fistula (a persistent opening between the vagina and the rectum). These tears are not common, occurring in only one per cent of births. They usually follow forceps or ventouse delivery for a first baby, persistent occipito-posterior positions or the delivery of a baby weighing more than 4kg (9lb).

EPISIOTOMY CUT

The medio-lateral cut for an episiotomy – in which the cut is angled down and away from the vagina and the perineum – is the preferred choice in the UK and most of the rest of the world. The cut is done at an angle between the vagina and the rectum. Research suggests that tearing is less likely with this procedure than with the midline episiotomy (in which the incision is made straight down into the perineum between the vagina and anus).

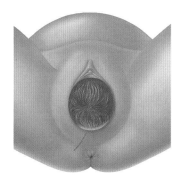

MEDIO-LATERAL The cut is angled down and away from the vagina and the perineum into the muscle.

The third stage of labour

The third stage of labour involves the delivery of the placenta and membranes. The minutes after the birth are invariably an emotional time and you and your partner will probably be aware only of the fact that you are finally cuddling your new baby.

Cutting the cord

Many women request that their baby is placed on their tummy immediately after delivery to start the bonding process. The cord will still be attached at this point and will continue to pulsate for one to three minutes. Unless the baby has been distressed during the delivery and is in need of prompt attention from the paediatric doctors, there is no hurry to clamp and cut the cord. Indeed, it is important to leave it for two to three minutes to allow blood to redistribute from the placental part of the circulation into the baby's. This provides the baby with a normal volume of blood and extra oxygen until the lungs start working properly. Also, without this blood transfer, the baby is more likely to have iron deficiency and develop anaemia.

The midwife will place two clamps in the middle of the long umbilical cord, 3–5cm (1–2in) apart, to prevent bleeding from the baby at one end and from the placenta at the other end. She will then cut the cord between the two clamps, or your partner can cut it. Later on, the cord will be trimmed further and a plastic clip will be attached to the stump near your baby's umbilicus. Over the next few days, this bit of remaining cord will shrink and the plastic clamp will either fall off or be removed, leaving the baby with a little knot of tissue at the umbilicus, or belly button, that will quickly disappear.

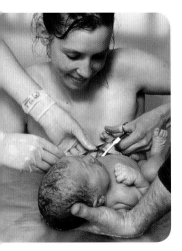

CUTTING THE CORD
This is a straightforward procedure. If your partner would like to do it, let your midwife know in advance.

Delivery of the placenta

Having cut the cord, the next thing your midwife will do (in addition to checking over your baby) is make sure the placenta is delivered correctly and promptly. After the baby is born, the continuing uterine contractions and the shrinking or retraction of the uterus reduces the size of the placental bed considerably. The placenta buckles inwards, tearing the blood vessels and attachments to the uterine wall. This results in a small haemorrhage behind the placenta which further helps it to separate. The process starts as soon as the baby is born and is usually complete within five minutes. However, the placenta is usually retained in the uterus for longer because the membranes take more time to strip away from the uterine wall. Once this placental separation has occurred the uterine muscular wall clamps down to strangle the blood vessels in the placental bed and encourages the formation of clots in the torn ends, thus reducing further blood loss.

Physiological management

When the placenta and membranes are allowed to separate on their own and no attempt is made to deliver them until clear signs of separation are seen, this is described as physiological management of the third stage. The signs are a gush of blood (the retroplacental haemorrhage), followed by contractions, which make the fundus of the uterus rise in the abdomen. There is also a lengthening of the umbilical cord visible outside the vagina, and you will experience an urge to bear down, which is the best sign that the placenta has separated and that the uterus is trying to expel it into the vagina. When these events have all occurred (which usually take about 20 minutes) the midwife will place her hand above your pubic bone to hold the uterus in place, and then ask you to push downwards to encourage the separated placenta to leave the vagina, followed by the membranes and the retro-placental blood clot. She will then massage the uterus firmly to "rub up" a further contraction, which helps to contract the uterus further and prevent any more bleeding. Further massaging of the uterus may be needed at regular intervals during the first hour after the birth to keep it firmly contracted.

If you are keen to have no medical intervention in the third stage, you can speed up the natural process and try to avoid heavy bleeding by placing the baby at your breast and encouraging suckling as soon as possible after birth. Suckling stimulates the release of the hormone oxytocin, which causes your uterus to contract and the placenta to separate from the uterine walls. Ensuring that your bladder is empty will also help to deliver the placenta promptly.

Active management

The reason why many units advise active management of the third stage is because bleeding after the delivery of the baby and placenta can be torrential. Indeed postpartum haemorrhage (see p.335) remains the most important cause of maternal death worldwide. During the antenatal period, your midwives will have discussed the third stage with you and explained that active management involves giving you an injection of Syntocinon or Syntometrine in

❝ ...you can speed up the natural process by placing your baby at your breast... ❞

your thigh muscle as soon as the baby's head and first shoulder have delivered. Syntometrine is a combination of Syntocinon and ergometrine: the ergometrine makes the uterus contract rapidly and the syntocinon ensures that the contraction is prolonged or sustained, although it is rather slower to start working. The combination of both drugs helps to contract the uterus firmly, to separate and start to expel the placenta and membranes, and then maintain the uterine contraction without any relaxation for a period of about 45 minutes. Having waited for the uterus to contract firmly, your midwife will place a protective hand above your pubic bone to prevent the uterus being pulled downwards when she gently pulls on the umbilical cord. This is called controlled cord traction (CCT) and usually ensures prompt delivery of the placenta and membranes. Undue force can lead to uterine inversion – the uterus is literally turned inside out.

Your physical response

Immediately before or after the delivery of the placenta, it is common for mothers to experience strange reactions in response to the enormous effort of giving birth. You may find yourself shivering and shaking uncontrollably and your teeth chattering violently, as if you have suddenly been exposed to extreme cold. This is frequently accompanied by intense nausea, which is often a side effect of the syntometrine injection and may make you physically sick. Since you are likely to have an empty stomach, this will probably amount only to retching of bile and watery fluids. Rest assured that all these reactions are entirely normal and common. Your midwife will not be at all surprised and will help you and your partner to deal with them.

CHECKING THE PLACENTA AND MEMBRANES

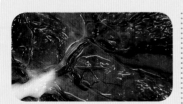

FETAL SURFACE This smooth side of the placenta has blood vessels radiating out from the umbilical cord.

As soon as the placenta and membranes are delivered, they will be checked to ensure that they are complete. A healthy term placenta weighs about 500g (1lb 2oz), measures about 20–25cm (8–10in) in diameter, and looks like a spongy disc. Any unusual appearances will prompt your midwife or doctor to send it to the pathology laboratory for analysis. In the vast majority of cases, the placenta will be unremarkable and, after weighing it and recording all the observations in your notes, it will be disposed of by the hospital. You may want to see this extraordinary lifeline before this happens, or you may even want to take it home with you.

When problems arise

Occasionally, complications can arise during the third stage of labour.

A retained placenta is one that remains within the uterus for more than one hour after delivery of the baby. Approximately 1 per cent of deliveries are complicated by this and it is more likely to occur after very premature births because the umbilical cord is thinner and may snap more easily during cord traction. Since a retained placenta is almost always associated with postpartum haemorrhage, prompt action is needed to remove it. This is usually done manually in the operating theatre.

Primary postpartum haemorrhage (PPH) is defined as the loss of 500ml (about one pint) of blood from the uterus or vagina within 24 hours of delivery of the baby. About 6 per cent of deliveries in the UK are complicated by a PPH, but it is more likely to follow a prolonged labour or a forceps, ventouse or Caesarean delivery. The incidence of PPH has fallen over the last 50 years because of improved awareness of the situations that are likely to cause it and either preventive management or prompt treatment when it occurs. Active management of the third stage of labour is an important preventive measure that has contributed to the reduction, but antenatal diagnosis of placenta praevia (see p.428), improved anaesthetic techniques, and the realization that prolonged or difficult labours are more likely to lead to a PPH have also made a contribution.

When a serious primary postpartum haemorrhage does occur, strict labour ward protocols, involvement of senior obstetricians and anaesthetists, improvements in intensive care, readily available blood transfusions, better antibiotics, and a major reduction in the number of women who become severely anaemic during pregnancy has meant that the number of maternal deaths has been greatly reduced.

Secondary postpartum haemorrhage is defined as any sudden loss of blood from the uterus or vagina, regardless of the volume of blood, from 24 hours to six weeks after the delivery. Secondary PPH occurs after 1 in 50–200 births, and is usually because of retained pieces of placenta or membranes in the uterus. These frequently become infected when they are left in the uterine cavity, and the inflammation that accompanies the infection further contributes to the bleeding. Usually the mother complains of feeling unwell, with pain and tenderness in the lower abdomen and develops a temperature and a smelly vaginal discharge. The problem needs to be identified quickly and treated with antibiotics. The removal of the retained tissues under general anaesthetic is also usually required to resolve most secondary PPHs.

> 66
> ...active management of the third stage has contributed to the reduction in PPH.
> 99

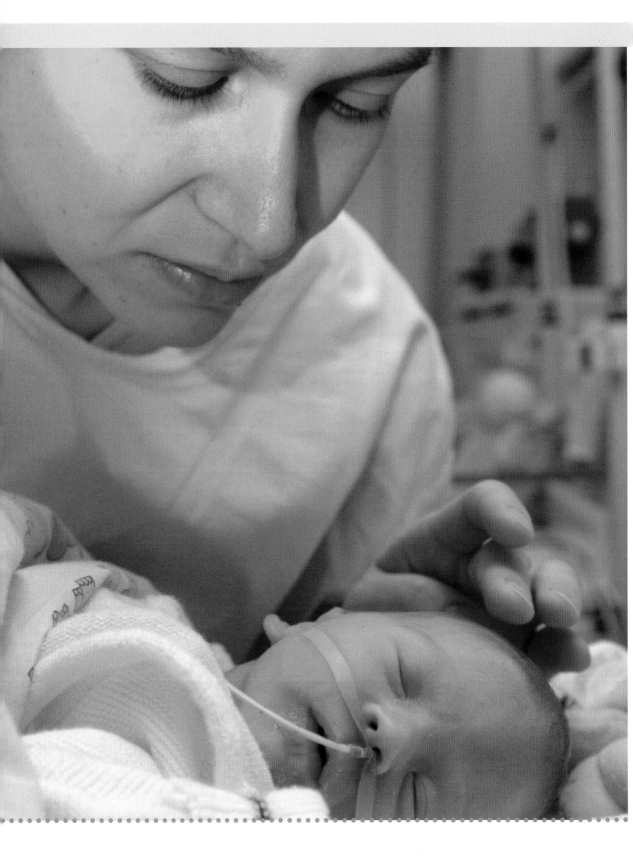

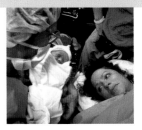

When help is needed

Although all women and their carers hope for a full-term pregnancy and an uncomplicated delivery, when events make this difficult or impossible, extra medical help will be needed to ensure the safety of both mother and baby. If this should happen to you, being aware of what can occur during labour and birth and the possible outcomes will help you make informed decisions along the way.

CONTENTS

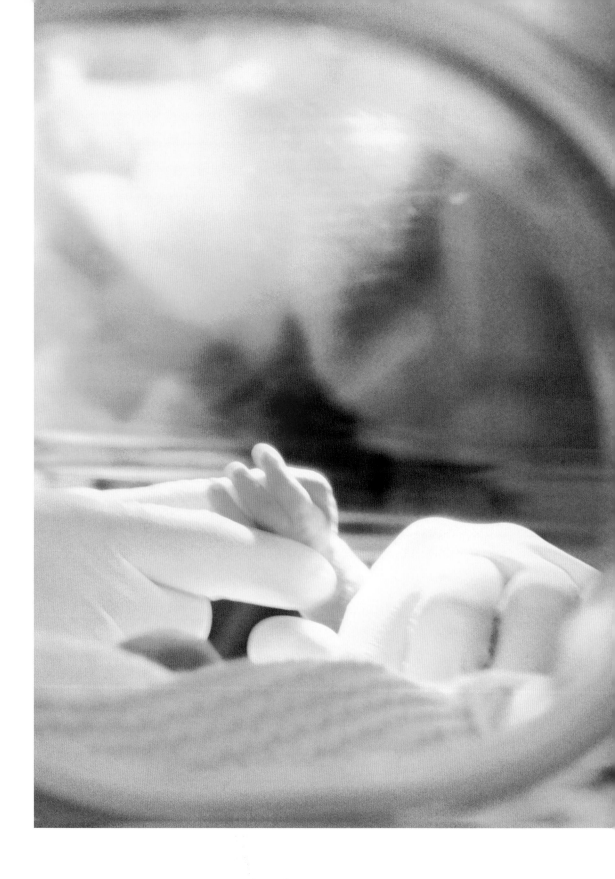

Premature labour

AROUND 10 PER CENT OF BIRTHS IN THE UK are classified as premature because they occur before 37 weeks. However, thanks to the enormous advances that have been made in neonatal care over the past 10 years, babies born after 30 weeks who have not had serious complications in utero are unlikely to experience major long-term developmental problems.

The most important thing to remember here is that the longer a healthy normal baby stays in utero and the greater its birth weight, the lower the chances are of that baby experiencing problems after delivery and the shorter the time that he or she will have to spend in a special care baby unit. The chance of survival without handicap for a baby born at 23 weeks is only one per cent, but as each week follows the chance of survival improves significantly so that at 26 weeks nearly one quarter will survive unharmed, and by 30 weeks the risk of handicap is very small. This is why every effort will be made to keep your baby in utero for as long as possible, provided there are no problems that suggest it would be better cared for in the outside world. It is also important to understand that only about 1.5 per cent of all births occur prematurely before 32 weeks, and below 28 weeks the figure is less than 1 per cent.

Much time is spent in antenatal clinics trying to identify those pregnant women who are at greater risk of going into premature labour. In the Journey section of this book I have included many mentions of the possible symptoms that may help you, your midwife, and doctor to recognize that you are at risk of delivering your baby prematurely.

> 66 ...every effort will be made to keep your baby in utero for as long as possible... 99

Causes of premature labour

There are many reasons why babies are delivered prematurely, but despite all the research to try to predict why a pregnant woman might go into premature labour or why her membranes may rupture weeks before the due date, we are still unable to prevent the vast majority of preterm births. Indeed, we do not know exactly what triggers labour itself, let alone what the exact mechanisms are that set this trigger off too early. One theory focuses on the role of hormones secreted by the baby, the mother or the placenta; another suggests that the levels of a protein in the vagina and cervix called fetal fibronectin increase markedly when a woman is about to go into labour. Infection appears to play a part in 20–40 per cent of preterm births, and if you have already had a premature baby you are more likely to have another premature birth. However, babies sometimes have to be delivered early for medical reasons. These include pre-eclampsia, high blood pressure, diabetes, placental abruption or bleeding from placenta praevia (see pp.426–8), all of which may recur in your next pregnancy.

Signs of premature labour

If your waters break before 37 weeks or you experience abdominal pain, vaginal bleeding or start to develop uterine contractions, contact the labour ward and arrange to be examined by a midwife or doctor urgently. They will check whether your uterus is contracting and the baby's position and then perform an internal examination to assess the cervix, determine the presenting part, and ensure that the umbilical cord has not prolapsed (see p.430). They will also be looking for signs of infection if the protective membranes have gone, and may want to induce or augment uterine contractions with a syntocinon drip (see p.297) in order to deliver your baby promptly. This may need to be by Caesarean section if your baby is showing any signs of distress, the presentation and lie of the baby are not ideal or your cervix is very unripe.

Even if your waters have not broken, if you think you are getting contractions, or have had a show, you must contact the labour ward urgently. You will almost certainly be advised to come straight in for complete bed rest and close monitoring. So long as there are no contraindications, you may also be given a tocolytic drug in an attempt to stop the uterine activity. Nifedipine (a calcium channel blocker) is the cheapest drug available and can be given by mouth, but may cause some maternal side effects. Atosiban (a selective oxytocin receptor blocker) is more expensive and must be given as an IV infusion. It is usually reserved for women with uterine contractions and a positive fetal fibronectin test (see box, left) whose delivery needs to be delayed while they complete a course of steroids to help mature the baby's lungs (see p.342) or undergo transfer to another hospital with a special care baby unit. If your baby is less than 32 weeks gestation, you will also be given a bolus dose of magnesium sulphate, which is a neuroprotectant and helps reduce the risk of the baby developing cerebral palsy.

FETAL FIBRONECTIN TEST (fFN)

▶ **Indications**
Threatened Preterm Labour (PTL)
Baby 24 to 34 weeks
Membranes intact
Cervix < 3cm dilated
Healthy fetus
▶ **Method**
Take vaginal swab from mother
Place swab in test fluid
Machine reads Fibronectin + or −
▶ **Interpretation of results**
Positive (+): 1 in 6 women will deliver within next 14 days.
Action: start treatment with tocolytics, steroids, arrange in utero transfer.
Negative(−): 1 in 25 women will deliver in next 14 days.
Action: reassure mother, discharge home if contractions settle.

If your contractions are only mild, bed rest alone may halt the beginnings of labour and you will probably be able to go home when your uterine activity ceases, although you will need to take it easy for the remainder of the pregnancy and avoid having sex. However, if your contractions are established and your cervix has begun to dilate, it is difficult, even with the use of drugs, to delay delivery by much more than 48 hours. Before 36 weeks, the advantages of the baby remaining in utero are usually greater than those of being delivered, so you may be advised to take one of the drugs mentioned earlier, in an attempt to stop or reduce the uterine contractions. However, it is important to understand that tocolytic drugs may prolong the pregnancy but they do not make the babies healthier.

Giving birth to a premature baby

When delivery becomes inevitable or is the preferred option, you will either progress in labour to a vaginal delivery or if there are any signs of fetal distress, a Caesarean section will be performed. The good news is that your labour is likely to be shorter than that for a full-term baby, since your baby's head and body are a bit smaller, which can speed up their journey down the birth canal. The smaller head also means you are less likely to suffer a perineal tear. However, you are likely to have an elective episiotomy if your doctor decides to apply forceps to cradle the baby's head and control the speed of delivery as it reaches the perineum. A premature baby's skull is softer than that of a full-term baby and needs protecting from sudden expulsion from the vagina. You will probably be advised to avoid pethidine for pain relief, since this can depress your baby's respiratory system and cause problems after the delivery.

It is unlikely that you will be advised to attempt a vaginal birth if your baby is breech, and you will be offered a Caesarean even if you are already in labour (see p.356). The exception to this rule is for babies with a gestational age of less than 26 weeks, when a vaginal breech delivery is usually preferable to a Caesarean section. Similarly, if you have developed an additional complication, such as placental abruption or pre-eclampsia, vaginal delivery will be considered too dangerous for your premature baby. Whether you have a vaginal or abdominal delivery, you will be attended by a paediatrician, midwife, and obstetrician. As soon as the baby is born, he will be assessed and given assistance with breathing if needed. Hopefully you will have the opportunity to hold your baby briefly before he is taken to the special care baby unit. If this is not available at your hospital, you will either be transferred to the nearest suitable maternity unit before the delivery or your baby will be transferred there in a special ambulance (neonatal flying squad) immediately after the birth.

> 66
> ...a preterm labour is likely to be shorter than that for a full-term baby.
> 99

Problems your baby may encounter

Most healthy babies born at or before 35 weeks will need help from a specialist baby care unit (SCBU), because they are likely to experience breathing difficulties and require help with feeding. The breathing problems result from the fact that their lungs are not yet sufficiently developed and elastic enough to breathe unaided.

As discussed in the Journey section (see p.232), the fetal lungs continue to develop more tiny airways and alveoli well into the third trimester of pregnancy and only start to produce surfactant from about 26 weeks. This substance coats the developing alveoli, allowing them to remain open and available for oxygen exchange after birth. When there is little surfactant present, the lungs are rigid and collapse down easily, which makes every breath the newly born premature baby takes more difficult. This is why a mechanical ventilator is often needed to push the air into and out of the immature lungs, and the neonatal doctors may suggest spraying some artificial surfactant into the baby's lungs. After 35 weeks, there is usually enough surfactant available to make full ventilation unnecessary, although your baby may require some little tubes placed in his nose for a short time to ensure that sufficient oxygen is readily available.

If you have to be delivered at or before 35 weeks, you will be given an injection of steroids (either betamethasone or dexamethasone) to speed up the production

IN SAFE HANDS
Don't be alarmed by the equipment you encounter in the special care baby unit. The machinery and tubes are there to monitor your preterm baby and to help her breathe and feed until she is able to do so for herself.

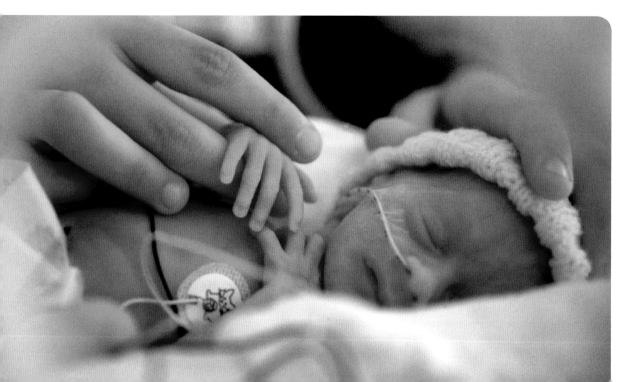

of surfactant in the baby's lungs. The steroids need 24 to 48 hours to reach their full effect, so in cases of threatened preterm labour, the doctors will always try to delay the delivery for enough time to allow the steroids to work. Similarly, your baby's sucking reflex is poorly developed before 35 weeks (see p.231) and the digestive system is often too immature to cope with large liquid feeds. This is why many premature babies need to be tube fed with small quantities of milk (preferably expressed breast milk) at very regular intervals. They soon get used to larger meals and I often find myself telling anxious mothers who have a baby in the special care baby unit that when their baby can deal with 60ml (2fl oz) of tube feed every three to four hours, she is likely to be discharged from SCBU very soon. This is a clear indication that she will now be capable of suckling on her mother's breast or from a formula milk bottle.

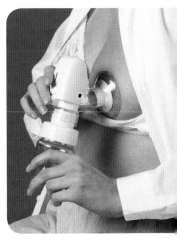

EXPRESSING MILK
A positive way of getting involved with helping to care for your premature baby is to express milk. You will be providing her with the best nutrition available.

After the birth

Rest assured that, although the birth of a premature baby is invariably very medicalized, it is vital to assemble all the machines, equipment, and staff required to ensure that your baby is given the best care possible at this delicate stage in her life. The medical staff attending the birth will be well aware of how upsetting the whole situation usually is for parents – particularly first-time parents with no previous experience of childbirth – and they will do their best to make things easier for you. They will take a photograph of your baby within minutes of birth, so that you can put it beside your bed and get to know your baby's face. They will also give you all the time you need to ask questions, both during and after the birth, and will do everything in their power to reassure you and to explain the situation clearly.

On pages 404 to 405, I provide more detailed information on caring for premature babies, particularly during their stay in the special care baby unit. Remember, though, that however distressing the early days and weeks can be, the vast majority of premature babies go on to become strapping toddlers who are every bit as healthy as their full-term peers.

My daughters were delivered by emergency Caesarean section after I went into premature labour at 33 weeks. They were both a reasonable size for twin babies of their gestational age and had not had any problems antenatally. Nonetheless, they both needed help with breathing and feeding and were in the special care baby unit for four weeks. The paediatricians were very careful to ensure that they had carried out numerous checks on them before they allowed me to take them home. It took only a month or two for them to catch up in their growth, and by the time they started nursery school they were taller and heavier than their classmates, which I found very reassuring.

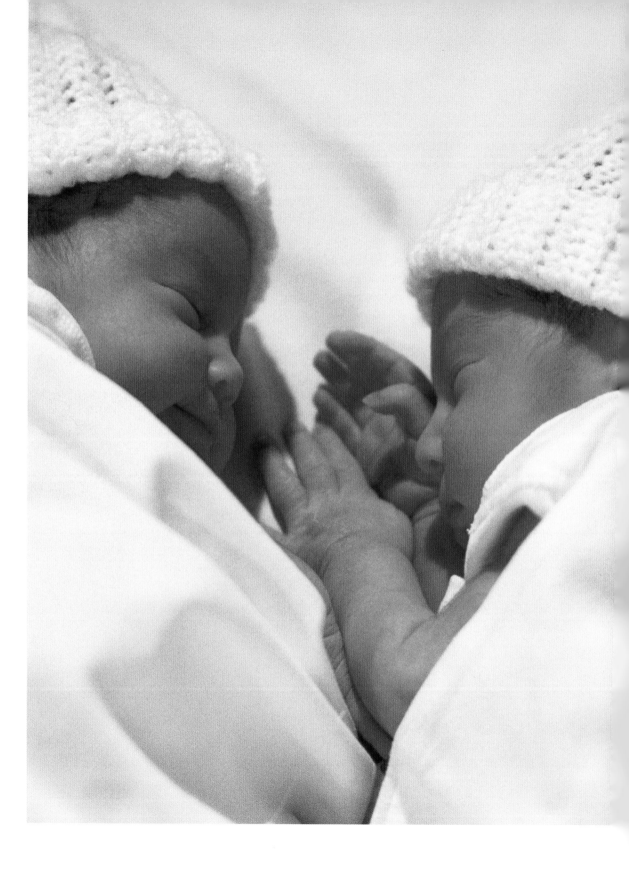

Multiple births

THE NUMBER OF TWIN AND TRIPLET PREGNANCIES has increased over the last 10 to 20 years and currently about 15 in every 1,000 deliveries in the UK are multiple births. This rise is mainly due to the wider availability of assisted fertility treatments, which increase the chances of more than one egg being fertilized at the time of conception. Another important factor is that more women are embarking on pregnancies later in life, and rising maternal age increases the incidence of non-identical (dizygotic) twin pregnancies.

Multiple pregnancies are at greater risk of a variety of complications, in particular premature delivery, fetal growth restriction, pre-eclampsia, anaemia, placenta praevia (see pp.424–9), and twin-to-twin transfusion syndrome (see p.346). Furthermore, the incidence of cerebral palsy is dramatically higher after multiple births compared to singletons. As a result, antenatal care for mothers with a multiple pregnancy is more closely monitored, and the delivery is usually planned in a hospital unit where emergency help is always available.

Even if the pregnancy has been uncomplicated, 50 per cent of twins will be born prematurely, before 37 weeks, and these babies are more likely to need admission to a special care baby unit. This is because they tend to be smaller than singleton babies and, irrespective of their actual birthweight, also behave less maturely than singletons and often require some assistance with breathing and feeding during the first few days or weeks of their lives.

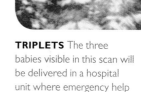

TRIPLETS The three babies visible in this scan will be delivered in a hospital unit where emergency help is readily available.

Delivering twins

The main concern in a vaginal twin birth is the delivery of the second twin. Even if the first baby is head down and the labour starts spontaneously and progresses smoothly, there is no way of knowing how the second twin will cope with the mechanics of a hasty descent through the birth canal until the first twin has been delivered. No woman wants to go through labour and the vaginal delivery of her first twin, only to be told that she needs to undergo an emergency Caesarean section to deliver her second baby. As a result, an increasing number of twin and all triplet (and higher number) pregnancies are now delivered by Caesarean section. This may be an emergency procedure if the labour is very premature or if complications develop during labour, or an elective procedure if the risks of a vaginal delivery are generally considered to be too great. If there are no maternal or fetal reasons to perform the elective Caesarean section sooner, delivery should be delayed until 37–38 weeks to avoid neonatal respiratory problems. A Caesarean delivery of twins is likely to be planned when:

• the mother requests this rather than vaginal delivery

• the first twin is not presenting head first

• placenta praevia is diagnosed on an ultrasound scan

• intrauterine growth restriction (see p.429) is identified

• the birthweight of the second twin is estimated to be 500g (1lb) greater than that of the first

• one or both of the twins has a physical abnormality

• twin-to-twin transfusion syndrome is present. This disorder in the blood supply to identical twins only affects monochorionic pregnancies and has serious consequences because the blood vessels in the shared placenta favour one twin over the other – early delivery is usually required to save the life of the smaller twin.

• the babies are conjoined, or Siamese, twins. An attempt to separate them surgically may be attempted after delivery, depending on which organs they share.

Induction of labour for twin pregnancies in which the first twin is cephalic may be performed at 37–38 weeks, since many women find the discomfort of late twin pregnancy difficult to deal with. Complications are also more likely to develop after this date. Recent studies have shown there is no significant increase in the rate of emergency Caesarean section or reduction in the likelihood of delivering a healthy baby if an induction of labour is carried out at 37 weeks.

Vaginal delivery of twins

If you are planning a vaginal delivery for your twins, you will be carefully reviewed in the early stages of labour, to ensure that nothing has happened since the last clinic visit to suggest the plan should be revised. The labour ward staff will monitor both babies and will also perform an ultrasound to check their sizes and positions. If you have a scar in your uterus from a previous Caesarean section or surgery, a vaginal delivery may be possible if the first twin is a cephalic presentation.

Since there will need to be a lot of people on hand during a twin delivery (one or more obstetricians, an anaesthetist, two midwives, and two paediatricians), you will be cared for in a larger than normal delivery room equipped to carry out emergency procedures. You will most probably be advised to have an epidural anaesthetic so an emergency Caesarean can be carried out without delay at any stage. A good epidural block is particularly important during the second stage of labour when external or internal manipulation to turn the second twin into a longitudinal lie may be required.

During the labour, continuous electronic fetal monitoring (see p.292) is advisable and attaching a scalp clip to the first twin ensures that the tracings from the abdominal monitor on the second twin can be read without confusion. The first stage of labour is often a little shorter than for a singleton. If progress is slow, this is usually seen as an ominous sign prompting Caesarean delivery. The use of syntocinon to augment labour is rarely considered to be the best option. The second stage of labour, before the delivery of the first twin, is essentially the same as for a single baby, but there will always be an anaesthetist and senior obstetrician present in addition to the midwives and paediatricians. Immediately after the delivery of the first twin, the umbilical cord is clamped in two places (near the baby and at the end of the cord leading to the placenta) to prevent the transfusion of placental blood away from the second twin, who may remain in utero for some time.

> The first stage of a twin labour is often a little shorter than for a singleton.

Delivery of the second twin

The obstetrician will now palpate your abdomen to establish the lie of the second twin. If it is transverse, gentle external pressure will be applied to achieve a longitudinal lie (the baby lying parallel to your spine), and the midwife will be asked to maintain this position by gentle manual pressure.

If there is any uncertainty as to whether the presentation is cephalic or breech, a quick ultrasound scan can be performed. External cephalic version (turning a baby from presenting breech to head first, see p.271) for a breech presentation of a second twin is not common practice as this often results in further complications, which may then necessitate an emergency Caesarean section. A smooth assisted breech delivery (see pp.356–9) is preferable.

There are no strict rules as to how long the second stage for twin two should be allowed to continue, but if delivery cannot be achieved within 30 minutes it is highly likely that an emergency Caesarean section will be needed. Because the uterine contractions frequently diminish after the delivery of the first baby, most obstetricians will already have a syntocinon infusion in place and this will be started as soon as a longitudinal lie has been confirmed, in order to help drive the presenting part of twin two into your pelvis.

Ideally, the membranes around your second baby are left intact until the baby has descended further through your cervix and into the vagina, which helps prevent the cervix from closing. If the membranes rupture and there is a delay in the delivery, the obstetrician will insert a hand into your vagina and up into your uterus to guide the head downwards (towards the helping hands of a pair of forceps or a ventouse cup) or grasp hold of the breech or legs and assist the vaginal delivery. Occasionally, it may be better to perform an internal version or manipulation in the uterine cavity, turning a breech presentation through 180 degrees, but more usually the delivery continues as an assisted breech (see pp.357–9). Because of the limited experience of modern-day obstetricians, the incidence of Caesarean section for twin two has increased.

Third stage of a twin birth

Active management of the third stage of labour (see p.333) is particularly important in twin births since the risk of postpartum haemorrhage is higher because the uterus is more distended. As soon as your second twin is delivered, the doctors will increase the oxytocin infusion and you will be given an intramuscular injection of syntometrine. The infusion may need to be continued for some time after the delivery to ensure that your uterus remains well contracted.

TWIN BIRTHS These can be more complicated than singleton births, but they are also very special with the end result invariably being the safe delivery of two perfect babies.

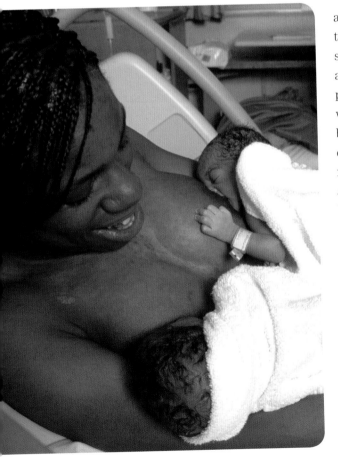

Twin births are special. I speak here as a mother and an obstetrician, having been blessed with twin daughters. Since the birth is not always straightforward and often involves babies that are premature and small for dates, the paediatricians will monitor them carefully and will not hesitate to admit them to the special care baby unit if they have any concerns. This is distressing and alarming for parents, but do remember that in the vast majority of cases this is a short, almost routine visit and the outcome is a happy one. Rest assured that the paediatric staff will be keen to keep you fully informed about your babies' progress and will be anxious to reunite them with you as soon as possible.

Support for the parents of multiple pregnancies is important, and detailed information and practical support to help them prepare for caring for their babies is best started in antenatal classes. After the birth, joining a local twin club will offer the great advantage of being put in touch with experienced parents who are undoubtedly one of the best sources of advice for others in the same situation (see p.438).

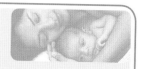

BIRTH STORY

Deborah, 32, first pregnancy
Nicholas and Patrick, born 37 weeks + 5 days,
Nicholas weighed 2.25kg (5lb), Patrick weighed 3.15kg (7lb)

I discovered I was carrying identical twins at my 12-week scan and, after recovering from the shock, my pregnancy progressed well. I was seen regularly by my consultant from 28 weeks onwards and everybody told me that there was no reason why I could not attempt a vaginal delivery.

My 36-week scan showed that the babies were growing well. But the following scan, at 37 weeks + 4 days, showed that one twin had stopped growing. This was because, like all identical twins, the babies were sharing a placenta, but had separate amniotic sacs. In other words, they were monochorionic but diamniotic twins. The scan took place at 4pm and I was immediately booked in for a Caesarean section the following morning. There was no question of inducting a vaginal birth, especially as the consultant could see from the scan that one baby was lying transverse. Nobody could know what would happen during labour. My biggest fear all along had been that I might have one baby vaginally, only to end up with a Caesarean section for the second twin. I had one over-riding feeling: I wanted both babies out safely and it didn't matter to me how they came out. I had been present at my cousin's vaginal birth and I couldn't see what was so appealing about all that pain. As a result, I was very happy at the prospect of the Caesarean section.

The birth itself was very straightforward and calm. My husband was in the operating theatre with me, and both babies came out without any problems. Little Nicholas was born first and it turns out he had been cephalic and very much ready to come out. But he was the one who had stopped growing. Patrick was lying transverse, with one hand nonchalantly behind his ear, and he was born five minutes later. I don't think he felt like leaving his warm home. I asked to see the placenta: Nicholas' side was all crusty and dried up, while Patrick's was red and healthy. It was clear what had happened and I'm so grateful that the doctors spotted the problem and were able to act on it at once.

All the staff were fantastic, although I was more or less turfed out of hospital after four days because they were short of beds. After two months, I have learned to be very organized. I breastfed for one month but it was very difficult, so I now bottle-feed and the twins almost sleep through the night. Nicholas' weight is catching up with his younger, heavier brother and I feel blessed to have them both in such good health.

❝ I had one over-riding feeling:
I wanted both babies out safely and it
didn't matter how they came out. **❞**

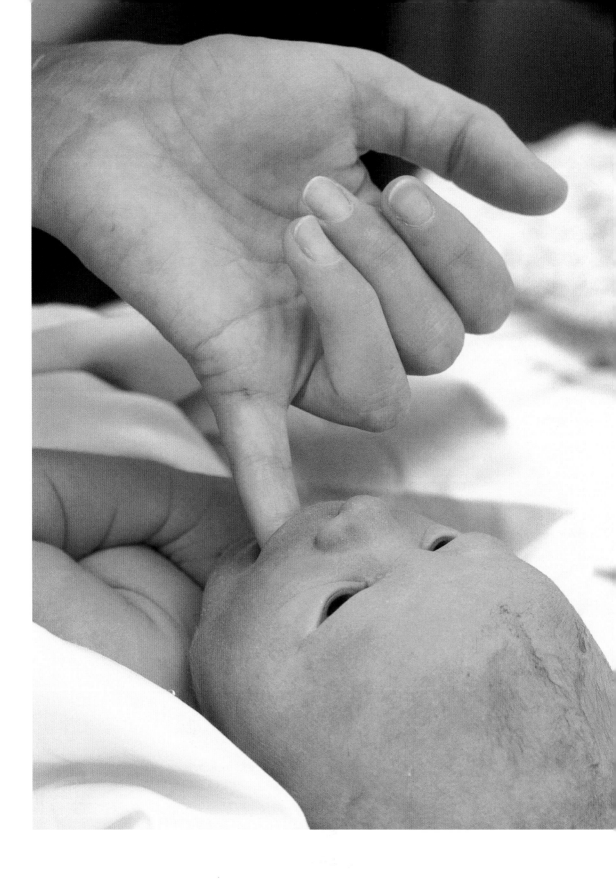

Assisted deliveries

THE TERM ASSISTED OR INSTRUMENTAL DELIVERY can sound rather frightening and I want to remind you that the vast majority of babies are still delivered vaginally without any need for assistance or medical intervention. However, if the labour has been prolonged or the second stage is not progressing smoothly, it may be necessary to assist the vaginal delivery with the use of instruments such as forceps or a vacuum extractor (ventouse).

It is important to understand that the aim of an assisted delivery is to guide the baby out of the birth canal with the help of your uterine contractions pushing the baby from above. The forceps or vacuum equipment are not designed to pull the baby out on their own. Most assisted deliveries are performed by an experienced obstetric doctor, but in some units, senior midwives have received special training and are able to perform ventouse deliveries and low lift-out forceps (see p.354). For either a forceps or a ventouse delivery your doctor or midwife will request that you are in the lithotomy position, with your legs supported by stirrups so they have maximum visibility and access to your baby during the delivery. Whether or not you need an episiotomy will depend on individual circumstances and considerations (see pp.330–1). Generally speaking, most forceps deliveries will require an episiotomy, but if you are having a vacuum extraction you may not need one.

Effects of instrumental deliveries

Babies born by assisted vaginal delivery often bear the marks of the instruments after the birth, but don't worry because these usually disappear within a few days. After a ventouse, there will always be a swelling on the scalp where the suction cup was placed and this can sometimes lead to extensive bruising and may even cause the baby to become jaundiced. With forceps, the skull or face may be bruised and appear slightly misshapen at the sites where the blades were placed. However, it is important to remember that a baby's skull is designed to cope with being put under pressure or compressed in some way during the birth, so these instruments are highly unlikely to pose any serious threat to your baby's long-term wellbeing.

> 66
> A baby's skull is designed to cope with pressure during birth.
> 99

Vacuum extraction

The use of the ventouse or vacuum extractor has become increasingly popular over the past few years and, in many obstetric units, this is now the instrument of choice for assisted vaginal deliveries, virtually replacing the use of forceps.

How the ventouse works

Ventouse equipment essentially consists of a cup made of metal or soft plastic that has a chain or a handle. The cup is attached to a tube, which connects with suction apparatus. The cup is positioned over the crown (occiput) of the baby's head and is held firmly against the scalp while a vacuum is gently built up, using a hand or electrical pump. This sucks some of the scalp tissue into the cup and the chignon, or swelling, that develops on the baby's head effectively produces a firm attachment.

...the ventouse is often the instrument of choice for assisted vaginal deliveries...

When a suitable vacuum has been achieved, the edges of the suction cup are checked to ensure that no maternal tissues have been trapped. Traction is applied by pulling on the chain or plastic handle attached to the cup, while the mother bears down during a contraction. Once the head has crowned, the vacuum is released and the cup is removed. After allowing time for the baby's head to rotate externally, delivery of the shoulders and body proceeds as normal. The principle of vacuum extraction is that the line of traction should follow the mother's pelvic curve, since this is the pathway of least resistance for the baby's head as it descends through her birth canal.

Advantages and disadvantages

The greatest advantage of the ventouse is that, if the baby's head is not directly in the occipito-anterior position, it can still rotate automatically as it descends through the maternal pelvis. Hence it is easier for the diameters of the head to negotiate the various diameters of the maternal pelvis (see p.328). Another important advantage of the ventouse is that it takes up less space in the vagina than forceps would. As a result, there is less risk of damage to the vagina and perineum compared to a forceps delivery and some women may not require an episiotomy. In addition, the requirements for pain relief are usually less, although, in an ideal world, an effective regional block should always be in place before an instrumental vaginal delivery is attempted. The disadvantage of the ventouse is that the delivery tends to be slower, because time is required to set up the equipment and achieve a good vacuum and also because the cup can become dislodged. However, in experienced hands, a good vacuum application and chignon can usually be developed in about two minutes, about the same as the gap between contractions during the second stage of labour. If careful attention is paid to the positioning of the cup, the number that become dislodged is reduced and the number of smooth, swift ventouse deliveries increases.

If the baby's head has not been delivered after three or four good contractions, or after the cap has been in place for a total of 15 minutes, an alternative means of delivery needs to be considered. A smaller ventouse cap made of very soft rubber is now available, called a KIWI.

Possible complications

Although maternal complications after ventouse delivery are uncommon, fetal complications, including superficial scalp injuries, bruising, and bleeding into the head, can occur even after an apparently simple procedure but are more likely when the cap has become dislodged or the delivery is prolonged. A chignon, or scalp swelling, is always present after a vacuum extraction and is usually more extensive when a metal cup has been used. It invariably subsides in a few days with no harmful effects.

VENTOUSE The cup is attached to the baby's head and a vacuum is built up within it. Then, in synchrony with the mother's contractions, the baby is helped down the birth canal.

Superficial scalp injuries occur in about 12 per cent of ventouse deliveries and again it is rare for them to lead to any long-term complications. However, cephalohaematomas (a collection of blood beneath the top layer of the skull bones) develop in about 6 per cent of vacuum extractions. The haematomas usually resolve by themselves within two weeks but, if they are extensive, may cause jaundice in the baby and presumably result in a nasty headache!

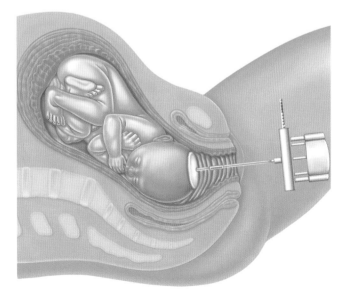

Bleeding into the head (intracranial haemorrhage) is uncommon (about 1 in 300–400 cases) but is potentially extremely serious. However, recent studies have shown that this figure is no greater than the figure for babies delivered by forceps or emergency Caesarean section during labour, suggesting that the abnormal labour is the cause of the problem rather than the ventouse application itself.

Forceps delivery

Forceps have been used by obstetricians for nearly 400 years. Until the latter half of the 20th century, Caesarean section was a dangerous operation and forceps prevented many mothers and babies from succumbing to life-threatening events during delivery.

Nowadays, thanks to the enormous medical advances that have been made in anaesthesia and the routine availability of antibiotics, blood transfusion, and adult and neonatal intensive care units, Caesarean section is a relatively safe procedure and, as a result, the potential complications of a difficult forceps delivery are considered to be a greater threat to the mother and her baby.

There are three types of forceps: lift-out, straight traction, and rotational. Forceps deliveries can be described as high, mid, low, and outlet, depending on where the baby's head is positioned in the pelvic cavity when the forceps are applied. High-cavity forceps deliveries are no longer performed because of the significant risk of causing maternal and fetal damage.

Lift-out (outlet) forceps are used to lift the baby's head out when the scalp is visible at the mother's vulva, which means that the whole of the baby's head has already reached the pelvic floor and is distending the vagina, but the perineal muscles are holding it back. They are only appropriate if the baby's head is positioned directly occipito-anterior (see p.270) or slightly rotated to the left or right. An injection of local anaesthetic into the perineal tissues or the pudendal nerve (see p.316) may be all that is needed for a lift-out forceps delivery. An episiotomy is not always necessary.

Straight traction forceps are longer and are used for low- and mid-cavity deliveries when the baby's head has engaged and descended to more than 2cm (1in) below the ischial spines (low) or just above this station (mid-cavity). (See p.302 for a diagram of stations and head descent.) The forceps lock together easily to form a protective cradle

FORCEPS DELIVERY
The curved blades of the forceps are inserted one at a time and cradled around the baby's head. They are then used, in time with your contractions, to help draw the baby down the birth canal and deliver it.

around the baby's head. At the height of a contraction, the operator applies gentle downwards traction. The head descends with each pull even if it slips backwards again between contractions. Delivery is usually achieved with three good contractions and moderate traction, but if there is no obvious head descent by this time it suggests that there may be a degree of disproportion present and the decision as to whether to proceed with a vaginal delivery should be reviewed. Because the forcep blades take up additional room in the vagina, an episiotomy is often required to prevent uncontrolled perineal tearing as the baby's head stretches the perineum. An epidural or spinal block should be used for this type of forceps delivery to ensure that the mother does not experience pain or discomfort when the blades are inserted and during the traction, delivery, and subsequent repair of the perineum.

Rotational forceps are rarely used nowadays to turn the baby's head in the mid-cavity from a transverse or occipito posterior position to direct occipito anterior, following which downwards traction on the long handles of the forceps allows the smooth descent of the baby's head and the delivery is then completed as for straight forceps. The application of rotational forceps requires considerable skill and experience and this type of delivery is likely to be carried out in an operating theatre so that, if any difficulties are encountered, a Caesarean section can be done immediately. It is essential for the mother to have an effective epidural or spinal block in place, not just for the delivery, but also afterwards so that her vagina and cervix can be carefully examined for any potential tears or damage that the rotational forceps may have caused.

> 66
> ...forceps have prevented many mothers and babies from succumbing to life-threatening events...
> 99

Forceps or ventouse?

Despite the current trend favouring the use of ventouse over forceps, there is still debate as to which is the best method of instrumental delivery. It is generally thought that the use of the vacuum results in less damage to the mother's vagina and perineum. On the other hand, the vacuum may be more traumatic for many babies compared to a smooth forceps delivery, because it leaves a swelling on the baby's head where the cup was placed.

There are pros and cons to each type of instrument, and I think it is more useful to consider the two methods as complementary, designed for different circumstances, rather than rivals to each other. The final choice should be determined by the circumstances that have led to the need for an attempted instrumental vaginal delivery and the experience and skills of the individual who performs the delivery.

Breech births

The number of babies presenting as breech (bottom first) is closely related to their gestational age. At 28 weeks, some 20 per cent of all babies are breech, but most of them turn of their own accord during the third trimester to become cephalic (head-down) presentations, leaving less than 4 per cent of babies in a breech position at term.

If your baby is breech, it will be in one of three positions: a frank breech in which the bottom presents to the cervix and the legs are extended upwards along the baby's body; a complete breech in which the bottom is still lowest but the thighs are extended upwards, and the knees are flexed so that the legs are folded against the baby's body; or a footling breech in which the legs are presenting below the baby's bottom.

Vaginal breech deliveries are more prone to risks and complications, the most important being that the largest diameter of the baby (the head) is the last to deliver. Furthermore, the breech does not fit into the mother's pelvis as well as a head, so there is always the risk that the umbilical cord will prolapse or fall through the cervix alongside the bottom or the legs (see p.430). Invariably, a prolapsed cord results in acute fetal distress because when the umbilical cord is exposed to air, it constricts or closes down, cutting off the oxygen supply to the baby.

BREECH PRESENTATIONS ·

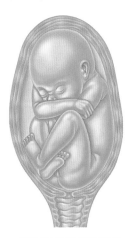

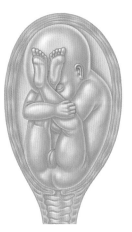

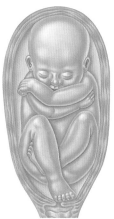

COMPLETE BREECH The buttocks are presenting but the thighs are extended upwards and the knees are flexed.

FRANK BREECH The baby's buttocks are presenting and legs are extended upwards against the baby's body.

FOOTLING BREECH The legs present below the baby's bottom. They drop down once the membranes have ruptured.

COMPLETE BREECH **FRANK BREECH** **FOOTLING BREECH**

Trial of labour

A vaginal breech birth is most likely to be considered if your baby is in a frank breech position with the back of his bottom (the sacrum) positioned anteriorly in the birth canal. It is always considered as a trial of labour and will be allowed to continue only if no problems develop. The doctor and midwife will want you to be monitored continuously, either with an external monitor or by an internal monitoring electrode clipped onto the baby's bottom (see p.292). They may also advise you to have an epidural anaesthetic in place early in your trial of labour, so that any necessary interventions can be performed speedily. The other advantage of an epidural is that it protects you from the urge to push before the cervix is fully dilated.

Breech labours are often slower than cephalic labours because the presenting part, the baby's bottom, is softer and does not exert the same downwards pressure on the cervix. The first stage of labour can be longer and more tiring, and since most obstetricians will be reluctant to use syntocinon augmentation when progress is poor, it is quite possible that you will be advised to have a Caesarean section during the first stage.

> 66
> ...the first stage of a breech labour can be longer and more tiring for the mother...
> 99

Second stage

Assuming that all has gone well and that you have now reached full dilatation, the mechanics of the second stage of a breech labour are best thought of as the reverse of a cephalic delivery. The bottom and legs travel through the pelvis first, followed by the trunk and shoulders. A senior obstetrician and midwife will always be present during the second stage of a breech labour. They will request that you have your legs in stirrups so they can ensure they have easy access to your emerging baby. They will also want to ensure your epidural is well topped up so that they can rotate your baby, apply forceps to the baby's "after-coming head", or resort to a Caesarean section if the delivery proves to be difficult.

The buttocks will be delivered first with the help of your contractions and pushing efforts. The obstetrician will then gently guide the delivery of the two legs. This frequently involves rotating the baby's buttocks to the left or the right to allow the doctor to insert a finger into the vagina and hook it around the first and then the second leg, to encourage their smooth entry into the world.

When the buttocks and legs have been delivered, the baby's back and trunk are then allowed to emerge up to the shoulders, in their own time. The shoulders usually need rotating to one side and then the other, so that once again the obstetrician can insert a finger into the vagina and hook a finger around the upper limbs to aid delivery of the arms. The key to a successful

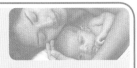

BIRTH STORY

Nathalie, 34, has one daughter, aged four
Second baby Enzo, born 40 weeks + 4 days, weight 3.8kg (8lb 6oz)
Length of labour from start of contractions: 21 hours

My 34-week scan *had shown the baby to be transverse, but at subsequent examinations I was told he had turned and was cephalic, although his head never engaged, even at term. The day before my labour started, I remember a registrar getting me to feel the baby's bottom high up in my abdomen.*

My labour started *at around 1am with regular, period-like cramps that were generally perfectly bearable, so much so that I was able to get some sleep. By midday, the cramping stopped completely and only started again at around 3pm. I decided to go shopping with my husband for some last-minute food items, even though the contractions were now coming every 10 minutes or so. At 5pm I had a show, so I called the hospital but was told to wait until the contractions were longer and closer together. By 5.30,*

my waters broke; the contractions were coming every five minutes and were more painful so we left soon after for the hospital.

A midwife examined me on arrival *and, palpating my abdomen, remarked on how hard the place was where the baby's bottom should be. I was taken to a delivery suite and waited while things progressed. At around 7pm, a doctor came and did a scan and revealed that in fact the baby was breech. What we had assumed was his firm little bottom had obviously been his head. We were shocked. He explained to us what a breech vaginal birth entailed and informed us of the risks, and left us to digest the information. By now the contractions were very strong and I was still using only gas and air.*

At 8pm, a new doctor came in, *did an internal examination and told us we*

needed to hurry up and make a decision as I was already 3cm dilated. He strongly advised me to have a Caesarean as the baby was big. Not only were we really disappointed, but we were also still coming to terms with the turn of events. Soon after, we agreed to a Caesarean delivery, simply because I did not want to risk my baby's health for the sake of misguided hesitation and stubbornness.

Enzo was finally born at 10pm *and, although the birth itself went fine, I had to be given morphine regularly for the first couple of days. I was frustrated and depressed not to be able to look after him properly because of the pain from the incision. I was also exhausted, partly because of the inevitable noise on the ward. After three days, I discharged myself, as I knew I would get more rest (and better food!) at home.*

> 66 ...the doctor explained what a breech vaginal birth entailed...he strongly advised me to have a Caesarean. 99

vaginal breech delivery is that it should not be hurried and there should never be any pulling or tugging of the baby, just guidance and gentle rotation as the baby emerges.

Delivering the head

If all is going well, the weight of the baby's body will help with the remainder of the delivery, encouraging the neck to be well flexed, which results in the head being best positioned to be smoothly and safely delivered. If the baby's neck remains extended, with the face looking upwards into the uterine cavity (called star gazing) it is highly likely that problems will develop in delivering the "after-coming head". The baby's head is the largest part of its body, and when the neck is extended an even wider diameter is presenting to the cervix, which may not yet have been fully dilated by the delivery of the buttocks, trunk, and shoulders. Performing a Caesarean section in this situation is traumatic for everyone concerned. This is why everyone involved in your delivery will have been careful to heed earlier signs that a breech labour may not be progressing well and will advise changing to a Caesarean delivery if it is thought the head may get stuck at the last moment.

On a more positive note, if all continues to go well, your obstetrician will now gently sweep the baby's body upwards, over your pubic bone and may insert a finger into the baby's mouth and gently pull downwards, further flexing the head and helping it to emerge smoothly. At this point, it is often best to apply a pair of lift-out forceps to the breech baby's head to guide it out in a controlled manner as it escapes the constrictions of the lower part of the birth canal. As you will now realize, several pairs of hands are needed to deliver a breech baby vaginally and an episiotomy is usually performed.

Vaginal or Caesarean breech delivery

In the last decade, several studies have been published that have changed most obstetricians' views about the best way to deliver a breech baby. Caesarean section is now recommended as the optimal way to deliver a term breech baby in a first-time mother, if attempts to turn the baby (see external cephalic version, p.271) have failed. The risk of your baby dying or having a serious problem is reduced by a planned Caesarean section compared to planned vaginal birth. However, some 10 per cent of women with a breech presentation who are scheduled for a Caesarean section will deliver vaginally because labour starts earlier than expected and is already well advanced when they arrive at hospital. In addition, a small number will find themselves in an advanced stage of labour before it is realized they have a breech baby – the undiagnosed breech.

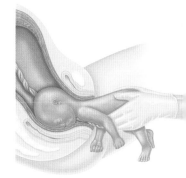

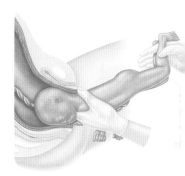

DURING A BREECH DELIVERY The baby's buttocks are delivered first, followed by the legs. The baby then turns so the shoulders can be delivered. The baby's weight draws the head down and the legs are lifted to allow safe delivery of the head.

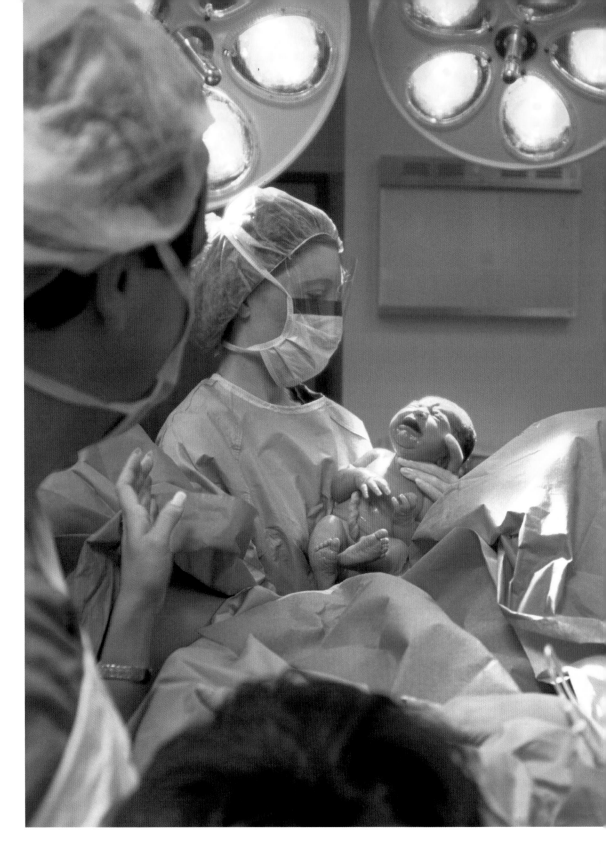

Caesarean birth

I AM VERY CONSCIOUS OF THE FACT that most antenatal classes, pregnancy books, and media publications focus much of their attention on what labour will be like. Yet the reality is that a sizeable percentage of women (at least one in five births in Britain) now deliver their babies by Caesarean section and this is why I have included a detailed account of what you can expect to happen if you turn out to be one of them.

Despite the marked increase in the numbers of babies born by Caesarean section, there are many individuals in our society who continue to view this mode of delivery as the poor relation in childbirth. Indeed, some people appear to feel that it is the method of last resort. Of course, they are entitled to their viewpoint, but my concern is that all too frequently this leaves some women who have needed a Caesarean delivery feeling that they have in some way failed or not done their bit for natural childbirth.

I feel strongly that pregnant women should not be subjected to pressure or disapproval about the way their baby is delivered. There is no way that even the most experienced midwife or doctor can accurately predict what will happen to a woman in labour, so to suggest that, "if all else fails you will have to be subjected to a Caesarean section" is, in my opinion, insensitive and unkind. Every labour is different, and it is impossible to consider yourself a failure when you have successfully nurtured a baby in your womb for nine months then delivered a healthy baby into the outside world. If this mode of delivery allows more women a guarantee of going home with healthy babies, then Caesarean sections have to be a good thing and quite the opposite of a "failed" birth. I really do believe that the route by which you deliver your baby is of secondary importance, as long as you are both safe.

A Caesarean section may be performed electively – meaning that this method of delivery was decided before labour started – or it may be an emergency procedure carried out after labour has already began. Of course, the operation itself is exactly the same, whether it is performed electively or as an emergency, but the underlying reasons for the Caesarean section may be different.

> 66
> ...women should not be subjected to disapproval about the way their baby is delivered.
> 99

Elective or emergency sections

There are a wide variety of reasons why a Caesarean section may be advised or chosen. It is important to remember that only a few of these are absolute indications; most are relative, depending on individual labours and circumstances.

Most "elective" Caesarean sections are performed when there are existing medical reasons to indicate that a vaginal birth is potentially risky, for the mother and/or her baby. That is not to say that a vaginal birth cannot be attempted, but in the opinion of the mother and her antenatal carers, Caesarean section is the safer option. This may be the case when the baby is presenting breech or in another position that may make vaginal delivery difficult; if you have a placenta praevia; if you are expecting twins or more; if you are suffering from an illness such as kidney, lung or heart disease or diabetes; or if you have developed pre-eclampsia or severe high blood pressure in pregnancy.

The term "emergency" Caesarean section may give the impression that the baby needs to be delivered in a matter of minutes, if not seconds, in order to avoid a catastrophe. Very occasionally this is the case, but more often it means that it has become obvious to everyone involved that a Caesarean section is required during the next hour or so.

The indications for an emergency Caesarean section are dependent on many complex factors, which include unpredictable events that occur in labour, such as prolapse of the umbilical cord or signs of fetal distress; maternal and medical perceptions of the progress of that labour; and practical considerations such as the staffing and expertise available to achieve the safe delivery of a healthy baby.

> ❝ ...elective Caesarean sections are performed when a vaginal birth is considered potentially risky... ❞

Safety of operative deliveries

Caesarean section is now considered to be a relatively safe procedure. When complications develop they are almost always due to the fact that the Caesarean is performed under emergency circumstances or because an underlying maternal or fetal problem is present. Thanks to the medical advances in anaesthetics, antibiotics, blood transfusion, and adult and neonatal intensive care facilities, the risks for the mother have become a secondary consideration in the vast majority of cases, and the risk of physical damage to the baby during the delivery is small.

However, any surgical procedure is associated with a degree of risk and there are factors that significantly increase the risk associated with Caesarean section. When the pregnant woman is seriously overweight, a smoker, has a personal or

THE RISE IN THE RATE OF CAESAREAN SECTIONS

The number of Caesarean deliveries has increased dramatically over the last 10 to 15 years and I think the most useful way to understand this change is to consider all the contributory factors.

ADVANCES IN GENERAL MEDICAL CARE

These have meant that some women with medical problems that were previously thought to preclude them from having children are now getting pregnant and, with specialist help, are remaining healthy during pregnancy. However, the underlying medical disorder may mean that a planned Caesarean section is the safest way to deliver the mother and her baby. Similarly, mothers-to-be who develop severe diabetes or pre-eclampsia may require early delivery by Caesarean section to protect their health.

ADVANCES IN OBSTETRIC CARE

Antenatal and intrapartum (labour) care have become so much more sophisticated. The routine availability of ultrasound scanning has resulted in our being able to identify many mothers and babies who are likely to experience problems in labour, before they are exposed to serious complications. The widespread introduction of regional anaesthesia (see pp.311–6) for Caesarean deliveries needs a special

mention here, since it allows the woman to remain conscious throughout the operation, supported by her partner, and avoids the significant risks of a general anaesthetic. There are three other obstetric reasons that have contributed to the increase in the Caesarean section rate. The first is that the number of babies born prematurely has risen significantly over the last decade. Secondly, the increase in the numbers of older women giving birth makes an additional contribution to the Caesarean section rate, since these women experience more complications during labour. Thirdly, the use of high-cavity obstetric forceps in the second stage of labour has virtually disappeared over the last five to 10 years, and an emergency Caesarean section is usually performed instead.

SOCIAL CHANGES, VIEWPOINTS, AND PERCEPTIONS

The views that pregnant women now hold about the way in which they would prefer to deliver their babies have also made a significant contribution to the increased rate of

Caesarean sections. Many of the women I meet in antenatal clinics have already developed clear views about the method of delivery they want. Some are passionate about achieving a vaginal delivery. Others are equally clear that they want to be delivered by Caesarean section. Most recently, the trend for celebrity mothers to opt for a Caesarean section (invariably in the private sector) because they want to dovetail their baby's birth into a busy work schedule, has resulted in the procedure being perceived as a fashionable option or the must-have accessory in childbirth. It must be emphasized that all Caesarean sections carry an element of risk.

MEDICOLEGAL CONSIDERATIONS

On some occasions when complex vaginal deliveries have resulted in babies suffering brain damage or other physical injuries, expensive and lengthy legal cases have followed. Inevitably, this leaves doctors more likely to err on the side of caution when there is a choice to be made between a Caesarean section or a complicated vaginal delivery.

family history of thrombosis, has a pregnancy-related problem such as pre-eclampsia, or is unable to have an epidural anaesthetic, her risks of developing complications because she has undergone pelvic surgery are markedly higher.

Vaginal delivery versus Caesarean section

It is difficult to make direct comparisons of the likely post-delivery complications experienced by women who have delivered vaginally and abdominally, but recent figures show that, on the whole, the increased risks associated with elective Caesarean deliveries are marginal. The risk of postpartum haemorrhage is only slightly increased, as is the risk of endometrial or urinary infection. Breastfeeding is often quicker to establish after a vaginal birth, but there is no difference in the mother's risk of postnatal depression or pain with intercourse after three months. After a Caesarean birth you will need to stay in hospital for longer, and recovery from major surgery will take longer than recovery from a vaginal delivery. In addition, there is a slightly increased risk of being admitted to an adult intensive care unit and of needing further major surgery, such as a hysterectomy, after a Caesarean section. On the other hand, the incidence of urinary incontinence is greater after a vaginal birth, as is the incidence of uterovaginal prolapse in later life. So, overall, there are advantages and disadvantages to both types of delivery.

Vaginal birth after Caesarean delivery (VBAC)

In the past, most Caesarean sections were performed using a vertical incision in the uterus leaving the muscle weakened along its whole length, and as a result doctors were reluctant to advise an attempt at subsequent vaginal delivery. Nowadays the majority of Caesarean sections are performed using a transverse or horizontal incision in the lower segment of the uterus, which is much thinner and usually heals more effectively and is less likely to rupture during a subsequent labour. Nevertheless, the risk of uterine rupture is higher in a vaginal birth after a Caesarean, and significantly increased if an induction of labour is performed. Generally speaking, if a woman chooses to have a trial of labour after a previous Caesarean section performed for a non-recurring cause, she can be reassured that she has a more than 70 per cent chance of achieving a successful vaginal birth after Caesarean delivery (VBAC). The single best predictor of vaginal delivery is a previous vaginal birth and is associated with a 87–90 per cent success rate.

Similarly, the old adage that a woman could undergo a maximum of two Caesarean sections has been overturned. Although the uterus is inevitably weakened by scar tissue, theoretically, there is no limit to how many pregnancies a woman can have delivered by Caesarean, so long as every case is individually assessed.

> *Nowadays the majority of Caesarean sections are performed using a horizontal incision...*

What to expect in theatre

Once the decision has been made to deliver your baby by Caesarean section, your midwife will help you prepare for the operating theatre. If you are not already in a loose hospital gown, you will be asked to change into one.

You will also be asked to remove your jewellery, apart from any rings that cannot be taken off easily. These will be covered by sticky tape to ensure that they do not act as a conductor of heat, since the surgeon will probably use diathermy during the operation – an electrical instrument that cauterizes bleeding blood vessels – and uncovered pieces of metal next to your skin could result in you experiencing a superficial burn or skin blister. You will probably be asked to remove your face make-up and nail polish as well, so that in the unlikely event of you becoming unwell during the operation, the anaesthetist will be able to assess your true skin colour immediately. If your partner wishes to be with you, he will be given a theatre pyjama suit, a disposable hat, and overshoes.

WHO WILL BE PRESENT DURING THE BIRTH?

I know that many women are surprised and a bit shocked by how many people are present in the operating theatre for a Caesarean birth. However, every one is there for a specific purpose: to ensure that you and your baby are safely delivered. This is the usual cast list, which may increase if you are delivering twins or triplets:

▶ anaesthetist
▶ operating department assistant (ODA) – to help the anaesthetist
▶ obstetrician – who performs the operation
▶ assistant surgeon
▶ sterile theatre nurse or midwife – to pass instruments, sutures, and such like to the surgeons
▶ non-sterile midwife/runner – to fetch all of the above
▶ midwife – to collect the baby when delivered
▶ paediatrician
▶ porter – to transfer you to and from a ward elsewhere in the hospital
▶ medical and/or nursing students – you may request that they leave, but do remember that the only way these people can be trained is by practical experience.

Your partner can stay beside you and hold your hand, to provide comfort and reassurance throughout the procedure.

The only time he will be asked to leave is if you have to undergo a general anaesthetic. In this situation you will be unconscious and your partner cannot communicate with you, which means that he becomes an extra person taking up space in a crowded room, not to mention the fact that he may start to feel distressed by being unable to contribute to the procedure. It is important that you realize that the request that he leaves the theatre is not because anything is being hidden and that you both fully understand and agree with the proposal.

> ...the anaesthetist will do everything possible to make you feel at ease and to explain what is going on, so you are sufficiently relaxed.

If this is an elective Caesarean you will probably walk into the operating theatre and lie down or sit on the operating table, in readiness for the epidural/spinal anaesthetic to be inserted (see p.313). If you are already in labour, you will be wheeled into the operating theatre on your delivery room bed and, once in theatre, you will be transferred onto the operating table. Looking around the theatre, you will see lots of pieces of equipment, much of it on mobile stainless-steel trolleys. There will be an anaesthetic machine at the head of the operating table you are lying on, covered in instruments, monitors, dials, cylinders of different types of gases, and drawers full of useful bits and pieces.

There will be a baby resuscitation trolley in the room, equipped with an overhead heater to keep him or her warm, a piped oxygen supply, and lots of drawers containing equipment that the paediatrician may need. As you lie there, the theatre nurse or midwife will be opening up sterile packs of instruments onto several trolleys that will move into position beside the operating table when they are needed. The walls of the operating theatre will be covered by open shelves containing sterile packs of instruments, gloves, gowns, syringes, needles, swabs, and sutures.

Caesarean anaesthesia

Once in theatre, the anaesthetist will insert an intravenous drip into your arm so that you can receive fluids during the operation, and start to perform the epidural or spinal block. It is common at this stage for women to get anxious about the whole situation. Some start to hyperventilate and to feel light-headed and nauseous. Others start to shake with nerves, not necessarily at the prospect of the operation, but more at the thought of the needle going into their spine. They can also worry about the anaesthetic not working properly and being in pain during the operation. Let me reassure you on all these fronts. The anaesthetist will be used to the physical signs of anxiety and, if you let him or her know you are feeling faint, you will be given oxygen through a mask. Any obstetric anaesthetist will be skilled at inserting the needle, with or without maternal shakes. Indeed, they will do everything possible to make you feel at ease and to explain what is going on, so you are sufficiently relaxed throughout.

If you are having an elective Caesarean, the anaesthetic will take effect in a few minutes a but the positioning of an additional epidural catheter (to provide you with pain relief after the operation) will take further time, usually around 20 minutes. If you are having an emergency Caesarean section, you may already have an epidural in place, in which case you will need only a top-up dose of anaesthetic, which usually requires only a few minutes to take effect. As for the idea of the epidural or spinal block not working properly, the anaesthetist will make sure that it has been 100 per cent successful by making a few checks: he or she will spray your body above and below the skin line where the anaesthetic has been introduced and will only be satisfied that you are properly anaesthetized when you confirm that you cannot feel the cold of the spray.

Final preparations

When the anaesthetist is happy that you are completely pain-free, a urinary catheter will be placed into your bladder. This has a dual purpose. First, it ensures that your bladder remains empty during the operation and does not get in the way of delivering your baby. Second, because it will be left in for 24 hours or so after the operation, it will eliminate the need for you to get out of bed and struggle to the toilet during those first few uncomfortable hours after the operation.

The next thing to happen is that your pubic hair will be shaved away from the site of the planned skin incision. Your abdomen will be thoroughly cleaned with an antiseptic solution and sterile sheets will then be draped over your upper abdomen and legs, leaving uncovered just the space where the incision will be made. The top end of the sterile sheets nearest your head will be hooked up to the anaesthetist's drip stands to form a screen, so that you will not have to see what is going on during the operation, unless you tell the midwife that you want to be able to watch.

Caesarean delivery

Once everything is in place, the doctor will make an incision through the skin on your lower abdomen, at the top of where your pubic hair used to be, so that the scar will be mostly hidden once the hair has grown back. Incisions vary slightly in shape and length but, generally speaking, they are about 20cm (8in) long and are either straight or slightly curved, like a smile. The surgeon will then cut through several layers of fat and fibrous and muscular tissue before making an incision into the lower part of the uterus.

Once the uterus is opened, the membranes will be ruptured (if they have not already done so) and the amniotic fluid will come pouring out. For practical reasons, most of the fluid will be suctioned away before delivering the baby, so that all of the sterile sheets, not to mention the surgeon's clothes and feet, are not completely soaked with liquor. The surgeon will then check the exact position of the baby's head and insert a hand into the uterus, around the top of the head, and gently disengage it from the pelvic brim, in order to deliver the

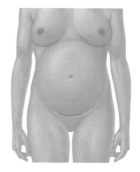

CAESAREAN INCISION
The cut will be made just above the line of your pubic hair (bikini line). When the incision heals the scar is very discreet.

head through the uterine incision. This is often a tight fit and the assistant surgeon may be asked to apply some pressure at the top of the uterus, to help the delivery. Sometimes small forceps will also be required, particularly if the baby's head is in an awkward position.

If this is an emergency section, performed during the second stage of labour, it may even be necessary for another assistant to examine you vaginally and help push the baby back up the birth canal, to deliver the head smoothly through the incision. This may seem a bit alarming to the parents, but I promise you that it is not dangerous for the baby. As the head gently emerges from the uterus, the baby's mouth and nose are immediately suctioned to clear all the mucus and liquor, and then the shoulders, followed by the trunk, are delivered very quickly.

After the birth

Most babies have started crying and protesting before their legs are free of the uterine cavity. Indeed, the baby positively bursts into the world during a Caesarean section. The cord is clamped and cut and the baby is then free – to be shown to the expectant parents for a first kiss and then quickly wrapped in towels to dry all the liquor and prevent her from becoming cold. It is very likely that the midwife or paediatrician will choose to move the baby to the warmed resuscitaire machine for a short time, in order to check her breathing and heart rate, clean all the vernix off her face and body, and perform the Apgar scores (see pp.375–6). They will then bring your swaddled baby over to you and your partner to cuddle, unless of course there is a problem that means that your baby has to be moved straight to the special care baby unit. If this is necessary, you will still be shown your baby beforehand.

Many partners choose to move in front of the screen so they can watch the delivery and take photographs of the birth. Others will want to remain

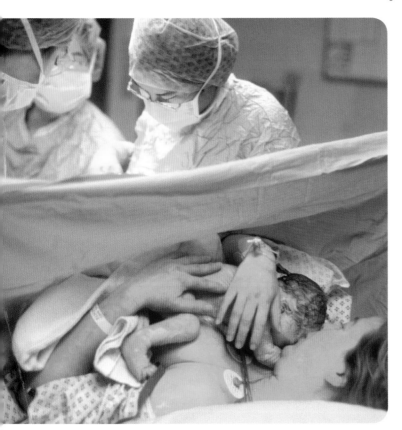

FIRST CUDDLE Your newborn baby will be handed to you to cuddle while the surgeon stitches together all the layers of tissue that were cut to reach the uterus.

shielded from the view of the operation and the delivery. For the mother, the Caesarean delivery will be a strange and sometimes rather amusing experience. There won't be many times in your life when you have no sensation of pain, but are conscious of the fact that someone is rummaging around in your tummy.

As soon as the baby is delivered, the anaesthetist will give the mother an injection of syntometrine to contract the uterus and help to deliver the placenta. Just like in a vaginal delivery, active management of the third stage of labour helps to reduce bleeding from the uterus or placental bed (see p.333). The placenta will be carefully checked to ensure that it is complete. Meanwhile, the surgeon will clean the uterine cavity before starting to repair the uterine incision with one or two layers of stitches. They will then start to stitch up all the layers of tissue that were cut through to reach the uterus, using soluble stitches, and finishing with the skin stitches or staples. The skin suture material will be removed during the next three to five days.

From the time the anaesthetic is given to the time when the stitching is complete, a Caesarean will take around one hour, of which only five minutes involves the actual delivery of your baby. The rest of the time is taken up by anaesthetizing you and stitching you up afterwards.

> ❝ ...the procedure takes about one hour, of which only five minutes involves the delivery of your baby. ❞

Classical Caesarean sections

A classical section, in which the uterine incision is made vertically into the muscles in the upper segment of the uterus, is performed only rarely nowadays. This is because horizontal lower segment incisions are preferred for most Caesarean deliveries, since the uterine muscle heals better and the skin incision also heals more quickly and is less unsightly. However, there are occasionally reasons to perform a classical incision, most usually for a premature baby of less than 30 weeks, when the lower segment may be so narrow and poorly developed that trying to deliver a fragile and already compromised baby through such a small aperture will undoubtedly lead to physical trauma for that baby.

When a baby is in a transverse lie and the membranes have ruptured it may be impossible for the surgeon to manipulate the baby to deliver through a lower segment incision without risking serious trauma to the uterus or baby. Similarly, when the lower segment cannot be approached easily because of large uterine fibroids or dense adhesions from previous surgery, it may prove necessary to perform a classical uterine incision. Because the risks of uterine rupture in a subsequent labour are high, individuals who have undergone a classical section will be advised not to have a trial of vaginal delivery in future pregnancies.

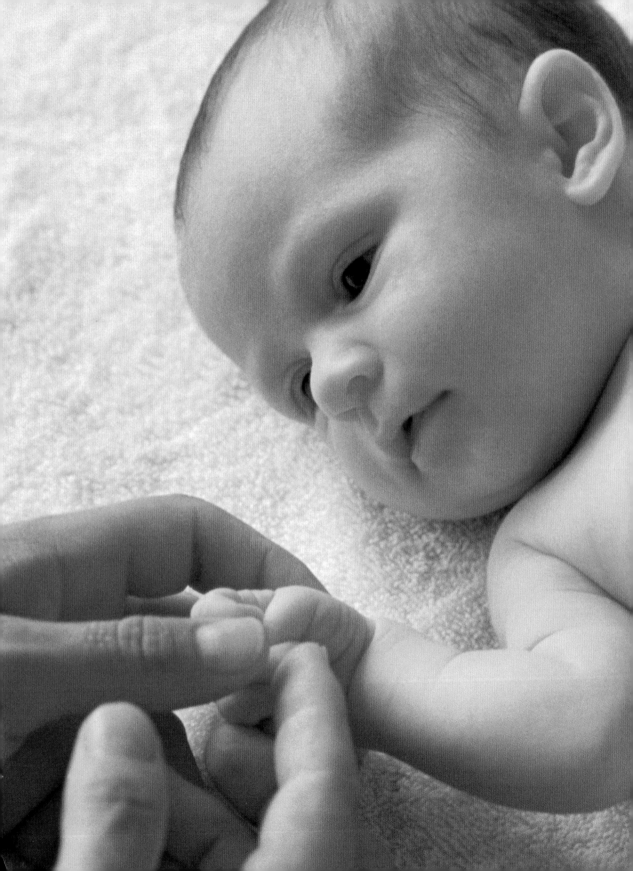

Life After Birth

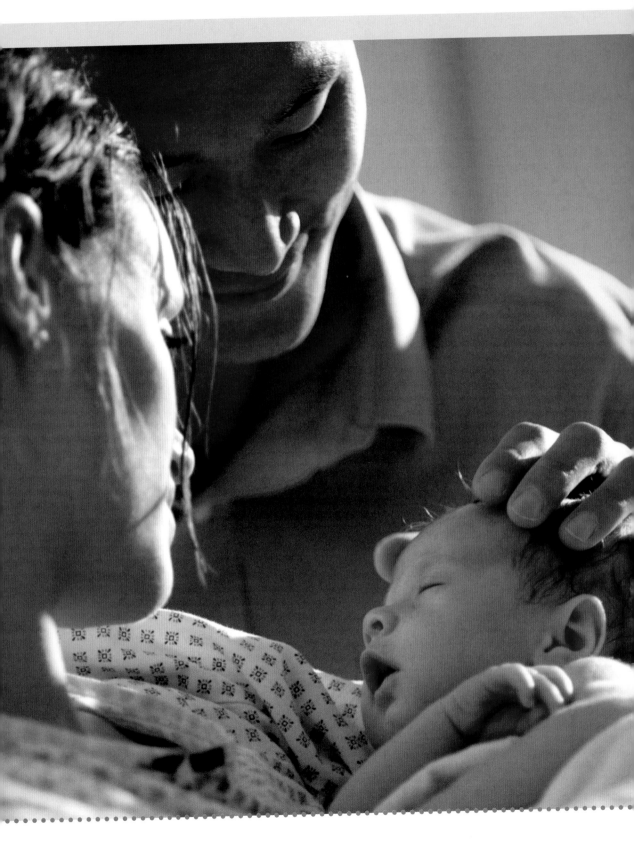

Your newborn baby

The busy hours you spent in labour and giving birth are often followed by a brief period of reflective calm. The staff who have been involved in your delivery melt away and you and your partner are left to savour and marvel at the arrival of your beautiful new baby. It is an emotional time since, after nine months of anticipation, you now meet the tiny new person you have created together.

CONTENTS

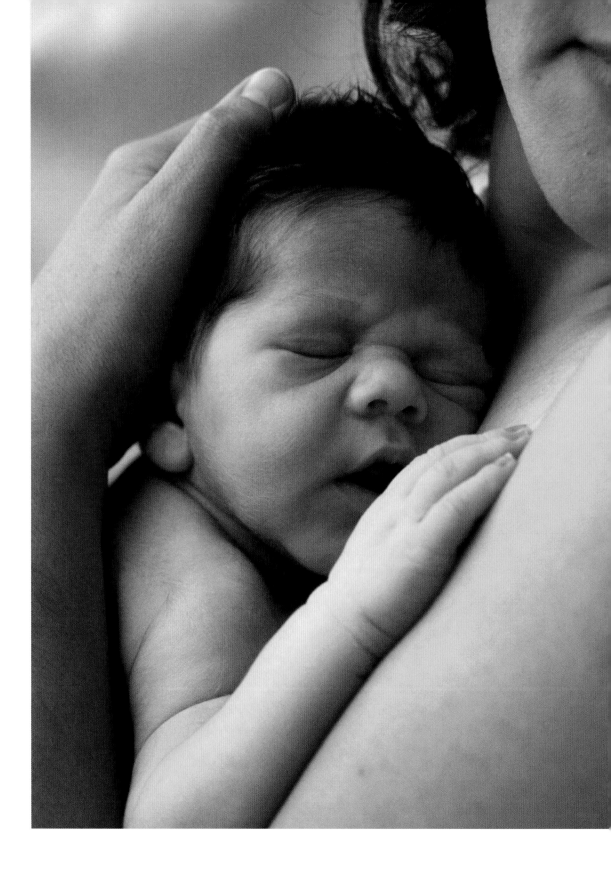

The hours after birth

MOST TERM BABIES WILL TAKE THEIR FIRST BREATH or gasp within 30–60 seconds of the head emerging from the birth canal and before the umbilical cord is cut. This gasp is stimulated by the light and colder temperature of the delivery room compared to that of the environment in the uterus. It is an extraordinary event, since the baby's chest is often still trapped in the pelvic cavity. Nevertheless, this first gasp is usually strong enough to start inflating the lungs.

As your baby takes his first breath, your midwife may need to ensure that his upper airway is clear by suctioning mucus and amniotic fluid from the mouth and nose. Once the baby's cord has been cut, the fact that there is no longer an oxygen supply from the mother acts as a further stimulus to establish breathing.

Successful inflation of the baby's lungs is achieved by the presence of surfactant in the alveoli or air sacs. Surfactant determines the stability of the lungs after birth by lowering the surface tension in the alveoli, thereby allowing efficient gas exchange. Without enough surfactant, the alveoli become completely airless at the end of each breath and the baby then has to struggle against the continuing high surface tension to draw in the next breath. A short time after birth, the baby's breathing rate increases, the nostrils flare, expiratory grunting is noted, and the tissue between the ribs is pulled in with each breath. This is respiratory distress syndrome (or surfactant deficient respiratory disease, SDRD) and occurs in 1 in 100–200 of all deliveries, but is usually mild. Premature babies frequently require help with breathing since they often have insufficient surfactant in the alveoli of their lungs and may need to be given surfactant to reduce the surface tension (see p.342).

Apgar scores

The doctor or midwife will assess your baby's overall condition one minute after birth and again after a five-minute period of observation, using the Apgar scoring system. This is a simple and highly effective tool developed by an American doctor, Virginia Apgar, after whom it is named. The maximum score is 10, two points being given for each of the signs that are assessed: skin colour, breathing, heart rate, muscle tone, and reflexes (see table, p.376). In black or Asian babies, the colour of the mouth, palms of the hands, and soles of the feet is checked. A score of seven

> "…your baby's overall condition will be assessed using the Apgar scoring system."

APGAR SCORING SYSTEM

Apgar score	2	1	0
Skin colour	Pink all over	Body pink; extremities blue	Pale/blue all over
Breathing	Regular, strong cry	Irregular, weak cry	Absent
Pulse/heart rate	Greater than 100 bpm	Less than 100 bpm	Absent
Movements/muscle tone	Active	Moderate activity	Limp
Reflexes after given certain stimuli	Crying or grimacing strongly	Moderate reaction or grimace	No response

or more at one minute indicates a baby in good condition; a score between four and six usually means that the baby will need help to breathe; and a first score of less than four means that resuscitation and life-saving procedures are required. At the five-minute assessment, a score of seven or more indicates a good prognosis and a lower score means that the baby needs careful monitoring.

Apgar scores provide an excellent short-term diagnosis of the baby's wellbeing immediately after birth. However, they are of little help in assessing a baby's long-term development, so don't worry if your baby's first score is low, as it invariably picks up by the second assessment. Even if this is not the case, it is unlikely that your baby will have any serious long-term problems.

Measurements and identification

While the Apgar scores are being performed, your midwife will be busy cleaning off all the blood and liquor on your baby's skin. The body temperature of newborns falls by 1–1.5°C immediately after the birth, because they lose heat rapidly from their wet skin and also because they have a relatively large surface area to body weight. This is why it is so important to dry babies as soon as possible after delivery and ensure that they are warmly wrapped.

Next, your midwife will weigh your baby, measure the head circumference, and attach plastic identification bracelets to the wrists or ankles with your surname and the baby's hospital number and date of birth. It is essential that your baby can be clearly identified before leaving the delivery room so that there is never any confusion or baby mix-up fears at a later date. The baby's cot will also be clearly labelled, and some maternity units take footprints, from the baby which are then attached to the baby's notes. Some maternity units attach an electronic tag to the baby, which sets off an alarm if he is removed from the ward.

Physical checks

Your midwife will carry out a preliminary check to make sure that your baby has no obvious physical abnormality. She will look at the baby's face and tummy, listen to the heart and lungs with a stethoscope (a newborn baby's heart rate is normally about 120 beats per minute), turn him over and look at his back, run her fingers down his spine, check that his anus is open, note whether he has or has not passed urine, and count the number of fingers and toes present. At a later date, a paediatrician or a specially trained midwife will check your baby again and perform a more thorough physical examination before you go home (see p.387). It is quite common for newborn babies to have mild inflammation or conjunctivitis after the lengthy journey through the birth canal. If your baby has a sticky eye, you will be shown how to bathe the eyes with sterile water. In the UK, antibiotic eye drops are only given to newborns with an eye infection. After all the checks have been completed, your warmly wrapped baby will be handed over to you so you can start to get to know him.

> ...your midwife will check that your baby has no obvious physical abnormality.

Vitamin K

Soon after the delivery, your midwife will ask you if you would like your baby to receive a vitamin K supplement and, if you do, whether you prefer it to be given by injection or by mouth. Vitamin K, which is present in food, especially liver and some vegetables, is essential because it helps our blood to clot and prevents internal bleeding. However, newborn babies receive very little vitamin K because they are fed entirely on milk. Added to this, their livers, which are responsible for producing other essential blood-clotting substances, are relatively immature and, as a result, they run a small risk of developing vitamin K deficiency bleeding (VKDB), or haemorrhagic disease of the newborn. The Department of Health recommends that all babies receive vitamin K supplements after birth. There are two methods of giving vitamin K to your baby:

• by injection – one dose of intramuscular vitamin K (Konakion) prevents VKDB in virtually all babies. A single dose is given to your baby by the midwife soon after birth. This is the most effective method of administration.

• by mouth – oral vitamin K is as and effective as intra-muscular injection, but only if repeated doses are given. Two doses are administered in the first week of life for all babies regardless of whether they are breastfed or bottle-fed. Breastfed babies are advised to have a third dose at one month of age.

Formula milk is fortified with vitamin K, and as a result bottle-fed babies are at an even lower risk of VKDB. However, the advantages of breast milk are considered to far outweigh this marginal increase in risk.

Adaptations at birth

Throughout pregnancy, your baby receives a continuous supply of oxygen and nutrients from the placenta, which also removes all the baby's waste products. Within a few minutes of delivery, your newborn has to change from being completely dependent on the placenta to taking independent control of his entire metabolism.

The first thing to happen is that your baby's lungs need to receive blood to oxygenate and pass back to the left side of his heart to pump around all of the body organs. In utero, 90 per cent of the blood supply by-passed your baby's lungs because there was no need to oxygenate it and hence the right side of the heart and the pulmonary (lung) vessels were at a higher pressure than the left side. This ensured that blood returning to the heart was either shunted directly from the right to the left side through a hole (the foramen ovale) between the two upper chambers (atria), or passed via the lower right chamber of the heart (ventricle) into the pulmonary artery. Because of the high pressure in the lungs, the vast majority of this blood was forced to flow into a duct, the ductus arteriosus, which diverts blood into your baby's aorta to reach the rest of his body.

As your baby takes a first breath and fills his lungs with air, the pressure in the pulmonary blood vessels falls and the ductus arteriosus closes, which

CIRCULATION BEFORE AND AFTER BIRTH ·

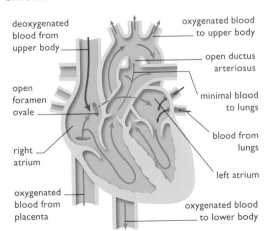

deoxygenated blood from upper body

oxygenated blood to upper body

open ductus arteriosus

open foramen ovale

minimal blood to lungs

blood from lungs

right atrium

left atrium

oxygenated blood from placenta

oxygenated blood to lower body

BEFORE BIRTH the baby's blood supply is shunted from the right to the left side of the heart through the foramen ovale.

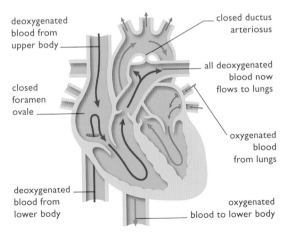

deoxygenated blood from upper body

closed ductus arteriosus

all deoxygenated blood now flows to lungs

closed foramen ovale

oxygenated blood from lungs

deoxygenated blood from lower body

oxygenated blood to lower body

AFTER BIRTH the blood supply passes through the lungs where it receives oxygen and begins to circulate around the body.

results in all of the blood from the right ventricle entering the lungs to receive oxygen. From the lungs, this massive increase in blood flow passes to the left side of the heart, ready for pumping around his body. At the same time, the flow of blood to the right side of the heart is reduced as the vessels in the umbilical cord start to constrict. As the pressure on the left side of the heart increases and the pressure on the right side reduces, it is no longer possible to shunt blood through the foramen ovale, which closes over like a flap. The baby now has an "adult" blood circulation (see diagram).

After all these cardiovascular changes are in place, your infant's liver receives much larger quantities of blood. As a result, the liver can start to metabolize the food or glycogen stores that it has built up over the last eight weeks of intrauterine life in order to meet the energy needs of the first few days of life until feeding becomes established.

The body temperature of most newborn infants falls by 1–1.5°C after birth (see p.376). Term babies have laid down brown fat, which they can now utilize for heat production without even needing to shiver.

How your newborn looks

Many couples are surprised by the appearance of their newborn baby. Their newly delivered infant can be a far cry from the cherub-like individual depicted in magazines. But it will only take a few days for the blemishes and visible signs of the traumas of delivery to disappear.

The first glimpse of your baby will arouse all sorts of different emotions, not all of which are necessarily positive.

All babies are born with blue eyes and the final colour of their eyes may not be evident until six months of age or more. The eyelids will probably look puffy – another consequence of the pressure effects of labour. Your baby may squint or appear to be cross-eyed for several months after birth, but this is rarely anything to worry about. Your baby's focus is poorly adjusted at birth, but when you hold him at about 20cm (8in) from your face he will be able to see you and start to absorb the details of your face.

The head often appears pointed or cone-shaped after a vaginal delivery, particularly if the labour was prolonged. This is because the bones of the skull mould together (overlap) to allow the head to be subjected to pressure and progress smoothly during the descent through the bony birth

> 66
> All babies are born with blue eyes. The final colour may not be evident until six months of age...
> 99

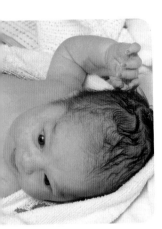

YOUR BABY'S HEAD
This may appear cone-shaped or pointed for a few days after a vaginal delivery.

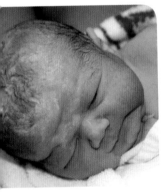

AT BIRTH Your baby may be covered by a thick greasy vernix, which has protected his skin from the watery environment of the uterus.

canal. Within a week, your baby's skull will have returned to its normal shape. Sometimes the pressure also causes swelling on the sides of the face, and if forceps or a vacuum extractor were needed, there may be some bruising on the face or scalp. You will notice a soft diamond-shaped area on the top of the head (the anterior fontanelle) where the baby's skull bones have not met together. This will not close completely until about 18 months of age.

Some babies are born with a thick coating of white greasy vernix caseosa, which has protected their skin from the watery environment in the uterus. Others will have none or just a few residual patches. Some midwives will clean it off the baby's skin soon after the delivery while others will leave it on to fall off or rub off in the next few days. Most newborn babies have quite blotchy skin, not just because of the rigours of labour but also because it takes some time for the circulation to the arms and legs to become well established. Dry, flaky areas of skin on the arms and legs are common. In the uterus, your baby was covered in fine, downy lanugo hair. At birth, some babies have lots of it left on the scalp and shoulders, whereas others have none. Any that remains rubs off during the next week or two. Small white spots on the face, called milia or milk spots, are very common. They are caused by blocked sebaceous glands that are designed to lubricate the skin. The spots will disappear quickly after delivery. The colour of your baby's scalp hair at birth may change over the next few months.

Some babies are born with long fingernails, and the problem with this is that they tend to lead to scratches on the face and elsewhere as the baby starts to explore his own body. Avoid cutting your baby's young nails with scissors, which can damage the nail beds. Instead, nibble the nails off gently and painlessly in your mouth. Placing protective cotton mittens on your baby's hands will help to prevent further scratches developing.

Birthmarks are skin blemishes caused by clusters of small blood vessels under the surface of the baby's skin. They do not usually require any treatment. Caucasians are commonly born with pink skin patches (called stork bites) on the nose, eyelids, forehead, base of the skull, and under the hairline on the neck. Most of them disappear within a year. Strawberry birthmarks (naevi) start off as small red dots on the skin and may continue to increase in size for a year after birth. The majority of them have disappeared by the age of five years. Most babies with dark skin tones have birthmarks called Mongolian spots. These are blue-grey patches of skin on the back or the buttocks. They are completely harmless and usually fade away in the first couple of years. Port wine stains are large reddish-purple skin marks usually found on the baby's face and neck. Since these are permanent birthmarks you may wish to seek expert advice from a skin specialist.

Babies of both sexes frequently have swollen breasts at delivery and may even leak a little milk. This is entirely normal and is a result of the mother's pregnancy hormones that take time to clear from the baby's body. The swelling and milk secretions will subside in a few days. Both girls and boys frequently have swollen genitals at birth. Once again, this is the result of maternal hormones engorging the tissues and will settle down quickly. In girls, the high oestrogen levels produced by the placenta can also cause the womb lining to become thickened while they are still in utero. You may notice that your baby daughter experiences some vaginal bleeding after delivery as the thickened womb lining breaks down. It will only last for a day or two. The testicles of a baby boy may still be in the groin at birth, but usually descend at a later date.

Putting your baby to the breast

There are enormous benefits of skin-to-skin contact with your baby in the first hour after birth as a method of promoting breastfeeding. While you are holding your new baby, it is a good idea to try putting him to your breast because the hormones oxytocin and prolactin are produced when the nipple is touched or stimulated. Oxytocin helps the uterus to contract, so even if you are planning to bottle-feed, it is useful to put your baby to the breast soon after the delivery. Prolactin makes the milk come in and, although you will be producing only colostrum for the first few days, the sooner you get the milk or "let-down" reflex working, the better. You are simply getting the baby used to being on the breast, so don't worry if he does not seem very interested in feeding. Most term babies already have a sucking or rooting reflex (see p.387), which means that if you touch the corners of their mouths with a finger or the nipple, they will turn to the stimulus and attempt to suckle.

Term babies already have food reserves built up when they are born. Many women feel anxious if their baby does not start to feed immediately, but the truth is, babies are often more interested in sleeping after the labour and delivery. However, premature babies need to be given small bottle or drip feeds of expressed milk or formula during the first 24–48 hours of life because they have less reserves and the sucking reflex is rarely developed before 35 weeks of gestation.

FIRST FEEDS These help your baby get used to the idea of breastfeeding as well as stimulating the release of hormones that cause the uterus to contract.

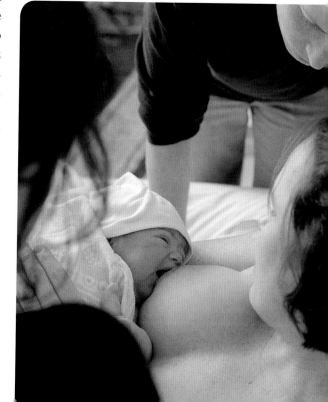

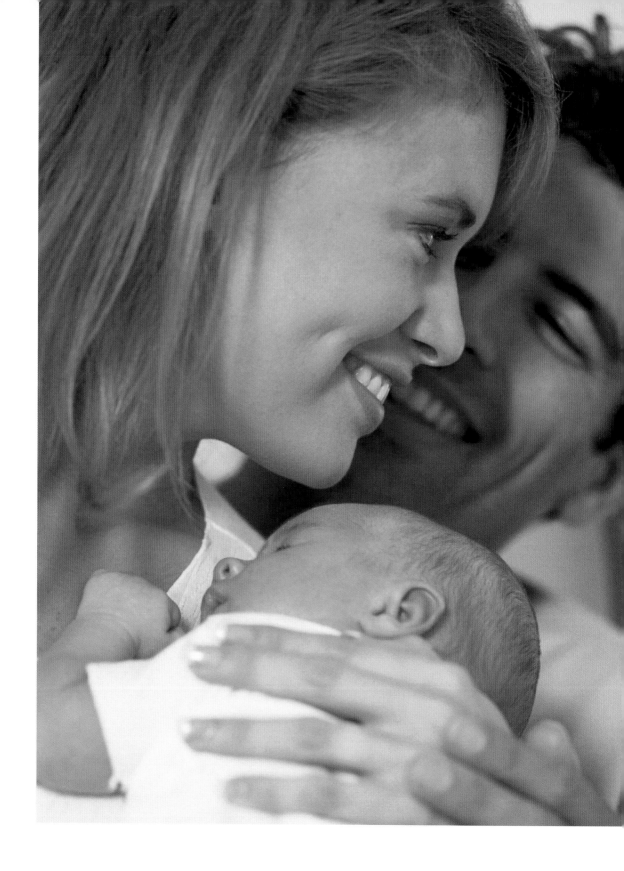

The first six weeks

AFTER NINE MONTHS OF ANTICIPATION, excitement, and probably some apprehension, you and your partner can now start on the next stage of this journey as you discover and explore your roles as parents. This section of the book will guide you through the first few weeks of your life after your baby's birth.

During this period of enormous change, you will inevitably experience a huge range of emotions. You will feel wonder and awe at the tiny person you have created and will be fascinated as you get to know the little quirks of her personality. You may also feel overwhelmed by her vulnerability and complete dependency on you.

In addition, you will be recovering from the physical effects of giving birth, as well as adjusting your relationship with your partner as you learn to accommodate your new family member. Getting to grips with the practical aspects of caring for your baby can also be challenging, especially when you still have all your usual household chores to do as well.

Adjusting to change

At times it may seem like there are a lot of balls in the air to juggle and the pressure on women nowadays not to drop any of those balls is probably greater than it has ever been. It seems to me that this is made worse by the media coverage of celebrity mums who, within 10 minutes of having their babies, are zipped back into their size 10 jeans, starring in their next blockbuster movie, and at the same time seem to be able to be the perfect mother. Faced with these sorts of images, many "normal" women dare not own up to having a difficult time during these first few weeks.

Becoming a mother is a time of great joy for both you and your partner, but it is also a time when the learning curve of parenting is steep. I hope that by being honest with you about what life after birth can be like, you will realize that all the physical and emotional changes you are experiencing are very common, and that whatever you are doing, or not doing, with your baby, you are nonetheless going to be a good mother.

> ...many women dare not own up to having a difficult time in the first few weeks of parenting.

Your physical recovery

The postpartum period is the six weeks following the birth of your baby. How you recover physically will depend on a variety of factors, including the type of labour and delivery you had, your general state of health, and your domestic support and social circumstances.

Here, I will discuss the most common physical after-effects of labour and delivery and some of the problems that can arise.

As your uterus starts to shrink back to its pre-pregnant state in the first few days after the birth, you will have a very heavy bloody vaginal discharge, called lochia. Lochia is made up of blood, mucus, and tissue debris, all of which needs to be expelled from the uterus. You will need extra-thick sanitary towels for the first few days and disposable knickers, because the blood loss is likely to be heavy. The flow usually calms down after the first week and the appearance of the blood gradually changes from bright red to a brown colour.

After-pains are the period-like pains that many women experience after delivery, particularly if they are breastfeeding. They are uterine contractions caused by the hormone oxytocin, which encourages the uterus to shrink back down into the pelvis more quickly. Since oxytocin is released when the baby suckles at the breast, it is common for women to experience after-pains or pass some small blood clots while they are breastfeeding. After-pains should last only a few days after the delivery, but if they are making you feel uncomfortable ask your midwife for a suitable form of pain relief. Depending on the type of delivery you have had and the extent of your discomfort, you can choose from injections, oral tablets or rectal suppositories.

Some degree of breast engorgement may occur as the milk starts to come into your breasts. The breasts become swollen, hard, and sore, and this normal inflammation commonly raises your temperature slightly. Fortunately, the problem usually resolves spontaneously in a day or two as breastfeeding becomes established (see p.398), but in the meantime can be helped by improved positioning and attachment (see page 397).

If you have stitches they will become tighter as the skin surrounding them swells and the wound starts to heal. This can make sitting down uncomfortable. Sitting on a rubber ring helps during the first few days, as this avoids any direct pressure being placed on the perineum. Similarly, maternity cool packs or local anaesthetic creams and sprays on the perineum can help.

> " After-pains are uterine contractions caused by the hormone oxytocin... "

You may also find that urinating produces a burning or stinging sensation as the urine flows directly over the wound. If possible, try to stand up or crouch over the toilet with your legs as wide apart as possible as this helps direct the flow of urine straight into the toilet. Gently wash the area with a cool sponge or flannel after you have finished and pat your wound dry. Bidets are a real bonus at this time, since you can bathe your perineum with soothing warm water while passing urine.

The bladder undergoes a particularly stressful time during labour and delivery, which can result in difficulties passing urine. If this happens to you, you may need to have a catheter inserted into your bladder to rest the muscles and allow them to regain their normal tone. The physical trauma of delivery can also encourage the development of a bladder infection. Prompt treatment with antibiotics and ensuring that you drink plenty of water usually resolve the problem.

Many women fear that opening their bowels for the first time after the delivery will be a painful experience. Rest assured that your stitches are unlikely to burst open even if you do find that you are straining to pass a motion. To help prevent constipation developing start drinking plenty of fluids (ideally water) as soon as possible and eat plenty of high-fibre foods such as cereals, fresh fruit and vegetables, and dried fruits. Gentle exercise will also help enormously.

POSTNATAL EXERCISES

It is important to perform pelvic floor exercises (see p.165) after a vaginal delivery, particularly if you had a long, drawn-out labour, which will have stretched the muscles considerably. Make sure you do these exercises for a short time on a regular basis. Try setting yourself the target of doing them by lunchtime every day, for example, which is much better than doing lots of them once a week. You can start by doing a few pelvic squeezes the day that you give birth, then gradually build up your regular exercise programme.

After giving birth, you can also use deep breathing to tone your lower back and abdominal muscles.

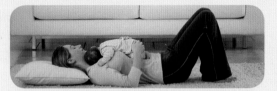

PELVIC FLOOR EXERCISE Pull in and tense your pelvic floor muscles as if you are holding back urine, hold for a few seconds then relax gradually. Repeat 10 times.

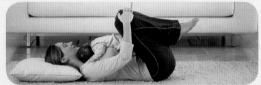

ABDOMINAL STRETCH Lie on your back with your hands clasping your bent knees. Breathe deeply, pulling your abdominal muscles inwards and upwards as you exhale.

Reducing the size of your abdomen as quickly as possible after the birth is probably a key concern. If you had a vaginal delivery, you can try gentle abdominal exercises during the first few weeks after delivery. If you had a Caesarean delivery, you may be advised to wait until after your six-week check-up before starting. My view is that you can try some gentle exercises soon after a Caesarean delivery, as long as they do not make you feel uncomfortable.

After a Caesarean section

The lochia is frequently less heavy after a Caesarean section, because the surgeon usually cleans out the uterine cavity with swabs before stitching up the walls of the uterus, thereby removing blood clots, pieces of membrane, placenta, and other debris. Nonetheless, you will have lochia for several weeks and may pass small blood clots and experience some after-pains when breastfeeding.

Most women will need strong and effective analgesia for the first 48 hours after the operation. Some hospitals offer patient-controlled analgesia (PCA) – hand-held pumps that allow you to give yourself small doses of intravenous morphine via a drip. Pain relief can come in the form of further intramuscular injections of morphine (which may leave you feeling rather hazy), rectal suppositories (which enter the blood stream quickly and are effective at numbing the pain while leaving your head clear) or tablets. Tablets are the slowest acting form of pain relief and are usually more suitable after the first couple of days.

Any person who has an abdominal operation and subsequently requires bed rest is at risk of developing thrombosis (see p.424). Pregnant women have additional risk factors because of their hormonal status and the fact that they have been carrying a heavy weight pressing on their pelvic and lower leg veins for many months. This is why your midwives and doctors will be encouraging you to get up and move around at the earliest possible opportunity after your Caesarean section. If your first attempt to stand up and walk leaves you feeling dizzy, just remember that in a few hours time you will be a lot stronger. The more active you are in the first few days, the shorter your overall recovery time will be.

Your abdominal wound will be covered by a sterile dressing that may remain in place for 48 hours to five days. You may not realize what type of stitches or clips have been used to close the skin layer until one of the midwives takes down the dressing to inspect the wound. Staples or clips are usually removed on about day three, whereas individual or continuous sutures are usually left in place until about day five. It is rare for the removal of the skin sutures to cause much more than a little discomfort, but if any problems are anticipated you will be given some pain relief beforehand.

> Most women will need strong analgesia for the first 48 hours after a Caesarean section.

EARLY POSTNATAL CHECK-UP

Before being discharged from hospital, both you and your baby will undergo a postnatal check-up. Many hospitals prefer to have a paediatrician carry out the check on your baby, but in some units specially trained senior midwives perform this task.

Your midwife will want to know how much lochia you are passing, whether you are experiencing any problems passing urine or opening your bowels, and how you are feeling emotionally. She will measure your temperature, pulse, and blood pressure, examine your breasts, check that your uterus is well contracted, inspect your perineum, and ensure that your calves are not tender or swollen. Your haemoglobin level will be measured and you will be given iron tablets if it is low. You will be offered a rubella vaccination if you are not already immune. Your midwife will make sure that you have enough painkillers to take home with you. She will also discuss your plans for contraception as the majority of women ovulate by six to eight weeks after giving birth, even if they are still breastfeeding.

YOUR BABY'S REFLEXES

Newborn babies have several important reflexes, which will be tested during their discharge examination:

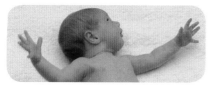

STARTLE REFLEX Your baby's arms and legs will stretch out when her head is allowed to flop backwards.

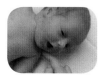

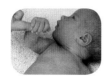

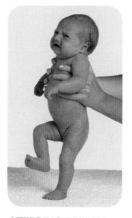

ROOTING REFLEX Your baby's head will turn towards a finger stroking her cheek, her mouth open ready to suck.

GRASP REFLEX Your baby's fingers and toes will be able to grasp your finger very strongly.

STEPPING REFLEX When supported under the armpits, your baby makes stepping movements.

YOUR BABY

Your baby's physical condition will be reviewed by examining her head, eyes, skin, limbs, breasts, and genitals. The heart and lungs will be carefully listened to with a stethoscope. Her hips will be checked for any signs of dislocation by gently bending the legs upwards and then rotating the hips outwards. The abdomen will be palpated to exclude enlargement of any organs and the baby's spine will be carefully checked to confirm that all of the vertebrae are complete. Your midwife will also be looking for more generalized problems, such as signs of infection, jaundice (see p.388) or low blood sugar. She will check your baby's temperature, skin colour, and muscle tone, and look for evidence of lethargy or irritability. All babies now undergo a routine hearing check before leaving hospital.

Your scar will appear rather red and raised at this stage and will also be tender to the touch. You may find it helpful to place a soft pad over it when you are dressed. However, the wound does not need to be covered all the time, and indeed being exposed to the air will help it to heal more quickly. It is also perfectly safe to have as many long soaks in the bath as you like – the warmth of the water can be very soothing. Always dry the wound gently with a clean towel.

You may find that the skin around the scar becomes dry and itchy after about a week – gently rubbing in some emollient cream helps to relieve this. The area of skin around the wound may be quite numb because the nerves that innervate the skin have been cut. This superficial numbness is normal and tends to continue for several months while the nerves grow back. Another cause of concern is that the upper edge of the scar tends to be rather bumpy and sometimes overhangs the lower edge when you are standing upright. Once again, this is normal and just reflects the fact that the surgeon cut through several muscle layers and these take time to knit together again and provide a flat muscular wall.

NEONATAL JAUNDICE

Jaundice is common in newborns because the excess red blood cells that the baby required in utero have to be broken down and eliminated. A yellow pigment called bilirubin is produced and needs to be processed by the liver before it can be excreted. When the bilirubin levels are high, the pigment is deposited in the skin and the whites of the eyes, which then appear yellow.

Physiological jaundice is very common, occurring in as many as 60 per cent of all newborns, particularly premature babies because their livers are immature. The yellow discolouration affects all the skin and is visible from 24 hours after the birth. The jaundice usually peaks on about day four and disappears without treatment within 10 days. However, if the levels of bilirubin become very high there is a risk that the pigment will be deposited in the brain causing permanent damage (called kernicterus). To prevent this, heel-prick samples will be taken to monitor bilirubin levels in your baby's blood. If they reach a certain threshold, ultraviolet light or phototherapy will be given for a few hours every day. The UV light breaks down the bilirubin in the skin, which can then be excreted in the urine without needing to be processed by the liver. You will be encouraged to carry on feeding regularly, since the calories and fluid intake will also help to resolve the problem. As soon as the bilirubin levels fall below the threshold levels, the phototherapy will be stopped.

Breast-milk jaundice affects about 5 per cent of breastfed babies who remain mildly jaundiced for up to 10 weeks, probably because hormones in the breast milk interfere with the liver's ability to break down bilirubin. The jaundice is not harmful and disappears if bottle-feeding is started, but there is no need to stop breastfeeding if your baby is otherwise well. After two to three weeks, your GP will advise that your baby has blood tests to confirm that her liver and thyroid function are normal. (For pathological jaundice see p.435.)

Leaving hospital

The length of your stay in the maternity unit will depend very much on the type of birth you have had. It can range from a few hours (six hours after giving birth is usually the earliest a woman will be allowed home) to more than a week if you have experienced complications. The average stay in hospital is one to two days after a normal vaginal delivery, and three to five days after a Caesarean section.

It is important to remember that the purpose of you being in the maternity unit is to be given advice and help on how to look after your newborn baby and also to ensure that you make a swift recovery from the labour and delivery. If you have opted to go home as quickly as possible, make sure that you feel confident about how to change a nappy and give your baby a bath and have talked to the midwives about obtaining practical help with feeding after you have left hospital.

The hospital will notify your community midwife and GP practice that you are about to be discharged from the maternity unit with your newborn baby and will provide details of your baby's postnatal progress and any concerns or problems that have occurred or may need special attention during the next few weeks. Arrangements will be made for your baby to have a newborn blood spot test about seven days after birth to exclude phenylketonuria (a rare metabolic disorder), cystic fibrosis, and thyroid deficiency. The tiny sample of blood is obtained by pricking your baby's heel.

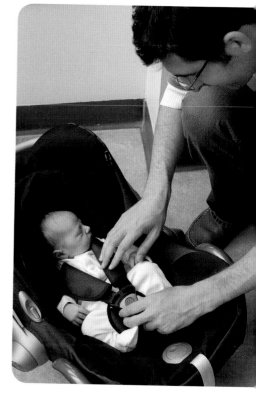

REAR-FACING CAR SEAT
A correctly fitted car seat is a must if you are driving your baby home from hospital.

On the road

If you are returning home by car, the law requires that your baby travels in a special baby car seat that needs to be facing the rear of the car. If you have a passenger-side airbag in the front, your baby seat must be fitted into the back seat of the car. Wrap up your baby warmly, because newborn babies are not good at maintaining or regulating their body temperature. As a rough rule of thumb, they should wear one more layer than you, plus a suitable hat and mittens in winter or a sun hat in summer.

If you had a Caesarean section, technically you should not drive for several weeks because your insurance company may take the view that, due to your abdominal wound, you are less capable of making an emergency stop. As a result, you are more likely to cause an accident or injure a third party. Contact your insurers to discuss your individual situation and needs.

Your emotional recovery

The dramatic changes in hormone levels that occur immediately after the birth of a baby frequently result in emotional peaks and troughs. So don't be surprised if, during the first few days and weeks, you find yourself bursting into tears for no obvious reason.

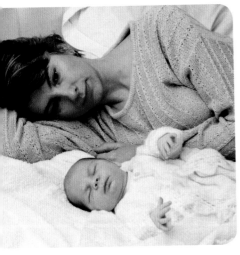

Giving birth is an enormous achievement and most women will be feeling physically and emotionally exhausted. Instead of being able to catch up on much-needed sleep and recover from the events in peace and quiet, you now find yourself on call day and night for your new baby. The realization that you are completely responsible for this helpless new human being hits you for the first time with a bang. These are powerful and difficult emotions to deal with, particularly for first-time mothers, and it is not at all surprising that they leave you feeling vulnerable and weepy. Let me reassure you that these feelings and responses are entirely normal and also temporary. They will start to subside in the next few days or weeks as your hormone levels become more stable and you adjust to the new demands of being a parent.

TIME FOR ADJUSTMENT The days and weeks following the birth of your baby are ones of major adjustment. Allow yourself time to get to know your baby and to adapt to your new responsibilities.

Bonding

Many new mothers I talk to are worried about whether they are bonding well with their newborn baby. I firmly believe that there is no right or wrong way to get to know and learn to love your baby. Some women fall immediately and unconditionally in love with their newborn, whereas others will be so shell-shocked by the delivery that it may take some time to adjust to the fact that they have just become a parent. Just because the so-called bonding process starts a little more slowly, this does not mean that they are going to be bad mothers or that their baby will suffer in the future. So please do not fall into the trap of feeling guilty or inadequate if this is the case for you. You will bond with your baby in your own time and much unnecessary anxiety and distress can be avoided if you keep reminding yourself of this fact.

Another common problem in the early postnatal period is that many women strive for "imaginary perfection" as soon as they reach home and then feel distressed and frustrated when they realize that this is virtually impossible to achieve. The reality of your new lifestyle is that it will be unpredictable. Young babies rarely understand how to fit in with your perception of an ideal daily routine, and it will take time and much patience to reach some sort of acceptable compromise for both of you.

Baby blues

The demands of an infant are endless and often tedious and many women, especially when they have their first child (less so with subsequent children), suddenly find that they are left, literally, holding the baby. In the past, women were surrounded by an extended network of female relatives who all helped out when a new baby arrived (and continued to do so throughout the subsequent years). Nowadays, women are much more isolated and, until they have made a few friends locally, they have to struggle on by themselves.

The vast majority of women experience some degree of the "baby blues" in the week following the birth of their baby. The baby blues usually start around day four or five, just when your breast milk is beginning to come in, and you are feeling particularly uncomfortable physically. However well prepared you may think you are for the postnatal period and no matter how many people have warned you about what is likely to happen, the baby blues will invariably take you by surprise. You are expecting to continue to feel euphoric and exhilarated that you have successfully delivered a healthy baby, but suddenly and inexplicably you find yourself weeping uncontrollably. I think the most disturbing aspect for most women is that they are powerless to do anything about these extraordinary surges of emotion. Make sure that you tell your midwife how you are feeling.

The period of baby blues usually resolves naturally within a couple of weeks. You start to recover physically, your hormone levels settle down, and you learn to look after your baby and find ways to ensure that you are not left coping on your own. Yet, for some mothers, these feelings of mild depression do not improve and postnatal depression can ensue.

Postnatal depression

Exactly how many women suffer from postnatal depression has always been difficult to establish. Depending on who you ask, the answer could be anything from 5–30 per cent of all women during the first year of their baby's life. I am sure that this uncertainty is because many women feel ashamed by their feelings of distress and are reluctant to own up to the problem and ask for help. It is also because their family,

SIGNS OF DEPRESSION

If you are experiencing some of the following feelings it may be that you are suffering from postnatal depression:
▶ overwhelming tiredness, disturbed sleep, and early-morning wakening
▶ persistent anxiety and low self-esteem
▶ lack of concentration
▶ weepiness
▶ your mouth is dry, you lose your appetite or suffer from constipation
▶ loss of libido
▶ rejection of your partner

"

...symptoms of postnatal depression can develop at any time during the first year after birth.

"

friends, doctors, and midwives are not very good at recognizing that early baby blues has now developed into a more serious problem. Postnatal depression is an illness, and when you are unwell it is difficult to be objective about the problems you are experiencing. As a result, you may not even be aware that you have it.

The symptoms of postnatal depression (see p.391) may not become apparent until after the six-week postnatal check and can develop at any time during the first year after the birth. Postnatal depression may be short-lived, lasting for just a few weeks, but if unrecognized or untreated, can persist for a long time and be seriously debilitating. Mothers who have had complicated deliveries or a multiple birth are more likely to develop postnatal depression. For mothers of twins or triplets, the diagnosis is often delayed because it is assumed that the woman's symptoms reflect the fact that she has even more reason to be tired, distressed, and experience difficulties in coping with life.

For milder cases of postnatal depression, treatment may simply be a question of making sure the woman is supported, both emotionally and practically, by those around her. However, severe cases may need to be treated with antidepressant medication (which is not contraindicated during breastfeeding). Counselling and psychotherapy with or without drug therapy have an important role to play in treatment.

No one knows exactly what causes postnatal depression. It may be that the sudden change in hormonal balance after the birth is important, but the fact that this affects some women more than others suggests that there are other triggers such as genetic and environmental factors. Women who have suffered from depression in the past are more likely to develop postnatal depression. Furthermore, of those women who have had postnatal depression following a previous birth, 1 in 4 are likely to have a recurrence after each pregnancy. Although not directly linked, it is important to remember that thyroid disorders are very common postnatally and that this may lead to symptoms that are very similar to those of postnatal depression. It is useful to perform postnatal thyroid function tests for women who become severely lethargic or hyperactive.

Puerperal psychosis

This is an acute psychotic illness that differs from severe postnatal depression because it usually appears within two weeks of delivery and involves schizophrenic or manic depressive symptoms. Puerperal psychosis is thought to affect 1 in 500 women, but if there has been a previous episode, the recurrence risk may be as high as 25–50 per cent. Occasionally, the mother is at risk of suicide or of harming her baby and will need to be cared for in a secure mother and baby unit.

COPING STRATEGIES

First and foremost, every mother needs to remind herself that she is doing her best and that there is no such thing – fortunately – as the perfect mother, whatever the alleged childcare experts and those around you might say.

If you do become depressed there are several things you can do to help yourself and make the illness as short-lived as possible. Start by reminding yourself that there is no such thing as the perfect mother. As long as you keep trying to do your best then that is all that anyone can reasonably expect of you at this difficult time.

The expectations placed on new mothers are often unrealistically high, but when the woman is seen to fall short of being the ideal mother, either in her emotional response or her practical everyday care of the new baby, she is often made to feel guilty, inadequate, and bewildered. It is not difficult to see how easily this can lead to the woman experiencing some or all of the symptoms for postnatal depression.

Next you should remember that you need to reserve some time for yourself during the postnatal period. Everyone is so focused on the new baby that the mother's emotional or physical health are often overlooked. Here are some tips to help you cope practically and emotionally with being a new mother.

▶ **Avoid becoming isolated** and try to get out of the house at least once every day.

▶ **Actively seek out other new mothers.** Many of them will be experiencing the same emotions as you and can provide a useful support network.

▶ **Ensure you receive as much domestic help as possible.** Pay for it, if necessary.

▶ **Don't suffer in silence.** Talk to your partner, friends, and family and make sure they understand your feelings and help support you practically and emotionally.

▶ **Seek medical help early.** Don't hesitate to talk to your doctor if you are feeling down. You may benefit from a short course of antidepressants (which do not interfere with breastfeeding) and/or seeing a counsellor.

▶ **Regular gentle exercise** and plenty of fresh air will do wonders for your sense of wellbeing.

▶ **Try to ensure that you eat regularly and sensibly.** This is particularly important in helping breastfeeding go smoothly.

▶ **Women, and mothers in particular, are very good at feeling guilty.** Don't. You are allowed to complain and to feel unhappy about your situation.

▶ **Arrange regular treats** or things to look forward to. Accept offers from family or friends to look after the baby, giving you some time to yourself.

▶ **Contact some of the organizations and support groups** that deal with postnatal depression, such as the Association for Post-Natal Illness or Meet-A-Mum Association (MAMA) (see Useful Contacts, pp.437–8).

❝ ...remember to reserve some time for yourself during the postnatal period. ❞

First days and weeks at home

Now that you are at home with your tiny baby, all sorts of anxieties may start to surface. Remember that babies are a lot tougher than they look. Short of accidentally dropping him, there is not much you can do that will actually harm your baby.

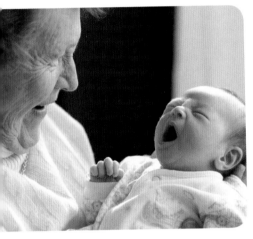

GRANDPARENTAL ROLE Accept any offers of help that come your way. Grandparents in particular are often enthusiastic supporters as you adjust to your new life.

During the first few weeks, try to find someone else to do the household chores, particularly those that involve lifting, carrying or bending, since you will need all your energy to care for your baby. The more help you can arrange, the quicker your recovery will be. You also must ensure that your return home does not result in your house becoming a hotel service or a coffee shop. Of course family and friends want to see the new baby, but ensure that they pull their weight when they visit.

Your community midwife will visit you at home during the first 10 days after delivery to check you and your baby are progressing. She will also be able to help you with any breastfeeding problems. Once she feels you are coping well, she will pass you on to your local health visitor, who will initially call on you at home to establish contact, following which you will be invited to attend the local health clinic on a weekly basis. Your baby will be weighed and measured at these visits and you will have the opportunity to ask the health visitors any questions you might have. Remember that you can also contact your midwife for the first four weeks after delivery.

Pace yourself

Many women find that once they have returned home they don't feel like venturing out again for some days. Indeed, for many women, caring for a newborn baby takes up all of their time and waking thoughts and the last thing they want to do is to expose themselves to the fast pace of life outside the front door. This is an entirely normal reaction and my advice is to aim to do only what you feel like doing, so that you can recover from the birth and get to know your baby in your own time. During the next few months you will experience much broken sleep and are likely to become tired as you provide round-the-clock care for your baby. So pace yourself from the beginning and instead of trying to do the housework while your baby is sleeping (he will be asleep for an average of 16 hours a day), use this time to grab some rest and much-needed sleep for yourself.

COMMON WORRIES ABOUT YOUNG BABIES

UMBILICAL CORD

The stump of the umbilical cord usually stays in place for about 10 days after birth, during which time it should be washed and carefully dried on a daily basis to avoid infection. If the cord becomes sticky or smells offensive, contact your midwife or doctor.

VOMITING

Young babies frequently bring up some of their feed (posseting), particularly when they are trying to get rid of wind. This is nothing to worry about unless the vomiting is forceful and occurs after every feed (see pyloric stenosis p.435), in which case you should talk to your midwife, health visitor or GP.

TRAPPED WIND

Trapped wind gives rise to abdominal cramps and pain and, not surprisingly, the baby cries and is difficult to settle after a feed. If simple measures such as placing your baby against your chest and massaging his back to encourage the wind to escape do not work, then ask your midwife or health visitor to recommend some medication to ease your baby's discomfort.

LOOSE STOOLS

Your baby should pass meconium (a sticky green-black mixture of bile and mucus) for the first 24 hours, after which the stools will turn yellow-brown. Breastfed babies commonly pass looser stools than bottle-fed babies,

but if your baby starts to pass watery green stools it is likely that he is suffering from diarrhoea. Young babies can quickly become dehydrated and this needs to be treated as a matter of urgency. Give your baby a little cooled, boiled water. If he has constant diarrhoea, develops a dry mouth, and a sunken anterior fontanelle, contact your doctor at once.

NAPPY RASH

The ammonia in urine irritates the baby's sensitive skin, so it is not surprising that most babies experience a degree of nappy rash, even if their nappies are changed regularly. However, nappy rash can be made worse by perfumed toiletries, creams, and wipes that are not hypoallergenic. It is best to wash your baby's bottom with water and non-perfumed baby soap and gently pat it dry. Zinc- and sulphur-based barrier creams smoothed onto the reddened area encourage the skin to heal and help to protect against further irritation.

STICKY EYES

This is usually due to a mild eye infection called conjunctivitis. It is common immediately after delivery when blood or other fluids may have come into contact with the eye. Gently wiping each eye with a fresh piece of cotton wool soaked in cooled boiled water usually resolves the sticky eyes, but if the problem continues your GP will prescribe you an antibiotic eye cream.

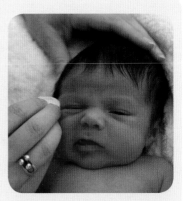

CLEANING A STICKY EYE Always wipe from the inside outwards.

FACIAL SPOTS

The small white spots (milia) that many babies are born with usually disappear in a few weeks without any treatment. If they become infected and red, bathe them in cooled boiled water before applying an antiseptic cream.

Contact your doctor promptly if your baby:

▶ is vomiting continually
▶ is passing watery green stools
▶ is very lethargic
▶ is irritable and feeding poorly
▶ starts to wheeze or develops a cough
▶ is breathing very quickly, very slowly or irregularly
▶ develops a high temperature
▶ shows signs of an infection or skin rash

Feeding your baby

Most women have developed views before the birth about whether they want to breastfeed or not. The decision is a personal matter and I believe that women should not be made to feel inadequate if, for whatever reason, they choose to bottle-feed from the outset.

It is important to be aware that you can offer your baby significant long-term health benefits by breastfeeding, even for a few weeks. Breastfed babies are likely to experience fewer respiratory, gastrointestinal, urinary or ear infections and are less likely to develop allergies and childhood obesity than bottle-fed babies. Furthermore, breastfeeding for a minimum of two months is thought to reduce a woman's risk of developing breast and ovarian cancer in later life. Breastfeeding can be undertaken at any time and in any place. Vitamin D supplementation (10mcg per day) is now recommended to breastfeeding mothers.

Breastfeeding

When a baby sucks on a nipple and areola two things occur. First, the mother's pituitary gland (at the base of the brain) is stimulated into releasing the hormone prolactin that produces milk. Secondly, the pituitary gland also releases oxytocin, which stimulates the alveoli to contract and forces the milk into the milk ducts and towards the nipple. This process is called the let-down reflex.

MILK PRODUCTION ···

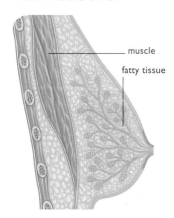

muscle

fatty tissue

BEFORE PREGNANCY

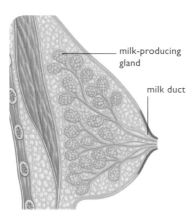

milk-producing gland

milk duct

DURING BREASTFEEDING

STRUCTURE OF THE BREAST
Your breast is made up of a mixture of adipose (fatty) and secretory tissue. Each breast contains about 15–25 lobes and each lobe is drained by a milk duct that leads to the nipple. The lobes are made up of individual alveoli (sacs) that swell up and contain the milk.

For the first few days after the birth your breasts will produce only small quantities of colostrum (about 3–4 teaspoonfuls daily). This is a concentrated clear yellow secretion, which provides your baby with all the water, protein, and minerals required until you are producing proper milk. Colostrum also contains high levels of maternal antibodies and a substance with natural antibiotic activity called lactoferrin, which helps to combat infection. If, for any reason, your baby is not with you in the days immediately after the birth, try to express any colostrum you can and ask that it be given to your baby. Even tiny amounts of colostrum are beneficial, especially for a premature baby or one who is in a special care baby unit.

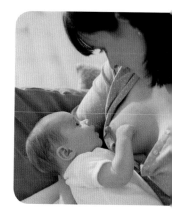

Your breasts start to produce white breast milk in increasing quantities from about day three onwards. Breast milk contains fat, carbohydrate, protein, and other nutrients in exactly the right proportions to ensure the healthy growth of your baby. After the milk comes in you may find you are feeding up to a dozen times over 24 hours. Soon, you will build up to around 20 minutes per feed every two to four hours.

How to breastfeed

When breastfeeding, the whole areola should be in your baby's mouth in order for him to "latch on" and feed correctly. If he is latched on correctly, he will have his mouth wide open and you should feel a suction effect over the whole area. His top lip is turned upwards and creased over and you will see his ears and jaw moving rhythmically as he sucks. If he is not latched on correctly, start again. Do not leave him to suck on just your nipple as it will become sore and cracked. Your baby should empty one breast each feed to ensure he gets both the dilute and thirst-quenching foremilk and the thicker, more nutritious hindmilk.

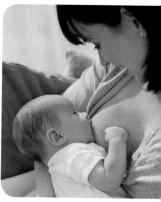

It is essential to be comfortable when you are feeding. Support your back properly and put a pillow under your baby so you are not bending down. Your baby should lie facing you, rather than just with his head turned towards your breast. You can also try lying down with your baby alongside you.

Expressing breast milk

You can express your milk by hand or with a breast pump, although expressing by hand can take longer. Breast pumps have a funnel that you place over your areola, which then forms an airtight seal. Pumps can be either hand- or battery-operated. Before starting to express you will need to sterilize the collecting bottle. You can then keep the milk in the fridge at 4°C for 3–5 days or freeze at -20°C in a sterile freezer bag, where it will keep for up to three months.

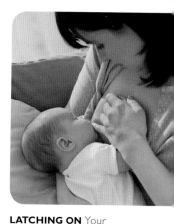

LATCHING ON Your baby should have all of your nipple and as much of the areola as possible in his mouth, which then forms a tight seal. As he squeezes the nipple against the roof of his mouth, milk will be drawn out.

BREASTFEEDING

Q&A

▶ **My breasts are very engorged and painful. What should I do?**
When the milk starts to come in, between the third and fifth day after delivery, it is common for the breasts to swell and become engorged due to over-production. Finding yourself with a temperature and swollen, rock-hard breasts can be a painful experience, but it is entirely normal and usually settles down within 24 hours or so. As your baby starts to feed regularly and empty your breasts more effectively, your body will adapt to producing the right quantities of milk needed to nourish him.

If you develop breast engorgement, it is essential that you try to drain the milk from your breasts regularly, to prevent the milk seeping into the surrounding breast tissue, which can lead to mastitis (see breast infection pp.433–4). There are several things you can do to drain swollen breasts and prevent severe engorgement.

• Feed your baby a little and often to drain your breasts regularly.
• Express a little milk before you start to feed – this will soften the nipple and will help your baby to latch on.
• Even if you have a cracked nipple, you must try to drain that breast – try using a nipple shield or express milk regularly from it.

• If your baby is not feeding very well, express the milk and either store it or discard it. Milk production works on a supply and demand basis, so if you do not empty a full breast regularly, future production will be poorer.

▶ **How can I cure blocked ducts?**
If a red, tender patch develops on the breast, then you have a blocked milk duct. This is extremely common, but to prevent it developing into mastitis:
• start each feed from that breast, because your baby's suction is strongest at the beginning of a feed
• place a warm flannel or a cold cabbage leaf inside your bra over the red patch
• feed your baby on all fours, so that your breasts hang down directly over him – this allows the breast to drain much more quickly
• express milk from that breast to help clear the blockage.

▶ **My nipple is cracked and really sore. What should I do?**
Force yourself to keep feeding on that breast to avoid engorgement. If necessary, express milk from that side while your nipple recovers and feed your baby from the other side. After a feed, smear a little milk or saliva on the nipple and let it dry naturally.

Expose your breasts as much as possible to the air and change breast pads after each feed to help heal your nipples.

▶ **I don't think my baby is putting on as much weight as he should. What can I do?**
Breastfed babies often put on weight at a slower rate than bottlefed babies and the growth chart you will be shown at the health centre gives a wide spectrum for so-called "normal" weight. If your health visitor is worried about your baby's weight gain ask yourself the following questions:
• Are you eating enough? Successful breastfeeding requires an extra 500 calories per day, 1,000 for twins, for your body to produce enough milk.
• Are you drinking enough? Plenty of fluids are needed to aid milk production. Aim to add an extra litre (1¾ pints) a day of water to your normal intake.
• Are you resting enough? If you are tired your milk supply will be lower.

If you are experiencing breastfeeding problems seek advice from your midwife or health visitor or contact an organization such as the NCT or La Leche League (see pp.437–8).

Bottle-feeding

Bottle-feeding does offer some advantages, not least that your partner can help to feed your baby. Infant formula feeds are made with cow's milk and are fortified with essential vitamins and minerals and are a close imitation of human milk. Soya alternatives are not recommended since they contain phytoestrogens and are more likely to result in lactose intolerance for your baby.

If, like many women, you breastfeed first then switch to bottle-feeding, the switch should be gradual, starting with one bottle a day, so that your baby gets accustomed to a teat and to the taste of formula milk. In this way, you will also prevent your breasts from becoming engorged. If you have been able to express breast milk into a bottle while breastfeeding, you should find the switch to formula relatively effortless. If your baby complains, it can sometimes help if someone other than you gives the bottle.

If you bottle-feed from the start, you will probably find that your milk does not come through very strongly and that it gradually dries up. Formula-fed babies invariably need fewer feeds a day and wake less during the night. This is because cow's milk forms a much more solid curd, which takes longer to digest, hence the strong tendency for formula-fed babies to go longer between feeds.

It is important to be hygienic and organized when bottle-feeding. Wash the bottles thoroughly before sterilizing them. Use boiled water cooled to 70°C to make the feeds. Cool the feed further before giving it to your baby. To reduce the risk of gastrointestinal problems, it is best to make up bottles as and when you need them rather than storing them for many hours. Bottle-fed babies need to drink extra water, as the feeds are not as thirst-quenching as breast milk. Once again, boiled cooled water is best. The temperature of formula milk is a matter of habit, with some babies happy to drink cold milk straight from the fridge. If you do warm it up, always test it on the inside of your wrist, and if you heat it up in a microwave, shake the bottle to disperse the heat before testing the temperature.

WINDING YOUR BABY
Sit him on your lap using one hand to support his neck and prevent his head from slumping down while you use your other hand to rub his back firmly.

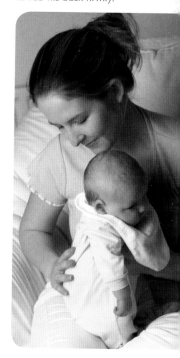

Winding your baby

Breastfed babies take in very little air during a feed, particularly once they have learnt to latch on correctly. Bottle-fed babies, on the other hand, tend to take in more air – their mouths form a less airtight seal around a teat – so may need more winding. The two main positions for burping a baby are over the shoulder and sitting on your lap. When your baby is sitting on your lap, make sure the head does not slump down. The oesophagus (feed pipe) needs to stay relatively straight in order for the air to escape easily. Rub rather than pat your baby's back and place a muslin cloth under your baby's chin to catch any milk that is brought up with the burp. You will soon work out the most effective way to deal with wind.

Family adjustments

However much you vowed – as many first-time parents do – that your baby would not change your life, the reality will be very different. Having a first baby causes an enormous emotional, practical, and financial change in your lives.

Partners

Fathers are often overlooked during the adjustment period after the birth, because the baby and mother are usually receiving most of the attention. Yet your partner is probably feeling physically tired, too, and is expected to be supportive and understanding of you and appear delighted by the demands that a new baby has suddenly placed on his lifestyle. I am sure that the key thing here is to ensure that you both communicate clearly about your individual needs.

Do try to get your partner involved in the care of the new baby, since this will help him to understand some of the difficulties that you may be experiencing and prevent him from feeling excluded. This will probably require you to step back a bit and allow him to do things in his own way, even if this is slightly different from how you do them. Try to resist the temptation of continually criticizing his nappy changing or dressing technique. Babies are very adaptable and the last thing you want to do is undermine your partner's ability to help you look after his baby.

Your partner may find that he ends up feeling physically distanced from you during the first few weeks, particularly if you are breastfeeding. It is not difficult to understand how this can become another source of resentment. You are locked into a close relationship with your new baby and seem to have an endless supply of cuddles and kisses for him, but not enough energy left for anyone else. It is easy for your partner to start feeling neglected. This situation will change in time, but recognizing that your partner may need some reassurance that he is not going to be left out in the cold permanently is an important consideration and one that you need to make sure you convey.

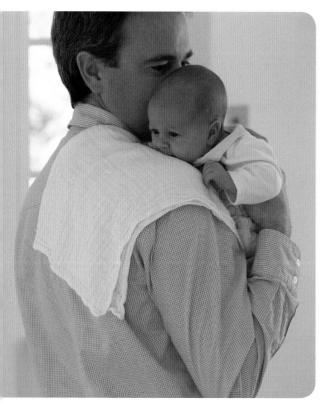

BEING A DAD Allow your partner to be as involved as possible in the care of his new baby – even if his way of doing things is slightly different to yours.

RESUMING YOUR SEX LIFE

Sex is an issue that is rarely discussed openly by new parents or their doctors. However, it is estimated that more than 50 per cent of couples have not returned to their pre-pregnancy sexual activity one year after the birth of their first child.

This fact suggests that it is common for couples to experience a significant change in desire, frequency, and the quality of their sexual relationship at this time. There are many factors that could account for this change. An appreciation of the most likely reasons may help you and your partner to discuss and hopefully improve the situation.

▶ **Many mothers are so exhausted** by the birth and by the continuous demands of their baby that the only thing they are interested in doing in bed is sleeping until the next time their baby wakes them for a feed.

▶ **An episiotomy scar** (or perineal tear) can make penetrative sex painful for weeks after the birth.

▶ **Vaginal dryness** is a consequence of breastfeeding (the result of high levels of prolactin and low levels of oestrogen) and can make sex painful.

▶ **Some women feel they have become unattractive** to their partner because they have gained weight during pregnancy, because their lactating breasts leak milk as soon as they are touched, or because they now have a large red abdominal scar after having a Caesarean delivery.

▶ **Women often feel unsupported,** lonely, worried or taken for granted after having a baby, all of which can result in a lack of libido. Postnatal depression is much more common than most people realize (see p.391) and mothers may experience symptoms for up to a year following the birth, which will invariably have an adverse effect on their sex lives.

▶ **Men, too, can suffer a temporary loss of desire.** This may simply be caused by tiredness, or the fact that they are adjusting to their new role as a father, but it may have a more deep-rooted cause. For example, some men now view their partner more as a mother than a lover, or they feel distressed having witnessed their partner's difficult vaginal delivery and the pain she suffered.

It is important to understand that you are not unusual or alone if you find your desire for sex has deserted you in the weeks or months after the birth. It is also important that you discuss the physical or emotional problems you are experiencing with your partner at the earliest opportunity. You will both need to be open with each other to prevent resentment and anger from further complicating a sensitive and potentially explosive situation.

Most couples will find that they are much better able to cope with the situation if they receive regular reassurances that they are still loved and valued. Staying in regular physical contact, albeit only with cuddles and kisses, during the first months after the birth can help to reinforce the fact that this is not a permanent state of affairs.

Eventually, you will resume your sex life, but it may take time and it may not be with the same frequency. However, many couples discover that the change in their relationship and lifestyle results in a greater level of sexual intimacy in the long term.

Siblings

The arrival of a new baby in the house can be an unwelcome shock for other young children, who may find it difficult to accept the permanence of this new situation. Preparing a child psychologically and trying to involve him in the practical preparations for the arrival of the baby can be helpful. Friends and family can also ease the situation by bringing a little gift for siblings as well as for the new baby, playing with them or taking them out for a trip.

In the weeks following the birth, try to provide as much continuity as possible in the lives of other siblings, so that they don't feel that family life now revolves completely around the new baby. Keep up with playgroups and after-school activities, invite friends round to play, and in particular try to continue the normal bedtime routine – including reading a story – whenever possible.

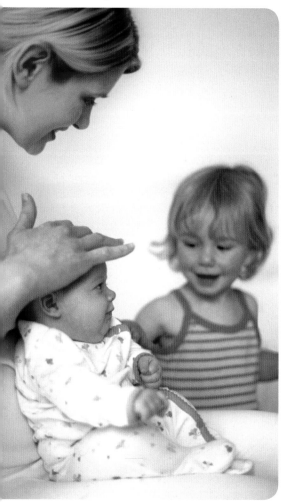

NEW ARRIVAL In the weeks following the arrival of a new addition to the family, try to involve older siblings as much as you can.

Coping with jealousy

Many children will go in for attention-seeking behaviour by being more clingy, whingy or naughty in the early weeks. There is no doubt that the addition of a new baby to the family frequently causes feelings of jealousy in other siblings and this needs to be addressed rather than swept under the carpet. With older children, encouraging them to talk about their feelings and telling them that you love them just as much as before will help to reassure them. However, with younger children it is likely that plenty of extra cuddles and some time spent alone with you each day will also be needed. Your partner and close family friends can really help by looking after the new baby for you while you offer your other children some individual and much-needed attention.

Don't be surprised to hear your young children talk about putting the baby in a dustbin or returning him to the hospital or back into mummy's tummy. You also need to be aware of the fact that it is common for young children to "accidentally" attempt to harm the new baby, by pinching or hitting them, when they think your back is turned. These are all entirely normal and predictable responses and I can assure you that your older children will come round to loving their new sibling in time. Nevertheless, you do need to take the precaution of never leaving your baby unattended with a young child in the room.

The six-week postnatal check

You and your baby will be seen by your hospital doctor, GP or paediatrician about six weeks after the birth. This provides an important opportunity for you to talk about any concerns you have about yourself or your baby.

Your baby's check will involve a full physical examination, together with an assessment of his developmental progress since birth, including:

- growth – size, length, and weight, which will be plotted on a growth chart
- head circumference and assessment of the anterior and posterior fontanelles
- eyes, ears, and mouth (sight and hearing will be formally assessed at later visits)
- heart, chest, and breathing
- abdominal organs and genitals
- hip alignment and stability
- reflexes – degree of head control, grasp reflex, and muscle tone.

The health clinic staff will ask about your baby's general wellbeing, feeding, and toilet habits and discuss with you the recommended times for vaccinations. If you have worries about these, talk to your doctor or health visitor or obtain up-to-date information from the Department of Health (see p.437). Many of the scare stories relating to vaccinations have been refuted, and recent innovations, such as the five-in-one jab, promise even greater safety, yet there are still babies at risk as a result of mothers deciding against some vaccinations.

Your examination will ensure you have fully recovered from the delivery.

- Your blood pressure will be measured.
- Your urine will be tested to ensure that there is no protein or blood present.
- You will be weighed and advised about diet if needed.
- Your breasts and nipples will be checked.
- Your abdomen will be examined to check that the uterus is well contracted, and if you had a Caesarean section, the scar will be examined.
- A pelvic examination will be performed if you had an episiotomy or perineal tear to check that the vagina is well healed and that you have no pain or discomfort. After a Caesarean section or complicated vaginal delivery an internal examination may be carried out to check that the uterus is well contracted, not tender, and that you have no vaginal bleeding or discharge.

Now is the time to discuss any problems you may have with pain, bleeding, bowels or bladder. You will also be reminded to think about contraception.

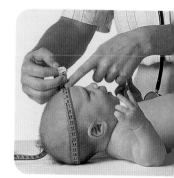

THE HEAD CIRCUMFERENCE of your baby will be noted.

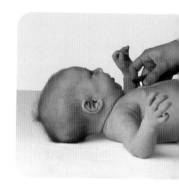

YOUR BABY'S HEART RATE and breathing will be monitored.

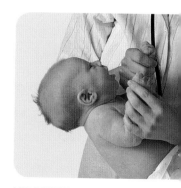

HIS DEGREE OF HEAD CONTROL will be checked.

CARING FOR A PREMATURE BABY

Around 10 per cent of babies are born before the 37th week and are classified as being premature. Many of these babies, although smaller than a full-term baby, can be cared for like a normal newborn and do not need any special care. A further 2–3 per cent of babies are born at term but with a low birthweight relative to their gestational age and need special care.

Generally speaking, any baby whose birthweight is less than 2kg (4lb 7oz), either because they are premature or small-for-dates, will be taken to the Special Care Baby Unit (SCBU). Other premature babies may be above this weight but may have other problems. Usually, they simply need more time to grow or for their lungs to mature so that they can breathe unaided.

THE SPECIAL CARE BABY UNIT

This specialist unit cares for vulnerable babies in the best possible environment. The unit protects your baby from infection by limiting access to all but essential people – medical staff, parents, and the immediate family of the baby. There is also a high ratio of carers to babies. While in the unit the babies are constantly monitored to ensure that any problem is dealt with immediately. The staff always encourage parents to participate in the care of their baby and they take care to explain what is going

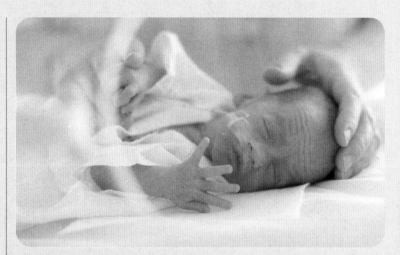

TOUCH IS VERY IMPORTANT Studies have shown that cuddling and touching premature babies can help them to gain weight and grow.

on, so that the parents understand and feel involved. Additionally, all SCBUs have counsellors for parents to talk to, and many have baby feeding advisers to help with breastfeeding.

If your baby is taken to an SCBU, she may well be placed in an incubator and attached to various monitors and wires. She may be ventilated to enable her to breathe.

The first visit to an SCBU is invariably a shock for parents. It is difficult to see your tiny baby lying helplessly in an incubator, surrounded by high-tech machinery and a tangle of wires. The medical staff will always be on hand at this time to reassure you and provide answers to any questions you might have. They will show you how to express milk and feed your baby, how you can stroke her inside the incubator, and will encourage you to talk to her. In addition, even the smallest baby can usually be cuddled, so they will help you take your baby out of the incubator. Gradually, you will learn how to care for her, including changing her nappy, giving her a bath, and helping with her feeds. Once she is stronger and no longer ventilated, you will be able to spend as long as you want holding her. There is no such thing as visiting hours in an SCBU and, right from the start, parents can spend as much time as they want with their babies.

COPING EMOTIONALLY

One of the major hurdles to overcome when your baby spends more than a few days in special care is the realization that you will be going home without her. This can be a severe blow, particularly if you are leaving behind a very

premature or sick baby. Yet, it is vital not to feel guilty – although I realize that this is easier said than done. It is unlikely that anything you have done has actively contributed to the premature birth and you can rest assured that your baby will now receive the best care available to enable her to thrive and go home as soon as possible.

When you go home make the most of this opportunity to regain your strength and to make the emotional and practical adjustments to having a baby that you and your family were perhaps not able to do because of the unexpected early birth.

Furthermore, you do not have to stay at the hospital every waking hour, particularly if you have other children. This could lead to feelings of resentment on their part once the baby is back home. The time that your new baby spends in hospital can be a useful adjustment period

for other children, and although you may not be spending more than a few hours a day with your baby in the SCBU, there is not a shred of evidence to suggest that this will impact negatively on your ability to love your child.

GOING HOME

Generally speaking, a baby will go home when she is able to feed fully, either with breast milk or formula, when she weighs at least 2kg (4lb 7oz), when she is more than 34 weeks gestation, gaining weight, and maintaining her own body temperature.

When the time to go home is imminent, many units like the mother to come in and stay for at least one night – they have special bedrooms available for this purpose. This gives mothers the confidence to look after their baby fully once they are both back home.

Premature babies are usually home within two to three weeks of the time they were due. By then, unless there is an underlying health problem, the baby should be treated as any full-term newborn. She should be given plenty of cuddles to make her feel secure and it is unlikely she will display any differences in behaviour from a full-term infant.

The stages of development and weight gain of a premature baby are calculated from the date that the baby was due. By the time he is two years old, he will have caught up developmentally and physically with full-term children.

LOOKING AFTER A SPECIAL-CARE BABY

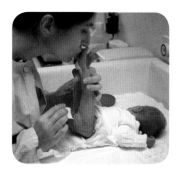

BABY CARE You will be encouraged to care for your premature baby, including changing her nappies.

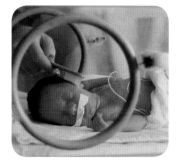

MAKING CONTACT There are many ways to interact with your baby while she is in the incubator.

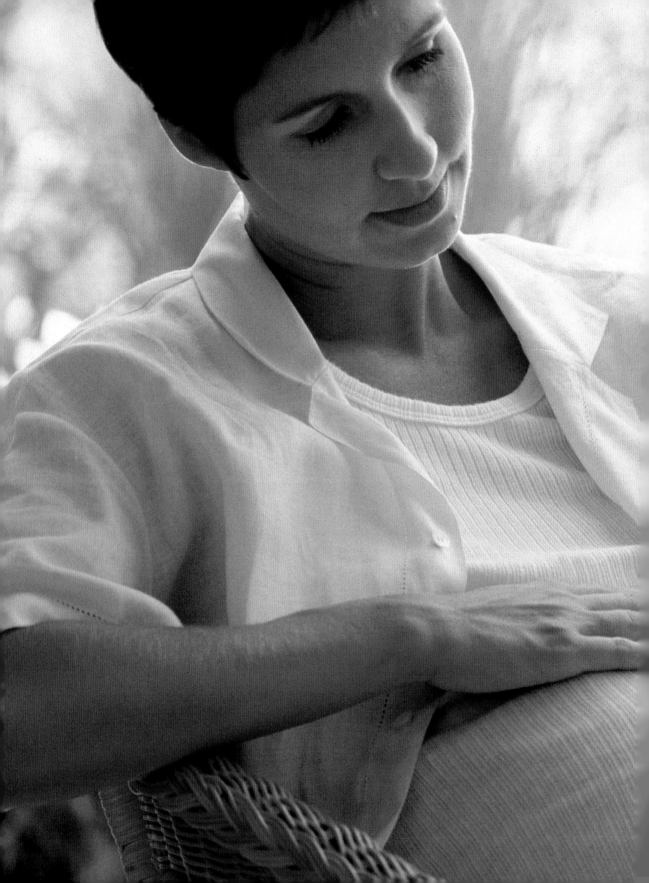

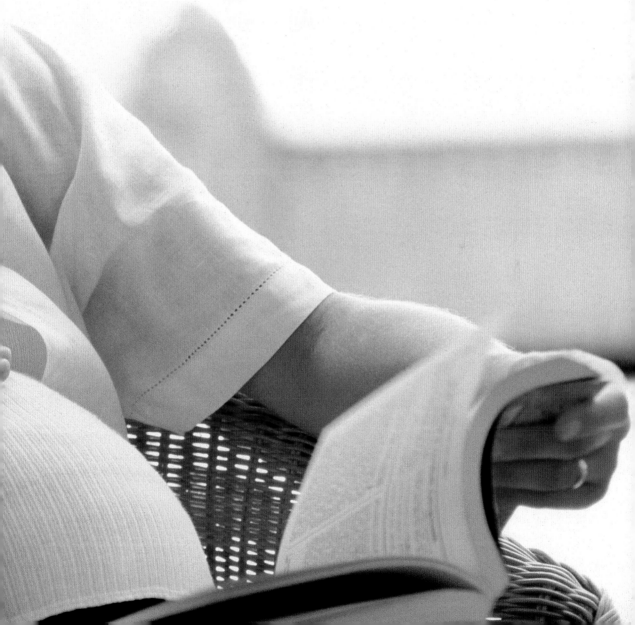

Concerns and Complications

Existing medical conditions

This section includes most of the disorders that I encounter on a day-to-day basis and those that I am asked about most frequently. If you know you have a medical condition or are diagnosed with one in pregnancy, it is important to make sure that you get specialized medical help.

Epilepsy

If you suffer from epilepsy, it is particularly important that you are under close medical supervision when you are trying to become pregnant and during the pregnancy itself. Some anti-epileptic drugs (particularly sodium valproate and carbamazapine) can cause abnormalities in the baby, such as heart and limb defects, mental retardation, and CLEFT LIP AND PALATE, and are best changed to a different type of drug. Your doctor will advise you of the best drug to be taking and, early in pregnancy, will arrange for you to have a specialist ultrasound scan to detect any fetal abnormalities. Pregnancy can change the way anti-epileptic drugs are metabolized in the body and you may need a higher dose to ensure that you do not have an epileptic fit. Some anti-epileptic drugs may reduce your folic acid levels and hence you need to take high-dose folic acid supplements before becoming pregnant and during the first 12 weeks of pregnancy to minimize the risk of having a baby with a neural tube defect such as SPINA BIFIDA. Since the drugs induce your liver enzymes, you will be advised to take vitamin K supplements daily from 36 weeks onwards.

Any fit in a pregnant or postpartum woman needs to be carefully assessed to establish whether it is due to epilepsy or eclampsia. Breastfeeding is safe, although some drugs (phenobarbitone and primidone) may have a sedative effect on the infant.

Diabetes

There are two types of diabetes in pregnancy: pre-existing diabetes mellitus and GESTATIONAL DIABETES (pregnancy induced). Diabetes mellitus affects 3 per cent of the population and, since pregnancy usually exacerbates the disorder, specialist antenatal care is needed to minimize the maternal and fetal complications associated with diabetic pregnancy. Women with pre-existing diabetes mellitus should aim for optimal control of their blood sugar levels before they become pregnant, since hyperglycaemia at conception and during the period of embryogenesis increases the risk of miscarriage and may cause major fetal abnormalities including cardiac, skeletal, and neural tube defects. High-dose folic acid (5mg) supplements should be prescribed for all diabetic women planning to become pregnant and continued until they reach the second trimester. A careful search for fetal abnormalities will be performed at the 20-week ultrasound scan.

Careful control of the mother's sugar levels needs to continue throughout pregnancy because maternal glucose, but not insulin, crosses the placenta. If your diabetes is usually managed with oral hypoglycaemic drugs you may need to change or add in insulin injections. The additional demands of pregnancy will make it more difficult to accurately control your blood sugar levels, on drugs alone, since they are long-acting, less predictable than insulin, and cross the placenta. Maternal hyperglycaemia prompts the secretion of additional insulin from the fetal pancreas, which results in macrosomia (big babies), polycythemia (too many red blood cells), poor lung maturation, and problems for the newborn including hypoglycaemia, respiratory distress syndrome, jaundice, and poor temperature control. Babies exposed to high and low blood sugar levels in utero are at risk of intrauterine death and stillbirth. Ultrasound scans for fetal growth and wellbeing will be performed regularly. It is important to remember that babies of some diabetic mothers are growth restricted.

Women with diabetes are more prone to developing pregnancy-induced hypertension, pre-eclampsia, polyhydramnios, and urinary tract and vaginal candida infections. You will be advised to have an eye check since retinopathy worsens in pregnancy. A combination of careful dietary measures and regular adjustments of the mother's insulin dosage is usually needed to maintain stable blood sugar levels in later pregnancy. You will be shown how to check your own blood sugar levels and you will also be asked to check your urine regularly for ketones. The timing of delivery, which should be performed in a unit with neonatal facilities, will be dictated by the presence or absence of fetal and maternal complications. Most women will require intravenous insulin infusions during labour and delivery.

Asthma

Some 3 per cent of pregnant women will have symptoms of asthma, which may be missed because most pregnant women develop a degree of breathlessness. Asthma is often triggered by allergies to foods, chemicals, dust, pollen, and smoke or follows a viral chest infection. Wherever possible, pregnant women should avoid exposure to these triggers. It tends to improve in pregnancy due to the increased production of maternal cortisone. Inhaled steroids and bronchodilator drugs have no effect on the fetus, but women who require oral steroids during pregnancy have a greater risk of developing PRE-ECLAMPSIA and having a baby with IUGR. During labour and delivery, which need to be covered with IV steroids, epidural and entonox are the best options for

pain relief. Breastfeeding should be encouraged because it reduces the risk of the baby developing future allergies (atopy).

Inflammatory bowel disease (IBD)

Inflammation of the small intestine (Crohn's disease) and large intestine (ulcerative colitis) usually causes profuse diarrhoea, with blood and mucus in the stools, and is accompanied by severe abdominal pain. Pregnancy does not usually alter the course of IBD, but women with IBD have higher rates of preterm delivery and low birthweight infants. A flare during pregnancy is most likely if your disease is active at the time of conception, so you will be advised to avoid pregnancy until your symptoms are well controlled so the amount of steroid medication needed during pregnancy is minimal. High dose folic acid, vitamin D and B12 supplements are all recommended. Vaginal delivery is preferable since women with this disease are at greater risk of post-operative complications.

Coeliac disease

This is a common disorder in which gluten-containing foods (wheat, barley, and rye, but not oats) trigger inflammation of the small intestine, which improves when gluten is excluded from the diet. The symptoms are variable and include tiredness, malaise, anaemia, diarrhoea, abdominal pain or bloating, weight loss, mouth ulcers, and vitamin deficiencies. Coeliac disease affects 1 in 70 pregnant women. The diagnosis should always be considered in

pregnant women with iron-deficiency anaemia or unexplained folate, B6 or B12 deficiency, and is confirmed by the finding of antibodies to gliadin or endomysin. Untreated coeliac disease is associated with high rates of miscarriage, IUGR, premature birth, and maternal anaemia. Gluten-free dietary control together with folate and vitamin B supplements should be started preconceptually.

Gallstones

Gallstones are a common finding in pregnant women and acute inflammation of the gall bladder (cholecystitis) complicates 1 in 1000 pregnancies. High oestrogen levels increase the secretion of cholesterol and raised progesterone makes the drainage of bile into the small intestine more sluggish. Conservative management with bed rest, fluids, and antibiotics is the first option to avoid the risks of miscarriage and preterm labour associated with surgery in the first and third trimesters respectively. However, many pregnant women relapse and may require definitive surgery at a later date.

Heart disease

Maternal heart disease during pregnancy is uncommon but potentially serious and should always be cared for in units with specialist expertise. Rheumatic heart disease used to be the most likely underlying cause of heart disease in pregnant women, but nowadays this is rare. However, there are now a significant number of women of childbearing age who underwent surgery for congenital heart disease as a child. The dramatic improvement in the life expectancy of these women has meant that many of them are now requesting help to achieve successful pregnancies of their own. Detailed management is beyond the scope of this book, but preventing sudden blood loss, controlling blood pressure, ensuring that the second stage of labour is short, and that delivery is covered by antibiotics are all important issues.

It is increasingly common to see older pregnant women with ischaemic heart disease. It is essential that lifestyle changes are encouraged, such as eating healthily and stopping smoking. Some types of heart disease are associated with very high mortality, such as pulmonary hypertension; these women may be advised not to conceive.

Essential hypertension

Pre-existing high blood pressure (essential hypertension) needs to be under good control when you are planning to become pregnant. The risk of developing PRE-ECLAMPSIA (toxaemia) and other severe problems such as kidney damage are greater if your blood pressure is high at the start of your pregnancy. About 3 per cent of pregnant women are taking anti-hypertensive drugs, but some are not suitable for use in pregnancy, so ensure that you have talked to your doctor about your plans to become pregnant well in advance, or as soon as the pregnancy test is positive. You may be advised to take low-dose aspirin to reduce your risk of developing pre-eclampsia.

Renal disease

Occasionally renal disease presents for the first time during pregnancy, triggered by the extra filtering load placed on the kidneys and additional problems of HIGH BLOOD PRESSURE and PRE-ECLAMPSIA. Women with existing renal disease need to understand that pregnancy can result in a marked deterioration in their renal function and an earlier requirement for dialysis. If the disease is progressive it is best to embark on pregnancy sooner rather than later. In a relapsing disease, it is better to aim for a remission before getting pregnant. Pre-pregnancy counselling should include advice on the risks of various medications to the fetus and the woman's fertility, the need for early booking and a possible change in medication, strict blood pressure control, together with details of the obstetric problems that may be encountered (premature delivery, pre-eclampsia, IUGR). Women with good kidney transplant function can usually achieve a successful pregnancy with specialist help. Immunosuppressive drugs do not significantly increase the risk of fetal abnormalities but early delivery by Caesarean section is commonplace. Women with transplants should also be warned that they run an increased risk of an episode of graft rejection after pregnancy. These pregnancies need careful team management by renal physicians and obstetricians.

Connective tissue disorders

Improved medical care for women with CT disorders has led to a dramatic increase in the number of women embarking on pregnancy and achieving successful outcomes. However, these pregnancies require specialist antenatal care by a multidisciplinary team since the risks of PRE-ECLAMPSIA, IUGR, ABRUPTION, and prematurity are increased and may be exacerbated by the steroid medication that many of these women need to continue taking during pregnancy.

SYSTEMIC LUPUS ERYTHEMATOSUS (SLE)

This is a multi-system disease that may affect the kidneys, skin, joints, nervous system, blood, heart, and lungs. Pregnancy increases the risk of flares, which are most common in late pregnancy and postpartum, particularly in women with active or new onset disease. If the mother carries anti Ro or La antibodies, the fetus is at risk of congenital heart block and neonatal lupus. In antiphospholipid syndrome, the presence of cardiolipin antibodies or lupus anticoagulant leads to RECURRENT MISCARRIAGE, late pregnancy complications, and an increased risk of maternal THROMBOSIS. Treatment with aspirin and heparin significantly improves pregnancy outcome.

SCLERODERMA

Women with scleroderma usually deteriorate during pregnancy and are at risk of serious maternal complications if the disease affects their heart, lungs, or kidneys, as well as poor fetal outcome.

RHEUMATOID ARTHRITIS (RA)

Rheumatoid arthritis usually improves during pregnancy but frequently relapses postpartum. Unlike other CT disorders, RA has no adverse effects on pregnancy and does not increase the risk of miscarriage. The main concern during pregnancy is the safety of medication used to control the disease. Steroids are preferable to non-steroidal anti-inflammatory drugs for management of pain.

Thyroid disease

If you suffer from an under- or over-active thyroid it is unlikely that you will get pregnant until your thyroid function is controlled. Women with thyroid disease need careful supervision during pregnancy because alterations in their thyroid function can be masked by the symptoms of pregnancy. If you are taking drugs for your thyroid, your doctor may advise you to switch to another type when you fall pregnant and the doses may need to be altered as the pregnancy progresses. Women with Graves' disease who have undergone thyroidectomy will be taking thyroxine replacement, but they may still have thyroid antibodies present that can affect the fetus. Scans will be needed to check for fetal goitre (enlarged thyroid gland). Hypothyroidism in the baby results in cretinism (a severe form of mental retardation), which is why all babies in the UK have a blood spot test during the first week of life (see p.389).

Skin disorders

ECZEMA

Atopic eczema affects 1–5 per cent of the population and is the commonest cause of an itchy rash during pregnancy. It is treated with regular topical applications of emollients and use of bath additives. Hand and nipple eczema are a common postpartum irritation.

ACNE

Acne usually improves during pregnancy, but can flare in the third trimester, and acne rosacea often worsens. Drug treatment with vitamin A (retinoids) and tetracycline antibiotics can cause abnormalities in the unborn baby and should be discontinued before you try to conceive. If you find yourself pregnant unexpectedly, stop the treatment immediately. Oral or topical erythromycin is safe to use.

PSORIASIS

This chronic autoimmune disorder affects 2 per cent of young adults and behaves unpredictably during pregnancy. It tends to improve or remain unchanged, but for 15 per cent of women the symptoms deteriorate. Many treatments are harmful to the fetus, so careful pre-conception planning is important. Topical steroids can still be used during pregnancy.

Psychiatric disorders

Mental health problems affecting pregnant women can be divided into psychotic and depressive illnesses. Schizophrenia affects 1 in 1,000 individuals and presents problems for pregnant women since they are usually single, socially isolated, and likely to be heavy cigarette, alcohol, and drug users. The effect of antipsychotic drugs on the fetus, the capacity of the woman to give informed consent for procedures, and the likelihood that she will relapse postpartum all have serious safety implications for mother and baby. These problems are increasing because antipsychotic drugs no longer reduce fertility. Bipolar affective disorder, or manic depression, is usually controlled with a combination of drugs (lithium, carbamazepine, and sodium valproate) all of which have well-recognized teratogenic effects on the developing baby. If the illness is stable, reducing the dose or replacing these drugs with an antidepressant may reduce the risk of serious relapse. A postpartum relapse will occur in half of all women with bipolar disease and their drugs should be restarted immediately after delivery.

At least 1 in 10 women will suffer some form of depression in their lifetime, and women with serious depressive illness often experience a deterioration during pregnancy or the postpartum period, which is worsened if their medication is withdrawn or reduced suddenly. Depression has a negative impact on pregnancy outcomes, affecting diet, attendance for antenatal care, levels of smoking, alcohol consumption, self harm, and domestic violence. It is possible that depression directly impacts on placental function and predisposes to IUGR and preterm birth. Women are at greatest risk of mental health problems during the postpartum period, which is when most maternal suicides take place. Some 15–30 per cent of women will experience a depressive episode, and for 1 in 10 this will be a major illness. Although postnatal depression is no longer a taboo subject (see p.391), pre-existing psychiatric disease in pregnant women remains stigmatized and poorly cared for. Most importantly, women who develop psychiatric problems during pregnancy are highly likely to need mental health services in later life.

Infections and illnesses

I am regularly asked by pregnant women about the possible effects of an infectious illness on their own health and that of their baby. Common illnesses such as colds and flu are unlikely to cause harm (see p.33), but others can have damaging effects. Information on these is provided here.

Chickenpox

Chickenpox is caused by varicella zoster virus and is transmitted by droplets spread at the time of face-to-face contact. The incubation period is between 10 and 21 days during which a fever usually develops along with an itchy rash of watery blisters that burst and crust over in a few days. An individual with chickenpox is infectious for 48 hours before the blisters appear until they crust over. Contact with chickenpox in pregnancy is common, but only 1 in 300 women will become infected because 90 per cent of children have had chickenpox before they reach adolescence.

If you are not immune, you can be given an injection of varicella zoster immune globulin (VZIG) up to 10 days after exposure to the virus. If you do develop your first chickenpox infection between 0 and 8 weeks of pregnancy it is unlikely to cause a miscarriage, but if you catch it between eight and 20 weeks your baby may develop the congenital varicella syndrome with abnormalities affecting the limbs, eyes, skin, bowel, bladder, and brain, together with growth problems in later pregnancy – but the risk is small (1–2 per cent). If you are over 20 weeks pregnant and have

chickenpox, you will be given the antiviral drug acyclovir if you are seen within 24 hours of symptoms developing. Between 20 and 36 weeks your baby will not be affected, but the virus will remain in the body and may show up as shingles in the first years of life. However, if you develop chickenpox after 36 weeks and up to 21 days after the delivery, your baby may develop chickenpox. This may be a severe infection (neonatal chickenpox) if it starts within five days of delivery or within the next three weeks, because the newborn baby's immune system is not mature enough to deal with the virus. If you are over 36 weeks pregnant and have chickenpox or have been exposed, your baby will be given VZIG at the time of delivery, which reduces the severity of the attack if given before symptoms appear. Acyclovir may reduce the symptoms if it is started within 24 hours of the rash appearing.

Rubella

Ninety per cent of pregnant women are immune to rubella because they have been previously infected or vaccinated as children. Only a few women will be infected for the first time in pregnancy, but this has serious implications for

the fetus who may develop congenital rubella syndrome. Rubella is spread by breathing infected air particles. Maternal symptoms develop two to three weeks after exposure – a rash of flat pink spots on the face and ears that spread to the trunk, together with pain, joint swelling, fever, and swollen glands. Infected individuals can infect others for one week before symptoms begin and a few days after they have passed. If you develop a rash in pregnancy, your doctor will do a blood test to establish whether you have rubella and repeat it two weeks later to see whether you have developed an antibody response. If rubella is confirmed before 12 weeks, your baby has an 80 per cent risk of congenital abnormalities ranging from eye cataracts, deafness, heart defects, and learning difficulties. Between weeks 13 and 17, a primary rubella infection may result in a baby with deafness. After 17 weeks there is no risk to your baby. Babies born with congenital rubella may have a low birthweight, skin rash, enlarged liver and spleen, and jaundice and may remain contagious for months. If you are rubella susceptible, you need to be vaccinated after the birth and you should use contraception for three months.

Parvovirus (fifth disease)

In adults, the mild flu-like symptoms of infection with parvovirus B19 may go unrecognized. In children it often causes a characteristic rash known as "slapped cheek disease". Parvovirus is spread by droplets (coughing and sneezing) and contact with bedding, clothes, and carpets. This virus does not cause congenital abnormalities and most infections during pregnancy are followed by healthy live births. It is most common in pregnant women who work with children. It may cause late miscarriage and intrauterine death, which is usually associated with fetal anaemia leading to HYDROPS, and can be seen on an ultrasound scan.

Cytomegalovirus (CMV)

CMV is one of the herpes viruses and is so common in young children that 60 per cent of women are immune when they become pregnant. The infection may cause a flu-like illness with sore throat, mild fever, aching limbs, and fatigue. It is usually acquired by close physical contact or from infected blood, urine, saliva, mucus or breast milk. Only a few susceptible women will experience a primary CMV infection during pregnancy and among these women the chance of transmitting the virus to the baby is about 30 per cent. These babies are at risk of congenital CMV, which may result in mental retardation and hearing, sight, and developmental problems. There is no treatment to halt or reverse the effects of CMV, but new antiviral drugs are being investigated. Since CMV is the commonest infectious cause of mental retardation in the UK the search for a vaccine is ongoing, but routine screening for CMV is not recommended. CMV is spread by droplets and excreted in the urine. At-risk groups (hospital, laboratory, and nursery workers) need to take aseptic precautions, such as handwashing, when pregnant.

Toxoplasmosis

Most of the population are immune to toxoplasmosis due to a previous infection, which may have been so mild that the symptoms of a flu-like illness with low-grade fever and swollen glands went unnoticed. Infection for the first time during pregnancy is rare (2 in 1,000) but can cause serious problems for the baby. During the first three months of pregnancy, the risk of the baby becoming infected is low, but the risk of injury is high and includes early or late miscarriage and live-born babies with severe neurological problems (HYDROCEPHALY, cerebral calcification, and damage to the eyes). Near delivery, the baby is more likely to become infected, but congenital toxoplasma infection is less likely to cause neurological damage.

In the UK, pregnant women are not routinely tested for toxoplasmosis, but if a blood test suggests that a woman is infected she will be offered antibiotic treatment to reduce the risk of transmission to the baby. If an abnormal ultrasound scan suggests the baby has been infected, amniocentesis will confirm the diagnosis and some women will opt for termination of pregnancy.

Tuberculosis

TB infection used to be extremely rare in pregnancy since the prevalence of pulmonary (chest) TB in developed countries is low and in underdeveloped countries more widespread disease involving the pelvis frequently led to infertility. However, increasingly mobile populations have resulted in a significant number of pregnant women who have pulmonary TB living in the UK. Furthermore, individuals with HIV infection are more susceptible to infection with TB due to alterations in their immune response. Active TB in the first half of pregnancy is usually treated with isoniazid antibiotic, but after 20 weeks it is safe to use rifampicin. If the mother's TB is inactive at the time of delivery, the baby needs to be vaccinated with BCG, does not need to be isolated, and can be breastfed.

Listeria

Listeria is a food-borne bacteria. Infection during pregnancy is uncommon but can have serious consequences for the baby, including late miscarriage and intrauterine death. During pregnancy, women have lowered resistance to listeria, which multiplies rapidly in the placenta. Typically the mother experiences a brief flu-like illness with malaise, nausea, diarrhoea, and abdominal pain. Penicillin antibiotics are a rapid cure, but the best way to avoid problems during pregnancy is to take careful measures to prevent any exposure to infection.

Streptococcus B

Some 25 per cent of women carry this bacterium in their vagina.

Most have no symptoms although it can produce a vaginal discharge or urinary tract infection. If the infection is present during labour the baby may be affected. Only 1 per cent of at-risk babies develop strep B infection by swallowing or inhaling vaginal secretions, but this neonatal infection can be fatal. Classically, signs of septicaemia and meningitis develop some two days after birth. Premature babies are at greater risk of infection, particularly if the mother's membranes are ruptured. Antenatal screening for strep B is not undertaken routinely in the UK. However, if you have had a previously affected baby or threaten to go into premature labour you will be offered testing, since the use of IV antibiotics during labour and four hours before the delivery is the best way to protect the baby from neonatal infection.

Malaria

Malaria is a parasitic infection transmitted by female mosquitos. Pregnant women are more likely to catch malaria and develop a severe case of the disease with cerebral complications due to the plasmodium falciparum species. It is far more dangerous for you and your baby to risk catching malaria than it is to take anti-malarial drugs to prevent or treat an infection: the high fever places you at risk of miscarrying and your baby is more likely to be of low birth weight, premature or even stillborn. The parasites may be found in the placenta in large numbers and pregnant women may develop severe anaemia with haemolysis leading to jaundice,

and heart and renal failure. Expert advice should always be sought promptly regarding the best choice of drug for an established infection and the risks of teratogenicity balanced against the poor prognosis for the mother and baby if inadequately treated.

Sexually transmitted diseases (STDs)

HERPES

There are two types of herpes infection. Type 1 (HSV1) causes cold sores of the mouth or lips. Type 2 (HSV2), or genital herpes, causes painful ulcers of the vulva, vagina or cervix. If a mother develops her first genital herpes infection within the six weeks prior to delivery, there is a 10 per cent risk that the baby will become infected during the delivery. The consequences of this can be severe, including herpes encephalitis or meningitis, which is why Caesarean section is advised and after delivery the baby will be given antiviral drugs. Following her primary infection the mother produces antibodies, which protect a future fetus but do not prevent her from suffering further attacks. Secondary genital herpes infection during pregnancy may be unpleasant for the mother but only rarely causes the baby any problems. A vaginal birth is the best option.

GONORRHOEA

Gonorrhoea is a highly contagious bacterial infection of the cervix, urethra, rectum or throat. It is often accompanied by CHLAMYDIA, TRICHOMONAS, and SYPHILIS infection. Unprotected sex with an infected individual leads to

transmission of the infection in 90 per cent of cases. The infection may be asymptomatic or accompanied by vaginal discharge, pain, and urinary discomfort. It is an important cause of pelvic inflammation, which damages the Fallopian tubes, leading to ECTOPIC PREGNANCY and infertility. Infection during pregnancy is associated with premature rupture of membranes and pemature delivery. The risk of postpartum pelvic inflammatory disease and systemic spread (painful joints and skin rash) is increased. The diagnosis is best made from culture of cervical swabs and effectively treated with penicillin antibiotics. Although the baby is not at risk of infection during pregnancy, exposure to the organism during delivery may cause neonatal conjunctivitis and occasionally a septicaemia requiring intensive treatment.

CHLAMYDIA

Chlamydia trachomatis is the most common STD in the UK. Some 40 per cent of infected men complain of penile discharge, testicular inflammation, and urinary discomfort, but only 15 per cent of infected women have symptoms such as vaginal discharge, pelvic pain or urinary problems. Infection may be present in the vagina, cervix, uterus, anus, urethra or eyes and can have serious consequences. Damage to the Fallopian tubes increases the risk of ectopic pregnancy and may lead to infertility. If present at the time of delivery, 40 per cent of babies will become infected. Chlamydia is the leading cause of neonatal conjunctivitis, which may result in blindness or pneumonia. Early diagnosis is important because the infection can be effectively treated with antibiotics.

SYPHILIS

Syphilis infection is caused by *Treponema pallidum* and was rare in pregnant women in the UK. The incidence has increased in the last 10 years among some ethnic groups, and damage to the baby can be prevented by early treatment with penicillin. This is why all pregnant women undergo routine screening for syphilis. In the primary stage of infection, an ulcer (chancre) appears, which is similar to herpes but less painful and lasts three to six weeks. Untreated, the infection progresses in a few months to secondary syphilis with fever, rash, swollen glands, weight loss, and tiredness. Without treatment, tertiary syphilis develops some years later with damage to the brain, nerves, and heart. The bacteria are able to penetrate the placenta after 15 weeks and 70 per cent of infected women will transmit the infection to the fetus, with 30 per cent being stillborn. If the fetus survives, it will be in the second stage of the illness at birth, and a further 30 per cent of these babies will be born with congenital syphilis and suffer from fits, developmental delay, skin and mouth sores, infected bones, jaundice, anaemia, and microcephaly. Penicillin usually cures the maternal infection and prevents fetal infection. At birth the baby will be given further antibiotics. Diagnosing syphilis should prompt an additional search for chlamydia, gonorrhoea, HIV, and hepatitis B and C infections.

HIV INFECTION

HIV infection is most commonly transmitted through sexual contact, the use of contaminated needles or infected blood and blood products. In Western countries, most cases of HIV infection are found in homosexual/bisexual males and heterosexual drug users. In central London, the prevalence of HIV infection in pregnant women is less than 1 per cent, but in some African countries the antenatal prevalence is as high as 40 per cent and is an important cause of infant death.

Routine antenatal screening and treatment of HIV-positive pregnant women has dramatically reduced the risk of transmission to the baby and development of full-blown AIDS in the mother thereby increasing her life expectancy. HIV transmission to the baby can be reduced from 25 per cent to less than 2 per cent by treating positive pregnant women with a combination of antiretroviral drugs antenatally, and during delivery of the baby by elective Caesarean section, avoidance of breastfeeding, and actively treating the new baby for four to six weeks. Sadly, the majority of pregnant women with HIV live in countries where the high cost of drugs and medical interventions excludes them from being offered life-saving treatment.

TRICHOMONIASIS

This infection is caused by the organism *Trichomonas vaginalis*, which inhabits the urinary tract and vagina and is frequently accompanied by chlamydia and gonorrhoea. It may be symptomless or cause a thin, frothy, yellow-green vaginal discharge with a fishy smell, together with inflammation and pain in the vagina and urethra. Infection during pregnancy is occasionally responsible for pneumonia in the newborn baby. The diagnosis can be made on a cervical smear or vaginal swab. Infections should be treated with metronidazole antibiotic, which is safe to use in late pregnancy and during breastfeeding.

BACTERIAL VAGINOSIS (BV)

This is a common cause of vaginal discharge, affecting 10–20 per cent of women, but may also be symptomless. The discharge is usually thin, grey-coloured and non-itchy, with a strong fishy odour. It is diagnosed by the presence of clue cells on a vaginal smear test. In pregnancy, the altered hormonal environment in the vagina is less acidic, favouring the growth of the many organisms that are present in bacterial vaginosis. BV infection during pregnancy has been strongly linked with late miscarriage and premature birth. Although treatment with clindamycin or metronidazole antibiotics clears the infection in a few days, recurrence in pregnancy is common. Screening and treating all infected pregnant women has not reduced the preterm birth rate. It appears that pregnant women with a history of premature delivery are particularly susceptible to this infection and may benefit from regular screening and antibiotic treatment when the infection is present.

Fetal abnormalities

Congenital abnormalities are present at birth and are often due to genetic causes. Others are acquired as a result of environmental factors during pregnancy or occur for no known reason. You will find more on how these abnormalities develop on pages 144–47.

CHROMOSOME ABNORMALITIES

These abnormalities are due to a fault in the baby's complement of 23 pairs of chromosomes, either because there are too many, too few or one chromosome is abnormal. The most common chromosomal disorder, Down's syndrome, is discussed in detail on page 147.

Trisomies

PATAU'S SYNDROME (TRISOMY 13)

In Patau's syndrome, which occurs in 1 in 10,000 live births, three copies of chromosome 13 are present. The majority of affected babies miscarry early in pregnancy, but of the 20 per cent that are liveborn, most die within a few days of birth. Those that survive have severe mental handicap. Microcephaly and severe facial abnormalities, too many fingers and toes, EXOMPHALOS and HEART AND KIDNEY DEFECTS are characteristic and are usually identified during pregnancy on an ultrasound scan.

EDWARD'S SYNDROME (TRISOMY 18)

In Edward's syndrome, three copies of chromosome 18 are present. This occurs in 1 in 7,000 live births, and the physical malformations include IUGR, strawberry-shaped head, CHOROID PLEXUS CYSTS, HEART AND KIDNEY DEFECTS, DIAPHRAGMATIC HERNIA, EXOMPHALOS, small receding jaw, low-set ears, shortened limbs, clenched hands, and feet with a curved sole described as "rocker bottom", all of which may be seen on the 20-week scan. The integrated screening test (see p.138) will identify 60 per cent of babies with Edward's syndrome. Severe mental retardation is usual and most of these babies die within the first year of life.

Triploidy (69XXY or XYY)

The presence of an extra set of 23 chromosomes is called triploidy and may result from an egg being fertilized by more than one sperm or the fertilized egg failing to divide. Triploidy occurs in about 2 per cent of conceptions, but these pregnancies usually miscarry (20 per cent of all chromosomal miscarriages are triploidies). When the extra set of chromosomes comes from the father, the embryo does not develop but the placental tissues grow rapidly in an uncontrolled manner and the pregnancy rarely continues beyond 20 weeks (see HYDATIDIFORM MOLES p.423). When the extra chromosomes come from the mother, the pregnancy may continue into the third trimester. The placenta is normal but the fetus usually has severe asymmetrical growth retardation. Triploidy is not influenced by maternal age.

Translocation

Translocation occurs when a piece of one chromosome becomes attached to the end of another. Individuals carrying a balanced translocation appear normal because the normal chromosome counteracts the effect of the abnormal one. However, if this man or woman becomes a parent, there are three possible outcomes: the baby may have entirely normal chromosomes; it can inherit the balanced translocation; or it may inherit an unbalanced translocation, which invariably leads to miscarriage or a severe abnormality in the baby. Translocations may be reciprocal or Robertsonian and are a cause of RECURRENT MISCARRIAGE. New translocations can arise that are not inherited from either parent.

Sex chromosome abnormalities

TURNER'S SYNDROME (45X)

This occurs in 1 in 2,500 live births; one of the two X chromosomes is completely missing. These girls have normal intelligence, but their growth is seriously affected, and they have no menstrual periods and are therefore infertile. Other characteristics are webbing of the neck and cubitus valgus (a wide carrying angle at the elbows). A high percentage of fetuses with a single X chromosome miscarry or are identified by prenatal diagnosis. Abnormalities detected on ultrasound include cystic hygroma (large fluid-filled sac behind the neck), CARDIAC DEFECTS, particularly coarctation of the aorta, HYDROPS FETALIS, and horseshoe kidneys. Turner's syndrome can also exist in mosaic form, meaning that the girl has two different cell lines – 46XX and 45X. If her egg cells contain a normal set of chromosomes, she will not necessarily be infertile.

KLINEFELTER'S SYNDROME (47XXY)

When boys have an extra X sex chromosome, this is known as Klinefelter's syndrome and occurs in 1 in 1,000 live births. In adult life, these men tend to be tall with a reduced head circumference and lower levels of intelligence, but are not usually classified as being mentally retarded. Men with Klinefelter's syndrome are infertile and more susceptible to auto-immune disease, malignancy, and cardiovascular disease in adult life.

TRIPLE X (47XXX)

Women with an extra X sex chromosome have normal fertility and there is a wide variation in mental capacity. Some may have lower intelligence than normal, but rarely suffer from mental retardation. This occurs in 1 in 1,000 live births.

SUPERMALES (47XYY)

Some boys have an extra Y chromosome. They have normal appearance, mental development, and fertility. In adult life they have an increased incidence of language and reading difficulties, hyperactivity, and impulsive and aggressive behaviour. This occurs in 1 in 1,000 live births.

Dominant disorders
FAMILIAL HYPERCHOLESTEROLAEMIA

This common dominant genetic disease affects 1 in 500 people in the UK, although men tend to be more severely affected than women. High blood cholesterol levels and narrowing of major blood vessels lead to heart attacks at an early age and fatty skin deposits around the eyelids. In parents who have a history of early heart disease, blood from their baby's umbilical cord can be tested for high cholesterol levels at birth. This allows the diagnosis to be made at birth and offers the possibility of preventative lifestyle measures to reduce the severity of the disease.

MARFAN'S SYNDROME

This syndrome affects 1 in 5000 people and is inherited as an autosomal dominant so there is a 50 per cent chance of the baby being affected. A mutation of the fibrillin protein gene on chromosome 15 gives rise to variably weak and stretchy connective tissue in the eye, heart, blood vessels, joints, and skin. Classically, a person with Marfan's is tall, thin, with very long digits, flat feet, spinal curvature, hypermobile joints, and an

abnormal aortic heart valve. In pregnancy, which needs to be managed by specialist teams, the biggest fear is that the dilated root of the aortic valve ruptures or dissects, which is fatal in 50 per cent of cases. There is also a risk of miscarriage, cervical weakness, preterm labour, and postpartum haemorrhage.

VON WILLEBRAND'S DISEASE

The most common inherited bleeding disorder (prevalence of 1 per cent) is due to a reduction in the quantity or quality of von Willebrand's factor in the blood. Although pregnancy usually increases the levels of the factor, this does not compensate sufficiently in severe cases and pregnant women are at risk of postpartum haemorrhage, which should be managed with IV desmopressin treatment.

HUNTINGDON'S DISEASE

This dominant disease affects 1 in 20,000 and has an insidious onset in middle life, starting with personality changes and progressing to uncontrolled movements, aggressive sexual behaviour, and dementia. Huntington's disease has full penetrance so that children of an affected parent have a 50 per cent risk of the disease, which never skips a generation. Affected individuals and their families often try to hide the early onset of symptoms, but the sufferer is usually only too aware of the problems lying ahead. Recent linkage studies show that the abnormal gene is on chromosome 4 and analysis of fetal DNA obtained from CVS samples provides accurate prenatal diagnosis and prediction of late onset disease. Genetic counselling for affected families is essential.

Recessive disorders

TAY-SACHS DISEASE

This is a fatal recessive disorder common in Ashkenazi Jewish families and French Canadians. It is caused by a deficiency in the enzyme hexosaminidase A, which results in fatty material being deposited in the nerve cells of the brain. Babies with the disease appear normal at first, but by six months have started to develop progressive motor weakness and mental disability. The child becomes blind, deaf, unable to swallow, and suffers increasingly severe fits before dying at the age of three to five years. Carriers of the disease can be identified by a simple blood test before or during pregnancy. If both parents are carriers, there is a 25 per cent chance in each pregnancy of their having an affected baby. Amniocentesis or chorionic villus sampling will be offered to confirm the diagnosis. Because there is no treatment for this disease, many couples choose to terminate an affected pregnancy.

CYSTIC FIBROSIS (CF)

This is the most common recessive genetic disease in Caucasians affecting 1 in 2,500 live births. The disorder is due to an abnormality in sodium transport, which makes the secretions of the lungs, digestive system, and sweat glands too thick and sticky. Mucus accumulates in the lungs leading to severe chest infections and, since the pancreas and liver are also affected, the normal flow of digestive enzymes in the gut is compromised. This causes malnutrition if life-long daily enzyme supplements are not started promptly. The severity of the disease is variable, ranging from death in the first year of life to poor health in middle age. Regular physiotherapy can help to improve the lung problems. Males with cystic fibrosis are infertile, due to blockage of their sperm transport tubes (vas deferens). One in 22 Caucasians are carriers for the most common gene mutation responsible for CF (AF508), which is located on chromosome 7, making it possible to screen prospective parents and undertake prenatal diagnosis on DNA samples from a fetus at risk of the disease. However, there are many different mutations in the CF gene and current screening techniques can only identify 85 per cent of carriers. Carrier detection for CF is offered to individuals with a history of CF, partners of identified CF carriers, parents of a fetus with echogenic bowel detected on an ultrasound scan, and sperm donors. It is important that couples who undergo screening receive detailed genetic counselling and are aware of the limitations of the tests.

PHENYLKETONURIA (PKU)

This recessive genetic disease is present in 1 in 12,000 UK births. It is caused by a defective gene that results in a deficiency of the enzyme that converts the essential amino acid phenylalanine into tyrosine. The build-up of high levels of phenylalanine in the bloodstream is toxic to the developing brain. If a special diet with low phenylalanine is started in the first few weeks of life the irreversible brain damage and learning disabilities can be avoided. All babies are tested for PKU six days after birth (see p.389).

SICKLE CELL ANAEMIA AND THALASSAEMIA

If you are of Mediterranean or African origin, you will be offered a special electrophoresis test of your haemoglobin to determine whether you have sickle cell or thalassaemia traits (see p.425). If you carry the sickle cell trait, it is important that your partner's sickle cell status is established early in your pregnancy, because there is a chance that your baby could inherit a double dose of the trait and develop full-blown sickle cell disease. This leads to severe anaemia, infections, pain, and eventually heart and kidney failure. Similarly, if you carry the A or B thalassaemia trait, you will need to arrange for your partner to be tested, too. A baby with full-blown thalassaemia suffers from severe anaemia and iron overload leading to multiple organ failure. If both parents are sickle cell carriers they may choose to undergo an invasive test such as amniocentesis or chorionic villus sampling to find out whether the baby has inherited the disease. Prenatal diagnosis is also offered when both parents carry the alpha or beta thalassaemia trait.

Sex-linked disorders

DUCHENNE'S MUSCULAR DYSTROPHY (DMD)

This is the most common sex-linked disorder and affects 1 in 4,000 boys. The child may appear normal in infancy, but, between the ages of four and 10 years, loses his ability to walk due to muscular weakness and is usually confined to a wheelchair soon after. Identifying female carriers of DMD used to depend on finding increased blood levels of the muscle enzyme creatinine kinase. This was an unreliable test and most couples carrying a male fetus were therefore offered a termination of pregnancy. The DMD gene has now been identified. In approximately two-thirds of families, a deletion is present on the short arm of chromosome X. Hence most female carriers can be identified before pregnancy. Prenatal diagnosis can also be performed on fetal DNA samples during pregnancy, to establish whether the baby is affected by DMD.

HAEMOPHILIA
This X-linked recessive disorder affects 1 in 10,000 males and is due to a deficiency in blood coagulation factors that makes the blood clot too slowly. There are two types of haemophilia. The most common is haemophilia A in which low levels of

factor VIII are present. In haemophilia B there is a deficiency in factor IX (also called Christmas disease). The symptoms of both are prolonged bleeding from wounds and into joints, muscles, and other tissues following minor trauma. The severity of the disease depends on how much clotting factor is present in the blood.

Both haemophilia A and B can be treated by injections or transfusions of plasma containing the missing clotting factors and sufferers can lead a more normal life. Since carrier females may have normal or low levels of the clotting factors, diagnosis was unreliable before DNA testing became available. In families with a history

of haemophilia, female carriers can now be accurately identified before pregnancy and fetal DNA testing during pregnancy can establish whether a male baby is affected.

FRAGILE X SYNDROME
This X-linked disorder is the most common form of inherited mental retardation (1 in 1,500 males and 1 in 2,500 females). Mental impairment is variable in carrier females, but DNA testing to confirm the suspected diagnosis of Fragile X or carrier status is now possible. Genetic counselling should be offered to all women and their families with a history of mental retardation, since as many as 1 in 200 women carry the gene mutation.

OTHER CONGENITAL ABNORMALITIES
This section includes fetal abnormalities for which there is no known specific genetic cause although some, such as neural tube defects, tend to run in families. The list includes most of the abnormalities that sometimes become apparent on ultrasound scans.

Neural tube defects (NTDs)
These are one of the most common and serious congenital abnormalities and are due to a combination of genetic and environmental factors. In the absence of antenatal screening about 1 in every 400 babies will be affected. The embryonic neural tube fails to close properly during the first four weeks of pregnancy, resulting in incomplete development of the brain and spinal cord and varying degrees of permanent neurological damage. The most severe forms are anencephaly (the skull bones are incomplete and the brain is

underdeveloped) and encephalocoele (brain tissue projects through a hole in the skull). These babies are rarely liveborn. In spina bifida (myelomeningocoele), the spinal cord is not protected by the bony spinal column and may be closed (covered by protective membranes) or open (no covering membranes). The degree of paralysis, weakness, and sensory disability is variable depending on the level of spinal defect. This can range from a wheelchair existence and complete lack of bladder and bowel function to mild walking difficulties. However, babies with open spina bifida are often severely

handicapped, requiring frequent surgical procedures and prolonged hospitalization. The majority of severe cases develop HYDROCEPHALUS, resulting in mental retardation and learning difficulties. The mildest form of NTD is spina bifida occulta, a lesion in the lowest part of the sacral spine that usually goes unnoticed and is present in 5 per cent of healthy babies. Antenatal screening for open spina bifida has been greatly improved by routine ultrasound scanning. In addition to the bony defect in the vertebral column, most babies with a myelomeningocoele have scalloping of the frontal skull bones (called the lemon sign on an ultrasound scan) and a cerebellum that looks more like a banana than the normal dumbbell-shaped structure. Closed spina bifida has a better prognosis because the defect is more easily treated surgically after delivery, but is more difficult to detect antenatally.

Spina bifida can run in families, but 95 per cent of these babies are born to women with no family history. It is linked to poor diet and the risk of recurrence is 1 in 20 after a previously affected baby. Taking folic acid supplements for three months before pregnancy and during the first trimester prevents 75 per cent of cases. Women with a previous NTD or on antiepileptic medication should take high doses of folic acid before conception (see p.51).

Hydrocephalus

This condition (often referred to as water on the brain) is caused by too much cerebrospinal fluid. It is usually due to a blockage in the circulation of the fluid or because of an over-production or reduced absorption of the fluid. Hydrocephalus is often associated with SPINA BIFIDA or follows a brain haemorrhage in a premature baby. If the problem is present before birth it can be seen on an ultrasound scan. As the head swells, the brain tissue is compressed, the skull bones become thinner, the sutures of the head widen, and the fontanelles bulge. After delivery, if the hydrocephalus is due to a blockage it may be possible to insert a tube to drain the fluid from the ventricles of the brain into the abdominal cavity or heart. Occasionally, the hydrocephalus is inherited as a sex-linked recessive disorder in males and these families need genetic counselling.

Microcephaly

In these babies the bony skull and brain size are smaller than average. The babies are nearly always severely intellectually impaired. Recognized causes include rubella infection in the first trimester, CYTOMEGALOVIRUS, TOXOPLASMOSIS and SYPHILIS infections, severe irradiation, and maternal heroin and alcohol addiction. A few cases are inherited as a recessive genetic disorder, but in many cases no obvious cause can be found.

Choroid plexus cysts (CPC)

These cysts in the ventricles of the baby's brain are usually bilateral and seen in as many as 1 per cent of all 20-week screening ultrasound anomaly scans. Most CPCs are now thought to be benign structures and usually disappear by 24 weeks. However, since they are associated with TRISOMY 18, detailed counselling will be needed to help parents decide whether they should expose their pregnancy to the risk of an invasive diagnostic test.

Gut abnormalities

DUODENAL ATRESIA

In this disorder, the small gut between the bottom of the stomach and ileum is absent and is usually diagnosed by the "double bubble sign" on an ultrasound scan (bubble 1 is the normal stomach, bubble 2 results from the duodenum being unable to empty into the lower gut, which can also cause POLYHYDRAMNIOS). The blockage can be resolved by surgery immediately after delivery,

but in one-third of cases this abnormality is associated with Down's syndrome.

OESOPHAGEAL ATRESIA

In this disorder, the tube between the throat and stomach is partially absent, which leads to vomiting and excess dribbling immediately after delivery. It is often associated with a fistula (passage) between the oesophagus and trachea (windpipe). Hence POLYHYDRAMNIOS and the "double bubble sign" may not be evident on ultrasound scans. If a fistula is present there is a serious risk of food entering the lungs and choking the baby. Oesophageal atresia requires immediate surgery and sometimes multiple operations, but responds well to surgical correction if it is an isolated problem.

HYPERECHOIC FETAL BOWEL

If the bowel is seen to be very echogenic (white streaked) on an antenatal ultrasound scan, this may be secondary to a major chromosomal abnormality, CYSTIC FIBROSIS, bowel obstruction, fetal infection or GROWTH RESTRICTION. It can also occur in entirely normal fetuses.

Diaphragmatic hernia

This serious congenital abnormality affects 1 in 3,000 babies and can be diagnosed on the 20-week ultrasound scan. The muscular diaphragm separates the contents of the chest (heart and lungs) from the abdomen (liver, stomach, spleen, intestines). If a defect occurs in the development of the diaphragm, varying amounts of these abdominal organs can herniate into the chest cavity. In about 50 per cent of fetuses there are associated chromosomal abnormalities, genetic syndromes, and other structural abnormalities. At birth the baby will need immediate intensive care and ventilation before undergoing multiple surgical operations to replace the abdominal organs and reconstruct the diaphragm. In utero, surgery may be attempted in specialist centres to give the affected lung a better chance of developing normally.

Abdominal wall defects

OMPHALOCOELE (EXOMPHALOS)

Omphalocoele occurs in 1 in 5,000 babies and is due to a defect in the abdominal wall underneath the umbilicus, through which varying amounts of small bowel and liver protrude covered by the peritoneal membrane. Most of these babies are identified on an ultrasound scan during pregnancy and some 50 per cent have associated chromosomal, cardiac or bladder abnormalities. Karyotyping (chromosome analysis) and ultrasound scans are needed to assess the problem. If it is an isolated defect, surgical correction after birth has a good prognosis, although it may require multiple operations.

GASTROSCHISIS

In this condition, loops of bowel protrude through the abdominal wall defect and are not covered by the peritoneum membrane. In most cases the abnormality is isolated and there is no increased incidence of chromosomal abnormalities. The abdominal wall defect is usually small and can be repaired easily. Early delivery helps to avoid bowel damage and complications.

Cardiac abnormalities

Structural heart disorders are the most common severe congenital abnormality in newborn babies, affecting 8 in 1,000 live births. They are an important cause of perinatal and childhood death. The incidence of cardiac abnormalities is increased in babies who are premature, have Down's syndrome, are infected with RUBELLA virus or who have mothers with congenital HEART DISEASE, DIABETES, EPILEPSY or families with a history of cardiac abnormalities. In 30 per cent of babies with a cardiac defect another structural abnormality is found, and in 20 per cent a chromosomal disorder is present. Many heart defects can be diagnosed by ultrasound during pregnancy. This is why the 20-week anomaly scan routinely aims to obtain a view of the four-chamber heart. If an abnormality is suspected, further scans will be arranged. The option of fetal karyotyping (chromosome analysis) should be offered to parents since the results may influence the plan for management at the time of delivery. Some cardiac lesions may require immediate surgical correction, whereas others can be dealt with later on.

SEPTAL DEFECTS

These "holes in the heart" account for 50 per cent of all congenital heart defects. A hole in the septum (wall) dividing the two upper (atrial) or the two lower (ventricular) chambers of the heart, results in oxygenated and deoxygenated blood being mixed instead of separated. An atrial septal defect may result in few symptoms, but ventricular septal defects give rise to a loud heart murmur, and since the heart has to pump harder, it becomes enlarged. Untreated, the problem can be very serious, particularly when complicated by CYANOSIS (blue baby).

CYANOTIC DEFECTS (BLUE BABY)

These disorders account for 25 per cent of all congenital heart disease and require expert surgical and medical care. The outlook for the baby is often poor, depending on the severity of the lesion. In Tetralogy of Fallot (one of the most common forms of complex congenital heart defects), there is a large septal defect, abnormal aorta, and narrowing of the pulmonary valve. When the aorta and pulmonary artery are connected the wrong way round most of the blood receives no oxygen from the lungs and any oxygenated blood is sent back to the lungs rather than being pumped around the body.

PATENT DUCTUS ARTERIOSUS

Ten per cent of cases of congenital heart disease are caused by failure of the duct between the heart and lungs to close after birth. This is more common in premature babies. The duct usually closes on its own given time, but may require indomethacin drug treatment and occasionally surgery.

HYPOPLASTIC LEFT HEART

This is present in 10 per cent of babies with congenital heart disease and accounts for 25 per cent of all neonatal cardiac deaths. The left side of the heart is so under-developed that when the ductus closes at birth, the baby cannot obtain oxygenated blood. The postnatal prognosis is poor, and, when diagnosed antenatally, some parents choose to terminate the pregnancy.

Hydrops fetalis

This is present in a wide variety of fetal, maternal, and placental disorders. It is diagnosed on antenatal ultrasound scan when widespread accumulation of fluid in the body leads to oedema of the skin and effusions (pools of fluid) around the heart, lungs, and abdominal organs. Immune hydrops occurs in severe RHESUS SENSITIZATION (see p.128). Non-immune hydrops may be seen with fetal chromosomal, heart, lung, blood and metabolic disorders, some congenital infections, and malformations of the placenta and umbilical cord. The overall outlook for the baby is poor, with a mortality rate of 80–90 per cent depending on the cause. Despite investigations, including invasive fetal testing, the abnormality remains unexplained in one-third of cases.

Renal abnormalities

The fetal kidneys and bladder are visible at the 20-week scan. Severe renal problems are usually accompanied by OLIGOHYDRAMNIOS, or reduced amniotic fluid, because urine production is compromised.

POTTER'S SYNDROME

The fetal kidneys are absent (agenesis) or poorly formed and the lungs are underdeveloped as a result of the lack of amniotic fluid. The baby usually has facial abnormalities including widely spaced eyes, down-turned nose, low-set ears, and a small jaw. At birth, no urine is passed and the baby dies within a few hours from respiratory failure. The problem is rare but more common in boys.

HYDRONEPHROSIS

Enlarged kidneys are identified on an ultrasound scan in 2 per cent of all fetuses during the second trimester. They are usually due to narrowing or blockage of one or both of the ureters. When isolated, the finding is often insignificant. However, it may be associated with chromosomal abnormalities, in particular Down's syndrome. Severe hydronephrosis leads to kidney damage due to the pressure of retained urine on the normal kidney tissue, which may need to be drained by inserting a ureteric shunt to prevent kidney failure.

POLYCYSTIC KIDNEYS

This is a recessive genetic disorder with variable expression. Some fetuses will appear to have normal kidneys on an antenatal ultrasound scan and present with renal failure as a teenager. Others will be found at the 20-week anomaly scan because of absent liquor and grossly enlarged kidneys. Adult polycystic kidney disease is a dominant genetic disease which can present in utero with enlarged cystic kidneys. One of the parents usually has kidney cysts.

FETAL SURGERY

A few fetal abnormalities may be amenable to corrective treatment before birth. These procedures are only undertaken in specialist units by pioneering fetal surgeons. The most successful techniques to date are those that involve inserting needles or fine tubes through the mother's abdomen and into the uterine cavity or the fetus under ultrasound guidance. Intrauterine blood transfusions may be needed for severe Rhesus incompatibility, and drugs to correct irregularities of the fetal heartbeat or destroy life-threatening tumours can be directly injected into the fetus. Occasionally, fetal tissue samples may need to be obtained to make the diagnosis of a rare genetic disorder.

Other examples of ultrasound-guided fetal surgery are the insertion of drainage tubes into severe cases of HYDROCEPHALUS or HYDRONEPHROSIS.

Open fetal surgery is experimental and is usually only considered in situations where there is nothing to lose. The mother's abdomen is opened and an incision in the uterus is made to gain access to the fetus and conduct the surgery. Great care is taken to keep the baby warm, replace the amniotic fluid and avoid damaging the placenta. Even if the surgery can be successfully performed, the baby remains at risk of premature labour, infection and leakage of amniotic fluid. Diaphragmatic hernias and fetal tumours may be treated in this way.

Problems in pregnancy and labour

Although the majority of pregnancies and births are straightforward, there are inevitably instances when something does not go according to plan. Some of the problems that you may encounter are summarized here with information on the up-to-date methods of managing and treating them.

Ectopic pregnancy

An ectopic pregnancy develops outside the uterine cavity. In the UK this occurs in 1 in 200 pregnancies. Although some ectopics "miscarry" without complication (tubal miscarriage), there is a risk that the pregnancy may continue to grow and rupture through the walls of the Fallopian tube. The vast majority of ectopic pregnancies occur in the Fallopian tubes, but occasionally they may be found on the ovary or in the abdominal cavity.

The general symptoms are the same as those of early pregnancy, accompanied by a positive pregnancy test and lower abdominal pain, which almost always starts before any vaginal bleeding has occurred. If your doctor suspects an ectopic pregnancy you will be sent for an ultrasound scan. This will show that there is no pregnancy sac within the uterine cavity, although the lining of the uterus may be thickened. The ectopic may be removed by surgery. More and more hospitals are developing the expertise to do this by laparoscopy, avoiding the need for an open operation. If the ectopic has not ruptured and the hormone HCG levels are low, treatment with methotrexate may be possible.

Hydatidiform mole

Hydatidiform moles are the most common type of placental tumour. There are complete moles and partial moles. Complete moles are rare in Caucasian women (1 in every 1,200–2,000 pregnancies), but are much more common in women from South-East Asia.

Moles are derived entirely from the cells of the father, due to an accident that occurs at the time of fertilization. No embryo is present in the pregnancy sac, but the placental tissues develop rapidly in an uncontrolled fashion, resembling a bunch of grapes on an ultrasound scan. Persistent bleeding and severe nausea are often associated with the presence of these moles, and the size of the uterus is usually larger than would be expected for the menstrual dates. A complete mole may develop into an invasive cancer in a small percentage of cases, so specialist treatment is needed.

Partial moles are more common and usually mimic the appearance of an inevitable or incomplete miscarriage. The partial mole contains a fetus/embryo that has three sets of chromosomes instead of two (TRIPLOIDY). The placental cells swell and proliferate but not to the same degree as occurs in a complete mole. A partial mole may only be distinguished from a miscarriage when the pathologist examines the tissue removed from the uterus.

Fibroids

Fibroids are benign growths of the uterine muscle wall and can vary in size from a small pea to a large melon. What causes them to develop is not understood, but they tend to run in families and are more common in Afro-Caribbean women. Most pregnant women will have no problems with their fibroids, but if the embryo implants over a fibroid protruding into the uterine cavity, the risk of early miscarriage is increased.

Fibroids usually increase in size during pregnancy because of the high oestrogen levels and increased uterine blood supply. If they undergo red degeneration (the fibroid's blood supply is cut off causing it to turn red and die), late miscarriage or premature labour may result. Large fibroids distorting the uterine cavity may lead to abnormal presentations and positions. Occasionally, fibroids obstruct the birth canal, preventing a vaginal delivery, but they usually shrink in size post-delivery.

Incompetent cervix

The cervix usually remains tightly shut and sealed with a plug of mucus throughout pregnancy. An incompetent cervix starts to shorten and open during the fourth or fifth month of pregnancy, exposing the membranes to the risk of rupture and miscarriage. The condition is uncommon and may be caused by damage to the cervix during a previous labour, cervical operation or termination. If you are diagnosed with a weak cervix, you may be advised to have a cervical cerclage or suture inserted at 12–14 weeks in your next pregnancy to keep your cervix tightly closed until the end of pregnancy. The suture is usually removed a few weeks before term to allow a normal vaginal delivery.

Venous thromboembolism

Women are more likely to develop a blood clot or thrombosis in a pelvic or leg vein during pregnancy and the postnatal period. This is due to increased levels of clotting factors and decreased levels of anticoagulant factors that protect women from uncontrolled uterine bleeding during pregnancy and after the delivery. Venous thrombo-embolism (VTE) occurs in less than 1 in 1,000 births, but there are several important risk factors that increase the likelihood of VTE in pregnancy including age over 35 years, immobility, smoking, obesity, operative delivery, previous VTE, family history of VTE, severe varicose veins, PRE-ECLAMPSIA, dehydration, SICKLE CELL DISEASE, maternal illness, and infection. The thrombosis usually starts in the deep veins of the lower leg but may have extended up into the femoral or pelvic veins before it is detected. The danger is that part of the blood clot may break off and be swept off into the lungs where it blocks one of the major blood vessels. This is called pulmonary embolus (PE) and although the incidence is only about 1 in 6,000 births, it is potentially very serious. Any pregnant woman with signs of a DVT or PE should be started on anticoagulation treatment as a matter of urgency even before the diagnosis is confirmed.

The signs of a DVT are pain and swelling in the calf or thigh muscles, with localized redness and tenderness of the leg – inability to put your heel to the ground when walking is diagnostic. Once the DVT is proven, an elastic compression stocking should be fitted and you will be confined to bed with your leg elevated until fully heparinized and until the leg stops being tender.

The symptoms of a pulmonary embolus are shortness of breath, chest pain, coughing up blood, faintness, collapse, together with all the signs of a DVT. A chest X-ray and examination may show evidence of a PE and a ventilation perfusion scan of the lung and bilateral Doppler ultrasound leg studies should be undertaken urgently since two-thirds of deaths from PE occur within the first two to four hours. Women with a proven PE will be given warfarin treatment after delivery for three to six months. If you have had a previous VTE in pregnancy or the postnatal period, or have other risk factors, you may be offered prophylactic heparin injections before and after the delivery.

Obstetric cholestasis

This is a rare condition but can lead to complications in late pregnancy, including stillbirth. The main symptom is severe itching without a rash, usually most intensely on the palms of the hands and soles of the feet, caused by bile salts being deposited under the skin. A small percentage of women become jaundiced. The lower levels of bile leads to a reduction in the absorption of vitamin K, which increases the chances of mother or baby bleeding. Ursodeoxycholic acid treatment helps to reduce the itching and liver function abnormalities, and vitamin K tablets improve blood clotting. You will also be advised to have an induction of labour at 37–38 weeks to reduce the risks of late pregnancy complications.

Anaemia

The red cells in your blood contain haemoglobin (a complex of four protein chains attached to iron), which carries the oxygen around your body. During pregnancy women often become mildly anaemic, because their haemoglobin levels fall due to the demands of the growing baby and also because of the increased fluid content of the mother's blood, which "dilutes" the haemoglobin level. If your levels drop below 11g/dl you will look pale, feel tired, breathless or faint, and require iron and folic acid supplements. Mild iron-deficiency anaemia in pregnancy is not harmful to the baby, who will carry on helping itself to all the iron it requires from your stores. More serious anaemia puts you at risk of having a preterm or low birthweight baby, so if your haemoglobin levels do not improve after a few weeks of treatment, further blood tests will be performed to check for rarer causes of anaemia. Occasionally, it may be necessary to give injections of iron or even a blood transfusion.

SICKLE CELL ANAEMIA

Sickle cell anaemia (see p.418) is an inherited abnormality in the production of the protein chains that make haemoglobin. This results in a change in the shape of the red blood cells produced making it more difficult for them to navigate around the blood vessels smoothly. As a result they are easily damaged. The breakdown of the damaged cells results in haemolytic anaemia. Cell debris clogs up the blood vessels leading to strokes, infection, and pain in the bones, limbs, chest or abdomen. Pregnant women with sickle cell disease are at constant risk of a sickle cell crisis. This can be life-threatening for the mother and compromises placental function and fetal growth. They need to be cared for in centres with specialist expertise.

THALASSAEMIA

The thalassaemias (see p.418) are another group of inherited haemoglobin abnormalities. Alpha thalassaemia is common in South- East Asia, whereas beta thalassaemia is usually found among people living around the Mediterranean or in the Middle East, India, and Pakistan. Carriers of the trait are likely to develop more severe anaemia during pregnancy. Beta thalassaemia major results in severe anaemia and a life-long problem of trying to get rid of the excess iron in the circulation. This is why iron supplements should never be given to thalassaemics although folate treatment is often prescribed.

ABO incompatibility

ABO incompatibility may occur in babies with blood type A, B or AB born to mothers with blood type O. Type O women routinely have antibodies to blood types A and B, but they are too large to cross the placenta. However, during pregnancy a few fetal red cells will enter the mother's circulation and stimulate the formation of a smaller sized anti-A or B antibody, which may cross back to the baby's circulation and attack the baby's red cells. If many red cells are destroyed this will lead to jaundice after birth, which may need treatment with phototherapy or an exchange transfusion.

Maternal red cell antibodies

At the antenatal booking visit your blood group is checked and the presence of any atypical antibodies to your red blood cells is noted and you will be given a special card with details of them, which should be shown to your antenatal carers. Red cell antibodies usually develop as a result of a previous blood transfusion or pregnancy, but can occur naturally. They are not related to any illness or infection and are not harmful to your health. However, it is important to know about these antibodies during pregnancy, because if you need a blood transfusion, other blood groups as well as ABO and rhesus have to be taken into account during the cross matching. In addition, red cell antibodies may occasionally attack the baby's red blood cells leading to jaundice (see ABO incompatibility).

Rhesus disease

The rhesus factor is present on the surface of red blood cells. It is made up of three paired parts – C, D, and E – of which D is the most important because it can lead to rhesus isoimmunization (see p.128). About 85 per cent of Caucasian people carry the D antigen and are known as rhesus D positive, while the 15 per cent who lack it are rhesus negative. If you are Rh-negative, problems may arise if you are carrying a baby who is Rh-positive because there is a risk that you could develop antibodies that can cross the placenta and attack and destroy the baby's red blood cells. Although this is rarely a problem in a first pregnancy, you may develop antibodies as a result of exposure to your baby's Rh-positive blood during delivery, which can cause problems in a subsequent pregnancy.

Rhesus disease can largely be prevented by giving injections of anti-D to Rh-negative women during pregnancy and after delivery (see p.128) to mop up any Rh-positive fetal blood cells that may have entered your circulation and stop development of destructive

BLOOD PRESSURE PROBLEMS

Uncontrolled high blood pressure in pregnancy can result in serious problems for both mother and baby. The most common form is pregnancy induced hypertension – PIH (pre-eclampsia or toxaemia), but women with pre-existing hypertension or hypertension due to kidney disease are also at risk. Depending on history and risk factors, you may be offered low-dose aspirin and calcium supplements from 12 weeks until delivery.

PRE-ECLAMPSIA

Pre-eclampsia, or pregnancy-induced hypertension (PIH), complicates 5–8 per cent of all pregnancies. Most cases are mild and usually occur in first-time mothers during the second half of pregnancy, and are resolved soon after the birth. Severe cases can present earlier in pregnancy. Others may not arise until you are in labour or make a first appearance only after delivery with little warning.

Pregnant women are checked for symptoms of impending pre-eclampsia at every antenatal visit, during labour, and after birth. The classical signs are raised blood pressure, peripheral oedema (swelling of the hands, feet and legs) and the presence of protein in the urine. The only cure for pre-eclampsia is delivery of the baby. However, if the baby is very immature, it may be possible to buy some more time for the baby to continue growing in utero by giving the mother treatment.

Mild pre-eclampsia may have no significant effect on the growth and wellbeing of the baby. However, when placental blood flow and function are reduced there is always the risk of the baby developing IUGR and oxygen shortage (hypoxia). Regular ultrasound

and Doppler blood flow monitoring of fetal growth in pregnancies complicated by pre-eclampsia is now commonplace and plays an important role in deciding on the best time to deliver. In mothers with severe PIH, the baby is also at risk of premature delivery, placental abruption, and intrauterine death.

Normal blood pressure in a non-pregnant woman is less than 140/90mm of mercury. However, blood pressure measurements in pregnancy vary between individuals and at different stages of pregnancy. Hence it is more useful to compare the antenatal visit readings with the booking blood pressure measurements when assessing the risk of pre-eclampsia.

Mild PIH – the blood pressure (BP) rises to 140/100, with mild oedema and clear urine. The woman usually feels well but may require oral anti-hypertensive treatment if the BP is consistently raised.

Moderate PIH – the BP exceeds 140/100 and is accompanied by proteinuria and marked oedema. Most women will be admitted to hospital to bring the BP under control and assess the wellbeing of the baby.

Severe PIH – the BP exceeds 160/110 and heavy proteinuria is present. Sudden and intense swelling of the face and limbs may occur with marked weight gain. Immediate treatment is needed to lower the BP and prevent the onset of convulsions, which usually requires intravenous antihypertensive and sedative drugs, followed by urgent delivery of the baby, usually by Caesarean section.

The causes of pre-eclampsia are not clearly understood. There is no doubt that there is a genetic component since the problem tends

to run in families. Pre-eclampsia is more common in first-time mothers, twin and diabetic pregnancies, and in women with pre-existing hypertension or kidney disease. It also appears to be associated with poor maternal diet and vitamin deficiency. There is increasing evidence to suggest that pre-eclampsia involves an abnormal response of the mother's inflammatory and immune system to the baby and placenta. Women who have had pre-eclampsia are at increased risk of cardiovascular disease in later life.

ESSENTIAL HYPERTENSION

Essential hypertension complicates 1–3 per cent of pregnancies and is more frequent in women over the age of 35 years. It is defined as persistently raised BP greater than 140/90 before 20 weeks and may be diagnosed before pregnancy or identified at the first antenatal visit. Most women will already be taking an antihypertensive drug and need to be supervised by a physician to modify the dosages during pregnancy.

ECLAMPSIA

The signs of eclampsia are coma and convulsions and usually occur at the final stage of severe untreated PIH or essential hypertension accompanied by PIH. Eclampsia is now rare in the developed world, although it remains a potentially life-threatening obstetric emergency for mother and baby, since all of the maternal blood vessels go into spasm leading to kidney, liver and brain dysfunction together with a dramatic shortage of blood flow and oxygen to the fetus. Immediate measures are needed to sedate the mother's irritable brain, stabilize her BP, and deliver the baby, which invariably requires Caesarean section.

maternal antibodies. However, if antibodies are detected in your booking blood tests in a subsequent pregnancy, you will need specialist care during your pregnancy. You will be offered further blood tests every four weeks, and your baby will be monitored for signs of anaemia or heart failure. Severely affected babies may need multiple blood transfusions in utero to allow the pregnancy to continue until it is safe to deliver. At birth, the baby will undergo tests for haemoglobin, ABO and rhesus blood grouping, bilirubin levels, and a Coombs test (which detects the maternal rhesus antibodies). Jaundice often develops in the first 48 hours of life, requiring immediate treatment.

Amniotic fluid problems

POLYHYDRAMNIOS

This excess of amniotic fluid usually becomes noticeable when the volume is greater than two litres. You will develop a tense abdomen through which it is difficult to feel fetal parts clearly, and in severe cases, heartburn, breathlessness, and abdominal discomfort develop, particularly when the onset is sudden. Polyhydramnios can be caused by increased production of amniotic fluid because the placental surface is large (twins) or the fetal urine production is increased (poorly controlled diabetes). It may also result because a fetal malformation prevents the fetus from swallowing the fluid or absorbing it. Polyhydramnios almost always occurs in pregnancies affected by HYDROPS, because the fetus

develops heart failure or severe anaemia, but in many cases no specific cause is identified. Polyhydramnios increases the risk of premature labour, CORD PROLAPSE, and ABNORMAL PRESENTATIONS and may be relieved by amniocentesis to drain away some of the fluid.

OLIGOHYDRAMNIOS

A reduced amniotic fluid pool is most likely to be due to intrauterine growth restriction or ruptured membranes, but can also occur in healthy post-mature pregnancies. The amount of amniotic fluid in late pregnancy is a good measure of fetal wellbeing, which is why ultrasound measurements that show reduced liquor near to term usually prompt a decision to deliver the baby. Rarely, oligohydramnios is noted on the 20-week scan, which usually means that the fetus has an abnormality of the renal tract. Oligohydramnios in early pregnancy results in poor lung development and limb pressure deformities.

Gestational diabetes

Between 1 and 3 per cent of pregnant women develop gestational diabetes (glucose intolerance). The risk is greater in women who are obese, over 30, have a history of gestational diabetes, large babies, intrauterine death or stillbirth, or a family history of diabetes. During pregnancy the placenta produces hormones that block the effects of insulin. This insulin resistance usually begins at 20–24 weeks and increases until delivery. If your pancreas cannot produce sufficient

insulin to counteract this effect you will develop hyperglycaemia (high sugar levels) and will be diagnosed as having gestational diabetes. If you have risk factors or are found to have glycosuria on more than one occasion, you will be offered a glucose tolerance test between 24 and 28 weeks (see p.212). Most women diagnosed with gestational diabetes can be managed by dietary measures alone, but 10–20 per cent will also require oral hypoglycaemic agents and/or insulin treatment before the end of their pregnancy. Careful monitoring by a multidisciplinary team (dietician, specialist midwife, obstetrician, and endocrinologist) improves pregnancy outcome for mother and baby.

Gestational diabetes is not associated with an increased risk of miscarriage or congenital abnormality because the glucose intolerance starts later in pregnancy. However, later pregnancy complications are common because the fetal pancreas produces more insulin to cope with the high maternal sugar levels that cross the placenta. This may lead to abnormal presentations, macrosomia (fat baby), and POLYHYDRAMNIOS, all of which increase the risk of premature labour and complications during labour and birth, particularly shoulder dystocia. Hence you will be offered regular fetal growth scans and estimations of liquor volume and may be advised to undergo an induction of labour before term. Half of gestational diabetics will develop overt diabetes or high blood pressure in later life.

Antepartum haemorrhage

Antepartum haemorrhage (APH) is best defined as significant vaginal bleeding after the 24th week of pregnancy. Before this date the bleeding is called a threatened miscarriage. After 24 weeks the baby has a chance of survival, so it is particularly important to diagnose or exclude bleeding from the placenta (due to PLACENTA PRAEVIA or PLACENTAL ABRUPTION), which may require immediate delivery to protect you and your baby. Occasionally, the bleeding is from a cervical erosion or polyp. If you experience bleeding in pregnancy, you and your baby need to be assessed in hospital immediately.

Placental abruption

In this condition the placenta starts to separate from the wall of the uterus. The underlying cause is often unclear, but it is more common in multiparous women, cigarette smokers, cocaine and crack users, and women with poor nutrition, high blood pressure or thrombophilia (pro-clotting tendency). The bleeding that results may be "revealed" if some of the blood is able to escape from the uterus into the vagina or "concealed" when the blood is trapped between the wall of the uterus and placenta.

Placental abruption is invariably painful, because blood seeps into the muscles of the uterus causing irritation and contractions. If you experience a minor abruption, the baby is not distressed and your own condition is stable, it may be possible for you to go home after a few days observation in hospital. If the bleeding is severe, the build-up of blood behind the placenta leads to severe pain and further detachment of the placenta. If on examination, the uterus feels "woody" and is tender to touch then an emergency delivery will be needed, usually by Caesarean section.

Placenta praevia

One in 200 pregnancies at term is complicated by placenta praevia where the placenta is implanted in the lower segment of the uterus and lies in front of (praevia) the presenting part of the baby. If the placenta completely covers the internal part of the cervix, the cervical os (major praevia), the only option available is delivery by Caesarean section. In minor degrees of praevia where the baby's head is able to descend past the lower edge of the placenta, a vaginal birth may be possible.

It is common for the placenta to be reported as low-lying at the 20-week scan. However, by 32 weeks, the lower segment of the uterus has started to extend downwards and previously low-lying placentas now appear to be placed higher in the uterus. Placenta praevia is responsible for 20 per cent of cases of antepartum haemorrhage and is more common in multiparous women. The bleeding is characteristically painless, usually recurrent, and can be very severe, necessitating emergency delivery and a blood transfusion.

Abnormally adherent placenta

The placenta usually separates from the uterine wall some minutes after delivery. Occasionally it has invaded too deeply into the endometrial lining and the uterine muscle (placenta accreta – 1 in 1,500 births) or penetrates through the muscle wall to extend outside the uterus (placenta percreta – 1 in 2,500 births). In these cases, it cannot spontaneously separate and attempts to remove it manually may lead to postpartum haemorrhage (see p.335) and even UTERINE RUPTURE. Placenta accreta or percreta are more common in women with a placenta that has implanted in the lower uterine segment or who have a uterine scar. If surgical removal is not possible, the placenta will be left to slough off in time.

Uterine rupture

This usually follows an obstructed labour, inappropriate use of oxytocic drugs or the rupture of a previous Caesarean section or myomectomy (fibroid) scar, but occasionally occurs before labour in women with a uterine scar. A classical (vertical) Caesarean section scar is far more likely to rupture during labour than a lower segment scar, which is why elective Caesarean delivery before term is advised for these women. The rupture may be silent and painless, or present with severe pain and shock due to intra-abdominal bleeding together with acute fetal distress. Emergency hysterectomy may be required.

FETAL GROWTH IN PREGNANCY

INTRAUTERINE GROWTH RESTRICTION (IUGR)

In approximately 3–5 per cent of pregnancies the baby suffers from growth restriction, which is also referred to as fetal growth retardation, small for dates, small for gestational age or placental insufficiency. The best definition of IUGR is a baby whose birthweight is below the 5th centile for growth at that gestational age. IUGR is the third most important cause of perinatal mortality (after prematurity and congenital abnormalities). This is why trying to identify babies at risk of IUGR is part of routine antenatal care.

CAUSES OF IUGR

• General factors include racial variations, low socioeconomic status, high parity (many previous births), poor antenatal education, and a previous baby with unexplained IUGR.
• Maternal health issues include low maternal weight before pregnancy, weight gain of less than 10kg (22lb) during pregnancy, and poor nutrition. Smoking is an important and preventable cause of IUGR worldwide. Alcohol, amphetamines, heroin, and cocaine all have a powerful adverse effect on fetal growth. IUGR has a high risk of recurrence, suggesting that the problem runs in families.
• About 5 per cent of IUGR babies have a chromosomal abnormality such as Down's syndrome or a structural congenital abnormality of the heart, kidney or skeleton. Symmetrical growth IUGR should always raise the suspicion of a fetal infection with RUBELLA, CYTOMEGALOVIRUS, SYPHILIS or TOXOPLASMOSIS. Syphilis and

toxoplasmosis can be treated with antibiotics during pregnancy to reduce the damage to the fetus.
• Any disorder that reduces placental function or blood flow will result in IUGR because the supply of oxygen and nutrients to the fetus is reduced. This may be due to abnormalities in the early development of the placenta or because the placenta becomes less efficient in later pregnancy following placental bleeding or abruption. Women with poor nutrition or an underlying medical disorder are more likely to develop placental insufficiency. IUGR develops in 20 per cent of all twin pregnancies but is more likely in identical twins where there is a risk that one baby will receive a reduced share of the placental blood flow (see twin-to-twin transfusion syndrome, p.346).

SCREENING FOR IUGR

Awareness of the causes of IUGR and those mothers who are at greatest risk is an important part of screening for IUGR. Abdominal examinations will miss some 30 per cent of babies with IUGR, and menstrual dates are inaccurate in at least 1 in 4 pregnancies. This is why a dating scan in the first trimester of pregnancy is such a useful baseline measurement to have, particularly in pregnancies that later become complicated. Sequential ultrasound scans during the second and third trimester of pregnancy (see p.214 and p.257) are the best way to identify fetal growth problems and will distinguish between symmetrical and asymmetrical IUGR.

If a fetal chromosomal abnormality or infection is suspected, the mother will be advised to undergo an amniocentesis or infective screen

to confirm the diagnosis. The inclusion of Doppler blood flow measurements of the fetal cerebral, umbilical, and uterine vessels can help to assess the severity of the IUGR. Together with other tests of fetal wellbeing they will influence how the rest of your pregnancy is managed.

MANAGING AN IUGR PREGNANCY

If consecutive ultrasound scans show that your baby's growth has been static or that the liquor volume or blood flow to the baby is now reduced, it may be necessary to consider delivering your baby early. Of course, this will only be an option if your baby has reached a viable age and if your doctors feel that the baby would be better cared for in the outside world rather than left in utero.

Babies with IUGR are more likely to develop fetal distress and asphyxia during labour and be born with low Apgar scores, which is why you may be offered steroids prior to delivery. In severe cases, an elective Caesarean section may be the preferred method of delivery. Babies with moderate IUGR may require induction of labour, particularly when the amniotic fluid volume is reduced. If carefully managed, babies with mild IUGR are often delivered normally.

IUGR babies are more likely to experience postnatal complications and a paediatrician may be on hand at the time of delivery to assess the severity of the IUGR and the support that the newborn baby may require. IUGR babies usually show good catch-up growth after delivery unless the IUGR is due to a congenital abnormality or was very severe in early pregnancy.

Umbilical cord problems

CORD PROLAPSE

If the umbilical cord is positioned below the baby and the membranes rupture, the cord can slip or prolapse through the cervix. This occurs in 1 in 300 pregnancies and is more common in premature babies, breech presentations, transverse or oblique lies, and when there is POLYHYDRAMNIOS. Prolapsed cord is an obstetric emergency, because once exposed to cold air the umbilical blood vessels will go into spasm, cutting off the oxygen supply to the baby. Prompt delivery is needed.

CORD COMPRESSION

Mild, intermittent cord compression during a contraction occurs in about 10 per cent of labours. The CTG may show signs of mild fetal distress, but usually the baby has sufficient energy stores to recover quickly from the temporary lack of oxygen. Cord compression is often seen in the second stage of labour, particularly when the cord is short or wrapped around the baby's neck. Cord compression is more likely to lead to fetal distress and asphyxia in a baby that is already at risk because of IUGR or post-maturity, particularly if OLIGOHYDRAMNIOS is also present.

SINGLE UMBILICAL CORD ARTERY

The cord usually contains three blood vessels: two arteries and one vein. However, in about 5 per cent of babies only one artery and one vein are present, which may

be noted on an ultrasound scan. In 15 per cent of affected babies the abnormality is associated with other congenital abnormalities and IUGR, which is why the finding will prompt further investigations. The condition is more common in twins.

VELAMENTOUS CORD INSERTION

When the cord runs through the membranes before entering the placenta (vasa praevia) there is a risk that the vessels will be damaged when the membranes rupture, resulting in fetal bleeding. This condition is present in 1 per cent of term pregnancies and is more common in twins.

Abnormal fetal lie and presentation

A transverse lie, oblique lie or shoulder presentation are more common in women who have already had a baby because the uterus is more lax. These abnormal presentations are also associated with prematurity, multiple pregnancy, FIBROIDS, uterine malformations, POLYHYDRAMNIOS, and PLACENTA PRAEVIA. It may be possible to perform a gentle cephalic version (having excluded placenta praevia), but the baby often returns to the previous presentation. In late pregnancy the risk of cord prolapse may require admission to hospital to await labour, and delivery may have to be by Caesarean section.

Face presentations occur in 1 in 500 deliveries, usually by chance, but occasionally because the baby is anencephalic or has

a swelling in the neck or shortening of the neck muscles. There is little point in trying to diagnose the problem before labour or in early labour, because the face presentation may resolve spontaneously as it passes through the pelvis. The labour is usually prolonged and the facial swelling can be severe and take several days to settle down.

Brow presentation is the least common (1 in 1,500 births) and most unfavourable of all abnormal presentations, since the presenting part is too broad to be delivered vaginally. It can be associated with fetal abnormalities, particularly HYDROCEPHALY.

Shoulder dystocia

This is an obstetric emergency because the head has already delivered but the shoulders do not follow because they are wedged in the pelvis. Swift action is required to prevent the baby developing asphyxia. Placing the mother's legs in stirrups allows the midwife or doctor to apply firm downward traction on the baby's head and neck to encourage the anterior shoulder under the pubic symphysis. An extensive episiotomy and pressure applied above the pubic bone by an assistant helps the delivery. Shoulder dystocia is more common in obese and diabetic women, in babies weighing more than 4kg (9lb), and following a prolonged labour with good uterine contractions. If there is a history of shoulder dystocia, a senior obstetrician should always be present at the next delivery.

Miscarriage

Miscarriage – the spontaneous loss of a pregnancy before the fetus is able to survive outside the mother's womb – is the most common complication of pregnancy. It occurs in 15 per cent of recognized pregnancies, but we now know that some 50 per cent of fertilized eggs are lost, many of which never reach the stage of being visible on the US scan. The vast majority of random miscarriages occur early in pregnancy and are due to fetal chromosome abnormalities that are incompatible with further development. Miscarriage after 12 weeks of gestation is uncommon and affects only 1–2 per cent of pregnancies.

Miscarriage is a process, not a single event, so if you experience vaginal bleeding or pain in pregnancy there are several possible outcomes. In a threatened miscarriage there is no obvious problem on an ultrasound scan and the bleeding will stop after a few days or recur again, but the cervix remains closed. If the process continues and the cervix starts to open, usually accompanied by cramping abdominal pain, the miscarriage becomes inevitable. It may go on to be complete, in which case the uterus empties its contents entirely, or incomplete if some pregnancy tissues are left behind.

Removal of the remaining tissues using drugs or surgery to evacuate the uterus is usually advised to prevent haemorrhage and infection. Sometimes the pregnancy stops developing, but there are no obvious signs of a problem (missed miscarriage) until an ultrasound scan demonstrates that the fetus has died (embryonic miscarriage) or there is no evidence of a fetal pole within the early pregnancy sac (anembryonic pregnancy).

The risk of miscarriage increases with maternal age and also if the woman has experienced previous miscarriages. Recurrent miscarriage – usually defined as three or more consecutive pregnancy losses – is uncommon, affecting only 1 per cent of couples. Most couples experiencing this distressing problem wish to undergo investigations sooner rather than later in order to establish whether or not they have an underlying cause for their repeated miscarriages. In the majority of cases, no cause is found and these couples should be reassured that their prognosis for a successful pregnancy next time is excellent. Nonetheless, referral to a unit with a specialist interest in miscarriage is very valuable for these couples, since they will be offered the latest investigations and opportunities to participate in new treatment trials, not to mention the psychological benefits of knowing that they have done all they can to help prevent the miscarriages recurring.

I cannot overstate the value of joining a research programme if you are a recurrent miscarriage sufferer. Repeatedly, studies have shown that future pregnancy outcome is improved for women who are cared for in a specialist clinic by a dedicated team.

RECOVERY AND COUNSELLING

Losing a baby at any stage in pregnancy can be a devastating experience. We all react to and deal with grief in different ways, but when it comes to pregnancy loss the stages of acute grief, mourning, and healing can be lengthy processes and there are no shortcuts to be taken. The first stage invariably includes shock, disbelief, numbness, confusion, and sometimes denial. Next comes the angry stage often complicated by guilt, despair, depression, and physical symptoms of anxiety, such as insomnia, poor sleep, and loss of appetite.

With time, acute grief gives way to a deep sadness and later will be replaced by feelings of mourning, regret, and yearning for the baby you have lost. Eventually, you will become resigned and accepting of what has happened although this never completely takes away the emotional pain, but you will be able to deal with it in a more controlled way. You will need support during the recovery period and this may come from many different sources: family, friends, the hospital medical team, your GP, other parents who have had similar experiences, and local or national support groups. Most maternity units can put you in touch with specialist counsellors who have experience in helping couples cope with the aftermath of early and late pregnancy loss.

Stillbirth and neonatal death

Stillbirth (SB) follows the death of a baby in utero after 20 weeks. It may be anticipated because a serious congenital abnormality was identified during pregnancy, but 50 per cent of all SBs occur without warning.

The diagnosis may be suspected if the mother reports a lack of fetal movements. This can be confirmed on an ultrasound scan that reveals the absence of a fetal heartbeat. Labour usually starts spontaneously a few days after the baby's death, but you may prefer to have labour induced at the earliest opportunity and occasionally some women may choose to deliver their baby by Caesarean section. If delivery has not occurred within seven days you will be advised to undergo induction of labour, because after this time there is a risk that you could develop a serious blood-clotting abnormality if the fetal tissues remain in utero.

The risk of SB is increased in high-risk pregnancies. However, the SB rate has fallen dramatically as a result of improved maternal health, nutrition, and antenatal monitoring for problems such as high blood pressure, diabetes, growth restriction, cholestasis, and rhesus disease.

SB in labour is now rare (1 in 1,000), due to improved intrapartum monitoring, but still occasionally follows a massive placental abruption. Even when a detailed postmortem is performed, the cause of the SB

is not always understood, which is particularly distressing for the parents.

Neonatal death (NND) is the loss of a baby within four weeks of birth and affects 3–4 in 1,000 babies, most of them dying within the first week of life. In 25 per cent of NNDs the baby has a severe genetic or chromosomal abnormality, or a structural problem, most commonly affecting the heart. NND is also associated with early premature birth, and occasionally follows infection during pregnancy, or fetal distress and asphyxia during labour. If the baby dies after four weeks of life, it is called an infant death.

Sudden infant death syndrome (SIDS) – previously called cot death – is rare, affecting 1 in 1,600 babies, but is more common among premature babies, severely growth-restricted babies, boys and multiple births.

Termination (early and late)

The decision to undergo a termination of pregnancy for fetal abnormality is never an easy one (see p.138). If you find yourself in this distressing situation you will need some information about your options and what is likely to happen, and my patients tell me that this is a subject that most pregnancy books fail to include. Before 12 weeks of pregnancy, the termination can be performed surgically or medically, but after 12 weeks it is usually safer to induce labour using drugs and

deliver the fetus vaginally. The surgical approach involves clearing out the uterus using suction under general anaesthesia, which has the advantage of being quick and physically painless since the mother is unconscious. You should expect to have some vaginal bleeding for up to a week after the procedure and will probably be given a course of antibiotics to prevent infection.

The medical approach involves a combination of two drugs; the first is a single dose of an oral progesterone antagonist (an anti-hormone tablet); the second is a prostaglandin, which is usually given as a vaginal pessary 48 hours later. The prostaglandin can also be given orally, but this route can be associated with nausea and stomach upsets. The vaginal pessaries are repeated at regular intervals until the termination is complete, the number of doses required being related to how far advanced the pregnancy is. However, vaginal bleeding and cramping abdominal pains usually start before or soon after the first pessary is inserted and in the majority of cases the fetus is expelled within 24 hours. You will be given pain-killing drugs to help you cope with any discomfort and you can expect to have light vaginal bleeding for up to a week after the termination.

If it is suspected that some of the pregnancy tissues have been retained, you will be advised to have a surgical curettage under anaesthetic, but in the vast majority of cases this will not be necessary.

Concerns after birth

The days and weeks after birth are often dogged with minor problems. I have included general advice on many of these in Life After Birth (see pp.370–405) and so am concentrating here on maternal complications that may arise and also problems that may be present in newborns.

MATERNAL PROBLEMS

It is important to seek advice promptly if you notice symptoms of any of the following conditions that sometimes occur in the days and weeks after the birth. Most are only temporary and can be resolved speedily with appropriate treatment, although a few may need specialist help.

Puerperal pyrexia

Puerperal or postpartum pyrexia is defined as a rise in maternal temperature to 38°C (100.4°F) or more, from day 1 to day 10 post delivery and is usually caused by infection. Thanks to improved hygiene, obstetric care, and infection control in hospitals, the incidence of postpartum infection has now fallen to about 3 per cent and is rarely life-threatening. The most likely site of infection is the uterine cavity (endometritis) or perineum, but the urinary tract and breast are also common sites. THROMBOEMBOLISM may also cause a postpartum pyrexia and is more likely to develop after a Caesarean section, as are chest or wound infections.

UTERINE INFECTION

Most cases are caused by ascending infections from the cervix or vagina. The organisms infect the placental bed and any pieces of retained placenta or membranes left in the endometrial cavity. If the lochia begins to smell offensive or you start to develop lower abdominal pain and tenderness, it is likely that you have developed endometritis. This is important to diagnose and treat promptly to avoid complications such as damage to the Fallopian tubes, resulting in future difficulties becoming pregnant.

Your doctor will examine you internally and take some vaginal swabs for testing. If the examination suggests that there may be tissues left within the uterine cavity (cervix partly open and the uterus, enlarged, tender, and boggy), you will be started on a course of antibiotics and advised to undergo a uterine evacuation to remove the tissues. Since no one wants to give a woman who has just delivered a baby a general anaesthetic unless absolutely necessary, an ultrasound scan is often performed to confirm the examination findings.

URINARY INFECTION

Urinary infections are particularly common in women who have been catheterized during labour or have had a difficult delivery. Any rise in temperature after delivery should prompt your midwife to send a sample of urine to the laboratory to be tested and antibiotics are usually started immediately. It is important to check that the urine infection has been treated effectively by testing another urine sample after the course of treatment has been completed.

MASTITIS

Almost every mother develops some degree of breast engorgement as the milk starts to come into her breasts. The breasts become swollen, hard, and sore, and this commonly raises her temperature slightly. Fortunately, the problem usually resolves spontaneously in a day or two as breastfeeding becomes established. However, if you become feverish and start to feel unwell, your breasts need to be examined for signs of localized or patchy redness and induration (pitting hardness). This is called mastitis and can be exquisitely painful because one of the milk ducts has become blocked and the stagnant pool of milk in the blocked duct can quickly become infected. The organism is usually a staphylococcus present on your or your baby's skin, which then enters a cracked or sore nipple and spreads into the breast tissues.

Caught early, mastitis responds promptly to antibiotics, mild painkillers and keeping the breast milk flowing by continuing to breastfeed, or expressing the milk to relieve the pressure. However, if mastitis is not identified and treated quickly, it can develop into a full-blown breast abscess. In addition to feeling generally unwell with a high swinging temperature, there will be a hot firm lump in one of your breasts that contains pus and this will have to be surgically incized (opened) and drained in hospital.

Perineal problems

Approximately 69 per cent of women who give birth vaginally require some sort of stitching. If at any stage in the few weeks after the delivery your perineum starts to throb, look inflamed or produces any sort of discharge, consult your midwife or GP. You may have developed a wound infection, and this is usually treated simply and effectively with antibiotics. Sometimes it is judged best to remove one or two of the stitches to release the pressure in the inflamed area and make it easier to access the wound to clean it thoroughly. Occasionally, after a traumatic

vaginal delivery, a haematoma or collection of blood can swell up in the walls of the vagina. This needs to be removed surgically to relieve the pain, tie off the bleeding point, and prevent infection developing.

Some women continue to experience problems with their episiotomy or perineal wounds for several weeks, but there is no need to suffer in silence. Your GP and midwife will be able to check you over and make sure there is no sign of infection. They may suggest you consider having some specialist physiotherapy using ultrasound to help relieve the discomfort. Your maternity unit will also be able to refer you to the obstetric physiotherapists, who have expertise in helping women with postnatal problems involving the perineum, bowel, bladder, and vagina.

Stress incontinence

Women who have had a vaginal delivery often suffer mild, temporary urinary incontinence, because the bladder neck has been stretched and pulled downwards by the pressure of the baby's head passing through the birth canal. Usually this manifests itself as stress incontinence, where urine seeps out when you laugh, cough, sneeze or move quickly.

Pelvic floor exercises will improve your ability to regain full bladder control – the sooner you start on them, the quicker the benefits will be. However if, despite regularly performing these exercises, you are still suffering from urinary or urge

incontinence that disrupts your lifestyle (leaking persistently, unable to go out of the house because of the fear of accidents or not being able to find a toilet quickly enough), then you need to see your GP and arrange for some more specialist help.

Faecal incontinence

After a vaginal delivery, particularly those involving a prolonged second stage of labour and an extensive episiotomy or tear, some women may lose a degree of control over their bowels. This usually resolves soon after giving birth, with the help of some pelvic floor exercises. However, on the rare occasions when a woman develops full faecal incontinence and is simply unable to control her bowel movements, specialist help is needed, since it usually means that the anal sphincter and rectal skin have been torn.

Anaemia

Symptomatic anaemia after the birth may be due to acute blood loss (more common after prolonged labour, operative delivery, and postpartum haemorrhage) or because the mother's iron stores have been depleted during pregnancy because of poor nutrition, difficulties in absorbing iron, twin pregnancies or several pregnancies in quick succession. Blood transfusion may be required in severe cases, but iron and folic-acid replacement is usually sufficient. Treatment should be started promptly.

PROBLEMS IN BABIES

Most of these problems are detected only after the birth, usually during your baby's check-ups in hospital and at six weeks. However, cleft lip and palate is sometimes seen on ultrasound and fetal alcohol syndrome may be suspected if your baby has growth problems during pregnancy.

Cerebral palsy

Cerebral palsy (CP) describes a range of abnormalities in movement, muscle tone, posture, speech, vision, and hearing in young children, caused by damage to one or more areas of the brain. CP affects 1 in 400 children and is more common in pregnancies complicated by premature delivery, IUGR and infection. There are three types of CP depending on the area of the brain affected and affected children usually have a combination of two or more types. There is no antenatal test that can detect cerebral palsy.

Fetal alcohol syndrome

Regular alcohol consumption during pregnancy may result in teratogenic (early) and toxic (later) damage to the fetus depending on how much alcohol is consumed. The main features of fetal alcohol syndrome (FAS) are IUGR, failure to thrive after birth, damage to the nervous system, and poor childhood growth. Attention deficit disorder, language delays, and mild to moderate mental retardation gradually become evident. The characteristic facial appearance includes microcephaly, flattened nasal bridge, middle of the face underdeveloped, short upturned nose, and thin upper lip. Newborn babies are irritable, hyperactive, and have poor muscle tone. FAS affects at least 1 in 750 babies born in the UK and is an important and preventable cause of mental retardation and learning difficulties.

Pathological jaundice

Occasionally, neonatal jaundice (see p.388) may be a sign of a more serious underlying condition such as anaemia caused by blood group incompatibility, liver or thyroid disease, or an inherited enzyme disorder that weakens the red cells making them break down more readily. These rarer forms of jaundice are referred to as pathological jaundice and usually necessitate treatment with phototherapy and possibly even a blood transfusion. In severe cases, or when the baby is very premature, drugs to stimulate the liver to get rid of the excess bilirubin may need to be given.

Cleft lip and palate

The development of the upper lip and palate (roof of the mouth) in the fetus involves the joining together of tissues in the midline of the face. When this is incomplete, as occurs in 1 in 750 babies, a split in the lip (harelip) and/or the palate results. The defect can be seen on antenatal ultrasound scans. Babies with a cleft palate may have difficulties feeding and are at risk of choking, because the absence of a bony roof to the mouth interferes with sucking and swallowing. They are also likely to suffer recurrent ear infections and hearing difficulties. Corrective surgery will be planned after the birth. A cleft lip is usually closed at about three months, but surgery to close the palate may be delayed until at least 12 months, to ensure it has developed fully.

Pyloric stenosis

This affects 1 in 500 newborn babies and is more common in boys. It is caused by thickening of the pylorus muscle between the bottom of the stomach and the small intestine. As food builds up, the stomach contracts strongly in an attempt to force food into the upper intestine. The problem presents soon after birth with persistent projectile vomiting during or straight after a feed. As a result, the baby becomes hungry and irritable, and quickly develops dehydration and weight loss. Pyloric stenosis is diagnosed by feeling the contracted muscle on abdominal examination and confirmed with an ultrasound scan or barium swallow X-ray. Prompt surgery to loosen the muscle offers a complete cure.

Umbilical hernia

This is caused by a weakness in the muscles of the abdominal wall at the point where the umbilical cord entered your baby's abdomen. A small bulge around the baby's umbilicus containing a section of intestine is common, occurring in about 10 per cent of all babies, with a higher incidence in Afro-Caribbean children. It usually closes up of its own accord in time.

Inguinal hernia

This weakness in the lower abdominal wall in the groin region is caused by failure of the inguinal canal to close after birth in about 3 per cent of newborn babies and is often bilateral. During pregnancy, the testicles of a baby boy pass through the inguinal canal to reach the scrotum. Although girls do not have testicles, they do have an inguinal canal and so they too are susceptible to hernias.

Hernias are more likely in premature babies, babies with CYSTIC FIBROSIS, and baby boys with UNDESCENDED TESTICLES. As long as the contents of the bulge can be pushed back into the abdominal cavity, there is little cause for concern. However, occasionally, a loop of intestine becomes trapped in the hernia, so obstructing the bowel. These strangulated hernias are a surgical emergency and need to be dealt with promptly to save the bowel and repair the abdominal wall defect.

Hypospadias

This common abnormality is found in 1 in 500 baby boys. The external opening of the urethra is positioned on the underside of the penis instead of at the end.

The penis may curve downwards and the foreskin or prepuce appears hooded. Sometimes the urethral opening is far back in the scrotum or on the upper side of the penis (epispadias). Curative surgery is carried out at one year.

Undescended testes

This condition is found in 1 in 125 newborn boys. In 15 per cent of cases both testes are undescended. The majority have descended spontaneously by nine months of age, but if the problem persists after this time referral to a paediatric surgeon is recommended. If they remain undescended this can lead to testicular cancers, abnormal sperm production, and infertility.

Imperforate anus

The anus is closed, either because it is sealed by a thin membrane of skin over the external opening or because the passage between the rectum and anal canal has not developed (anal atresia). The baby's lower bowel becomes distended and swollen towards the end of pregnancy, which is visible on an ultrasound scan. All babies are examined at the time of delivery and undergo immediate corrective surgery if necessary.

Dislocated hips

This congenital abnormality is identified in as many as 1 in 200 babies at the routine postnatal check (see p.387). It is more common in girls, in the left hip, in multiple pregnancies, and in babies

that are born breech, or have another abnormality such as Down's syndrome or a NEURAL TUBE DEFECT.

The hip joint is unstable and will make a clicking sound when the knees are bent up towards the hips and the legs rotated outwards. The problem is usually curable with the use of orthopaedic manipulation and splints to hold the hip in the correct position during the first few months of life. Occasionally surgery may be required.

Talipes

This is a condition in which the baby's feet are turned inwards (equino varus) so that the soles are facing each other. Less commonly, the feet are turned outwards (calcaneo valgus). Talipes can be diagnosed on an ultrasound scan during pregnancy and often the problem runs in families.

The mildest form is caused by abnormal positioning of the feet during pregnancy and usually corrects itself during the first few months after birth. However, if the feet cannot be easily manipulated into the correct position, regular physiotherapy will be required and the baby will probably need to wear corrective splints for many months to ensure that his walking develops normally. Very severe forms of talipes may necessitate surgical correction at various points over several years.

Useful contacts

Active Birth Centre
Tel: 020 7281 6760
www.activebirthcentre.com

APEC (Action on Pre-eclampsia)
Tel: 020 8427 4217 (helpline)
www.apec.org.uk

ARC (Antenatal Results and Choices)
Tel: 0845 077 2290 (helpline)
www.arc-uk.org
Advice on antenatal tests and results

ASH (Action on Smoking and Health)
Tel: 020 7739 5902
www.ash.org.uk

Association of Breastfeeding Mothers
Tel: 0300 330 5453 (helpline)
www.abm.me.uk

Association for Improvements in the Maternity Services (AIMS)
Tel: 0300 365 0663 (helpline)
www.aims.org.uk

Association for Postnatal Illness
Tel: 020 7386 0868
www.apni.org

Association of Radical Midwives
Tel: 01865 428159
www.midwifery.org.uk
Organization committed to improving NHS maternity care

Birthworks
Tel: 0333 240 9710
www.birthworks.co.uk
Birthpool advice and hire

The Bladder and Bowel Foundation
Tel: 0845 345 0165 (helpline)
www.bladderandbowelfoundation.org
Advice on bladder and bowel problems

BLISS Baby Life Support System
www.bliss.org.uk
Support for parents of special-care babies

Blue Lagoon Birth Pools
Tel: 07949 016 877
www.bluelagoonbirthpools.co.uk

Breastfeeding Network
Tel: 0300 100 0210 (helpline)
www.breastfeedingnetwork.org.uk
Helpline for breastfeeding mothers

British Acupuncture Council
Tel: 020 8735 0400
www.acupuncture.org.uk

British Chiropractic Association
Tel: 0118 950 5950
www.chiropractic-uk.co.uk

British Homeopathic Association
Tel: 01582 408 675
www.britishhomeopathic.org

British Osteopathic Association
Tel: 01582 488 455
www.osteopathy.org

British Pregnancy Advisory Service
Tel: 08457 304030
www.bpas.org

British SPD Support Group
Tel: 0807 770 3236 (9am to 5pm)
www.spd-uk.org

Support for sufferers of symphysial pubic dysfunction

Child Bereavement Charity
Tel: 01494 568 900 (helpline)
www.childbereavement.org.uk

Cleft Lip and Palate Association (CLAPA)
Tel: 020 7833 4883
www.clapa.com

The Compassionate Friends
Tel: 0845 123 2304 (helpline)
www.tcf.org.uk
Support group for bereaved parents

Contact a Family
Tel: 0808 808 3555 (helpline)
www.cafamily.org.uk
Contact group for families with children with disabilities

Cruse Bereavement Care
Tel: 0844 477 9400 (helpline)
www.crusebereavementcare.org.uk
Bereavement counselling

Curative Hypnotherapy Register
Tel: 0115 970 1223
www.curativehypnotherapyregister.co.uk

Cystic Fibrosis Trust
Tel: 0300 373 1000 (helpline)
www.cftrust.org.uk

Department of Health
www.dh.gov.uk
Government health website, which includes advice for travellers

Diabetes UK
Tel: 020 7424 1000
www.diabetes.org.uk

Down's Syndrome Association
Tel: 0333 1212 300 (helpline)
www.downs-syndrome.org.uk

Family Planning Association
Tel: 0845 122 8690 (helpline)
www.fpa.org.uk

Fatherhood Institute
www.fatherhoodinstitute.org
Institute advocating involved fatherhood

**Foresight (The Association
for the Promotion of
Preconceptual Care)**
Tel: 01275 878953
www.foresight-preconception.org.uk
Advice on preconceptual health

FRANK (drugs helpline)
Tel: 0800 77 66 00 (freephone 24 hours)
www.talktofrank.com

**FSID (The Foundation for
the Study of Infant Deaths)**
Tel: 0808 802 6868 (helpline)
www.sids.org.uk
*Charity working to prevent infant deaths
and promote baby health*

Gingerbread
Tel: 0808 802 0925 (helpline freephone)
www.gingerbread.org.uk
*Local self-help groups for single parents and
their children*

The Hospital for Tropical Diseases
www.thehtd.org

Independent Midwives UK
Tel: 0845 460 0105
www.independentmidwives.org.uk

Infertility Network UK
Tel: 0800 008 7464
www.infertilitynetworkuk.com

La Leche League (Great Britain)
Tel: 0845 120 2918 (helpline)
www.laleche.org.uk
Breastfeeding advice and support

**MAMA (Meet-A-Mum
Association)**
Tel: 0845 120 3746 (helpline)
www.mama.co.uk

Maternity Action
Tel: 0845 600 8533
www.maternityaction.org.uk
*Promotes wellbeing of pregnant women,
new parents, and babies*

**MENCAP (Understanding
Learning Disability)**
Tel: 0808 808 1111 (helpline)
www.mencap.org.uk

**MIND (National Association
for Mental Health)**
Tel: 0300 123 3393 (information line)
www.mind.org.uk

The Miscarriage Association
Tel: 01924 200 799 (helpline)
www.miscarriageassociation.org.uk

Mumsnet
www.mumsnet.com

National Childbirth Trust
Tel: 0300 330 0772 (pregnancy
and birth helpline)
Tel: 0300 330 0770 (breastfeeding helpline)
www.nct.org.uk

NHS Direct
Tel: 0845 4647 (24 hours)
www.nhsdirect.nhs.uk

**NICE (National Institute for
Health and Clinical Excellence)**
www.nice.org.uk

QUIT
Tel: 0800 002 200 (helpline)
www.quit.org.uk
Practical help to stop smoking

RCOG Consumers' Forum
www.rcog.org.uk
*Royal College of Obstetricians and
Gynaecologists patients' forum*

The Recurrent Miscarriage Clinic
Tel: 020 3312 6666
www.st-marys.nhs.uk
*Specialist clinic for the investigation and
treatment of miscarriage*

Royal College of Midwives
Tel: 020 7312 3535
www.rcm.org.uk

**SANDS (Stillbirth and Neonatal
Death Society)**
Tel: 020 7436 5881 (helpline)
www.uk-sands.org

Save the Baby
www.savethebabyunit.org
*Charity based at St Mary's Hospital, London,
funding research into infertility, miscarriage,
and pregnancy and newborn complications*

**SENSE (National Deafblind
and Rubella Association)**
Tel: 0845 127 0060
Textphone: 0845 127 0060
www.sense.org.uk

**Shine (Association for Spina Bifida
and Hydrocephalus)**
Tel: 01733 555 988 (helpline)
www.shinecharity.org.uk

**TAMBA (Twins and Multiple
Births Association)**
Tel: 0800 138 0509
www.tamba.org.uk

Tommy's (The Baby Charity)
Tel: 0800 0147 800 (information line)
www.tommys.org
*Charity funding research into premature
birth, miscarriage, and stillbirth*

Turn2us
www.turn2us.org.uk
Benefits advice

Working Families
Tel: 0300 012 0312 (helpline)
www.workingfamilies.org.uk
Advice for working parents

Index

Acknowledgments

Author's acknowledgments

Writing this book has been an exciting and rewarding challenge. It has had a lengthy gestation period, during which I have had the pleasure of working with some very talented individuals. I want to acknowledge their contribution and thank them for their expertise, guidance, encouragement and practical support. There are too many to include each by name but some need a special mention. Maggie Pearlstine persuaded me to embark on the project and convinced me that it could, should and would be written. Debbie Beckerman, author and mother of two young children, has devoted countless hours to ensuring that we included all the issues that other pregnancy books have not addressed. That she is now a close personal friend is an unexpected bonus. Esther Ripley has contributed more than editorial skills to the project. Her enthusiasm for the subject matter is only surpassed by her ability to remain calm, patient and encouraging on every occasion that I was late meeting a deadline. Additional thanks to Angela Baynham, Liz Coghill and the creative team at Dorling Kindersley. I am also grateful to my colleague May Backos, who read through the entire manuscript, to all my medical and midwifery colleagues at St Mary's for their help and advice and the many patients who have so generously shared their feelings, thoughts, anxieties, fears and triumphs with me over the years. I hope that I have done justice to their requests for a new pregnancy bible.

Without the support of my family, this book would never have got off the starting block, let alone reached completion. My husband, John, deserves special recognition. I consider myself very fortunate to be able to rely on the fact that he is always supportive, constructively critical and tolerant, even when dinner is late yet again. A big thank you is also due to my twin daughters who have remained extraordinarily good humoured and understanding, despite my preoccupation. Clare and Jenny are a daily source of delight and wonder to me, which is without doubt, the inspiration and real reason for writing this book.

Publisher's acknowledgments

DK would like to thank Dr Mary Steen for her expert help in updating the new edition, and Claire Cross for proofreading.

For the 2005 edition
Project editors Esther Ripley, Angela Baynham
Art editor Nicola Rodway
Designers Briony Chappell, Alison Gardner
DTP designers Karen Constanti, Jackie Plant
Picture researchers Sarah Duncan, Anna Bedewell
Illustrator Philip Wilson
Production controller Shwe Zin Win
Managing editor Liz Coghill
Managing art editors Glenda Fisher, Emma Forge
Art director Carole Ash
Publishing manager Anna Davidson
Publishing director Corinne Roberts

Thanks to the following for their editorial support:
Julia Halford, Katie Dock, Isabella Jones

Additional photography Ruth Jenkinson
Additional illustrator Debbie Maizels
Additional DTP design Julian Dams, Grahame Kitto
Picture Research Administrator Carlo Ortu
Additional picture research Franziska Marking
Picture librarian Romaine Werblow
Proofreader Constance Novis
Indexer Hilary Bird

For the 2010 revised edition
Project editor Anne Yelland
Senior art editor Nicola Rodway
Production editor Ben Marcus
Production controller Hema Gohil
Creative technical support Sonia Charbonnier
Managing editor Penny Warren
Managing art editor Glenda Fisher
Publisher Peggy Vance

Picture credits
Most of the images in this book are of the embryo and fetus live in utero, pictured using endoscopic and ultrasound technology. When this has not been possible, images have been taken by reputable medical professionals as part of research or to promote educational awareness.

Dorling Kindersley would like to thank the following for their kind permission to reproduce their photographs: (abbreviations key: a=above, b=below/bottom, c=centre, f=far, l=left, r=right, t=top)

1 Prof. J.E. Jirasek MD, DSc.: CRC Press/Parthenon. **2–3 Corbis:** Ariel Skelley. **4 Corbis:** LWA-Dann Tardif (b); **Mother & Baby Picture Library:** Paul Mitchell (t); **OSF:** (m). **7 Photonica:** Henrik Sorensen.

8 Science Photo Library: Edelmann (tl). **9 Corbis:** Susan Solie Patterson (tr). **10–11 Getty Images:** David Oliver. **12 Getty Images:** Bill Ling. **13 Mother & Baby Picture Library:** Ian Hooton. **14 Science Photo Library:** Prof. P. Motta/Dept. Of Anatomy/University "La Sapienza", Rome (cla); D. Phillips (crb); VVG (clb). **15 Science Photo Library:** Edelmann (c); Prof. P. Motta/Dept. Of Anatomy/University "La Sapienza", Rome (cra). **Wellcome Library, London:** Yorgos Nikas (cfr). **16 Science Photo Library:** Richard Rawlins/Custom Medical Stock Photo. **18 Science Photo Library:** Professors P.M. Motta & J. Van Blerkom (bl); Prof. P. Motta/Dept. Of Anatomy/University "La Sapienza", Rome (br). **19 Science Photo Library:** Dr Yorgos Nikas (bl); D. Phillips (br). **20 Science Photo Library:** Edelmann (all). **24 Mother & Baby Picture Library:** Ruth Jenkinson. **26 Alamy Images:** Camera Press Ltd. **31 Mother & Baby Picture Library:** Ian Hooton. **33 Science Photo Library:** CNRI (tr); Moredun Scientific Ltd (crb); Dr Gopal Murti (cr). **36 Bubbles:** Lucy Tizard. **37 Mother & Baby Picture Library:** Ian Hooton. **38 Mother & Baby Picture Library:** Ian Hooton. **44 Getty Images:** Tom Mareschal (bl). **46 Getty Images:** Chris Everard (bl). **Prof. J.E. Jirasek MD, DSc.:** CRC Press/Parthenon (br). **47 Alamy Images:** foodfolio (bl); **Science Photo Library:** Ian Hooton (tl); TISSUEPIX (br). **51 Getty Images:** Anthony Johnson. **57 Mother & Baby Picture Library:** Ruth Jenkinson. **58 Mother & Baby Picture Library:** Ian Hooton. **60 Punchstock:** Blend Images **64 Getty Images:** Chronoscope. **66–67 Prof. J.E. Jirasek MD, DSc.:** CRC Press/Parthenon (all). **68–69 Prof. J.E. Jirasek MD, DSc.:** CRC Press/Parthenon (both). **70–71 Prof. J.E. Jirasek MD, DSc.:** CRC Press/Parthenon (all). **74 Science Photo Library:** Zephyr. **75 Getty Images:** Peter Correz. **76 Corbis:** Ariel Skelley. **80 Professor Lesley Regan. 83 Mother & Baby Picture Library:** Ian Hooton. **84 Science Photo Library:** Ian Hooton. **88 Mother & Baby Picture Library:** Ian Hooton. **89 Wellcome Library, London:** Anthea Sieveking. **90 Mother & Baby Picture Library:** Ian Hooton. **92–93 Prof. J.E. Jirasek MD, DSc.:** CRC Press/Parthenon (both). **Life Issues Institute** (bl); **Science Photo Library:** Edelmann (bc) (br). **96 Bubbles:** Jennie Woodcock (cl); **Mediscan:** Medical-On-Line (bl). **99 Getty Images:** Ericka McConnell. **105 Mother & Baby Picture Library. 106–107 Science Photo Library:** Edelmann (both). **108 LOGIQlibrary** (tl). **109 Science Photo Library:** GE Medical Systems (b). **110 LOGIQlibrary. 111 Science Photo Library:** BSIP (cla). **115 Getty Images:** Daniel Bosler. **118 Mother & Baby Picture Library:** Ian Hooton. **121 Mother & Baby Picture Library:** Ian Hooton. **123 Mother & Baby Picture Library:** Eddie Lawrence. **124 LOGIQlibrary. 125 LOGIQlibrary** (cl) (cr); **Patients and staff of St Mary's Hospital, Fetal Medicine Unit** (br). **126 Mother & Baby Picture Library:** Ian Hooton. **137 Professor Lesley Regan** (both). **141 Professor Lesley Regan** (r). **148 Mother & Baby Picture Library:** Ian Hooton. **149 Mother & Baby Picture Library:** Paul Mitchell. **150 Getty Images:** Steve Allen (l); **Prof. J.E. Jirasek MD, DSc.:** CRC Press/Parthenon (b). **150–151 Getty Images:** Ranald Mackechnie. **151 Prof. J.E. Jirasek MD, DSc.:** CRC Press/Parthenon (br); **Life Issues Institute** (tr). **152–153 Getty Images:** Steve Allen (both). **154 Science Photo Library:** Professor P.M. Motta & E. Vizza (cl); VVG (tl). **155 Science Photo Library:** GE Medical Systems (b). **158 Science Photo Library:** CNRI (bc); Edelmann (bl). **159 Alamy Images:** janine wiedel (bc); **Photonica:** Henrik Sorensen (bl). **162 Bubbles:** Angela Hampton. **163 Alamy Images:** Camera Press Ltd. **166–167 Science Photo Library:** Neil Bromhall (both). **168 OSF:** (bl); **Science Photo Library:** Neil Bromhall / Genesisi Films (br). **171 Science Photo Library:** DR P. Marazzi (cr); **Wellcome Library, London:** (br). **175 LOGIQlibrary** (l) (tl); **Professor Lesley Regan** (cr) (c). **176 Mother & Baby Picture Library:** Ian Hooton. **177 Alamy Images:** Camera Press Ltd. **179 Alamy Images:** Bubbles Photolibrary.

180–181 Prof. J.E. Jirasek MD, DSc.: CRC Press/Parthenon (both). **182–183 Prof. J.E. Jirasek MD, DSc.:** CRC Press/Parthenon (all). **185 Mother & Baby Picture Library:** Ruth Jenkinson. **187 Corbis:** Cameron. **189 LOGIQlibrary. 190 Mother & Baby Picture Library. 193 Alamy Images:** Bill Bachmann. **195 SuperStock. 197 Alamy Images:** Dan Atkin. **198 Corbis:** Jim Craigmyle. **199 Science Photo Library:** Ian Hooton. **200 LOGIQlibrary** (l) (c); **Science Photo Library:** Dr Najeeb Layyous (b). **200–201 Getty Images:** Jim Craigmyle. **201 LOGIQlibrary** (tr) (br). **202–203 Life Issues Institute** (both). **204 Science Photo Library:** BSIP, MARIGAUX. **205 Professor Lesley Regan** (bl). **211 Mother & Baby Picture Library:** Ian Hooton. **218 Oppo. 221 Mother & Baby Picture Library:** Ian Hooton. **223 Mother & Baby Picture Library:** Ian Hooton. **225 Alamy Images:** Camera Press Ltd. **227 Corbis:** Roy McMahon. **228 Getty Images:** Ross Whitaker. **230–231 Science Photo Library:** GE Medical Systems (both). **232 LOGIQlibrary** (br); **Science Photo Library:** GE Medical Systems (bl). **233 Alamy Images:** Nick Veasey x-ray. **236 Mother & Baby Picture Library:** Ian Hooton. **243 Alamy Images:** Stock Image. **246 Science Photo Library:** Colin Cuthbert. **248 Science Photo Library:** Mark Clarke. **249 Bubbles:** Moose Azim. **256 Mother & Baby Picture Library:** Caroline Molloy. **257 Professor Lesley Regan** (both). **260–261 Science Photo Library:** GE Medical Systems (both). **263 Science Photo Library:** Mehau Kulyk. **265 Mother & Baby Picture Library:** Ian Hooton. **271 Mother & Baby Picture Library:** Ian Hooton. **278–279 Alamy Images:** plainpicture/Kirch, S.. **280 Alamy Images:** plainpicture/Kirch, S.. **281 Corbis:** Jules Perrier. **282 Mother & Baby Picture Library:** Ian Hooton. **290–291 Science Photo Library:** BSIP, Laurent. **293 Mother & Baby Picture Library:** Ruth Jenkinson. **297 Mother & Baby Picture Library:** Ruth Jenkinson. **309 Mother & Baby Picture Library:** Ian Hooton. **314 Alamy Images:** Janine Wiedel. **322 Wellcome Library, London:** Anthea Sieveking. **324 Angela Hampton/Family Life Picture Library. 329 Wellcome Library, London:** Anthea Sieveking. **332 Mother & Baby Picture Library:** Moose Azim. **334 Science Photo Library:** CNRI. **336 Alamy Images:** Peter Usbeck. **337 Corbis:** Annie Griffiths Belt. **342 Corbis:** Tom Stewart. **343 Mother & Baby Picture Library. 344 Corbis:** ER Productions. **345 Professor Lesley Regan. 348 Mother & Baby Picture Library:** Indira Flack. **360 Alamy Images:** Yoav Levy. **368 Alamy Images:** Janine Wiedel. **370–371 Getty Images:** Kaz Mori. **372 Getty Images:** Rubberball Productions. **373 Alamy Images:** plainpicture/Kirch, S.. **374 Alamy Images:** Bubbles Photolibrary. **380 Alamy Images:** Shout (cl); **Mother & Baby Picture Library:** Ruth Jenkinson (tl). **381 PunchStock:** Brand X Pictures. **382 SuperStock. 390 Bubbles. 394 Corbis:** Don Mason. **399 Bubbles:** Loisjoy Thurstun. **402 Mother & Baby Picture Library:** Ian Hooton. **404 Alamy Images:** Janine Wiedel. **405 Alamy Images:** Peter Usbeck (l); Science Photo Library: Joseph Nettis (r). **406–407 Corbis:** Norbert Schaefer.

All other images © Dorling Kindersley
For further information see: www.dkimages.com

SPECIAL MESSAGE TO READERS

THE ULVERSCROFT FOUNDATION
(registered UK charity number 264873)
was established in 1972 to provide funds for
research, diagnosis and treatment of eye diseases.
Examples of major projects funded by
the Ulverscroft Foundation are:-

- The Children's Eye Unit at Moorfields Eye Hospital, London
- The Ulverscroft Children's Eye Unit at Great Ormond Street Hospital for Sick Children
- Funding research into eye diseases and treatment at the Department of Ophthalmology, University of Leicester
- The Ulverscroft Vision Research Group, Institute of Child Health
- Twin operating theatres at the Western Ophthalmic Hospital, London
- The Chair of Ophthalmology at the Royal Australian College of Ophthalmologists

You can help further the work of the Foundation
by making a donation or leaving a legacy.
Every contribution is gratefully received. If you
would like to help support the Foundation or
require further information, please contact:

THE ULVERSCROFT FOUNDATION
The Green, Bradgate Road, Anstey
Leicester LE7 7FU, England
Tel: (0116) 236 4325

website: www.foundation.ulverscroft.com

Born in Bedford, Ruth Hogan read everything she could get her hands on, from *The Lion, the Witch and the Wardrobe* to the backs of cereal packets and gravestones. She studied English and Drama at Goldsmiths College, and worked for ten years in local government, before a car accident left her unable to work full-time and convinced her to start writing seriously. Later, while undergoing chemotherapy and struggling to sleep at night, she passed the time by writing her debut novel, *The Keeper of Lost Things*. Ruth lives in a chaotic Victorian house with her partner and an assortment of rescue dogs. Her favourite word is 'antimacassar', and she still likes reading gravestones.

You can follow her on Facebook at
www.facebook.com/RuthMarieHogan
And on Twitter @ruthmariehogan

THE KEEPER OF LOST THINGS

Anthony Peardew is the Keeper of Lost Things. Forty years ago he carelessly lost a keepsake from his beloved Therese. That very same day, she died unexpectedly. Broken-hearted, Anthony sought consolation in rescuing lost objects — the things others have dropped, misplaced, or accidentally left behind — and writing stories about them. Now, in the twilight of his life, he worries that he has not fully discharged his duty to reconcile all the lost things with their owners. As the end nears, he bequeaths his secret life's mission to his unsuspecting housekeeper Laura, the one person he can trust to fulfil his legacy. But the final wishes of the Keeper of Lost Things have unforeseen repercussions that trigger a most serendipitous series of encounters . . .

RUTH HOGAN

THE KEEPER OF LOST THINGS

Complete and Unabridged

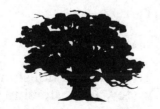

CHARNWOOD
Leicester

First published in Great Britain in 2017 by
Two Roads
An imprint of John Murray Press
London

First Charnwood Edition
published 2017
by arrangement with
John Murray Press
An Hachette UK company
London

A catalogue record for this book is available
from the British Library.

ISBN 978–1–4448–3320–1

Published by
F. A. Thorpe (Publishing)
Anstey, Leicestershire
Set by Words & Graphics Ltd.
Anstey, Leicestershire
Printed and bound in Great Britain by
T. J. International Ltd., Padstow, Cornwall

This book is printed on acid-free paper

To Bill, my faithful wingman,
and Princess Tilly Bean

But he, that dares not grasp the thorn
Should never crave the rose.

Anne Brontë

1

Charles Bramwell Brockley was travelling alone and without a ticket on the 14.42 from London Bridge to Brighton. The Huntley & Palmers biscuit tin in which he was travelling teetered precariously on the edge of the seat as the train juddered to a halt at Haywards Heath. But just as it toppled forward towards the carriage floor it was gathered up by a safe pair of hands.

★   ★   ★

He was glad to be home. Padua was a solid redbrick Victorian villa with honeysuckle and clematis framing the steeply pitched porch. The cool, rose-scented, echoing space of the entrance hall welcomed the man inside from the relentless glare of the afternoon sun. He put down his bag, replaced his keys in the drawer of the hall table and hung his panama on the hat stand. He was weary to the bone, but the quiet house soothed him. Quiet, but not silent. There was the steady tick of a long-case clock and the distant hum of an ancient refrigerator, and somewhere in the garden a blackbird sang. But the house was untainted by the tinnitus of technology. There was no computer, no television, no DVD or CD player. The only connections to the outside world were an old Bakelite telephone in the hall and a radio. In the kitchen, he let the tap run until the water was icy cold and then filled a tumbler. It was too early for gin and lime, and too hot for tea. Laura had gone home for the day, but she had left a note and a ham salad in the refrigerator for his supper. Dear girl. He gulped the water down.

Back in the hall, he took a single key from his trouser pocket and unlocked a heavy oak door. He retrieved his bag from the floor and entered the room, closing the door softly behind him. Shelves and drawers, shelves and drawers, shelves and drawers. Three walls were completely obscured and every shelf was laden and every drawer was full with a sad salmagundi of forty years gathered in, labelled and given a home. Lace panels dressed the French windows and diffused the brash light from the afternoon sun. A single shaft from the space between them pierced the gloom, glittering with specks of dust. The man took the Huntley & Palmers biscuit tin from his bag and placed it carefully on a large mahogany table, the only clear surface in the room. Lifting the lid, he inspected the contents, a pale grey substance the texture of coarse-grained sand. He had scattered the like many years ago in the rose garden at the back of the house. But surely these could not be human remains? Not left on a train in a biscuit tin? He replaced the lid. He had tried to hand them in at the station, but the ticket collector, cocksure that it was just litter, suggested that he put it in the nearest bin.

'You'd be amazed at the rubbish people leave on trains,' he said, dismissing Anthony with a shrug.

2

Nothing surprised Anthony any more, but loss always moved him, however great or small. From a drawer he took a brown paper luggage label and a gold-nibbed fountain pen. He wrote carefully in black ink; the date and time, and the place — very specific:

*Huntley & Palmers biscuit tin containing
cremation remains?
Found, sixth carriage from the front, 14.42
train from London Bridge to Brighton.
Deceased unknown. God bless and rest
in peace.*

He stroked the lid of the tin tenderly before finding a space on one of the shelves and gently sliding the tin into position.

The chime of the clock in the hall said time for gin and lime. He took ice cubes and lime juice from the refrigerator and carried them through to the garden room on a silver drinks tray with a green cocktail glass and a small dish of olives. He wasn't hungry but he hoped they might awaken his appetite. He didn't want to disappoint Laura by leaving her carefully prepared salad. He set the tray down and opened the window into the garden at the back of the house.

The gramophone player was a handsome wooden affair with a sweeping golden horn. He lifted the needle and placed it gently onto the liquorice-coloured disc. The voice of Al Bowlly floated up through the air and out into the garden to compete with the blackbird.

The very thought of you.

3

It had been their song. He released his long, loose limbs into the comfort of a leather wing-backed chair. In his prime, his bulk had matched his height, and he had been an impressive figure, but old age had diminished the flesh, and now skin lay much closer to bones. His glass in one hand, he toasted the woman whose silver-framed photograph he held in the other.

'Chin-chin, my darling girl!'

He took a sip from his drink and lovingly, longingly kissed the cold glass of the photograph before replacing it on the side table next to his chair. She was not a classic beauty; a young woman with wavy hair and large dark eyes that shone, even in an old black and white photograph. But she was wonderfully striking, with a presence that still reached out from all those years ago and captivated him. She had been dead for forty years, but she was still his life, and her death had given him his purpose. It had made Anthony Peardew the Keeper of Lost Things.

2

Laura had been lost; hopelessly adrift. Kept afloat, but barely, by an unhappy combination of Prozac, Pinot Grigio and pretending things weren't happening. Things like Vince's affair. Anthony Peardew and his house had saved her.

As she pulled up and parked outside the house, she calculated how long she had worked there — five, no almost six years. She had been sitting in her doctor's waiting room anxiously flicking through the magazines when an advertisement in the *Lady* had caught her attention:

Housekeeper/Personal Assistant
required for gentleman writer.
Please apply in writing to Anthony
Peardew — PO Box 27312

She had entered the waiting room intending to plead for more drugs to make her unhappy existence more bearable, and left it determined to apply for a position that would, it turned out, transform her life.

As she turned her key in the lock and stepped through the front door, the peace of the house embraced her as it always did. She went through to the kitchen, filled the kettle and set it on the hob. Anthony would be out on his morning walk. She hadn't seen him at all yesterday. He had been to London to see his solicitor. Waiting for the kettle to boil, she leafed through the neat pile of paperwork he had left for her to deal with: a few bills to pay, some letters to answer on his behalf and a request to make an appointment with his doctor. She felt a prickle of anxiety. She had tried not to see him fading over the past months, like a fine portrait left too long in harsh sunlight, losing clarity and colour. When he had interviewed her all those years ago, he had been a tall, muscular man with a full head of dark hair, tanzanite eyes and a voice like James Mason. She had thought him much younger than his sixty-eight years.

Laura had fallen in love with both Mr Peardew and the house moments after stepping through the door. The love she felt for him was not the romantic kind, but more the love of a child for a favourite uncle. His gentle strength, tranquil manner and immaculate urbanity were all qualities that she had learned, albeit a little late, to appreciate in a man. His presence always lifted her spirits and made her value her life in a way that she hadn't for a very long time. He was a comforting constant, like Radio 4, Big Ben and 'Land of Hope and Glory'. But always very slightly distant. There was a part of himself which he never revealed; a secret always kept. Laura was glad. Intimacy, both physical and emotional, had always been a disappointment to her. Mr Peardew was the perfect employer who had become Anthony, a dear friend. But one who never came too close.

As for Padua, it was the tray cloth that made

Laura fall in love with the house. Anthony had made her tea at her interview. He had brought it into the garden room; teapot with cosy, milk jug, sugar bowl and tongs, cups and saucers, silver teaspoons, tea strainer and stand. All set out on a tray with a tray cloth. Pure white, lace-edged linen. The tray cloth was definitive. Padua was clearly a house where all these things, including the tray cloth, were part of everyday life; and Mr Peardew was a man whose everyday life was exactly the kind that Laura longed for. When they were first married, Vince had teased her about her attempts to introduce such things into their own home. If he was ever forced to make his own tea, he abandoned the used teabag on the draining board, no matter how many times Laura asked him to put it in the bin. He drank milk and fruit juice straight from the carton, ate with his elbows on the table, held his knife like a pen and spoke with his mouth full. Each on its own was a small thing, like the many other small things he did and said that Laura tried to ignore, but nonetheless chafed her soul. Over the years, their accumulation in both number and frequency hardened Laura's heart and stymied her gentle aspirations for even modest fragments of the life she had once sampled in the homes of her school friends. When Vince's teasing eventually curdled into mocking, a tray cloth to him became an object worthy only of derision. And so did Laura.

The interview had taken place on the day of her thirty-fifth birthday and had been surprisingly brief. Mr Peardew had asked her how she

7

took her tea and then poured it. There had been precious few other questions from either party before he had offered Laura the job and she had accepted. It had been the perfect present, and the beginning of hope for Laura.

The whistle of the kettle pierced her reminiscence. Laura took her tea, along with a duster and some polish, through to the garden room. She hated cleaning at home, especially when she had shared a home with Vince. But here it was an act of love. When she had first arrived, the house and its contents were gently neglected. Not dirty or shabby, just vaguely overlooked. Many of the rooms were unused. Anthony spent most of his time in the garden room or his study, and never had any guests to stay in the extra bedrooms. Softly, gently, room by room, Laura had loved the house back into life. Except the study. She had never been in the study. Anthony had told her at the start that nobody went into the study except him, and when he wasn't in there it was kept locked. She had never questioned it. But all the other rooms were kept clean and bright and ready for anyone to enjoy, even if no one ever came.

In the garden room, Laura picked up the silver-framed photograph and buffed the glass and silver until it shone. Anthony had told her that the woman's name was Therese, and Laura knew that he must have loved her very much because hers was one of only three photographs on display throughout the whole house. The others were copies of a picture of Anthony and Therese together, one of which he kept on a small table next to his bed, and the other on the dressing table in the big bedroom at the back of the house. In all the years she had known him she had never seen him look as happy in life as he did in that photograph.

When Laura left Vince, the last thing she had done was to chuck the large framed photograph of their wedding into the bin. But not before she had stamped on it, grinding the smashed glass into his smirking face with her heel. Selina from 'Servicing' was welcome to him. He was a complete and utter arsehole. It was the first time she had really admitted it, even to herself. It didn't make her feel any better. It just made her sad that she had wasted so many years with him. But with an unfinished education, no real work experience and no other means of supporting herself, there had been little choice.

When she had finished in the garden room, Laura went through to the hallway and started up the stairs, stroking a golden gleam from the curved wooden banister with her duster as she went. She had often wondered about the study; of course she had. But she respected Anthony's privacy as he respected hers. Upstairs, the largest bedroom was also the handsomest and had a bay window that overlooked the back garden. It was the room Anthony had once shared with Therese, but now he slept in the smaller room next door. Laura opened the window to let in some air. The roses in the garden below were in full bloom; undulating ruffles of scarlet, pink and creamy petals, and the surrounding borders frothed with fluttering peonies punctuated with

9

sapphire lances of larkspur. The scent of the roses floated upwards on the warm air and Laura breathed deeply, taking in the heady perfume. But this room always smelled of roses. Even in mid-winter when the garden was frozen and asleep, and the windows sealed with frost. Laura straightened and stroked the already perfect bedcovers and plumped the cushions on the ottoman. The green glass dressing-table set sparkled in the sunlight, but was lovingly dusted nonetheless. But not everything in the room was perfect. The little blue enamelled clock had stopped again. 11.55 and no ticking. Every day it stopped at the same time. Laura checked her watch and reset the hands on the clock. She carefully wound the small key until the soft ticking resumed, and then returned it to its place on the dressing table.

The sound of the front door closing signalled Anthony's return from his walk. It was followed by the unlocking, opening and closing of the study door. It was a sequence of sounds with which Laura was very familiar. In the kitchen she made a pot of coffee that she set out on a tray with a cup and saucer, a silver jug of cream and a plate of digestive biscuits. She took it through to the hall and knocked gently on the study door and when it was opened passed the tray to Anthony. He looked tired; etiolated rather than invigorated by his walk.

'Thank you, my dear.'

She noticed unhappily that his hands shook slightly as he took the tray from hers.

'Is there anything in particular that you'd like

10

for lunch?' she asked coaxingly.

'No, no. I'm sure whatever you decide will be delicious.'

The door closed. Back in the kitchen, Laura washed up the dirty mug that had appeared in the sink — left, no doubt, by Freddy, the gardener. He had started working at Padua a couple of years ago but their paths rarely crossed, which was disappointing for Laura, as she had the feeling that she might like to get to know him better. He was tall and dark, but not so handsome as to be a cliché. He had a faint scar which ran vertically between his nose and top lip, and puckered his mouth a little on one side, but somehow its effect was to add rather than detract, giving his smile a particular lopsided charm. He was affable enough when they did bump into one another, but no more so than politeness demanded, giving Laura little encouragement to pursue his friendship.

Laura started on the pile of paperwork. She would take the letters home with her and type them on her laptop. When she had first worked for Anthony, she used to proofread his manuscripts and type them on an old electric typewriter, but he had stopped writing several years ago now and she missed it. When she was younger, she had thought about writing as a career; novels, or maybe journalism. She had had all sorts of plans. She was a clever girl with a scholarship to the local girls' school followed by a place at university. She could have — should have — made a proper life for herself. But instead she met Vince. At seventeen she was still

11

vulnerable, unformed; unsure of her own worth. She was happy at school, but the scholarship meant that she was always slightly displaced. Her factory worker father and shop assistant mother were so proud of their clever daughter. Money was found — scraped together — to buy every item of her expensive school uniform; unheard-of unnecessaries like indoor and out-door shoes. Everything had to be new. Nothing second-hand for their girl, and she was grateful, truly she was. She knew only too well the sacrifices that her parents had made. But it wasn't enough. Being bright and beautifully presented was never quite enough for her to slip seamlessly into the society of those who formed the rank and file of the school's assembly. Girls for whom holidays abroad, trips to the theatre, supper parties and sailing weekends were commonplace. Of course she made friends, girls who were kind and generous, and she accepted their invitations to stay at grand houses with their kind and generous parents. Grand houses where tea was served in pots, toast in racks, butter in dishes, milk in jugs and jam with a silver spoon. Houses with names instead of numbers that had terraces, tennis courts and topiary. And tray cloths. She saw a different kind of life and was enchanted. Her hopes were raised. At home, the milk in a bottle, the marge in a tub, the sugar in a bag and the tea in a mug were all stones in her pockets, weighing her down. At seventeen she had fallen into the space between the two worlds and there was nowhere left she truly belonged. And then she met Vince.

He was older; handsome, cocksure and ambitious. She was flattered by his attentions and impressed by his certainty. Vince was certain about everything. He even had a nickname for himself: Vince the Invincible. He was a car dealer and drove a red Jaguar E-Type; a cliché on wheels. Laura's parents were quietly distraught. They had hoped that her education would be the key to a better life for her; better than theirs. A life with more living and less struggling. They may not have understood about tray cloths, but they knew that the kind of life they wished for Laura was about more than just money. For Laura, it was never about the money. For Vince the Invincible, it was only ever about money and status. Laura's father soon had his own private nickname for Vince Darby: VD.

Unhappy years later, Laura often wondered what it was that Vince had seen in her. She was a pretty girl, but not beautiful, and certainly not the teeth, tits and arse combination he usually favoured. The kind of girls Vince normally dated dropped their knickers as naturally as they dropped their aitches. Perhaps he had seen her as a challenge. Or a novelty. Whatever it was, it was enough for him to think that she would make him a good wife. Eventually, she came to suspect that his marriage proposal was driven as much by his desire for status as it was by physical desire. Vince had plenty of money, but alone it wasn't enough to get him into the Freemasons or elected chair of the golf club. With her beautiful manners and private school education, Laura was intended to bring a sheen of social sophistication to his brass. He was to be bitterly disappointed. But not as much as Laura.

When she first found out about Vince's affair, it had been easy to blame him for everything; to cast him as some Austen-esque cad about town with Laura as the virtuous heroine left at home to knit spare toilet-roll covers or sew ribbons on her bonnet. But somewhere deep down Laura knew that that was really fiction. Desperate for refuge from an unsatisfactory reality she had asked her doctor for antidepressants, but he had insisted that she see a counsellor before handing over the drugs. For Laura it was a means to an end. She fully expected to run rings round a mousey, middle-aged, polyester Pamela to procure her prescription. What she got was a sassy, sharp-suited blonde called Rudi who forced her to face some rather unpalatable facts. She told Laura to listen to the voice inside her head; the one that pointed out inconvenient truths and raised uncomfortable arguments. Rudi called it 'engaging with her internal linguistics' and said that it would be 'a very gratifying experience' for Laura. Laura called it consorting with the Truth Fairy and found it as gratifying as listening to her favourite record with a deep scratch in it. The Truth Fairy had a very suspicious nature. She accused Laura of buckling under the weight of parental expectations, of marrying Vince in part to avoid going to university. In her opinion, Laura was afraid of going to university in case she failed; afraid to stand on her own two feet in case she fell flat on her face. She also raised the unhappy memory of

Laura's miscarriage and subsequent, almost obsessive and ultimately unsuccessful quest for a baby. In truth, the Truth Fairy unsettled Laura. But when she got her Prozac she had stopped listening.

The clock in the hallway struck one and Laura began gathering ingredients for lunch. She beat eggs and cheese together with fresh herbs from the garden, tipped the mixture into a hot pan on the stove and watched it froth and bubble and then settle into a fluffy, golden omelette. The tray was set with a crisp, white linen napkin, a silver knife and fork and a glass of elderflower cordial. At the door of the study, she swapped it with Anthony for the remains of his morning coffee. The biscuits had not been touched.

3

Eunice

Forty years earlier . . . May 1974

She had decided on the cobalt blue trilby. Her grandmother had once told her that one could blame ugliness on one's genes and ignorance on one's education, but there was absolutely no excuse whatsoever for being dull. School had been dull. Eunice had been a clever girl, but restless; too bored in lessons to do well. She wanted excitement; a life less lifeless. The office where she worked was dull, full of dull people, and so too was her job: endless typing and filing. Respectable, her parents called it, but that was just another word for dull. Her only escape was in films and books. She read as though her life depended on it.

Eunice had seen the advertisement in the *Lady*:

Assistant required for established publisher.
Wages woeful but work never dull!

The job was obviously meant for her and she applied the same day.

Her interview was at 12.15 p.m., and she had allowed herself plenty of time to get there, so now she could walk the remainder of the way at her leisure, gathering in the sights and sounds of the city to furnish future memories. The streets were crowded and Eunice drifted through the homogeneous flow of humanity, occasionally struck by a figure who, for some reason, bobbed above the surface of the indeterminate tide. She nodded at the whistling waiter sweeping the pavement outside The Swish Fish restaurant, and swerved to avoid an unpleasant collision with a fat and sweaty tourist too busy studying her *A–Z* to watch where she was going. She noticed and smiled at the tall man waiting on the corner of Great Russell Street because he looked nice, but worried. In the moment she passed him, she gathered in everything about him. He was well built and handsome with blue eyes and the bearing of a good man. He was anxiously checking his watch and looking up and down the street. He was clearly waiting for someone, and they were late.

Eunice was still early. It was only 11.55 a.m. She strolled on. Her thoughts drifted to the approaching interview and interviewer. She hoped that he would look like the man she had left waiting on the corner. But perhaps it would be a woman; a sharp, spiky unfolded paperclip of a woman with black bobbed hair and red lipstick. As she reached the glossed green door of the address she had been given on Bloomsbury Street she barely noticed the crowd gathered on the pavement opposite and the distant keen of a siren. She pressed the buzzer and waited; back straight, feet together, head held high. She heard the sound of footsteps bounding down stairs and

17

the door was flung open.

Eunice fell in love with the man as soon as she saw him. His physical components were individually unremarkable: medium height, medium build, light brown hair, pleasant face, two eyes and ears, one nose and mouth. But in composition they were magically transformed into a masterpiece. He grasped her hand as though to save her from drowning and pulled her up the stairs behind him. Breathless with exertion and enthusiasm he greeted her on the way up with: 'You must be Eunice. Delighted to meet you. Call me Bomber. Everyone does.'

The office that they burst into at the top of the stairs was large and light and very well organised. Shelves and drawers lined the walls and three filing cabinets stood beneath the window. Eunice was intrigued to see that they were labelled 'Tom', 'Dick' and 'Harry'.

'After the tunnels,' Bomber explained, following her gaze and registering the query on her face. The query remained.

'*The Great Escape*? Steve McQueen, Dickie Attenborough, bags of dirt, barbed wire and a motorbike?'

Eunice smiled.

'You *have* seen it, haven't you? Bloody marvellous!' He began whistling the theme music.

Eunice was resolute. This was definitely the job for her. She would chain herself to one of the filing cabinets if necessary to secure it. Fortunately it wasn't. The fact that she had seen *The Great Escape* and was a fan was apparently enough. Bomber made them a pot of tea in the

18

tiny kitchen that adjoined the office to celebrate her appointment. A strange rolling rattle followed him back into the room. The sound was made by a small tan and white terrier with one ear at half mast and a brown patch over his left eye. He was seated on a wooden trolley affair with two wheels and pulled himself along by walking with his front legs.

'Meet Douglas. My right-hand man. Well, dog.'

'Good afternoon, Douglas,' Eunice greeted him solemnly. 'Bader, I presume.'

Bomber thumped the table with delight. 'I knew right away that you were the one. Now, how do you like your tea?'

Over tea and biscuits (Douglas drank his from a saucer) Eunice learned that Bomber had found Douglas abandoned as a puppy after he had been hit by a car. The vet had advised that he be put to sleep, but Bomber had brought him home instead.

'I made the jalopy myself. It's more Morris 1000 Traveller than Mercedes, but it does the job.'

They agreed that Eunice would start the following week on a salary that was perfectly adequate rather than 'woeful', and that her duties would include just about anything that needed doing. Eunice was euphoric. But just as she was gathering her things to leave, the door burst open and the unfolded paperclip woman strode into the room. She was an inelegant zigzag of nose, elbows and knees; unsoftened by any cushioning flesh and with a face which had, over the years, sunk into a permanent sneer.

'I see that deformed little rat of yours is still

alive,' she exclaimed, gesturing at Douglas with her cigarette as she flung her bag down onto a chair. Catching sight of Eunice, a twisted smile flitted across her face.

'Good God, brother! Don't tell me that you've found yourself a paramour.' She spat the word out as though it were a grape pip.

Bomber addressed her with weary patience. 'This is Eunice, my new assistant. Eunice, this is my sister, Portia.'

She looked Eunice up and down with her cold grey eyes, but didn't offer her hand. 'I should say that I'm pleased to meet you, but it would probably be a lie.'

'Likewise,' Eunice replied. It was barely audible and Portia had already turned her attention to her brother, but Eunice could have sworn that she saw the tip of Douglas's tail wag. She left Bomber to his odious sister and tripped downstairs into the bright afternoon sunshine. The last thing she heard as she closed the door behind her was from Portia, in an altogether changed, but still unpleasant, wheedling tone:

'Now, darling, when are you going to publish my book?'

At the corner of Great Russell Street she stopped for a moment, remembering the man she had smiled at. She hoped that the person he was meeting hadn't left him waiting for too long. Just then, in amongst the dust and dirt at her feet, the glint of gold and glass caught her eye. She stooped down, rescued the small, round object from the gutter and slipped it safely into her pocket.

4

It was always the same. Looking down and never turning his face to the sky, he searched the pavements and gutters. His back burned and his eyes watered, full of grit and tears. And then he fell; back through the black into the damp and twisted sheets of his own bed. The dream was always the same. Endlessly searching and never finding the one thing that would finally bring him peace.

The house was filled with the deep, soft darkness of a summer night. Anthony swung his weary legs out of bed and sat shrugging the stubborn scraps of dream from his head. He would have to get up. Sleep would not return tonight. He padded down the stairs, their creaking wood echoing his aching bones. No light was needed until he reached the kitchen. He made a pot of tea, finding more comfort in the making than the drinking, and took it through to the study. Pale moonlight skimmed across the edges of the shelves and pooled in the centre of the mahogany table. High on a shelf in the corner, the gold lid of the biscuit tin winked at him as he crossed the room. He took it down carefully and set it in the shimmering circle of light on the table. Of all the things that he had ever found, this troubled him the most. Because it was not a 'something' but a 'someone'; of that he was unreasonably sure. Once again, he removed the lid and inspected the contents, as he had done every day for the past week since bringing it home. He had already repositioned the tin in the study several times, placing it higher up or hidden from sight, but its draw remained irresistible. He couldn't leave it alone. He dipped his hand into the tin and gently rolled the coarse, grey grains across his fingertips. The memory swept through him, snatching his breath and winding him as surely as any punch to the gut. Once again, he was holding death in his hands.

The life they could have had together was a self-harming fantasy in which Anthony rarely indulged. They might have been grandparents by now. Therese had never spoken about wanting children, but then they had both assumed that they had the indubitable tenure of time. A tragic complacency, as it turned out. She had always wanted a dog. Anthony had held out for as long as he could, blustering about damage to the rose garden and excavations in the lawn. But she had won him round in the end, as she always did, with a fatal cocktail of charm and sheer bloody-mindedness. They were due to collect the dog from Battersea the week after she died. Instead Anthony spent the day wandering through the empty house desperately gathering in any traces of her presence; the indent of her head on a pillow; Titian strands in her hairbrush and a smudge of scarlet lipstick on a glass. Paltry but precious proof of a life now extinguished. In the miserable months that followed, Padua fought to keep the echoes of her existence within its walls. Anthony would come into a room feeling that she had, only moments before, left it. Day after day he played hide-and-seek with her shadow. He heard her music in the garden room, caught her laughter in the garden and felt her kiss on his mouth in the dark. But gradually, imperceptibly, infinitesimally she let him be. She let him make a life without her. The trace that lingered, and still remained to this day, was the scent of roses in places where it could not be.

Anthony brushed the grey powder from his fingertips and replaced the lid on the tin. One day this would be him. Perhaps that was why the ashes troubled him so much. He must not be lost like this poor soul in the tin. He had to be with Therese.

* * *

Laura lay wide awake with her eyes clenched shut in fruitless pursuit of sleep. The worries and doubts that daytime activity kept at bay came sneaking back under cover of darkness, unpicking the threads of her comfortable life like moths on a cashmere sweater. The slam of a front door and loud voices and laughter from the neighbouring flat crushed any fragile hope of sleep that remained. The couple who had moved in next door enjoyed a busy and rowdy social life at the expense of their fellow residents. Within minutes of their return, accompanied by a dozen or so fellow party animals, the thin walls of Laura's flat began to pulse to the relentless throb of drum and bass.

23

'Sweet Jesus — not again!'

Laura swung her legs out of bed and drummed her heels against the side of the divan in frustration. It was the third time this week. She had tried reasoning with them. She had threatened them with the police. In the end, and rather to her shame, she had resorted to yelling expletives. Their response was always the same: gushing apologies laced with empty promises followed by no change whatsoever. They simply ignored her. Perhaps she should consider letting down the tyres on their Golf GTi or shoving horse manure through their letter box. She smiled to herself in spite of her anger. Where on earth would she get horse manure from?

In the kitchen, Laura warmed milk in one saucepan to make hot chocolate, and with another she beat an exasperated tattoo on the party wall. A chunk of plaster the size of a dinner plate dislodged and smashed onto the floor.

'Shit!'

Laura scowled accusingly at the saucepan still clenched in her hand. There was a hiss of burning milk as the contents of the other saucepan boiled over.

'Shit! Shit! Shit!'

Having cleared up the mess and heated some more milk, Laura sat at the table cradling her warm mug. She could feel the clouds gathering about her and the ground slipping beneath her feet. There was a storm coming, of that she was certain. It wasn't just the neighbours who were troubling her; it was Anthony, too. Over the past weeks something had changed. His physical decline was gradual; inevitable with age, but there was something else. An indefinable shift. She felt as though he was pulling away from her like a disenchanted lover secretly packing a suitcase, preparing to leave. If she lost Anthony, then she would lose Padua too, and together they offered her asylum from the madness that was the real world.

Since her divorce, the precious few bearings that had set her course through life had drifted away. Having given up university and the chance of a writing career to marry Vince, she had hoped for children and all that motherhood would bring and later, perhaps, an Open University degree. But none of these had happened. She had fallen pregnant just once. The prospect of a child had temporarily shored up their already crumbling marriage. Vince had spared no expense and completed the nursery in a single weekend. The following week Laura had miscarried. The next few years were spent doggedly trying to replace the child that was never born. The sex became grim and dutiful. They subjected themselves to all the necessary invasive and undignified medical interventions to determine where the problem lay, but the results were all normal. Vince became angry more than sad that he couldn't have what he thought he wanted. Eventually, and by then to Laura's relief, the sex stopped altogether.

It was then that she began to plan her escape. When she had married Vince, he insisted that there was no need for her to work, and by the time it became clear that she was not going to be

25

a mother, Laura's lack of experience and qualifications were a significant problem when she began looking for a job. And she had needed a job, because she needed money. She needed money to leave Vince. Laura just wanted enough to get a flat and be able to keep herself; to slip away one day when Vince was at work and then divorce him from a safe distance. But the only job she could get was part-time and low paid. It wasn't enough and so she started writing, dreaming of a bestseller. She worked on her novel every day for hours, always hiding any evidence from Vince. In six months it was complete and with high hopes Laura began submitting it to agents. Six months later, the pile of rejection letters and emails was almost as thick as the novel itself. They were depressingly consistent. Laura's writing had more style than substance. She wrote 'beautifully' but her plot was too 'quiet'. In desperation, she answered an advertisement in a women's magazine. It guaranteed an income for writers who could produce short stories to a specific format for a niche publication which was enjoying a rapidly expanding readership. The deposit for Laura's flat was eventually paid for by an embarrassing and extensive catalogue of cloying erotica written for *Feathers, Lace and Fantasy Fiction* — 'a magazine for hot women with burning desires'.

When she began working at Padua, Laura stopped writing. The short stories were, thankfully, no longer necessary to provide an income and her novel ended up in the recycling bin. She had lost all confidence to begin another. In her darkest moments, Laura wondered to what extent she had engineered her own failures. Had she become a habitual coward, afraid to climb in case she fell? At Padua with Anthony she didn't have to think about it. The house was her emotional and physical fortress, and Anthony her shining knight.

She poked with her fingertip at the skin forming on the surface of her hot chocolate as it cooled. Without Anthony and Padua she would be lost.

5

Anthony swirled the gin and lime round in his glass and listened to the ice cubes tinkling in the colourless liquid. It was barely noon, but the cold alcohol woke what little fire was left in his veins, and he needed it now. He took a sip and then set the glass down on the table amongst the labelled bric-a-brac which he had taken from one of the drawers. He was saying goodbye to the things. He felt small in the gnarled oak carver, like a boy wearing his father's overcoat, but aware as he was of his own diminution he was not afraid. Because now, he had a plan.

When he had started gathering lost things all those years ago, he hadn't really had a plan. He just wanted to keep them safe in case one day they could be reunited with the people who had lost them. Often he didn't know if what he had found was trash or treasure. But someone somewhere did. And then he had started writing again; weaving short stories around the things he found. Over the years he had filled his drawers and shelves with fragments of other people's lives, and somehow they had helped to mend his, so cruelly shattered, and make it whole again. Not picture perfect, of course not, after what had happened — a life still scarred and cracked and misshapen, but worth living nonetheless. A life with patches of blue sky amidst the grey, like the patch of sky he now held in his hand. He had

28

found it in the gutter of Copper Street twelve years ago, according to its label. It was a single piece of a jigsaw puzzle; bright blue with a fleck of white on one edge. It was just a scrap of coloured cardboard. Most people wouldn't even have noticed it, and those who did would have dismissed it as rubbish. But Anthony knew that for someone, its loss could be incalculable. He turned the jigsaw piece over in the palm of his hand. Where did it belong?

Jigsaw puzzle piece, blue with white fleck.
Found in the gutter, Copper Street,
24 September . . .

They had the wrong names. Maud was such a modest little mouse of a name, quite unlike the woman who owned it. To have called her strident would have been a compliment. And Gladys, so bright and cheery sounding; it even had the word 'glad' in it. But the poor woman it described seldom had any reason to be glad now. The sisters lived unhappily together in a neat terraced house in Copper Street. It had been their parents' house and the place where they had both been born and brought up. Maud had entered the world as she had meant to carry on in it: loud, unattractive and demanding attention. Her parents' firstborn, she had been indulged until it was too late to salvage any sensitivity or selflessness in her character. She became and remained the only person of any significance in her world. Gladys was a quiet, contented baby, which was just as

29

well as her mother could barely accommodate her basic needs whilst coping with the inexhaustible demands of her four-year-old sister. When, at eighteen, Maud found a suitor almost as disagreeable as herself, the family breathed a collective and only very slightly guilty sigh of relief. Their engagement and marriage were enthusiastically encouraged, particularly when it transpired that Maud's fiancé would have to relocate to Scotland for his business interests. After an expensive, showy wedding, chosen and then criticised by Maud and entirely paid for by her parents, she left to inflict herself upon an unsuspecting town in the far west of Scotland, and life at Copper Street became gentle contentment. Gladys and her parents lived quietly and happily. They ate fish and chips for supper on Fridays, and salmon sandwiches and fruit salad with tinned cream for Sunday tea. They went to the pictures every Thursday night and to Frinton for a week each summer. Sometimes Gladys went dancing at the Co-op with her friends. She bought a budgerigar, named him Cyril and never married. It wasn't her choice; simply a consequence of never being given the choice. She had found the right man for her, but unfortunately the right woman for him had turned out to be one of Gladys's friends. Gladys had made her own bridesmaid dress and toasted their happiness with champagne and salty tears. She remained a friend to them both and became godmother to their two children.

Maud and her husband had no children.

'Bloody good job too,' her father remarked quietly to Cyril if the topic were ever raised.

As her parents grew older and frailer, Gladys took care of them. She nursed them, fed and washed them, kept them comfortable and safe. Maud stayed in Scotland and sent the occasional useless gift. But when they eventually died, she found the funerals very upsetting. The contents of the Post Office savings account were divided equally between the two sisters, and in recognition of her devotion her parents left their home to Gladys. But the will had a catastrophic codicil. It stated that if Maud should ever become homeless, she could live in the house in Copper Street until her circumstances improved. It had been kindly meant to make provision for a circumstance that her parents had believed to be most unlikely, and more easily included for that reason. But 'most unlikely' is not impossible, and when Maud's husband died he left her homeless, penniless and speechless with rage. He had gambled away every asset they possessed and, rather than face Maud, he had then deliberately died.

Maud returned to Copper Street an old-woman-shaped vessel of vitriol. The peaceful, happy life that Gladys enjoyed was destroyed the moment Maud arrived at the front door demanding money from her sister to pay the taxi driver. Untempered by any trace of gratitude, Maud invited misery as a permanent house guest. With her accomplished repertoire of tiny tortures she tormented her sister at every turn. She put sugar in her tea, knowing full well that Gladys didn't take it, overwatered the house plants and left a trail of mess and chaos in her wake. She refused to lift a finger to help with any of the chores, and sat all day growing fat and flatulent, eating fudge, doing jigsaw puzzles and listening to the radio at full blast. Gladys's friends stopped coming to the house and she went out as often as she dared. But her return was always met with a punishment; a precious ornament 'accidentally' smashed or a favourite dress inexplicably burned with the iron. Maud even frightened away from the garden the birds that her sister had lovingly fed by leaving out scraps for the neighbour's cat. Gladys could never disregard her parents' wishes, and any attempts to reason or remonstrate with her sister were met with disdain or violence. To Gladys, Maud was a death-watch beetle; an unwelcome parasite who had invaded her home and turned her happiness into dust.

And she tapped. Just like a death-watch beetle she tapped. Pudgy fingers tapping on the table, the arm of the chair, the edge of the sink. The tapping became the worst torture of all: incessant and invasive, it haunted Gladys day and night. Macbeth may have murdered sleep, but Maud murdered peace. That day she sat at the dining-room table tapping as she contemplated the huge half-completed jigsaw puzzle in front of her. It was Constable's The Hay Wain — a monstrous reproduction of one thousand pieces and the largest she had ever attempted. It was going to be her masterpiece.

She squatted toad-like in front of the puzzle, a surplus of buttocks spilling over the edges of a chair groaning under her weight, and tapped.

Gladys closed the front door quietly behind her and set off down Copper Street, smiling as the wind whisked and twirled the crispy autumn leaves along the gutter. In her pocket her fingers felt around the edges of a small scrap of cardboard, machine cut, blue with a tiny fleck of white.

Anthony's fingers traced the edges of the jigsaw piece in the palm of his hand and he wondered whose life it had once been a tiny part of. Or perhaps not so tiny. Perhaps its loss had been disproportionately disastrous to its size, causing tears to flow, tempers to flare or hearts to break. So it had been with Anthony and the thing that he had lost so long ago. In the eyes of the world it was a gimcrack, small and worthless; but to Anthony it was precious beyond measure. Its loss was a daily torment tapping on his shoulder: a merciless reminder of the promise he had broken. The only promise that Therese had ever extracted from him, and he had failed her. And so he had started to gather the things that other people lost. It was his only chance for atonement. It had worried him greatly that he had not found a way to reunite any of the things with their owners. Over the years he had tried: advertisements in the local press and newsletters, and even entries in the personal columns of the broadsheets, none of which had produced any response. And now there was very little time left.

But he hoped that he had at last found someone to take over: someone young enough and bright enough to have new ideas; someone who would find a way to return the lost things to where they belonged. He had seen his solicitor and made the necessary adjustments to his will. He leaned back into his chair and stretched, feeling the hard wooden struts press into his spine. High on its shelf, the biscuit tin gleamed, burnished by early-evening sun. He was so tired. He felt that he had overstayed his time, but had he done enough? Perhaps it was time for him to talk to Laura, to tell her that he was leaving. He dropped the jigsaw piece onto the table and took up his gin and lime. He had to tell her soon, before it was too late.

6

Eunice

June 1974

Eunice dropped the keys of the petty cash tin back into their rightful place and closed the drawer. Her drawer. In her desk. Eunice had worked for Bomber for a whole month now, and he had sent her out to buy iced buns for the three of them so that they could celebrate. The month had flown past with Eunice arriving earlier and leaving later each day, stretching her time in a place and with company that made her feel ignited with exciting possibilities. In those four short weeks she had learned that Bomber was a fair and generous boss, passionate about his job, his dog and films. He was also her matinée idol. He had a habit of quoting lines from his favourite films and Eunice was beginning to follow suit. Her taste was more contemporary, but he was teaching her to appreciate some of Ealing Studios' finest, and already she had piqued his interest sufficiently for him to see a couple of newer releases at the local cinema. They agreed that *Kind Hearts and Coronets* was utterly marvellous and *Brief Encounter* tragic; *The Exorcist* was shocking but the spinning-head bit hilarious; *The Wicker Man* chilling, *The Optimists of Nine Elms* magical

35

and *Don't Look Now* atmospheric and haunting, but with rather excessive exposure of Donald Sutherland's naked buttocks. Eunice was even considering the purchase of a red duffle coat like the one worn by the dwarf in the film and doing some haunting of her own. And, of course, *The Great Escape* was perfection. Bomber said that the wonderful thing about books was that they were films that played inside your head. Eunice had also learned that Douglas liked to go for a little stroll at 11.00 a.m., particularly if it took him past the bakery that sold such delicious iced buns, and that he always ate the icing first and then the bun. And finally, she had learned that poisonous Portia was every bit as odious as a bowl of rotting offal.

Bomber was in the kitchen making the tea and Douglas was chivvying him along by dribbling on his conker-coloured Loake brogues in anticipation of an iced bun. From the window, Eunice watched the street below, today bustling with life, but only recently paralysed by a death; pedestrians and traffic stopped in their tracks by a heart stopping forever before their very eyes. According to Mrs Doyle in the bakery, Eunice had been there. But she hadn't seen a thing. Mrs Doyle recalled the exact date and time, and every detail of what had happened. As an ardent fan of police dramas on the television she prided herself on being an excellent potential eyewitness, should the occasion ever arise. Mrs Doyle inspected unfamiliar customers carefully, committing to memory lazy eyes, thin moustaches, gold teeth and left-sided partings, all of which she believed to be signs of a questionable moral character. And women with red shoes and green handbags were never to be trusted. The young woman who had died had had neither. Dressed in a powder-blue summer coat with matching shoes and handbag, she had collapsed and died right there outside the bakery against a backdrop of Mrs Doyle's finest cakes and pastries. It had happened on the day of Eunice's interview at 11.55 a.m. exactly. Mrs Doyle was sure of the time because she'd had a batch of Bath buns in the oven that was due out at twelve.

'They were burned to buggery hell,' Mrs Doyle told Eunice. 'I was too busy phoning the ambulance to remember the buns, but I don't blame her. It wasn't her fault that she went and dropped dead, poor love. The ambulance came quick enough, but she was already gone when it got here. Not a mark on her, mind you. Heart attack I 'spect. My Bert says it could have been an annualism, but my money's on a heart attack. Or a stroke.'

Eunice could remember a crowd gathered and a distant siren, but that was all. She was sad to think that the best day of her life so far had been the last day of someone else's, and all that had separated them had been a few feet of tarmac.

'Tea up!' Bomber plonked the tray down on the table. 'Shall I be mother?'

Bomber poured the tea and dished out the iced buns. Douglas settled down with his bun gripped between his paws and set to work on the icing.

'Now, my dear girl, tell me what you think of

old Pontpool's latest offering. Is it any good or shall we chuck it on the slippery slope?'

It was Bomber's name for the slush pile of rejected manuscripts. The scrap-heap of stories invariably grew so high, so quickly, that it avalanched onto the floor before anyone transferred it to the bin. Percy Pontpool was an aspiring children's author and Bomber had asked Eunice to look at his latest manuscript. Eunice chewed thoughtfully on her iced bun. She didn't need any time to decide what she thought, but simply how honest to be. However amiable Bomber was, he was still her boss and she was still the new girl trying to deserve her place. Percy had written a book for little girls called *Tracey Has Fun in the Kitchen*. Tracey's adventures included washing up with Daphne the dish-cloth, sweeping the floor with Betty the broom, cleaning the windows with Sparkle the sponge and scrubbing the oven with Wendy the wad of wire wool. Sadly, he had missed the opportunity of having Tracey unblock the sink with Portia the plunger, which might have proved to be some small redemption. Tracey had about as much fun as a pony in a coal pit. Eunice had a horrible feeling that Percy would be working on a sequel called *Howard Has Fun in the Shed*, with Charlie the chisel, Freddy the fretsaw and Dick the drill. It was a load of sexist codswallop. Eunice translated her thoughts into words.

'I'm struggling to envisage an appropriate audience for it.'

Bomber nearly choked on his bun. He took a

swig of tea and rearranged his face into a suitably serious expression.

'Now tell me what you really think.'

Eunice sighed. 'It's a load of sexist codswallop.'

'Quite right!' said Bomber as he snatched the offending manuscript from Eunice's desk and hurled it through the air towards the corner where the slippery slope skulked. It belly-flopped onto the pile with a dull thud. Douglas had finished his bun and was sniffing the air hopefully in case any crumbs remained on the plates of his friends.

'What's your sister's book about?' Eunice had been dying to ask ever since her first day, but before Bomber could answer, the downstairs door buzzer sounded.

Bomber leaped to his feet. 'That'll be the parents. They said they might pop in for a visit while they were up in town.'

Eunice was eager to meet the couple who had produced such contradictory offspring and Godfrey and Grace were a double delight. Bomber was a perfect mix of their physical characteristics, with his father's aquiline nose and generous mouth and his mother's shrewd grey eyes and colouring. Godfrey was resplendent in salmon pink jumbo corduroy trousers, teamed with a canary yellow waistcoat, matching bow tie and a rather battered but still decent enough panama. Grace was wearing a sensible cotton frock with a print that might have looked more appropriate on a sofa, a straw hat with several large yellow flowers attached to the brim and smart shoes with a small heel but comfortable for walking in. The brown leather handbag which was tucked firmly into the crook of her arm was large and sturdy enough to biff any would-be muggers, whom Grace was convinced were lurking in every alley and doorway of the city, waiting to pounce on country folk like her and Godfrey.

'This must be the new girl, then.' Grace pronounced 'girl' to rhyme with 'bell'. 'How do you do, my dear?'

'Very pleased to meet you.' Eunice took the hand that was offered; soft but with a firm grip.

Godfrey shook his head. 'Good God, woman! That's not the thing at all now with the young 'uns.' He grabbed Eunice with both arms and squeezed her tight, almost lifting her feet from the floor, and then kissed her firmly on both cheeks. She felt the scratch of whiskers he'd missed when shaving and caught a hint of eau de cologne. Bomber rolled his eyes and grinned.

'Pops, you're shameless. Any excuse to kiss the girls.'

Godfrey winked at Eunice. 'Well, at my age you have to take any chance you can get. No offence intended.'

Eunice returned his wink. 'None taken.'

Grace kissed her son affectionately on the cheek and then sat down purposefully to address him, waving away offers of tea and iced buns with a dismissive hand.

'Now, I promised that I would ask, but I refuse to interfere . . . '

Bomber sighed. He knew exactly what was coming.

'Your sister has apparently written a book that she would like you to publish. I haven't read it — haven't even seen it, come to that — but she says you're being deliberately mulish and refusing to give it proper consideration. What have you got to say for yourself?'

Eunice was agog and intrigued by the hint of a smile that skittered across Grace's mouth as she delivered her words in such a stern tone. Bomber strode across the room to the window in the manner of a defence barrister preparing to address the jury.

'The first point is undoubtedly true. Portia has written something that she calls a book and she does indeed want me to publish it. The second point is a wicked falsehood which I deny with every fibre of my being.'

Bomber slammed the palm of his hand onto his desk to emphasise his apparent indignation, before laughing out loud and slumping into his chair.

'Listen, Ma, I have read it and it's bloody awful. It's also been written by someone else first and they made a damn sight better fist of it than she did.'

Godfrey furrowed his brows and tutted in disapproval. 'You mean she's copied it?'

'Well, she calls it an 'ommage'.'

Godfrey turned to his wife and shook his head. 'Are you sure that you brought home the right one from the hospital? I can't think where she gets it from.'

Grace bowled a rather desperate attempt at a defence for her daughter's sticky wicket.

'Perhaps she didn't realise that her story resembled someone else's. Perhaps it was simply an unfortunate coincidence.'

It was a no-ball.

'Nice try, Ma, but it's called *Lady Clatterly's Chauffeur* and it's about a woman called Bonnie and her husband Gifford, who's been paralysed playing rugby. She ends up having an affair with her chauffeur, Mellons, a rough yet strangely tender northerner with a speech impediment who keeps tropical fish.'

Godfrey shook his head in disbelief. 'I'm sure that girl was dropped on her head.'

Grace ignored her husband but didn't contradict him and turned to Bomber.

'Well, that's cleared that up. Sounds perfectly dreadful. I'd chuck it in the bin if I were you. I can't abide laziness and if she can't even be bothered to think of her own story she can't expect anything else.'

Bomber winked gratefully at her.

'A boy's best friend is his mother.'

Grace stood up and re-armed herself with her handbag. 'Come along, Godfrey. It's time for Claridge's.' She kissed Bomber goodbye and Godfrey shook his hand.

'We always have tea there when we come up to town,' she explained to Eunice. 'Best cucumber sandwiches in the world.'

Godfrey tipped his hat to Eunice. 'The gin and lime's not bad either.'

7

The ruby droplet glistened on her fingertip before splashing onto the pale lemon skirt of her new dress. Laura cursed, sucked her finger angrily and wished she had worn her jeans. She loved filling the house with fresh flowers, but the beauty of the roses came at a price and the tip of the thorn was still embedded in her finger. In the kitchen, she stripped the lower leaves from the stems she had cut and filled two large vases with tepid water. One arrangement was for the garden room and one for the hall. As she trimmed and arranged the flowers, she fretted over the conversation that she had had with Anthony that morning. He had asked her to 'come and have a chat' with him in the garden room before she went home for the day. She checked her watch. She felt as though she had been summoned to the headmaster's office. It was ridiculous; he was her friend. But . . . What was the 'but' that kept prickling Laura's skin? Outside, the sky was still blue, but she could smell a storm in the air. She picked up one of the vases, took a deep breath and carried it out into the hall.

★ ★ ★

In the rose garden, it was hushed and still. But the air was heavy with the coming storm. In Anthony's study nothing moved or made a

43

sound. But the air was thick with stories. A blade of light from the cloud-streaked sun sliced through the barely breached curtains and fired a blood-red glint onto a crowded shelf just beside the biscuit tin.

Red gemstone
Found in St Peter's churchyard,
late afternoon, 6 July . . .

The smell of gardenias always reminded Lilia of her mother in her lilac Schiaparelli gown. St Peter's was awash with their waxy blooms and their perfume filled the cool air that welcomed friends and relations in from the fierce after-noon sun outside. At least the flowers had been Eliza's choice. Lilia was glad to sit down. New shoes were pinching her toes, but her vanity made no concession to arthritis and old age. The woman in the ridiculous hat had to be his mother. Half the occupants of the pew behind her would miss the entire wedding. An announcement from the vicar brought the rus-tling congregation to its feet as the bride arrived in her ugly mushroom of a dress, cling-ing desperately to her father's arm. Lilia's heart winced.

She had offered Eliza the Schiaparelli. She loved it, but the groom wasn't keen.
    'Good God, Lizzie! You can't get married in a dead woman's dress.'
    Lilia had never liked Eliza's intended. Henry. She could never trust a man who shared his

44

name with a vacuum cleaner. The first time they met, he had looked down his shiny, bulbous nose at her in a fashion that clearly intimated that women over sixty five don't count. He spoke to her with the exaggerated patience of someone housetraining a recalcitrant puppy. In fact, at that first family lunch, so lovingly prepared and so kindly intended, Lilia got the distinct impression that none of the family passed muster — except, of course, Eliza. And her greatest assets, in his eyes, were her beauty and her tractability. Oh, he was complimentary enough about the food. The roast chicken was almost as delicious as his mother's, and the wine was 'really quite good'. But Lilia watched him registering with disdain a slight mark on his fork and an imaginary smudge on his wine glass. Eliza was already, even then, gently explaining and excusing his behaviour, like an anxious mother with an unruly toddler. Lilia thought that what he needed was a jolly good slap on the back of his chubby legs. But she wasn't really worried, because she never dreamed it would last. Henry was an irksome addition to the family, but she could cope because he was temporary. Surely?

Eliza had been such a spirited child; determined to follow her own path. She wore her party frock with wellingtons to go fishing for newts in the stream at the bottom of the garden. She liked banana and tuna fish sandwiches and once spent the whole day walking everywhere backwards 'just to see what it feels like'. But everything changed when her mother,

Lilia's daughter, died when Eliza was just fifteen. Her father had remarried and provided her with a perfectly serviceable step-mother. But they were never close.

Lilia's own mother had taught her two things: dress for yourself, and marry for love. Her mother had managed the first but not the second, and regretted it her whole life. Lilia learned this lesson well. Clothes had always been her passion; it had been a love affair that had never disappointed. And so it was with her marriage. James was a gardener for her parents at their country house. He grew jewel-hued anemones, pompom dahlias and velvet roses that smelled of summer. Lilia was astonished that such a man, sinewy and strong, with hands twice the size of hers could coax into life such delicate blooms and blossoms. She fell in love. Eliza had adored her grandfather, but Lilia was widowed when she was still a little girl. Years later, she once asked Lilia how she had known that he was the man she should marry, and Lilia told her: because he loved her anyway. Their courtship was long and difficult. Her father disapproved and she was strong-willed and impatient. But no matter how ill her temper, how sunburned her face, how dreadful her cooking, James loved her anyway. They were happily married for forty-five years, and she still missed him every day.

When her mother died, Eliza's sense of purpose faded away and she became lost, like an empty paper bag being blown this way and that in the wind. And so she remained, until one

46

day the bag got caught on a barbed-wire fence: Henry. Henry was a hedge fund manager and everyone knew that that was not a proper job. He was a money gardener; he grew money. For Christmas, Henry bought Eliza cordon bleu cookery lessons, and took her to his mother's hairdresser. Lilia waited for it to be over. For her birthday, in March, he bought Eliza expensive clothes that made her look like someone else and replaced her beloved old Mini with a brand new two-seater convertible she was too afraid to drive in case it got scratched. And still Lilia waited for it to be over. In June he took her to Dubai and proposed marriage. She wanted her mother's ring, but he said that diamonds were 'so last year'. He bought her a new one set with a ruby the colour of blood. Lilia always felt it was a bad omen.

Eliza would be there soon. Lilia thought that they'd sit under the apple tree. It was shady there and she liked to listen to the sleepy buzzing of the bees and smell the warm grass, like hay. Eliza always had tea with Lilia on Saturday afternoons. Salmon and cucumber sandwiches and lemon curd tarts. Thank heavens the tuna fish and banana had fallen out of favour eventually. It was a Saturday afternoon when she had brought Lilia's wedding invitation, and she had asked Lilia then what her mother would have thought of Henry; would she have liked him and would she approve of their marriage! Eliza had looked so young in spite of her overdone hair and her stiff new clothes, so anxious for approval and so keen for someone to reassure her that this would be the 'happy ever after' that she was longing for. Lilia had been a coward. She had lied.

Henry turned and saw Eliza creeping nervously down the aisle and smiled. But there was no tenderness softening his face. It was the smile of a man taking delivery of a smart new car; not that of a groom melting at the sight of his beloved bride. As she arrived at his side and her father placed her hand in his, Henry looked smug; he approved. The vicar announced the hymn. As the congregation struggled through Guide Me, Oh Thou Great Redeemer, Lilia could feel the panic bubbling inside her like jam in a saucepan about to boil over.

Lilia always used the best china tea things on a Saturday, and the lemon curd tarts always perched on a glass cake stand. The sandwiches were ready and the kettle had boiled, ready to warm the pot. It was their own little tea party and they had been keeping this ritual since Eliza's mother died. Today Lilia had a present for her.

A hush is a dangerous thing. Silence is solid and dependable, but a hush is expectant, like a pregnant pause; it invites mischief, like a loose thread begging to be pulled. The vicar started it, poor chap. He asked for it. When Lilia was a little girl during the war, they had a house in London. There was an Anderson shelter in the

garden, but they didn't always use it. Sometimes they just hid under the table; madness,
she knew, but you had to be there to understand it. When the doodlebugs were raining
down, the thing they all feared most was not
the bangs and the crashes and the ear-splitting
explosions, but the hush. The hush meant that
that bomb was for you.

'If any person here present knows of any
reason why . . . '

The vicar launched the bomb. There was a
hush, then Lilia detonated it.

As the bride swept back down the aisle
alone, her face was lit by a beaming smile of
relief. She looked truly radiant.

Eliza had given him back the ring. But the ruby
had fallen out on the day of the wedding and
they never found it. Henry was livid. Lilia
imagined his face the colour of the lost stone.
They should be in Dubai now. Eliza would
have preferred Sorrento, but it wasn't swanky
enough for Henry. In the end, he took his
mother with him instead. And Eliza was
coming to tea with Lilia. On her seat was her
present. Nestled in silver tissue paper and tied
with a lilac ribbon was the Schiaparelli. He'd
never loved her anyway.

Anthony picked up the framed photograph from
Therese's dressing table and gazed at her image.
It had been taken on the day of their
engagement. Outside, lightning crazed the
charcoal sky. From the window of her bedroom,

he stared out at the rose garden, where the first plump raindrops were splashing onto velvet petals. He had never seen Therese wearing the dress, but over the long years without her he had often tried to picture their wedding day. Therese had been so excited. She had chosen flowers for the church and music for the ceremony. And, of course, she had bought the dress. The invitations had been sent. He imagined himself nervously waiting at the altar for her arrival. He would have been so happy and so proud of his beautiful bride. She would have been late, of that there was no doubt. She would have made quite an entrance in her cornflower silk chiffon gown; an unusual choice for a wedding dress, but then she was an unusual woman. Extraordinary. She had said that it matched the colour of her engagement ring. Now the dress was shrouded in tissue paper and buried in a box in the attic. He couldn't bear to look at it; nor could he part with it. He sat down on the edge of the bed and buried his face in his hands. He had still been in church on the day that should have been their wedding day. It was the day of Therese's funeral. And even now, he could almost hear her saying that at least his new suit had been put to good use.

★ ★ ★

Laura threw her keys onto the hall table and kicked off her shoes. Her flat was hot and stuffy and she opened the window in the poky sitting room before pouring herself a large glass of white wine, icy cold from the fridge. She hoped that the wine would soothe her dishevelled mind. Anthony had told her so many things that she hadn't known, and the knowledge had swept through her head like a wild wind through a field of barley, leaving it mussed and disarranged. She could picture him waiting there all those years ago, checking his watch and searching for Therese's face in the crowd or a glimpse of her powder-blue coat. She could feel the sickening panic blooming in his stomach like a drop of ink in a bowl of water, as the minutes ticked by and still she didn't come. But she could never know the blood-freezing, gut-twisting, breath-choking anguish he must have felt when he followed the wailing ambulance and found her crumpled and dead on the pavement. He had remembered every detail: the girl in the bright blue hat who had smiled at him on the corner of Great Russell Street; 11.55 a.m. on his watch when he'd first heard the siren; the smell of burning from the bakery, and the rows of cakes and pastries in the window. He could remember the sound of the traffic, the hushed voices, the white blanket that covered her face, and that even as the greatest darkness fell on him, the merciless sun kept shining. The details of Therese's death, once shared, forged an intimacy between Anthony and Laura that both honoured and unsettled her. But why now? Why, after almost six years, had he told her now? And there was something else, she was sure. Something that had been left unsaid. He

51

had stopped before he had finished.

★ ★ ★

Anthony swung his legs onto the bed and lay back, staring at the ceiling, remembering the cherished nights he had spent there with Therese. He turned onto his side and formed his arms in an empty embrace, willing himself to remember when the space had been filled with her warm, living flesh. Outside, the thunder cracked and growled as the silent tears he so rarely allowed streamed down his cheeks. He was finally exhausted by a lifetime of guilt and grieving. But he could not regret his life without Therese. He would a million times rather have spent it with her, but to give up when she died would have been the greatest wrong; to throw away the gift that had been snatched from her would have been an act of appalling ingratitude and cowardice. And so he had found a way to carry on living and writing. The dull ache of dreadful loss had never left him, but at least his life had a purpose which gave him a precious, if precarious, hope for what might follow it. Death was certain. Reunion with Therese was not. But now, at last, he dared to hope.

He had spoken to Laura that afternoon, but he still hadn't told her that he was leaving. He'd meant to, but one look at her worried face and the words had dissolved in his mouth. Instead, he had told her about Therese and she had wept for them both. He had never seen her cry before. It wasn't at all what he had intended. He wasn't looking for sympathy or, God forbid, pity. He was just trying to give her a reason for what he was about to do. But at least her tears were testament to the fact that he had made the right choice. She was able to feel the pain and joy of others and recognise their value. Contrary to the impression that she often gave, she wasn't a mere spectator of other people's lives; she had to engage. Her capacity to care was instinctive. It was her greatest asset and her greatest vulnerability; she had been burned and he knew it had left a mark. She had never told him, but he knew anyway. She had made a different life, grown a new skin, but somewhere there was a hidden patch, still red and tight and puckered, and sore to the touch.

Anthony stared at the photograph that lay on the pillow next to him. There were no smudges on the glass or frame. Laura saw to that. She cared for every part and piece of the house with a pride and tenderness that could only be born from love. Anthony saw all of this in Laura and knew that he had chosen well. She understood that everything had a value far greater than money; it had a story, a memory and, most importantly, a unique place in the life of Padua. For Padua was more than just a house; it was a safe place to heal. A sanctuary for licking wounds, drying tears and rebuilding dreams — however long it took. However long it took a broken person to be strong enough to face the world again. And he hoped that by choosing her to finish his task, it might set Laura free. For he knew she was in exile at Padua — one that was comfortable and self-imposed, but an exile nonetheless.

Outside, the storm was spent and the garden washed clean. Anthony undressed and for one last time crept beneath the cool embracing covers of the bed that he had shared with Therese. That night, the dream stayed away and he slept soundly until dawn.

8

Eunice

1975

Bomber grabbed Eunice's hand and gripped it tightly as Pam recoiled in horror at the rather unusual furniture. It appeared to be made from human bones. She turned to flee but the grumpy Leatherface caught her, and just as he was about to impale the poor girl on a meat hook Eunice woke up.

They had been to see *The Texas Chainsaw Massacre* at a local film club the previous evening and had both been truly horrified. But it wasn't a nightmare that had broken Eunice's sleep. It was a dream come true. She climbed out of bed and hurried to the bathroom, where she smiled happily at her slightly rumpled reflection. Bomber had held her hand. Only for a moment, but he had actually held her hand.

Later that morning, on the way to the office, Eunice warned herself to be careful. Yes, Bomber was her friend, but he was also her boss, and she still had a job to do. At the green door on Bloomsbury Street Eunice paused for a moment and took a deep breath before galloping up the stairs. Douglas rattled over to greet her with his usual enthusiasm, and Bomber called out from the kitchen, 'Tea?'

'Yes please.'

Eunice sat down at her desk and began sorting studiously through the post.

'Sleep well?'

Bomber thumped a steaming mug down in front of her, and to her horror Eunice felt herself blushing.

'That's the last time I let you choose the film,' he continued — oblivious to, or perhaps kindly ignoring, her embarrassment. 'I didn't sleep a wink last night, even though I had Douglas to protect me, and I kept the bedside lamp on!'

Eunice laughed as she felt her red face returning to its usual colour. Bomber always managed to make her feel comfortable. The rest of the morning passed as easily as usual and at lunchtime Eunice went out to fetch sandwiches from Mrs Doyle's. As they sat together eating cheese and pickle on granary bread and looking out of the window, Bomber remembered something.

'Didn't you say that it was your birthday next Sunday?'

Eunice suddenly felt hot again. 'Yes. It is.'

Bomber passed a piece of cheese to Douglas, who was drooling hopefully at his feet.

'Are you doing anything fabulous?'

That had been the original plan. Eunice and Susan, her best friend from school, had always said that to celebrate their twenty-first birthdays, which were only days apart, they would go to Brighton for the day. Eunice had never been fond of parties, and her parents were happy to pay for the trip instead of hiring a hall with a bar and hirsute disco DJ. But Susan had found herself a boyfriend, a David Cassidy doppelgänger who worked in Woolworths, and he had apparently planned a surprise for her birthday. She had been very apologetic, but chose new love over her oldest friendship nonetheless. Eunice's parents had offered to come with her instead, but that wasn't quite what she'd had in mind. Bomber was distraught on her behalf.

'I'll come!' he volunteered. 'That is, if you don't mind your aged boss tagging along.'

Eunice was thrilled. But tried very hard not to show it.

'Okay. I suppose I could cope with that.' She grinned. 'I just hope you'll be able to keep up with me!'

★ ★ ★

On Saturday morning Eunice went to the hairdresser for a cut and blow dry, and then for a manicure. In the afternoon, having checked Sunday's weather forecast for the umpteenth time, she tried on virtually every item of clothing in her wardrobe, in every conceivable combination. She eventually decided on a pair of purple high-waisted flared trousers, a flower-printed blouse and a purple hat with a huge, floppy brim to complement her newly purpled nails.

'How do I look?' she asked her mum and dad, as she paraded up and down the living room, intermittently blocking their view of *The Two Ronnies* on the television.

'You look lovely, dear,' her mum replied.

Her dad nodded in agreement but said nothing. He had learned, over the years, that it was wiser to leave opinions on fashion to the ladies of the house.

That night Eunice hardly slept at all, but when she did, she dreamed of Bomber. Tomorrow was going to be an extraordinary day!

9

It had seemed like a perfectly ordinary day. But in the weeks that followed, Laura scoured her memory, searching for missed clues and portents that might have gone unheeded. Surely she should have known that something terrible was going to happen? Laura often felt that she should have been a Catholic. She did guilt so well.

That morning, Anthony went for his walk as usual. The only thing that was different was that he didn't take his bag. It was a beautiful morning and when he returned Laura thought how happy he looked; more relaxed than she had seen him in a long time. He didn't go into the study, but asked Laura to bring his coffee to the garden where she found him chatting to Freddy about the roses. As Laura placed the tray down on the garden table she deliberately avoided catching Freddy's eye. Perhaps it was because she found him attractive that being in his presence made her uncomfortable. He had an easy confidence and was blessed with both charm and good looks, which Laura found rather unsettling. He was too young for her in any case, she thought, and then immediately ridiculed herself for even considering that it would ever be an issue.

'Morning, Laura. Lovely day.'

Now she had to look at him. He was smiling at her, and held her eyes in a steady gaze. Her embarrassment made her sound clipped and unfriendly.

'Yes, lovely.'

And now she was blushing. Not a flattering, rosy tint, but a vivid, scarlet mottling that made her look as if she had just had her head in the oven. She hurried back into the house. The cool, calm of Padua soon restored her equilibrium and she went upstairs to change the flowers on the landing. The door to the master bedroom was open, and Laura went in to check that everything was all right. The smell of roses was overpowering that day, even though the windows were closed. The clock downstairs in the hall began chiming midday, and Laura automatically checked her watch. The long-case clock had been gaining time, and she had been meaning to arrange to get it fixed. Her watch said 11.54 a.m. and suddenly a thought struck her. She picked up the blue enamel clock from Therese's dressing table and watched as the second hand ticked rhythmically round the dial. When it reached the twelve it stopped. Dead.

Anthony had his lunch in the garden room, and when Laura collected the tray she was delighted to see that he had eaten almost everything. Perhaps whatever it was that had been troubling him in recent months had been resolved, or perhaps his visit to the doctor had resulted in some improvement to his health. She also wondered if finally sharing his story about Therese with her had helped in some way. Whatever it was, she was glad. And relieved. It was wonderful to see him looking so well.

She spent the afternoon sorting through Anthony's accounts. He still received some royalties from his writing and would occasionally be asked to do a reading for some local book group or branch library. After a couple of hours poring over the paperwork, Laura leaned back in her chair. Her neck was sore and her back ached. She rubbed her tired eyes and made a mental note, for the hundredth time, to get them tested.

The lure of the study eventually proved irresistible for Anthony, and Laura heard him go in and shut the door behind him. She slipped the sheets of paper in front of her into their respective files and then went out into the garden to stretch her legs and feel the sun on her face. It was late afternoon, but the sun was still hot and the sound of bees on the honeysuckle throbbed in the sultry air. The roses looked magnificent. Blooms of every shape, size and hue combined to create a shimmering sea of scent and colour. The lawn was a perfect square of lush green and the fruit trees and bushes at the bottom of the garden burgeoned with the promise of late-summer bounty. Freddy clearly had a gift when it came to growing things. When Laura had first come to work for Anthony, the only part of the garden that was lovingly cared for was the rose garden. The lawn had been patchy and ragged with weeds, and the trees had been left to outgrow their strength, with branches too spindly to bear the weight of fruit. But in the two years since Freddy had come to work at Padua, the garden had been brought back to life. Laura sat down on the warm grass and hugged her knees. She was always reluctant to leave Padua at the end of the day, but on days like this it was even harder. Her flat held little attraction in comparison. At Padua, even when she was alone, she never felt lonely. In her flat she only ever felt that way.

Since Vince, there had been no other long-term relationships. The failure of her marriage had knocked her confidence and mocked her youthful pride. The wedding had been arranged so quickly that her mother had asked her if she was pregnant. She wasn't. She was simply swept away by a handsome Prince Charming who promised her the world. But the man she married was a flashy rogue who, instead of the world, delivered insipid suburbia. Her parents had done their very best to persuade her to wait; until she was older, knew better her own mind. But she'd been young and impatient, stubborn even, and marrying Vince had seemed like a shortcut to growing up. She could still remember the sad, anxious smile which her mother had fixed on her face as she watched her daughter walk down the aisle. Her father was less able to hide his misgivings, but fortunately most of the congregation assumed his tears were ones of happiness and pride. The worst thing of all was that, on her wedding day, she too had feared for the first time that she was making a mistake. Her doubts were buried in a barrage of confetti and champagne, but she had been right. Her love for Vince was a callow, fanciful love, formed as quickly as the silver-edged invitations had been issued and as frothy as the dress that she had worn down the aisle.

That evening, Laura picked at her supper in front of the television. She wasn't really hungry and she wasn't really watching the flickering screen. Giving up on both, she unlocked the door and stood out on the cramped balcony of her flat looking up at the inky sky. She wondered how many other people in the world were looking up at the same vast sky at that exact moment. It made her feel small and very much alone.

10

The midnight summer sky was a watercolour wash of darkness with a glitter of tiny stars thrown across it. The air was still warm as Anthony walked down the path towards the rose garden, inhaling the rich perfume of the treasured blooms that he had planted all those years ago for Therese, when they first moved into the house. He had been to the post box, his footfalls echoing softly through the empty streets of the village. The letter posted was the final full stop to his story. His solicitor would pass it on to Laura when the time came. And now he was ready to leave.

It had been a Wednesday when they had moved into the house. Therese had found it.

'It's perfect!' she had said.

And it was. They had met only months earlier, but they had not needed an 'approved' passage of time to bind them to one another. The attraction was instant; illimitable like the sky that hung above him now. At first it had frightened him, or rather the fear of losing it had. It was surely too potent, too perfect to last. But Therese had absolute faith. They had found each other and that was exactly as it was meant to be. Together they were sacrosanct. She was named after St Therese of the Roses and so he planted the garden as a gift to her. He spent October in Wellingtons trenching the ground in the new beds and digging in well-rotted manure, while Therese brought him cups of tea and unstinting encouragement. The roses arrived on a dank, foggy November morning, and their fingers, toes and noses froze as Anthony and Therese spent the day setting out and planting the garden around a perfect patch of lawn. But the washed-out palette that painted the November landscape was rainbow-tinted by the descriptions Therese read aloud from the labels that named every rose. There was pink and fragrant 'Albertine' to climb over the trellis archway leading to the sundial; the blood red velvet 'Grand Prix', the pure white 'Marcia Stanhope', the flushed copper 'Gorgeous', the silvery pink 'Mrs Henry Morse', the dark red 'Etoile de Hollande', 'Melanie Soupert' with pale yellow petals suffused with amethyst, and the vermilion and old gold of 'Queen Alexandra'. At the four corners of the lawn they planted weeping standard roses — 'Albéric Barbier', 'Hiawatha', 'Lady Gay' and 'Shower of Gold' — and when it was all done and they stood close together in the spectral drear of a winter twilight, she kissed him softly on the lips and placed something small and round into his cold-bruised hand. It was a picture of St Therese of the Roses framed in gold metal and glass in the shape of a medallion.

'It was a gift for my first Holy Communion,' she said. 'It's for you, to say thank you for my beautiful garden and to remind you that I will love you forever, no matter what. Promise me you'll keep it with you always.'

Anthony smiled. 'I promise,' he solemnly declared.

Tears scored Anthony's cheeks once again as he stood alone amongst the roses on a beautiful summer night. Alone and bereft as he remembered her kiss, her words and the feel of the medallion pressed into his hand.

He had lost it.

It had been in his pocket as he stood waiting for Therese on the corner of Great Russell Street. But she never came, and by the time he got home that day he had lost them both. He went back to look for the medallion. He searched the streets and gutters, but he had known that it was a hopeless task. It was as though he had lost her twice. It was the invisible thread that would have connected him to her even after she was gone, but now it was broken along with his promise to her. The contents of his study were testament to the reparation he had tried to make. But had he done enough? He was about to find out.

The grass was still warm and smelled like hay. Anthony lay down and stretched out his long, dwindled limbs towards the points of an imaginary compass, ready to set his final course. The scent of roses washed over him in waves. He looked up at the boundless ocean of sky above him and picked a star.

11

She thought he was asleep. Ridiculous, she knew, but the alternative was unthinkable.

Laura had arrived at her usual time and finding the house empty, assumed that Anthony had gone for his walk. But an insistent unease was tapping on her shoulder. She went to the kitchen, made coffee and tried to ignore it. But the tapping grew faster, louder, harder. Like her heartbeat. In the garden room, the door to the outside was open and she went out, feeling as though she were walking the plank. Anthony lay covered in rose petals, spread-eagled on the dew-soaked grass. From a distance he could have been asleep, but standing over him, there was no such comfort. His once blue eyes, still open, were milky veiled, and his mouth gaped breathless, hemmed by purpled lips. Her reluctant fingertips brushed his cheek. The tallow skin was cold. Anthony had gone and left behind a corpse.

And now she was alone in the house. The doctor and the funeral directors had come and gone. They had spoken in hushed voices and dealt with death kindly and efficiently. It was their livelihood after all. She found herself wishing that Freddy had been there, but it wasn't one of his regular days at Padua. She sat at the kitchen table watching another cup of coffee grow cold, her face scorched red and tight by angry tears. This morning her whole world had blown away like feathers in the wind. Anthony and Padua had become her life. She had no idea what she was going to do now. For a second time she was completely lost.

The clock in the hall struck six and still Laura could not bring herself to go home. She now realised that she was already home. The flat was just somewhere to go when she couldn't be here. Tears spilled down her cheeks again. She had to do something; a displacement activity, a distraction, however short-lived. She would do her job. She still had the house and everything in it to take care of. For now. She would keep doing it until somebody told her to stop. She started a tour of the house; upstairs first, checking everything was in order. In the main bedroom she smoothed the covers and plumped the pillows, dismissing as ridiculous her suspicion that the bed had recently been slept in. The scent of roses was overwhelming and the photograph of Anthony and Therese lay face down on the floor. She picked it up and returned it to its place on the dressing table. The little blue clock had stopped as usual. 11.55. She wound the key until the ticking started, like a tiny heartbeat. She passed the bay window without looking out at the garden. In Anthony's room she felt awkward in a way that she had never done when he had been alive. It seemed too intimate; an inappropriate intrusion. His pillow still smelled of the soap he always used. She pushed away unwelcome thoughts of strangers pawing through his things. She had no idea who his next of kin might be. Downstairs, she closed the windows in the garden room and locked the door to the outside. The photograph of Therese lay flat on the table. Laura picked it up and gazed at the woman for whom Anthony had lived and died.

'I hope to God you find each other,' she said softly before replacing the picture in its usual upright position. Laura wondered to herself if that counted as a prayer.

In the hall she stood by the study door. Her hand hovered above the doorknob, fearful, as though it might burn her if she touched it, then she dropped it back down by her side. She was desperate to see what secrets the room might hold, but the study was Anthony's private kingdom, and one which she had never been invited to enter. She couldn't yet decide if his death had changed that or not.

Daring herself, she stepped outside from the kitchen door and into the garden. It was late summer and the roses were beginning to shed their petals like fragile, worn-out ballgowns coming apart at the seams. The lawn was perfect again. It bore no imprint of a corpse. Well, what had she expected? Not this. As she stood in the middle of the grass in the ebb and flow of the sun-warmed, rose-scented air, she felt lifted; strangely reassured.

On her way back down to the house, the glint of setting sun on tilted glass caught her eye. It was the study window, left open. She couldn't leave it. The house would not be safe. Now she would have to go into the study. When she reached the door, she realised she had no idea where Anthony kept the key when it wasn't in his pocket. As she tried to think where it might be her fingers closed around the cool wooden handle. It turned easily at her touch and the door to the study swung open.

12

Shelves and drawers, shelves and drawers, shelves and drawers; three walls were completely obscured. The lace panels at the French windows lifted and fell in rhythm with the evening air which breathed gently through the crack in the frame. Even in the half-light Laura could see that every shelf was packed, and without looking she knew that every drawer was full. This was a life's work.

She walked around the room peering at its contents in astonishment. So this was Anthony's secret kingdom: a menagerie of waifs and strays meticulously labelled and loved. Because Laura could see that these were so much more than things; much more than random artefacts arranged on shelves for decoration. They were important. They really mattered. Anthony had spent hours every day in this room with these things. She had no idea why, but she knew he must have had a very good reason, and somehow, for his sake, she would have to find a way to keep them safe. She slid open the drawer nearest to her and picked up the first thing she saw. It was a large dark blue button which looked as though it belonged on a woman's coat. Its label noted when and where it had been found. Memories and explanations began to coalesce in Laura's consciousness; tentacles grasping for connections that she could sense but not yet substantiate.

She reached for the back of a chair to steady herself. Despite the open window and the draughts, the room was stuffy. The air was thick with stories. Was that what this was all about? Were these the things that Anthony had written his stories about? She had read them all and she distinctly remembered one about a blue button. But where had all these things come from? Laura stroked the soft fur of a small teddy slumped forlornly against the side of a biscuit tin on one of the shelves. Was this a museum for the missing pieces of people's real lives or the furnishings for Anthony's fiction? Perhaps it was both. She picked up a lime-green hair bobble that lay next to the teddy on the shelf. It would have cost only a few pence when new, and one of the flowers on the elastic was badly chipped, yet it had been carefully kept and properly labelled like every other object in the room. Laura smiled at the memory of herself as a schoolgirl with swinging plaits adorned with bobbles much the same as this one.

Lime-green hair bobble with plastic flowers. Found on the playing field, Derrywood Park, 2 September . . .

It was the last day of the summer holidays and Daisy's mum had promised her a special treat. They were going for a picnic. Tomorrow Daisy would start at her new school; big school. She was eleven now. Her old school had not been a success. Well, at least not for her. She was pretty enough, with beautiful long dark hair; clever enough, but not too clever; didn't wear glasses or braces on her teeth. But it wasn't enough to keep her camouflaged. She saw the world through a slightly different lens from other children; nothing too obvious, just a fraction out of kilter. The faintest fontanelle in her character. But Ashlyanne Johnson and her posse of apprentice bitches soon sniffed it out. They pulled her plaits, spat in her lunch, urinated in her school bag and ripped her blazer. It wasn't what they did that upset her the most; it was how they made her feel. Useless, weak, scared, pathetic. Worthless.

Her mum had gone mad when she had found out. Daisy had kept quiet for as long as she could, but when the bed-wetting started she had to come clean. But it only proved how pathetic she was; a big girl of eleven wetting the bed. Her mum went straight to the head-mistress and scared her half to death. After that, the school did what they could, which wasn't much, and Daisy set her sights on the end of term with gritted teeth and her hair cut short. She had chopped the plaits herself with the kitchen scissors and when her mum saw her she had cried. But over the summer her hair had grown again; not long enough for plaits, but just about for ponytails. And today she had new hair bobbles for them, bright green with flowers on. 'Daisies for Daisy,' her mother had said. As she sat admiring them in the mirror, her stomach lurched like the gears slipping on a bicycle. What if tomorrow her new classmates looked at the face of the girl in the mirror and didn't like what they saw?

Annie zipped the cool bag closed, satisfied that she had included all her daughter's favourites in their picnic: cheese and pineapple sandwiches (brown bread with seeds), salt and vinegar crisps, custard doughnuts, Japanese rice crackers and ginger beer to drink. She could still feel the need for physical violence smouldering inside her, stoked rather than soothed by the reaction of that idiot fairy-fart of a headmistress who could barely control a basket of sleeping kittens, let alone a school full of chipfed, benefits-bred kids, most of whom already believed that the world owed them a council flat, a baby and the latest pair of Nike trainers. After Daisy's dad had left, Annie had worked bloody hard as a single mother to bring Daisy up. She had two part-time jobs, and the flat they lived in might not be in the best area, but it was clean and homely and it was theirs. And Daisy was a good kid. But good was bad. In the world of school where Daisy had to survive, the things that Annie had taught her were not enough. Common decency, good manners, kindness and hard work were treated as peculiarities at best, but in gentle Daisy they were seen as weaknesses; faults for which she was cruelly punished. So Annie had one more lesson to teach her daughter.

The sun was already high and hot by the time they reached the park, and the grass was littered with groups of young women accessorised with pushchairs, wailing toddlers,

74

mobile phones and Benson & Hedges. Daisy's mother took her hand and they walked straight across the grass playing field towards the woods at the back of the park. They weren't just strolling, they were striding; going somewhere specific. Daisy didn't know where, but she could feel her mother's sense of purpose. The woods were another world; cool and quiet and empty, save for the birds and the squirrels.

'I used to come here with your dad.'

Daisy looked up at her mother with innocent eyes. 'Why?'

Her mother smiled, remembering. She put down the cool bag and looked up towards the sky.

'We're here,' she said.

The cool bag was at the foot of a huge oak tree, which was bent and twisted like an old man racked with arthritis. Daisy looked up through its branches, glimpsing flecks and flashes of blue through the flickering canopy of leaves.

Twenty minutes later she was sitting in the canopy looking down at the cool bag.

When her mother had announced that they were going to climb the tree, Daisy thought she must be joking. In the absence of a punchline or a laugh, Daisy took refuge in fear.

'I can't,' she said.

'Can't or won't?'

Daisy's eyes filled with tears, but her mother was resolute.

'You don't know you can't until you try.'

The silence and the stillness that followed

75

seemed eternal. Eventually her mother spoke.

'In this world, Daisy, we are tiny. We can't always win and we can't always be happy. But the one thing that we can always do is try. There will always be Trashcan Johnsons' — a twitch of a smile crossed Daisy's face — 'and you can't change that. But you can change how she makes you feel.'

Daisy wasn't convinced. 'How?'

'By climbing this tree with me.'

It was the scariest thing Daisy had ever done. But somewhere before they reached the top a strange thing happened. Daisy's fear blew away like feathers in the wind. At the bottom of the tree she was tiny, and the tree an invincible giant. At the top, the tree was still huge, but tiny though she was, she had climbed it.

It was the best day of the summer holidays. By the time they walked home across the playing field, the park was nearly empty and a man riding a mower was about to cut the grass. Her hair had come loose climbing the tree and she pulled out her hair bobbles and stuffed them into her pocket, but when she got home she realised one of them was missing. After the triumph of the afternoon she scarcely cared. When Daisy got ready for bed that night, with her new school uniform hanging on the wardrobe door, she noticed that the face in the mirror was a new face; happy and excited. Today Daisy had learned how to conquer a giant, and tomorrow she was going to big school.

Laura replaced the hair bobble on the shelf and came out of the study, closing the door behind her. Her reflection in the hall mirror was of the face that belonged to the old Laura before Anthony and Padua: hollowed out, defeated. The clock struck nine. She would have to go. She picked up her keys from the small Maling bowl on the hall table where she always left them. But there was one extra. Underneath her bunch of house and car keys was a large single internal door key. Suddenly Laura understood, and the face in the mirror was transformed by a slow smile. Anthony had left the door to his secret kingdom unlocked for her. His trust in her resurrected the resolve that his death had dissipated. Today she had been left a kingdom and tomorrow she would begin unravelling its secrets.

13

Eunice

1976

Arrogantly sprawled across Eunice's desk, Portia flicked cigarette ash into a pot of paperclips. Eunice had nipped across the road with Douglas to fetch doughnuts from Mrs Doyle's, and Bomber was seeing a client out. Portia yawned and then sucked greedily on her cigarette. She was tired, bored and hungover. Too many Harvey Wallbangers with Trixie and Myles last night. Or rather this morning. She hadn't got in until 3 a.m. She picked up a manuscript from the pile which she had carelessly toppled as she arranged her spiky limbs into a praying mantis posture.

''*Lost and Found* — a collection of short stories by Anthony Peardew*',* she read aloud, with sing-song derision. As she flipped over the title page it ripped free of its treasury tag.

'Oopsy!' she sneered, frisbee-ing it across the room. She peered at the first page as though she were sniffing milk to see if it had turned.

'Good God! What a load of drivel. Who wants to read a story about *a large blue button* which fell off the coat of a waitress called Marjory! And to think he wouldn't publish me, his own sister.'

She threw the manuscript back onto the desk with such violent disdain that it toppled a half-empty cup, soaking the pages with coffee-coloured scorn.

'Shag and shit a pig!' Portia cursed as she retrieved the soggy sheaf of papers and hastily hid it halfway down the precarious stack of the 'slippery slope' just before Bomber bounded back into the room.

'Absolutely tipping it down out there now, sis. You'll get soaked. Would you like to borrow an umbrella?'

Portia looked up and about as though trying to locate an irksome bluebottle, and then addressed the room in general.

'Firstly, do not call me 'sis'. Secondly, I don't do umbrellas, I do cabs. And thirdly, are you trying to get rid of me?'

'Yes,' called Eunice, bundling back up the stairs, a muddle of mackintosh, damp Douglas and doughnuts. She dumped Douglas on the floor, the doughnuts on Bomber's desk and hung up her dripping mackintosh.

'I think we might need a bigger boat,' she muttered, tipping her head ever so slightly in Portia's direction. Bomber bit back the laugh that threatened to escape. Eunice saw that he was teetering and started 'duh da-ing' the music from *Jaws*.

'What is that ridiculous girl going on about now?' Portia squawked from her perch.

'Just a cinematic reference to the inclement weather,' Eunice replied cheerfully.

Portia was unconvinced, but more concerned by the fact that Douglas had wheeled himself as close to her as he could manage and was about to shake his wet fur in her direction.

'Get that blasted rat away from me,' she hissed, retreating, and promptly fell backwards onto Eunice's desk, scattering pens, pots and paperclips in all directions onto the floor. Eunice swept Douglas into the kitchen and soothed his hurt feelings with a doughnut. But Portia's rudeness had finally toppled even Bomber's extraordinary equanimity. His customary geniality slipped from his face like a landslide after a storm. Thunderstruck, he grabbed Portia by the wrists and heaved her from Eunice's desk.

'Clear it up,' he commanded, gesturing at the mess she had made.

'Don't be silly, darling,' she replied, picking up her bag and searching inside it for her lipstick in an attempt to disguise her surprise and embarrassment. 'I have people to do that sort of thing.'

'Well, they're not here now, are they?' fumed Bomber.

'No, darling, but you are,' said his sister, applying a fresh slick of scarlet. 'Be a sweetie and call me a cab.'

Red-faced, she dropped her lipstick back inside her bag and clip-clopped downstairs in her ridiculous heels to wait for the car she knew her brother would order. Portia hated it when he was cross with her but she knew that she deserved it, and the fact that he was right made her worse. She was like a toddler stuck in an eternal tantrum. She knew that she behaved badly, but somehow couldn't seem to stop herself. She sometimes wished that they could go

80

back to when they were children and he was the big brother who doted on her.

As Bomber watched her go, he tried and failed to recognise in this brittle woman even the faintest trace of the affectionate little girl that he had once loved so dearly. For years now he had mourned the sister he had lost so long ago, who had hung on his every word, ridden on the crossbar of his bicycle and carried his maggots when he went fishing. In return he had eaten her sprouts, taught her to whistle and pushed her 'as high as the sky' on her swing. But she belonged to the distant past, and his present was poisonous Portia. He heard the cab door slam and she too was gone.

'Is it safe to come in?' Eunice poked her head around the kitchen door.

Bomber looked up and smiled apologetically. 'I'm so sorry about this,' he said, gesturing at the floor around her desk.

Eunice grinned. 'Not your fault, boss. Anyway, no harm done.'

They gathered the things up from the floor and restored them to their proper places.

'I spoke too soon,' said Eunice, cradling a small object in her hand. It was a picture of a lady holding flowers, and the glass inside the gold-coloured frame was smashed. She had found it on the way home from her interview and had kept it on her desk from her first day. It was her lucky charm. Bomber surveyed the damage.

'I'll soon have that fixed,' he said, taking the picture from her and placing it carefully in an envelope. He disappeared downstairs without another word. Eunice finished rescuing her things from the floor and swept up the cigarette ash. Just as the kettle boiled, Bomber returned both in body and spirit; soaking wet again, but his broad smile and good humour restored.

'The watchmaker on Great Russell Street has assured me that the glass will be replaced by tomorrow afternoon at the latest.'

They sat down to their very belated tea and doughnuts, and Douglas, finally assured of Portia's departure, wheeled himself back into the room hoping for seconds.

'She wasn't always like this, you know,' said Bomber thoughtfully, stirring his tea.

'I know it's hard to believe, but as a little girl she was really quite sweet; and for a little sister, tremendous fun.'

'Really?' Eunice was understandably sceptical. 'What happened?'

'Great Aunt Gertrude's trust fund.'

Elevated eyebrows registered Eunice's curiosity.

'She was my mother's aunt; rich, pampered and cantankerous as hell. She never married but always longed for a daughter. Unfortunately Ma wasn't her idea of a girl at all; couldn't be bought with expensive dolls and pretty dresses. Might have had more luck with a pony or a train set, but anyway . . . ' Bomber bit into his doughnut and squirted jam onto his chin.

'Portia was a different matter. Ma tried to intervene; withheld some of the more lavish gifts; remonstrated with the termagant Gertrude, face to gargoyle face. But as Portia grew up Ma's influence inevitably diminished. Furious at what she called Ma's jealous meddling, when the Great Gertie died she took her revenge. She left the lot to Portia. And it was a lot. Of course Portia couldn't touch it until she was twenty-one, but it didn't matter. She knew it was there. She stopped bothering to make a life for herself and started waiting for one to happen to her. You see Great Gertie's legacy was a tainted tiara; the worst gift of all. It made Portia rich, but robbed her of any sense of purpose.'

'Thank goodness I'm not filthy rich if that's what it does to a girl,' Eunice joked. 'Just how filthy, exactly?'

'Feculent.'

Eunice cleared away the tea things and went back to work.

Bomber was clearly still fretting over the effect of Portia's tantrum. 'I hope you're not sorry that you came to work here.'

Eunice grinned manically. 'I must be nuts to be in a loony bin like this office,' she said in her best Jack Nicholson voice.

Bomber laughed his relief as he picked up a loose sheet of paper from the floor by his desk and screwed it into a ball. Eunice leapt to her feet, arms in the air.

'Hit me, Bomber, I got the moves!'

They had been to see *One Flew Over the Cuckoo's Nest* that week for the third time. They spent so much time together now, both in and out of work, that Bomber couldn't imagine life without her. The film had made an indelible mark and the ending had had them both in tears. Eunice knew the script almost by heart.

'So you're not about to hand in your notice and leave me to the mercy of my sister?'

Bomber's eyes almost filled with tears again as she replied with a line from the end of the film.

'I'm not goin' without you, Bomber. I wouldn't leave you this way . . . You're coming with me.' And then she winked. 'Now, about my pay rise . . .'

14

The girl watched as the tiny scarlet dome on black legs crawled across the back of her hand towards the curl of her little finger.

'Ladybird, ladybird, fly away home, your house is on fire, your children have gone.

All except one, and she is called Anne, and sorry but she died.'

The ladybird opened her wings.

'It's not truth.' The girl spoke slowly, as though she were reciting a poem that she was struggling to remember. 'It's only a made-up sing-song.'

The ladybird flew off anyway. It was hot; September. The girl sat swinging her legs on the wooden bench that faced Padua from the small green. She had watched as the shiny black cars had arrived outside the house. The first one had big windows in the side and she could see a box for dead people inside with flowers growing out of its lid. A sad lady and an old man but not the man who lived there came out of the house. The girl didn't know who the old man was, but she had seen the lady lots of times before she was sad. The man in the black chimney-pot hat put them in the second car. Then he went to the front of the car with the box in and started walking. He had a stick, but not a limp. But he was walking slowly so perhaps he had a bad leg after all. She wondered who was in the box.

Thinking was something she did slowly. She was quicker at feeling. She could feel happy or sad, or angry or excited in a winking of the eye. And she could feel other things too which were more difficult to explain. But thinking took longer. Thoughts had to be put in the right order in your head and looked at properly so that your brain could do the thinking. Eventually she decided that it must be the man who lived in the house who was in the box, and she was sad. He had always been nice to her. And not everyone was. After a long time (she had a nice watch, but she hadn't quite worked out the time please Mr Wolf yet) the sad lady came back on her own. The girl scratched the back of her hand where the ladybird's feet had tickled. Now that the man was dead, the lady would need a new friend.

★ ★ ★

Laura closed the front door behind her and slipped out of her black court shoes. The cold tiles of the hall floor kissed her aching feet and once again the peace of the house enveloped her. She padded through to the kitchen and poured herself a glass of wine from the fridge. Her fridge. Her kitchen. Her house. She still couldn't quite believe it. The day after Anthony had died she had telephoned his solicitor, hoping he would know if there was anyone she should contact; a distant cousin that she didn't know about, or a designated next of kin. He sounded as though he had been expecting her call. He told her that Anthony had instructed him to

86

inform Laura immediately after his death that she was his sole heir; everything he had owned was now hers. There was a will, and a letter for her, the details of which would be revealed after the funeral. But Anthony's first concern had been that she shouldn't worry. Padua would remain her home. His kindness made his death all the more unbearable. She had been unable to continue the telephone conversation, her words choked by tears. It was no longer grief alone that overwhelmed her, but relief for herself, chased by guilt that she could feel such a thing at such a time.

She took her wine through to the study and sat down at the table. She felt a strange solace surrounded by Anthony's treasures. She was now their guardian and they gave her a sense of purpose, even though she was as yet unsure as to what that might be. Perhaps Anthony's letter would explain, and then she might find a way to deserve his extraordinary generosity towards her. The funeral had been a revelation. Laura had expected there to be only a handful of people, including herself and Anthony's solicitor, but the church was almost full. There were people from the publishing world who had known Anthony as a writer and others who had only known him to say 'Good morning' to, but it seemed as though he touched the lives of everyone he met and left an indelible mark. And then, of course, there were the busybodies: stalwart members of the local residents' association, WI, Amateur Dramatics Society and general purveyors of the moral high ground, led by Marjory Wadscallop and her faithful deputy, Winnie Cripp. Their 'heartfelt condolences' — offered a little too enthusiastically as Laura left the church — had been accompanied by sad, well-practised smiles and unwelcome hugs that left Laura smelling of damp dog and hairspray.

The large blue button that Laura had taken from the drawer on her first visit to the study was still on the table, resting on its label.

Large blue button, from woman's coat?
Found on the pavement of Graydown Street,
11 November . . .

Margaret was wearing her dangerous new knickers. 'Ruby silk with sumptuous cream lace' was how the saleswoman had described them, clearly wondering what business Margaret had buying them. They were not even distant cousins of her usual Marks & Spencer utility wear. Downstairs her husband waited expectantly. Twenty-six years they had been married, and he had done his best to let Margaret know how much he loved her for every one of those years. He loved her with his fists and his feet. His love was the colour of bruises. The sound of breaking bones. The taste of blood. Of course, no one else knew. No one at the bank where he was assistant manager, no one at the golf club where he was treasurer, and certainly no one at the church where, in the first year of their marriage, he had been born again a Baptist bedlamite. Beating the crap out of her was God's will. Apparently. But no one else knew; just him, God and Margaret. His respectability was like a neatly pressed suit; a uniform he wore to fool the outside world. But at home, in mufti, the monster reappeared. They'd never had any children. It was probably for the best. He might have loved them too. So why had she stayed? Love, at first. She had truly loved him. Then fear, weakness, desolation? All of the above. Body and spirit crushed by God and Gordon.

'Where the flick's my dinner!' a voice bawled from the sitting room. She could picture him, fleshy faced and florid; rolls of fat seeping over the belt of his trousers, watching the rugby on the television and drinking his tea. Tea that Margaret had made; milk and two sugars. And six Tramadol. Not enough to kill him; not quite. God knows, she had enough. The last time she 'tripped' and broke her wrist, that kind doctor in A&E had given her a whole box. Not that she wasn't tempted. Manslaughter with diminished responsibility thrown in seemed like a fair trade. But Margaret wanted him to know. Her left eye was almost swollen shut and the colour of the Valpolicella Gordon was expecting to swill with his dinner. Touching it, she winced, but then she felt the whisper of soft silk brushing against her skin and smiled. Downstairs, Gordon wasn't feeling quite himself.

When she entered the sitting room, she looked him straight in the eyes for the first time in years. 'I'm leaving you.'

She waited to make sure that he understood.

The rage in his eyes was all the confirmation she needed.

'Get back here, you stupid bitch!'

He tried to haul himself from his chair, but Margaret had already left the room. She heard him crash to the floor. She picked up the suitcase in the hall, closed the door behind her and walked down the drive without looking back. She didn't know where she was going, and she didn't care as long as it was away. The bitter November wind stung her bruised face. Margaret put down her suitcase for a moment to fasten the top button of her old blue coat. The worn-out thread snapped and the button spun through her fingers and onto the pavement. Margaret picked up her suitcase and left the button where it was.

'Sod it,' she thought. 'I'll buy a new coat. Happy Birthday, Margaret.'

Laura awoke to the sound of knocking. She had fallen asleep slumped over the table, and her cheek now bore the imprint of the blue button it had been resting on. Still befuddled with sleep, she slowly realised that the knocking was coming from the front door. In the hall she passed her suitcase still waiting to be unpacked. She had decided that tonight would be the first night that she would stay at Padua. It had somehow felt right to wait until after the funeral. The knocking began again, insistent but not urgent. Patient. As though the person would wait for as long as it took for someone to answer. Laura opened the door to a young girl with a serious and beautiful

90

moon face, set with almond-shaped eyes the colour of conkers. She had seen her many times before, sitting on the bench across the green, but never this close. The girl drew herself up to her full height of five feet and one and a quarter inches and then she spoke.

'My name is Sunshine and I can be your new friend.'

15

'When the sitter comes, shall I make the lovely cup of tea?'

Laura smiled. 'Do you know how?'

'No.'

It had been two weeks since Anthony's funeral and Sunshine had called every day apart from on Sundays when her mum had stopped her.

'Give the poor woman a day off, Sunshine. I'm sure she doesn't want you pestering her peace and quiet all the time.'

Sunshine was unfazed. 'I'm not a pester. I'm her new friend.'

'Hmm . . . whether she likes it or not,' her mum muttered as she peeled the potatoes ready for Sunday lunch. Her mum worked long hours as a carer for the elderly and was rarely at home during the day, and her dad worked on the trains. Sunshine's older brother was supposed to keep an eye on her, but he rarely noticed anything that didn't take place in high definition on a screen the size of a kitchen table that obscured most of his bedroom wall. Besides, she was nineteen. They couldn't keep her locked up like a child. To be honest she was pleased that Sunshine had found something else to do other than sit on a bench all day. But she was always anxious about the response of strangers to her daughter's sudden and enthusiastic attachments. Sunshine was fearless and trusting, but her courage and good nature made her vulnerable. Her virtues were often her most serious handicap. Her mum had popped round to see the woman — Laura, she was called — who owned the big house, to check whether or not she minded Sunshine's visits. She also wanted to satisfy herself that Sunshine wouldn't come to any harm. The woman seemed nice enough, if a little stand-offish, and said that Sunshine was very welcome. But it was the house itself that reassured her the most. It was very beautiful, but more than that, it had a lovely feeling about it that she struggled to describe to her husband, Bert.

'It just feels *safe*,' was the best she could do to explain why she was happy to approve her daughter visiting Padua. For Sunshine, it was the highlight of her day, and now she sat at the kitchen table waiting patiently for Laura's answer. Laura paused, kettle in hand, and looked into Sunshine's serious face.

'I suppose I could show you how.'

Some days she found Sunshine an unwelcome intruder into her new and as yet uncertain life; a determined gatecrasher. Of course, she would never have admitted it. She had even told Sunshine's mum that she was very welcome. But some days Laura pretended not to be in, leaving Sunshine on the doorstep, patiently but persistently ringing the bell. Once she had even hidden in the garden behind the shed. But Sunshine had eventually found her and her beaming smile of delight had made Laura feel like a prize-winning idiot and a cold-hearted bitch.

Anthony's solicitor was coming today with the will and the letter. Laura had explained this to Sunshine, but could never be sure exactly how much she understood. She was watching Laura intently now as she set the kettle on the hob and took a fresh tray cloth from the drawer. Mr Quinlan was due at 2.30 p.m. Before that, Sunshine managed to squeeze in five practice runs, including the washing-up, and Laura, as Mr Quinlan's stand-in, had been forced to tip the last three cups into the aspidistra for the sake of her bladder.

Mr Quinlan arrived on time. Sunshine recognised him as the old man who had come out of the house with Laura on the day of Anthony's funeral. He was wearing a charcoal grey pinstripe suit and a pale pink shirt, and a gold watch chain could just be seen disappearing into his waistcoat pocket. He looked important. Uncertain how to greet a person of such standing, Sunshine bobbed a little curtsey and offered him a high five.

'I'm delighted to meet you, young lady. I'm Robert Quinlan, and who are you?'

'I'm Sunshine, the new friend for Laura. People sometimes call me Sunny for short.'

He smiled. 'Which do you prefer?'

'Sunshine. Do people ever call you Robber?'

'It's an occupational hazard, I'm afraid.'

Laura led them through to the garden room and Sunshine made sure that the sitter had the best chair. She looked at Laura meaningfully.

'Shall I go and make the lovely cup of tea now?'

'That would be very helpful,' Laura replied, secretly wishing that she had nipped to the loo just one more time before Mr Quinlan had arrived.

Mr Quinlan read the contents of the will to Laura while Sunshine was in the kitchen. It was clear and simple. Anthony thanked Laura for her work and friendship, but most particularly for her loving care of the house and everything in it. He wanted Laura to inherit all that he owned on the condition that she lived in the house and kept the rose garden exactly as it was. He knew that Laura loved the house almost as much as he had, and he had died content in the knowledge that she would continue to care for it and 'take the best possible advantage of all the happiness and peace it had to offer'.

'And so, my dear, it's all yours. As well as the house and its contents, there's also a sizeable sum in the bank, and any royalties from his writing will now come to you.' Mr Quinlan peered at her over the top of his hornrimmed spectacles and smiled.

'Here's the lovely cup of tea.' Sunshine barged the door open with her elbow and inched her way into the room like a tightrope walker. Her knuckles were white from the weight of the tray she was carrying, and the tip of her tongue poked out of her tiny rosebud mouth in agonised concentration. Mr Quinlan leapt to his feet and relieved her of her burden. He set the tray down on a side table.

'Shall I be mother?' he asked.

Sunshine shook her head. 'I've got a mum. She's at the work.'

'Quite right, young lady. I meant shall I pour the tea?'

Sunshine considered carefully for a moment. 'Do you know how?'

He smiled. 'Perhaps you'd better show me.'

Three expertly poured cups of tea and two custard creams later, all consumed under Sunshine's unswerving observation, Mr Quinlan's visit was drawing to a close.

'Just one more thing,' he said to Laura. 'The third condition of the will.'

He handed Laura a sealed white envelope bearing her name in Anthony's handwriting.

'I believe this explains it in greater detail, but it was Anthony's wish that you should endeavour to return as many of the things in his study to their rightful owners as you possibly can.'

Laura recalled the groaning shelves and packed drawers and balked at the enormity of the task. 'But how?'

'I can't begin to imagine. But Anthony clearly had faith in you, so perhaps all you need is a little faith in yourself. I'm sure you'll find a way.'

Laura was less sure than hopeful. But then hope went well with faith, didn't it?

'She had wonderful red hair, you know.' Mr Quinlan had picked up the photograph of Therese.

'Did you ever meet her?' Laura asked.

He traced the outline of the face in the photograph wistfully with his finger.

'Several times. She was a magnificent woman. Oh, she had a wild streak, and a fiery temper when roused. Still, I think every man who met her fell just a little bit under her spell.'

Clearly reluctant to let her go, he put the photograph back on the table. 'But Anthony was the only chap for her. He was my friend as well as a client for many years and I never saw a man more in love. When she died it crushed his soul. It was the saddest thing . . . '

Sunshine sat quietly, listening to every word and gathering them all in so that she could try to sort them into the proper story later.

'Let me guess,' said Mr Quinlan, getting up and going over to the gramophone. ' "The Very Thought of You', Al Bowlly?'

Laura smiled. 'It was their song.'

'Of course. Anthony told me the story.'

'I'd love to hear it.'

Since Anthony's death, Laura had been increasingly saddened by the realisation that she knew so little about him, and in particular about his past. Their relationship had been firmly fixed in the present, forged by daily routines and events and not by sharing the past or planning for the future. So now Laura was keen to find out anything she could. She wanted to better know the man who had trusted her and treated her with such kindness and generosity. Mr Quinlan returned to his seat in the best chair.

'One of Anthony's earliest and most precious memories was when he was a little boy dancing to that tune. It was during the Second World War and his father was home on leave. He was an officer in the RAF. That evening his parents were going to a dance. It was a special occasion and his father's last night so his mother had

97

borrowed a beautiful lilac evening gown from a friend. It was a Schiaparelli, I believe. There was a photograph Anthony had . . . Anyway, they were having cocktails together in the drawing room when Anthony came in to say goodnight. They were dancing to that Al Bowlly song — his dashing father and elegant mother — and they gathered him up into their arms and danced with him between them. He said he could still remember the smell of his mother's perfume and the serge of his father's uniform. It was the last time they were together, and the last time he saw his father. He returned to his air base early the next morning before Anthony was awake. Three months later he was captured behind enemy lines and was killed attempting to escape from Stalag Luft III. Many years later, not long after they met, Anthony and Therese were having lunch in a wine bar in Covent Garden that favoured deco over Donny Osmond and David Cassidy. The pair of them always did seem to belong to another age. The Al Bowlly song started playing and Anthony told Therese the story. She took his hand and stood up and danced with him then and there, as though they were the only ones in the room.

Laura was starting to understand. 'She sounds like an amazing woman.'

Mr Quinlan's reply was heartfelt. 'Indeed she was.'

As he began packing his paperwork into his briefcase, the silent Sunshine stirred. 'Would you like the lovely cup of tea again?'

He smiled gratefully but shook his head. 'I'm

afraid I must go or else I shall miss my train.' But in the hall he paused and turned to Laura.

'I wonder if I might use the loo before I go?'

16

The paper knife was solid silver with a handle in the form of an Egyptian pharaoh. Laura slid the blade between the folds of thick white paper. As the envelope split open she imagined Anthony's secrets escaping like a cloud of whispers into the air. She had waited until Sunshine had gone home before bringing the letter into the study. The garden room was more comfortable, but it felt more fitting to read it surrounded by the things it concerned. The mild summer evenings had slipstreamed imperceptibly into crisp autumn twilights and Laura was half tempted to light the fire in the grate, but instead she pulled the sleeves of her cardigan down to cover her knuckles and slid the letter out of the envelope. She unfolded the stiff sheets of paper and spread them on the table in front of her.

My dear Laura,

Anthony's deep and gentle voice sounded in her ears and the black writing disappeared into a blur, washed away by the tears which filled Laura's eyes. She sniffed loudly and wiped her eyes on her sleeve.

'For God's sake, Laura, get a bloody grip!' she admonished herself, and was surprised by the smile that hijacked her lips.

My dear Laura,

By now you will know that Padua and everything in it is yours. I hope that you will be very happy living here and will forgive my foolish sentimentality about the rose garden. You see I planted it for Therese, who was named after St Therese of the Roses. When she died, I scattered her ashes amongst the roses so that I could always be near to her, and if you could possibly bring yourself to do it, I should like mine to be scattered there too. If you find it too gruesome, perhaps you could ask Freddy to do it. I'm sure he wouldn't mind; he has the constitution of a concrete cockroach, dear boy.

And now I must tell you about the things in the study. Once again, it starts with the rose garden. On the day I planted it, Therese gave me a gift. It was her first Holy Communion medal. She told me that it was to say thank you for the rose garden, and to remind me that she would love me forever, no matter what. She made me promise to keep it with me always. It was the most precious thing that I have ever owned. And I lost it. On the day that Therese died. I had it in my pocket that morning when I left Padua, but by the time I returned it was gone. It felt as though the last remaining thread that bound us together had been broken. Like a clock, unwound, I stopped. I stopped living and began existing. I breathed, ate, drank and slept. But only as much as I had to, and that was all.

101

It was Robert who eventually brought me to my senses. 'What would Therese think?' he said. And he was right. She had been so full of life and it had been stolen from her. I still had life, but was choosing a living death. She would have been furious. 'And heartbroken,' said Robert. I began walking; visiting the world again. One day I found a glove; ladies', navy-blue leather, right hand. I took it home and labelled it — what it was, and when and where I'd found it. And so it began, my collection of lost things. Perhaps I thought that if I rescued every lost thing I found, someone would rescue the one thing left in the world that I really cared about and one day I might get it back and so restore my broken promise. It never happened, but I never gave up hope; never stopped gathering in the things that other people had lost. And those tiny scraps of other people's lives gave me inspiration for my stories and helped me to write again.

I know it is likely that most of the things are worthless, and no one will want them back. But if you can make just one person happy, mend one broken heart by restoring to them what they have lost then it will have all been worthwhile. You may wonder why I kept all this secret; kept the study door locked for all those years. I hardly know myself except perhaps it was that I was afraid of being thought foolish or even a little insane. And so this is the task I leave you with, Laura. All I ask is that you try.

I hope that your new life is everything that you wish for and that you find others to share it with. Remember, Laura, there is a world outside of Padua and it is well worth a visit now and then.

One final thing — there is a girl who often sits on the bench across the green from the house. She seems to be something of a lost soul. I have often wished that I could do more for her than a few kindly words, but unfortunately it is difficult for an old man to help a young lady nowadays without being sadly misconstrued. Perhaps you could 'gather her in' and offer a little friendship? Do what you think is best.

With fondest love and grateful thanks,
God bless,
Anthony

By the time Laura stirred from her chair in the study, her limbs were stiffened by cold. Outside, in a black sky, hung a perfect pearlescent moon. Laura sought warmth in the kitchen and set the kettle to boil as she pondered Anthony's requests. The scattering of his ashes she would do gladly. Returning the lost things was not so simple. Once again she felt those stones in her pocket, reminding her of who she really was. Laura's parents had been dead for some years now, but she had never been able to shake the feeling that she had let them down. They had never said as much, but in all honesty what had she ever done to repay their unfailing love and loyalty and make them proud? She had

103

dodged university, her marriage had been a disaster and she had failed to give them a single grandchild. And she had been eating fish and chips in Cornwall when her mother died. The fact that it had been her first holiday since she had left Vince wasn't any kind of excuse. When her father had died just six months later, Anthony filled some of the void that had remained, and perhaps now the task that he had left her would be her chance to make some sort of amends? Perhaps this was her opportunity to finally succeed at something.

And then there was Sunshine. In this, at least, she was ahead of Anthony, but she couldn't take any credit for it. It was Sunshine who had offered her friendship first and even then Laura had been — was still — reluctant to reciprocate. She thought about all the times that she had seen Sunshine before Anthony had died, and done nothing. Said nothing. Not even 'Hello'. But Anthony had done what little he could even after his death. Laura was disappointed in herself, but she was determined to try and change. She took her tea upstairs to the rose-scented bedroom she had claimed for her own. Or rather that she had chosen to share with Therese. Because she was still there. Her things were still there. Not her clothes, of course, but her dressing-table set, the photograph of her with Anthony, which was inexplicably face down once more, and the little blue enamel clock. 11.55. Stopped again. Laura put down her cup and wound the clock until its gentle ticking resumed. She went to bed leaving the curtains wide open, and outside the perfect moon veiled the rose garden in a ghostly damask of light and shade.

17

Eunice

1984

'At Christmas time we da, di, da and we vanish shade . . . '

Mrs Doyle was in fine voice as she served the man in front of Eunice with two sausage plaits and a couple of squares of Tottenham cake. She paused for breath to greet Eunice.

'He's a great bloke, that Bob Gelding, getting all those pop singers to make a record for those poor blighters in Ethio . . . ' the rest of the word slipped away from Mrs Doyle's lexical grasp. ' — in the desert.'

Eunice smiled in agreement. 'He's almost a saint.'

Mrs Doyle began putting doughnuts in a bag. 'Mind you,' she continued, 'it's not as though that Boy George and Midget Ure and the like can't afford to do a bit of charity. And those Bananas — lovely girls, but not a hairbrush between them, by the looks of things.'

Douglas was undisturbed by Eunice's returning footsteps up the stairs. His grey and grizzled muzzle twitched and his front paws flicked gently as he dreamed of who knows what. But it must have been a happy dream, Eunice thought, because the corners of his mouth were turned up in a smile. Bomber was watching him from his desk like an anxious child from a window watching his snowman begin inevitably to melt. She wanted to reassure him, but there was nothing she could say. Douglas was getting old. His days were growing shorter in length and in number. He would die and hearts would break. But for now he was warm and content, and when he eventually woke, a cream doughnut would be waiting for him. The switch from jam to cream (which was actually jam *and* cream) was an effort to keep Douglas's old bones padded with a little of the flesh that seemed to mysteriously dissolve with each passing year.

Bomber, however, was experiencing the exact opposite. In the ten years or so that Eunice had known him he had eventually managed to grow a very modest tummy to add a little softness to his still rangy frame. He patted it affectionately as he said for the umpteenth time, 'We must stop eating so many doughnuts.' A comment completely unaccompanied by any sincerity or intent, and duly ignored by Eunice.

'Are your parents coming into town this week?'

Eunice had grown very fond of Grace and Godfrey and looked forward to their visits, which were unfortunately becoming less and less frequent. It was all too apparent that old age was an unforgiving wingman. Godfrey in particular was becoming less solid in both body and mind; his reason and robustness inexorably stealing away.

'No, not this week. They're feeling a bit out of

sorts. Stoked up the Aga, stocked up on the single malt and secured the portcullis, I shouldn't wonder.' Bomber was frowning at a manuscript that was open on his desk.

'Why? What's up?' Eunice was concerned.

'Well, one of their good chums was caught up in that bomb in Brighton, and then there was the fire in the tube station a couple of weeks ago and that's on their normal route. I just think that they feel, in the words of that classic song favoured by teddy bears, 'it's safer to stay at home'.' Bomber slapped the manuscript shut. 'Probably just as well. I think that Ma might have felt duty bound to enquire about this.'

He waggled the manuscript at Eunice as though it were a rotting fish. Douglas finally stirred in his corner. He took in his surroundings through aged, opalescent eyes, and finding them safe and familiar summoned the energy to gently wag the tip of his tail. Eunice rushed over to kiss his sleep-warm head and tempt him with his doughnut, which was already cut and plated to his exacting requirements. But she hadn't forgotten the rotting fish.

'What is it?'

Bomber heaved an exaggerated sigh. 'It's called *Big Head and Bigot*.'

'Sounds intriguing.'

'Well, that's one word for my darling sister's latest *livre terrible*. It's about the five daughters of a bankrupt football manager. Their mother is determined to marry them off to pop stars or footballers or anyone who's rich. She parades them at the local hunt ball, where the eldest,

108

Janet, is asked to dance by the special guest, a young, handsome owner of a country house hotel called Mr Bingo. Her sister, Izzy, is rather taken with his enigmatic friend, Mr Arsey, a world-famous concert pianist, but he thinks that the antics of the Young Farmers in attendance are rather vulgar and refuses to join Izzy in a karaoke duet. She calls him a snob and goes off in a bit of a huff. To cut a long and strangely familiar story short, the youngest daughter runs off to Margate with a second-rate footballer where they get matching tattoos. She falls pregnant, is dumped and ends up in a bedsit in Peckham. After some well-intentioned but rather pompous interference from Mr Arsey, Janet eventually marries Mr Bingo, and after his agent forbids it, Mr Arsey ends up making sweet music with Izzy.'

Eunice had given up trying to keep a straight face by now, and was howling with laughter at Portia's latest literary larceny. Bomber continued regardless.

'The girls' cousin, Mr Coffins, a religious education teacher at an extremely expensive and completely incompetent private girls' school, offers to marry any of the sisters who will have him, but, to their mother's despair, none of them will on account of his bad breath and protruding belly button, and so he marries their other cousin, Charmaine, on the rebound. Charmaine is happy to have him as she has a slight moustache, and is on the shelf at twenty-one and a half.'

'Poor Charmaine. If she has to settle for bad

breath and a protruding belly button at twenty-one and a half, what hope is there for me at almost thirty-one?'

Bomber grinned. 'Oh, I'm sure we could find you a nice Mr Coffins of your own if you really want one.'

Eunice threw a paperclip at him.

Later that evening, she wandered round the garden of Bomber's rambling flat while he cooked their supper, closely supervised by Douglas. She would never marry. She knew that now. She could never marry Bomber and she didn't want anybody else, so that was an end to it. In the past there had been the occasional date with some hopeful young man; sometimes several. But for Eunice it always felt dishonest. Every man came second best to Bomber, and no man deserved to be forever runner-up. Every relationship would only ever be friendship and sex, never love, and no friendship would ever be as precious as the one she shared with Bomber. Eventually she gave up dating altogether. She thought back to her birthday trip to Brighton all that time ago. It was almost ten years now. It had been a wonderful day, but by the end of it her heart had been broken. On the train home, sitting next to the man she loved, Eunice had fought back the tears, knowing that she would never be the right girl for Bomber. There would never be a right girl for Bomber. But they were friends; best friends. And for Eunice, that was infinitely better than not having him in her life at all.

As he stirred the Bolognese sauce in the

kitchen, Bomber thought back to their earlier conversation. Eunice was a striking young woman with a fierce intelligence, a ready wit and an astonishing assortment of hats. It was unfathomable that she had never been courted or set one of her rather spectacular caps at any particular deserving young man.

'Does it bother you?' He was thinking aloud, albeit a little carelessly, rather than actually posing the question. It seemed a bit blunt to ask.

'Does what bother me?' Eunice appeared in the doorway waving a breadstick in the air like a conductor's baton and sipping a glass of red wine.

'Not having some handsome chap with a red sports car, a Filofax and a flat in Chelsea?'

Eunice bit the end off the breadstick decisively. 'What on earth would I want with one of those, when I have you and Douglas?'

18

'The lady doesn't want it back.'

Sunshine placed the cup and saucer on the table in front of Laura.

'You should keep it for the lovely cup of tea.'

The delicate cream bone china was almost translucent, and hand painted with deep purple violets speckled with gold. Laura looked up at Sunshine's serious face; into her treacle-dark eyes. She had brought Sunshine into the study that morning and explained in broad terms the content of Anthony's letter.

'He said that you and I should take care of each other,' she paraphrased.

It was the first time that she had seen Sunshine smile. Curious and eager, she had handled the things in the study without seeking permission, but with a gentleness and reverence which would have delighted Anthony as much as it reassured Laura. She cradled each object in her soft hands as though it were a baby bird with a broken wing. Laura's attention returned to the cup and saucer and its cardboard label. It was certainly a strange thing to lose.

'But we don't know that, Sunshine. We don't know whom it belonged to.'

Sunshine's conviction was immutable. 'I do. It was the lady and she doesn't want it back to her.'

Her words were delivered without a whisper of

arrogance or petulance. She was simply stating a fact.

'But how do you know?'

Sunshine picked up the cup and held it close to her chest. 'I can feel it. I don't think it in my head, I just feel it.' She put the cup back in its saucer. 'And the lady had a bird,' she added, for good measure.

Laura sighed. The fate of the lost things hung over her; heavy, like a drowning man's clothes. Anthony had chosen her as his successor and she was proud and grateful, but also terrified of failing him; and if the cup and saucer were anything to go by, Sunshine's 'feelings' might prove to be more of a hindrance than a help.

Bone china cup and saucer.
Found on a bench in the Riviera Public
Gardens, 31 October . . .

Eulalia finally stirred in her armchair, taking in her surroundings through age-opaqued eyes. Finding them familiar and herself quick rather than dead, a broad smile split her wrinkled brown face, revealing a haphazard assortment of still-white teeth.

'Praise Jesus for one more day this side of Heaven's gates,' she thought. 'And curse him too,' as arthritis shot shards of pain through her bony legs when she tried to stand up. Alive she might be, but quick she certainly wasn't. She had taken to sleeping downstairs in her chair more of late. Upstairs was fast becoming unattainable territory. Which was why she was

moving. Sheltered accommodation they called it. She called it surrender. A defeated display of the lily-livered flag. But it couldn't be helped. One room with en-suite, a communal lounge, shared kitchen and meals prepared if you wanted. Plastic mattress cover in case you wet the bed. Eulalia shuffled through to her kitchen, sliding in her slippers and gripping her sticks like a geriatric cross-country skier. Kettle on and teabag in the mug, she opened the back door and let the sunshine in. She had once been proud of her garden. She had planned and planted it, nurtured and cherished it for all these years. But now it had outgrown her, like an unruly teenager, and ran wild. The magpie appeared at her feet as soon as the door was opened. He looked as though he was having a bad feather day; a near miss with next door's cat, perhaps. But his eyes were bright and he chuck-chucked softly to Eulalia as he tipped his head this way and that.

'Good morning, Rossini, my friend' — it was their little joke — 'you'll be wanting your breakfast, I suppose.'

He hopped into the kitchen behind her and waited patiently for her to take a handful of raisins from a tin on the draining board.

'What will you do without me?' she asked, as she threw a couple onto the kitchen floor. The bird gobbled than up and looked to her for more.

'Outside now, my friend,' she said, scattering the rest of the raisins onto the doorstep.

She took her tea back into the sitting room,

114

making precarious progress with a single stick, and gingerly lowered herself into her chair. The room was full of pretty things; weird and wonderful baubles and ornaments. Eulalia had been a magpie all her life, surrounding herself with sparkle and glister, twinkle and velvet, the magical and the macabre, But now the time had come to let them go. These were her treasures and she would decide their fate. She couldn't take them with her, but neither could she bear the thought of her precious things being picked over by a white van driver called Dave — 'House Clearances: no job too big or too small'. Besides, some of the things could get her into trouble. Some of the things weren't exactly . . . legal. Well, not here, anyway. There were skeletons in her cupboards. Truly.

By the time she had filled her tartan shopping trolley with the chosen objects it was almost midday, Her ratchety limbs, lubricated by activity, moved more freely now as she headed towards the public gardens by the park. She would give her things away. She would leave them where others would find them; as many things as she had been able to drag in her trolley. And as for the rest, no one would have them. It was a school day and the park and gardens were deserted save for a couple of dog walkers and a poor unfortunate soul still asleep in the bandstand. Eulalia was unobserved as she placed four snow globes, a rabbit's skull and a gold pocket watch on the little wall that encircled the ornamental fountain. Further into the park, two silver church candlesticks, a stuffed weasel and a set of gold-plated dentures were secreted in the niches of the war memorial statue. A mummified pig's penis and the ormolu music box from Paris were left on the steps by the pond, and the china bride doll with empty eye sockets on the seat of one of the children's swings. Back in the gardens the crystal ball wallowed in a stone bird bath and the bowler hat with a cockade of crow's feathers was perched on top of the sun-dial. The ebony cursing bowl was placed at the foot of a sycamore tree whose leaves were a molten kaleidoscope of scarlet, orange and yellow. And so she continued until, almost emptied, the trolley bounced along behind her on skittish wheels. She sat down on the wooden bench facing the park and breathed a sigh of contentment. A job well done — almost. The final item on the wooden slats beside her was a bone china cup and saucer painted with gold and violets. It rattled in the aftershock of an explosion two streets away that killed a postman and seriously injured a passer-by. A thick pall of smoke smudged a dark column into the afternoon sky and Eulalia smiled as she remembered that she had left the gas on.

★ ★ ★

'Put the gas on under the kettle, tea to the teapot, milk to the jug.'

Back in the kitchen Laura smiled as Sunshine talked herself through the tea-making as she

116

always did with any task that required concentration. There was a knock at the back door and, without waiting for a reply, Freddy came in. Laura had spoken to him the night before to let him know that his job was still there if he wanted it, and to invite him for tea in the kitchen, rather than drinking it alone in the garden as he usually did. He had been away since the funeral, and when he had left the situation at Padua had still been uncertain.

She had surprised herself by issuing the invitation, but reasoned that the more often she came into contact with him, the less flustered she might be when she did. Because she couldn't help but find him rather increasingly attractive.

'Two sugars, please,' he said, winking at Sunshine, who blushed deeply and found something fascinating to look at on the teaspoon she was holding. Laura knew how she felt. There was something intriguing about this laconic man who tended the garden with such care, and did odd jobs around the place with quiet efficiency. Laura had learned scarcely anything about his life away from Padua; he gave so little away and she hadn't yet found the courage to ask. But she was building up to it, she promised herself. The only information he seemed to require was what needed doing, and if there were any biscuits.

'Freddy, this is Sunshine, my new friend and assistant. Sunshine, this is Freddy.'

Sunshine tore her gaze away from the teaspoon and tried to look Freddy in the eye.

'Hi, Sunshine. How's it going?'

'How's what going? I'm nineteen and I'm dancing drome.'

Freddy smiled. 'I'm thirty-five and three quarters and I'm a Capricorn.'

Sunshine placed a cup of tea in front of Freddy and then the milk jug and sugar bowl. Then a teaspoon and a plate of biscuits. And then a fork, a bottle of washing-up liquid, a packet of cornflakes and an egg whisk. And a box of matches. Freddy's slow smile split his handsome face, revealing a perfect set of white teeth. The smile burgeoned into a deep, throaty laugh. Whatever Sunshine's test was, he had passed it. She sat down next to him.

'Saint Anthony has left all the lost things to Laura and we have to get them back at the right people. Except the cup and saucer.'

'Is that right?'

'Yes it is. Shall I show you?'

'Not today. I'll finish my tea and washing-up liquid first, and then there's a job I have to go to. But next time I'm here, it's a date.'

Sunshine almost smiled. Laura was beginning to feel a little superfluous. 'Anthony was certainly a very good man, Sunshine, but strictly speaking, he wasn't a saint.'

Freddy drained his cup. 'Well now, he could have been. Have you never heard of Saint Anthony of Padua, the Patron Saint of Lost Things?'

Laura shook her head.

'I kid you not. It's true. Five years at Sunday school,' he added by way of explanation.

Sunshine smiled triumphantly. Now she had two friends.

19

Laura was throwing away her old life. It was going to be a messy business. She tipped a boxful of junk into the bin and slammed the lid shut, blowing a puff of dust and dirt into her face in the process. She had been sorting through the last of the things she had brought with her from the flat, many of which hadn't been unpacked since she had moved from the house she had shared with Vince. If she hadn't needed them in the last six or so years, she reasoned, she wasn't likely to need them now. The local charity shop might have been glad of some of her 'junk', but that would involve a trip into town which Laura wasn't keen to make. 'I'm too busy for that at the moment,' she convinced herself. Before the ink could dry on her words of excuse they were smudged with guilt as she remembered Anthony's letter: *there is a world outside of Padua and it is well worth a visit now and then.* 'Another day,' she promised herself.

She wiped the grime from her face with her hands, and then wiped her hands on her jeans. God, she was filthy; time for a shower.

'Hello. Do you work here?'

The question came from a leggy blonde who appeared down the path at the side of the house in skin-tight jeans and pale pink suede loafers which boasted tell-tale Gucci horse-bit trims and matched perfectly with her cashmere sweater.

Laura's dumbfounded expression clearly caused the young woman to assume that she was either foreign, simple or deaf. She tried again, speaking very slowly and a little too loudly.

'I'm looking for Freddo — the groundsman.'

Thankfully, at that moment, the man himself appeared, sauntering down the garden carrying a wooden crate of freshly dug potatoes that he set down at Laura's feet.

'Darling Freddo!'

The young woman flung her arms around his neck and kissed him enthusiastically on the lips. Freddy gently untangled himself and took her hand.

'Felicity, what in God's name are you doing here?'

'I've come to take my darling boyfriend out to lunch.'

Freddy grinned. He looked a little uncomfortable. 'Felicity, this is Laura. Laura, this is Felicity.'

'So I gather.' Laura nodded, but didn't offer her hand, which was just as well because Felicity wasn't in the habit of shaking hands with 'the help'. The happy couple trotted off arm in arm and Laura took the potatoes into the kitchen and banged the crate down on the table.

'Sodding cheek!' she fumed. 'Do I look like I work here?'

Catching sight of herself in the hall mirror, Laura was forced to reconsider. With her unkempt hair scragged back under a spotted bandana, grime-streaked face and baggy, shapeless sweatshirt, she looked like a modern-day scullery maid.

'Bugger!'

She stomped upstairs and had a long hot shower, but afterwards, as she sat on her bed swathed in a towel, it was clear that the water had only succeeded in washing away the dirt and not her anger. She was jealous. She was mortified to admit it, but she was. The sight of that wretched woman kissing Freddy had thoroughly annoyed her. Laura raised her eyebrows at her own reflection in the dressing-table mirror and smiled sheepishly.

'*I* can go out to lunch if I like.'

That was it. She *would* go out to lunch. Anthony had wanted her to go out, and so she would. Today. Right now.

The Moon is Missing was a 'smart casual' pub with black-tie aspirations. Its proximity to St Luke's meant it was popular for post-funeral pick-me-ups and pre-wedding loin-girders. Laura ordered a whisky and soda, and 'herb-crumbed goujons of cod served with hand-cut wedges of King Edwards and a lightly frothed tartare sauce', and took a seat in one of the booths that lined the wall facing the bar. Her bravura had deserted her almost as soon as she had left the house, and what should have been a treat had become something to endure, like a visit to the dentist or a crawl through rush-hour traffic. Laura was glad she had arrived early enough to bag a booth, and that she had remembered to bring a book with her to hide behind, just in case anyone tried to talk to her. On her way here, it had suddenly and rather worryingly occurred to her that Freddy and the frisky Felicity might also be lunching in this particular pub, but much though the thought horrified her, she was too stubborn to turn back. And so here she was, drinking in the middle of the day, which was unheard of, and pretending to read a book she wasn't really interested in, whilst waiting for a lunch that she didn't really want. All in order to prove a point to herself and not let Anthony down. And to think that she could have been at home cleaning the cooker . . . Even Laura couldn't help but crack a wry smile at her own ridiculousness.

The pub was filling up and just as the waitress brought her posh fish fingers and chips, the booth next to Laura's was occupied with a great deal of huffing and puffing and shedding of coats and shopping bags. As her new neighbours began reading aloud from the menu, Laura recognised the imperious alto of Marjory Wadscallop accompanied by the dithering descant of Winnie Cripp. Having decided upon and ordered two 'poussin and portobello potages', the pair chinked their glasses of gin and tonic and began discussing the production of *Blithe Spirit* currently in rehearsal by their amateur dramatics group.

'Of course, technically, I'm far too young to play Madame Arcati,' asserted Marjory, 'but then the part does require an actor of extraordinary range and subtlety, so I suppose, considering the 'dramatis personae' at Everard's disposal, I was the only real choice.'

'Yes, of course you were, dear,' agreed Winnie, 'and Gillian's an absolute pro at costumes and make-up, so she'll have you looking old in no time.'

Marjory was unsure whether to be pleased about this or not. 'Well, she absolutely looks like a 'pro' with the amount of slap she normally wears,' she replied tetchily.

'Naughty!' giggled Winnie and then fell guiltily silent as the waitress arrived with their chicken and mushroom soups accompanied by 'an assortment of artisan bread rolls'. There was a brief hiatus while they salted their soups and buttered their bread.

'I'm a bit nervous about playing Edith,' Winnie then confessed. 'It's the biggest part I've had so far and there's an awful lot of lines to remember, as well as all that carrying of drinks and walking on and off.'

'You mean 'stage business' and 'blocking', Winnie. It's so important to use the correct terminology.' Marjory took a large bite from her granary roll and chewed on it thoughtfully before adding, 'I shouldn't worry too much, dear. After all, Edith is only a housemaid, so you won't be required to do very much real acting.'

Laura had finished her lunch and asked for the bill. Just as she was gathering her things to leave, the mention of a familiar name caught her attention.

'I'm sure Geoffrey will be a perfectly serviceable Charles Condomine, but in his younger days Anthony Peardew would have been ideal for the role; tall, dark, handsome and so very charming.' Marjory's voice had taken on an almost wistful tone.

'And he was a writer in real life too,' added Winnie.

Marjory's tongue sought to dislodge a grain from her roll, which had become caught under her dental plate. Having succeeded, she continued, 'It does seem rather odd that he left everything to that rather prickly housekeeper of his, Laura.'

'Mmmn. It's a funny business, all right.' Winnie loved a side order of scurrilous gossip with her lunch. 'I shouldn't wonder if there wasn't a bit of *funny business* going on there,' she added knowingly, delighted at her double entendre.

Marjory drained the last of her gin and tonic and signalled to the waitress to bring her another one.

'Well, I expect she did a little more for him than just the dusting and hoovering.'

Laura had intended to try and sneak past them without being seen, but now she turned and faced them with a brazen smile.

'Fellatio,' she announced. 'Every Friday.'

And without another word, she swept out.

Winnie turned to Marjory with a puzzled expression. 'What's that when it's at home?'

'Italian,' said Marjory, dabbing at her mouth with a napkin. 'I had it in a restaurant once.'

20

Sunshine set the needle onto the spinning liquorice disc and was rewarded with the mellifluous tones of Etta James, hot and rich like smoked paprika.

In the kitchen, Freddy was sitting at the table, and Laura was making sandwiches for lunch.

'She's got great taste.' Freddy tipped his head in the direction of the music.

Laura smiled. 'She's choosing the music for when we scatter Anthony's ashes. She says it's like the film where the dog gets a bone and the clocks stop because Saint Anthony's dead, but he'll be together forever with Therese. But she calls her 'The Lady of the Flowers'. And your guess is as good as mine.'

She sliced cucumber into translucent slices and drained a tin of salmon.

'She wants to make a speech as well, although I'm not sure we'll make head or tail of it.'

'I'm sure we'll make it out just fine.' Freddy spun a teaspoon that was idling on the table. 'She just has her own way of saying stuff, that's all. She knows the words that we all use, but I suppose she just likes hers better.'

Laura licked a smudge of butter from her finger. She wasn't used to having actual conversations with Freddy. His way of saying stuff was usually a combination of nods, shrugs and grunts. But Sunshine wasn't having any of that. With her solemn eyes and soft, fluty voice she coaxed the words from him like a snake charmer.

'But isn't she just making life harder; setting herself further apart . . . '

Laura's voice trailed off along with her train of thought, stymied by political correctness. Freddy weighed her words carefully and without judgement.

'Further apart from 'normal' people, you mean?'

It was Laura's turn to shrug. She didn't really know what she meant. She knew that Sunshine had made few friends at school, and had been mercilessly taunted by the feral teenagers who hung around in the local park drinking cheap cider, vandalising the swings and having sex. Were they normal? And if they were, why should Sunshine want to be like them? Freddy balanced the neck of the teaspoon on the tip of his index finger. Laura went back to the sandwiches and began cutting them viciously into triangles. Now he would think she was a . . . A what? Bigot? Idiot? Maybe she was. The more she saw of Freddy, the more it mattered what he thought of her. Laura's idea of inviting Freddy to take his breaks in the kitchen in order to facilitate a more relaxed relationship between them could not yet be deemed a success, but the time they spent together was the part of the day she looked forward to most.

Freddy placed the teaspoon carefully down in front of him and leaned back in his chair, rocking the two front legs off the floor. She fought the urge to tell him to sit properly at the table.

'I think it's a sort of camouflage' — he rocked back onto four legs — 'the way she speaks. It's like a Jackson Pollock. There's so many specks and splashes of paint, that if one of them happens to be a mistake, no one can tell. If Sunshine does get a word wrong, we'll never know.' He shook his head, smiling to himself. 'It's genius.'

At that moment, the genius came into the kitchen looking for her lunch. Laura was still thinking about what Freddy had said. A gardener using the art of Jackson Pollock as a linguistic metaphor was a little unexpected, and another intriguing insight into the kind of man he really was. It made Laura both eager and determined to find out more.

'By the way,' said Freddy to Laura, 'the film. It's *Four Weddings and a Funeral*.'

Sunshine grinned and sat down next to her newest friend.

After lunch, they all went through to the study. Sunshine was desperate to show Freddy Anthony's museum of missing things, and Laura was toying with the idea of asking if he had any bright ideas about returning them to their rightful owners. Each time she came into the study it seemed to Laura that the room was filling up; less space, more things. And she felt smaller; shrinking, sinking. The shelves seemed to groan, threatening collapse, and the drawers creak, dovetails about to fly open and burst. She feared she would be buried under an avalanche

127

of lost property. For Sunshine it was a treasure trove. She stroked and held and hugged the things, talking softly to herself — or perhaps to the things themselves — and reading their labels with obvious enchantment. Freddy was appropriately astonished.

'Who'd have thought it?' he whispered, peering at his surroundings. 'So that's why he always carried his bag.'

The frail October sunlight struggled to permeate the trellis of flowers and leaves on the lace panels and the room was dark and stained with shadows. He drew back the lace, shooting a meteorite shower of shimmering dust motes spinning across the room.

'Let's throw a bit of light over things, shall we?'

Sunshine showed him round, like a curator proudly sharing a collection of fine art. She showed him buttons and rings, gloves, teddy bears, a glass eye, items of jewellery, a jigsaw puzzle piece, keys, coins, plastic toys, tweezers, four sets of dentures and a doll's head. And these were the contents of only one drawer. The cream cup and saucer painted with violets was still on the table. Sunshine picked it up and handed it to Freddy.

'It's pretty, isn't it? The lady doesn't want it back to her so Laura's going to keep it for the lovely cup of tea.'

Laura was about to contradict her, but Sunshine's face was set with such absolute certainty that the words died in Laura's mouth.

'That'll be yours, then.'

128

As Laura took the cup and saucer from him, his fingers brushed against her hand, and he held her gaze for just a moment before turning away and sitting down in Anthony's chair.

'And you're to try and get all the rest of this,' he said, sweeping his arms around the room, 'back to wherever it is that it belongs?' His equable tone gave no quarter to the enormity of the task.

'That's the idea,' Laura replied.

Sunshine was distracted by an object that had fallen out of the drawer she had opened. She picked it up from the floor but immediately dropped it again, howling in pain.

Ladies' glove, navy-blue leather, right hand. Found on the grass verge at the foot of Cow Bridge, 23 December . . .

It was bitter. Too cold for snow. Rose looked up at the black sky pierced with a tracery of stars and a sharp sickle moon. She had been walking briskly for twenty minutes but her feet were numb and her fingers frozen. Too sad for tears. She was almost there now. Thankfully there had been no passing cars; no one to distract or intervene. Too late to think. Here now. This was the place. Over the bridge and then just a shallow, grassy bank. She took off one glove and pulled the photograph from her pocket. She kissed the face of the little girl who smiled back at her. Too dark to see, but she knew she was there. 'Mummy loves you.' Down the grassy slope her gloveless hand clutched at razor frozen grass. At the bottom, shale underfoot. 'Mummy loves you,' she whispered again, as the distant lights pricked the darkness and the rails began to hum. Too hard to live.

'Too hard to live. The lady died.' Sunshine was shaking as she tried to explain.

Freddy pulled her close and squeezed her tight. 'I think that what you need is the lovely cup of tea.'

He made it, under Sunshine's strict supervision. Two cups of tea and a Jammie Dodger later, she tried to tell them a little more.

'She loved her little girl, but the lady was very sad,' was the best that she could do.

Laura was strangely unsettled. 'Sunshine, maybe it would be better if you didn't go into the study any more.'

'Why?'

Laura hesitated. Part of her didn't want Sunshine becoming too involved. She knew it was selfish, but she was desperate to find a way to make Anthony and maybe even her parents proud of her. Posthumously, of course. It was her chance to finally do something right and she didn't want any distractions.

'In case there are other things in here that upset you.'

Sunshine shook her head determinedly. 'I'm okay now.'

Laura looked unconvinced, but Sunshine had a point to make.

'If you never get sadness, how do you know

what happy is like?' she asked. 'And by the way, everybody dies.'

'I think she has you in checkmate there,' Freddy murmured.

Laura conceded defeat with a reluctant smile.

'But,' continued Freddy, 'I may have the very thing to cheer you up. I have a plan.'

21

Sunshine stood waiting by the sundial, a solemn figure in a pink duffle coat and silver sequinned baseball boots. The dank October afternoon was already seeping away, the edges of an empty sky tinged with the rhubarb flush of a looming sunset. On Sunshine's signal Freddy started the music and took his place next to Laura to walk down the 'aisle' of flickering tea lights to where Sunshine was waiting to start the ceremony. Freddy was carrying Anthony's ashes in a plain wooden urn, and Laura held a fancy cardboard box full of real rose petal confetti and the photograph of Therese from the garden room. Laura fought the urge to giggle as she walked as slowly as she could to the inevitable accompaniment of Al Bowlly.

Sunshine had planned everything down to the last detail. The gramophone had been conveniently positioned so that Freddy could reach it by leaning in the window, and the confetti and rose-scented candles for the tea lights had been ordered especially. Sunshine had originally wanted to wait until the roses were in bloom again, but Laura couldn't bear the thought of Anthony's ashes languishing on a shelf for the next nine months. She couldn't keep him from Therese any longer. The rose-scented candles and confetti had been a hard-won compromise. Freddy and Laura reached Sunshine just as Mr

132

Bowlly was beginning his final verse and she listened, really listened to the words for perhaps the first time.

It could have been written for Anthony and Therese. Sunshine left a pause just long enough for it to be dramatic before consulting the piece of paper she was clutching.

'Dreary beloved, we are gathered here in the sight of God and in the fate of this complication, to join together this man, Saint Anthony' — she tapped the top of his urn — 'and this woman, The Lady of the Flowers' — gesturing towards the photograph with an upturned palm — 'in holy macaroni which is the honourable estate. Saint Anthony takes The Lady of the Flowers to be the lawful wedding wife, to have and to hold from this day forward, for better for worse, richer or poorer, to love and to perish with death now you start. And it still rhymes,' she added proudly to herself.

She paused again, long enough this time for it to be almost uncomfortable, but no doubt with the intention of underscoring the sanctity of the occasion.

'Earth to earth, ashes to ashes, funky to punky. We know Major Tom's a monkey. We can be heroes just for today.'

She leaned forward and addressed Freddy and Laura in a stage whisper. 'Now you throw the ashes, and you throw the confetti,' and then, as an afterthought, 'Follow me!'

They made an odd little procession filing round the rose garden, Sunshine leading them in and out of the desolate-looking bushes whose summer finery had been reduced to a ragbag of sodden, yellowing leaves stubbornly clinging on. Freddy followed Sunshine, emptying the urn as delicately as he could, with Laura behind him, trying to avoid any backdraught as she scattered confetti on the wispy grey trail of Anthony's remains. The 'scattering of ashes' had always sounded like such an ethereal act to Laura, but in reality, she reflected, it was more akin to emptying a vacuum-cleaner bag. When the urn was finally empty, Sunshine consulted her piece of paper once again.

'He was her north, her south, her east, her west; her working week and Sunday vest.

'She was his moon and stars and favourite song; they thought that love would last forever: they weren't wrong.'

Freddy winked at her, smiling broadly. 'And it still rhymes,' he mouthed.

Sunshine wasn't to be distracted. 'I now announce you husband and wife. Those whom God, and Sunshine, have joined together let no man steal their thunder.'

She nodded at Freddy, who scampered off in the direction of the gramophone.

'And now it's time for the bride and groom's first dance.'

As the dying sun stained the ice blue sky crimson and a blackbird's call echoed through the gathering dusk, warning of a prowling tabby, Etta James proclaimed 'At Last'.

As the final note smouldered into the chilly air, Laura looked across at Freddy. He was gazing straight at her and when her eyes met his he smiled. Laura went to gather the tea lights. But Sunshine wasn't quite finished. She rattled her piece of paper and cleared her throat.

'I am the resurrection and the light, saith the Lord: he that believeth in me, though he were dead, yet shall he live. And it's goodnight from me and it's goodnight from him.'

★ ★ ★

When Laura went up to bed that night the room felt different somehow. Perhaps it was warmer. Or maybe that was just the wine she had shared with Freddy and Sunshine to celebrate Therese and Anthony's reunion. The things on the dressing table were all in order and the little blue clock had stopped at 11.55 as usual. She wound it up so that it could stop at the same time again tomorrow, drew the curtains and turned to get into bed.

There were petals of rose confetti on the bedcovers.

22

Eunice

1987

Bette trotted along just ahead of them, surveying the park for undesirables. Every now and then she would turn to check that they were following her obediently, her velveteen face crumpled into a comical frown. She was named after the film star to whom she bore an unnerving resemblance, but they had taken to calling her Baby Jane after one of her namesake's most memorable characters.

Bomber had been freeze-framed by Douglas's death. He had held the little dog in his arms until long after his final breath had sighed 'the end', and his soft fur had grown cold and strange. Eunice had howled an eruption of pain, but Bomber sat rigid and dry-eyed as an ash cloud of grief settled over him and choked his tears. The Douglas-shaped space in the office hurt every day. They were a man down and a doughnut too many, but Eunice kept going; on automatic pilot at first, but onwards nevertheless. Bomber crashed and burned. He drank away his pain and then he slept away the drink.

In the end only one man could reach him. It was difficult to say who had fallen for Tom Cruise the hardest, Bomber or Eunice, as he swaggered from bike to bar to plane in his Ray-Bans. They had seen *Top Gun* three nights in a row when it had opened at the Odeon the previous year. Three weeks after Douglas died Eunice stormed Bomber's flat with her spare key and kicked his grieving arse out of bed. As he sat at the kitchen table, tears finally released and dripping down his face and into the mug of black coffee Eunice had made, she took his hand.

'God, he loved flying with you, Bomber. But he'd have flown anyway . . . without you. He'd have hated it, but he would've done it.'

The following day, Bomber came into the office sober, and the following week Baby Jane arrived from Battersea Dogs Home; a bossy bundle of black and blonde velvet. Baby Jane didn't like doughnuts. The first time she was offered one, she sniffed at it disdainfully and turned away. It might as well have been a turd tartlet. Baby Jane liked Viennese whirls. For a stray, she had expensive tastes.

As the diminutive pug nosed an empty crisp packet on the grass, Eunice looked up at Bomber and almost recognised him again. His grief was still smudged under his eyes and pinched into his cheeks, but his smile was limbering up and his shoulders unfurling from their disconsolate stoop. She was never going to be a replacement, but she was already a distraction, and if Baby Jane had her way, which she usually did, Eunice had no doubt whatsoever that she would eventually prove to be a superstar in her own right.

Back in the office, Eunice put the kettle on

while Bomber went through the post. Baby Jane settled herself onto her cushion and rested her head on her front paws, gathering herself for the arduous task of eating her cake. When Eunice came through with the tea Bomber was waving a slim volume of short stories in the air that had just arrived from a rival publisher.

'*Lost and Found* by Anthony Peardew. Hmm, I've heard of this. It's doing rather well. I wonder why old Bruce has sent it to me.'

Eunice picked up the accompanying compliments slip and read it. 'To gloat,' she answered.

' 'Bomber',' she read, ' 'please accept a copy of this hugely successful collection with my compliments. You had your chance, old chap, and you blew it!' '

Bomber shook his head. 'No idea what he's talking about. If this Peardew fellow had sent it to us first we'd have snapped it up. It's an excess of hairspray. It's addled his brains.'

Eunice picked up the book and flicked through the pages. The author's name and title together, like two flints, sparked a vague memory; a manuscript? Eunice racked her brain for the answer but it was like bobbing for apples; just when she thought she'd got it by the skin of her teeth, it slipped away. Baby Jane sighed theatrically. Her cake was *en retard* and she was weak with hunger. Eunice laughed and ruffled the soft rolls of velvet on her head.

'You're such a diva, young lady! You'll get fat and then no more cakes for you. Just jogging round the park and the occasional stick of celery. If you're lucky.'

Baby Jane stared up at Eunice dolefully, her black button eyes framed by long dark lashes. It worked every time. She got her cake. At last.

Just as she was licking her lips in an optimistic search for remaining flecks of cream, the phone rang. Each pair of rings was followed by an imperious bark. Since her arrival, Baby Jane had quickly assumed a managerial position and she ran a very tight kennel. Bomber answered.

'Ma.'

He listened for a moment. Eunice watched his face and knew immediately that this was not good news. Bomber was on his feet.

'Do you want me to come over? I'll come now if you like. Don't be daft, Ma, of course it's no trouble.'

It would be about Godfrey. The lovely, kind, funny, gentlemanly Godfrey, whose dementia was casting him adrift. A once majestic galleon whose sails had worn thin and tattered, no longer able to steer its own course but left to the mercy of every squall and storm. Last month he had managed to flood the house and set fire to it at the same time. He had started to run a bath and then forgot about it, going downstairs to dry his shirt, which he left on the hotplate of the Aga before setting off for the village to buy a paper. By the time Grace had come in from the greenhouse, the water leaking through the kitchen ceiling had put out the fire started by the shirt. She hadn't known whether to laugh or cry. But she refused to accept that she needed help. He was her husband and she loved him. She had promised 'in sickness and in health'. Till death

139

do us part. She couldn't bear to think of him in a home where the interior design included armchairs with built-in commodes. And yet . . . This time he had run away. Well, wandered off, more like. After an hour of frantically searching the village, Grace had come home to telephone the police. She was met at the gate by the local vicar who, on his way to visit a parishioner, had found Godfrey walking in the middle of the road, with a broom held up against his shoulder like a rifle and Grace's red beret stretched onto his head. He told the Rev. Addlestrop that he was returning to his regiment after a weekend pass.

Bomber dropped the phone back into its cradle with a resigned sigh.

'Do you want me to come with you, or stay here and hold the fort with Baby Jane?'

Before he could answer the buzzer went.

Portia received the news of her father's latest escapade with horrible tranquillity. She refused to join Bomber and go and see her parents, let alone offer any kind of help or support. Bomber tried in vain to crack the surface of her callous composure.

'This is serious, sis. Ma can't be expected to watch over him every minute of the day and night, and he's a danger to himself. And before long, God forbid, he may be to her as well.'

Portia inspected her scarlet fingernails. She'd just had them done and she was quite pleased. She'd even tipped the girl a pound.

'Well? What do you expect me to do about it? He belongs in a home.'

'He *is* in a home,' Eunice hissed. 'His home.'

'Oh, shut up, Eunuch. It's none of your business.'

'Well at least she gives a damn!' snapped Bomber.

Stung by Bomber's painful reprimand and secretly terrified by her father's illness, Portia responded in the only way she knew how to: with insults.

'You heartless bastard! Of course I care about him. I'm just being honest. If he's dangerous, he needs to be locked up. At least I've got the guts to say it. You always were completely spineless; always sucking up to Ma and Pa and never once standing up to them like me!'

Baby Jane could see that things were getting out of hand, and she wasn't having her friends spoken to in that manner. A low growl rumbled her displeasure. Portia sought out the source of the admonishment and found the feisty little pug preparing for battle.

'Is that revolting-looking cushion-pisser still here? I should have thought you'd have had enough when that other little monster finally died.'

Eunice glanced across to where Douglas's ashes sat safe in a box on Bomber's desk and offered a silent apology. She was just wondering how to inflict appropriate and excruciating pain on this execrable woman, when she realised that Baby Jane had already decided. Leaving her cushion with the prowling menace of a lion who has just spotted a dithering gazelle, she fixed Portia with her fiercest stare and turned up the volume until her whole body vibrated. Her lips curled back revealing a small but businesslike set of teeth. Portia flapped her fingers ineffectually at her, but Baby Jane continued her advance, eyes fixed firmly on her prey and growl now punctuated by dramatic snarls.

'Shoo! Shoo! Sit! Down!'

Baby Jane kept coming.

Halfway across the floor, Portia capitulated with an undignified retreat and an unladylike barrage of expletives.

Bomber began gathering his things.

Eunice repeated her offer of help. 'I'll come with you if you want me to.'

He smiled gratefully but shook his head. 'No, no. I'll be fine. You stay here and look after madam,' he said, reaching down to fondle Baby Jane's ears while she gazed up at him adoringly.

'At least we know now that it's true,' he added with a mischievous grin.

'What's that? That Portia's a complete waste of hot air and high heels?'

He shook his head and gently lifted a blonde paw in his hand.

'Nobody puts Baby Jane in a corner!'

Eunice hooted with laughter.

'Get out of here, Patrick Swayze!'

23

'*Lost and Found* by Anthony Peardew. I knew there was a copy somewhere in the house!'

Laura came into the kitchen triumphantly waving a slim volume of short stories. Freddy looked up from the laptop he was hunched over on the kitchen table. He took the book from her and flicked through it.

'Is it any good?'

'It depends what you mean by 'good'.' Laura sat down in the chair facing him. 'It did very well. Apparently Anthony's publisher at the time was very happy. He was a peculiar little man, I seem to remember. He came to the house once or twice. Used far too much hairspray.'

'Too much!' Freddy expostulated. 'I should think that any is too much. Unless you're Liberace. Or a ballroom dancer.'

'It's called 'male grooming',' Laura smiled. 'But I wouldn't exactly call that your specialist subject,' she added, looking at the unruly mop of dark curls that crept over the collar of his shirt and the stubble that shaded the contours of his face.

'No need,' he replied, winking at her. 'I'm naturally handsome.'

He was, Laura silently agreed. Oh God! She hoped it had been silent. But maybe she'd nodded. She could feel a tell-tale flush creeping up her neck. Bugger! Maybe he would just think it was her age. Double bugger! Maybe he *would* just think it was her age. Middle age. Ready for big knickers, hot flushes and winceyette nighties. And she absolutely wasn't. In fact, she was going on a date.

'But did you think it was any good?'

Freddy was speaking.

'Sorry. Miles away. What was that?'

Freddy waved the book at her. '*Lost and Found* — what did you think?'

Laura sighed and spread her hands on the table in front of her.

'I thought it was safe. It was beautifully written, as always, but the content had lost a little of his usual edge. It was a bit too 'happy ever after' for me. It was almost as though if he wrote enough happy endings for other people, he'd get one for himself.'

'But it never came?'

Laura smiled sadly. 'Until now.'

Fingers crossed.

'Is that why he stopped writing?'

Laura shook her head. 'No. He wrote several volumes of these short stories — based on the things he found, I now assume. At first they were optimistic tales; congenial and commercial. Bruce the peculiar was delighted with them and, no doubt, the money they brought in. But over time the stories grew darker, the characters more ambivalent; flawed, even. The happy endings gradually gave way to uncomfortable mysteries and unanswered questions. All this was before my time, of course, but when I eventually read them, I thought they were much better and they were certainly more like his earlier work, crediting his readers with both imagination and intelligence. Anthony told me that Bruce had been furious. He just wanted more of the 'nice' stories; literary lemonade. But Anthony had given him absinthe. Bruce refused to publish them and that was that.'

'Didn't Anthony look for another publisher?'

'I don't know. By the time I started working for him, he seemed to be writing them more for himself than for anyone else. Eventually he stopped giving me anything to type at all, apart from the odd letter.'

Laura picked up the book from the table and tenderly stroked its cover. She missed her old friend.

'Maybe that's what we should call the website — 'Lost and Found'?'

The website had been Freddy's plan. At first Laura had been unsure. For so many years Anthony had resisted the intrusion of technology into his tranquil home, and to throw open the doors to the behemoth Internet and all its goblin relatives so soon after his death somehow felt like a violation. But Freddy convinced her.

'The only thing Anthony asked you not to change was the rose garden. He left the house to you because he knew that you would do the right thing. It's your home now but it came with a covenant on its coat-tails and Anthony trusted you to use whatever method you saw fit to get those things back to the people who are missing them.'

The website would be a huge, virtual 'lost

property' department where people could browse the things that Anthony had found and then re-claim items that belonged to them. They were still working on the details, including the name.

''Lost and Found'. Too boring.' Sunshine had wandered in from the study, looking for biscuits.

'Shall I make the lovely cup of tea?'

Freddy rubbed his hands together in exaggerated delight.

'I thought you'd never ask. I'm as dry as James Bond's Martini.'

Sunshine filled the kettle and set it carefully on the hob.

'How can the drink, which is wet because it's the drink, be dry?'

'That's a good question, kiddo,' said Freddy, thinking *to which I'm buggered if I know the answer*.

Laura saved him. 'How about The Kingdom of Lost Things?'

Sunshine wrinkled her nose in disapproval. 'Saint Anthony kept all the lost things safe. He was the Keeper, and now you are. We should call it The Keeper of Lost Things.'

'Brilliant!' said Freddy.

'Where's the biscuits?' said Sunshine.

★   ★   ★

Laura arrived back from the hairdresser's salon just as Freddy was leaving for the day.

'You look different,' he said, almost accusingly. 'Have you got a new jumper?'

146

She could, quite cheerfully, have kicked him. Her jumper was several years old and bore a generous sprinkle of pilling to prove it. But she had just spent the best part of two hours and seventy quid having her hair cut and coloured with what her stylist, Elise, had described as burnished copper lowlights. When she left the salon, tossing her glossy chestnut mane like a frisky show pony, she had felt like a million dollars. Now, for some reason, she felt like she'd wasted her money.

'I've just had my hair done,' she muttered through gritted teeth.

'Oh, right. That must be it then,' he said, rummaging through his rucksack for his car keys. Finding them, he gave her a quick grin and headed for the door.

'I'll be off then. See you tomorrow.'

The door closed behind him and Laura gave the bamboo umbrella stand a petulant kick, toppling its contents onto the floor. As she gathered up the scattered umbrellas and walking sticks, she told herself that her new hair wasn't for Freddy's benefit anyway, so it hardly mattered if he hadn't noticed.

Upstairs, Laura admired the new black dress hanging on the front of the wardrobe. It was elegant and tasteful but with a hint of sexy, exposing just the right ratio of legs to cleavage for a woman of her age, according to the saleswoman who had taken Laura's credit card. Laura thought it was a bit tight and bloody expensive. She would have to eat only a little and be sure not to spill anything down the front of it.

Her date was called Graham. He was Vince's area manager and she had bumped into him in the car park of The Moon is Missing after her lunch there. She had met him many times at dealership Christmas dinners and numerous other social trials while she was married to Vince and he was married to Sandra. But now she wasn't, and neither, since quite recently, was he, and so he had asked her out. And fresh from meeting Felicity for the first time she had thought 'why not?' and said yes.

But now she wasn't so sure. As she wriggled into her dress and checked her hair yet again in the mirror, she was beginning to have doubts. According to Elise, whose salon chair doubled as a confessional for most of her clients, Laura was currently the favourite topic of conversation with the locals. In life, Anthony had attained the status of a minor celebrity on account of him being a published author. In death, therefore, it automatically followed that his affairs should remain squarely, if a little unfairly, in the public domain. His public's assessment of Laura apparently ranged from 'a conniving coffin-chaser' and 'a gold-digging tart' to 'a faithful friend and deserved beneficiary' and 'former traditional Irish dancing national champion'.

'But I think Mrs Morrissey might have got you muddled up with someone else there,' Elise had to admit. 'Well, she is nearly eighty-nine and only eats cabbage on a Thursday.'

Perhaps, thought Laura, she shouldn't be going out at all. People might think she was enjoying herself too soon after Anthony's death.

In her new dress, with her new hair, it might look as if she were flaunting her inheritance; dancing on his grave before the earth had a chance to settle. Except, of course, he'd been burned and scattered, so technically there wasn't one. Well, it was too late now. She checked her watch. Graham would be almost there. He had always seemed like a nice man. A gentleman.

'You'll be fine,' she told herself. 'It's only dinner.'

But by the time her taxi came, she wasn't feeling hungry at all.

Graham was indeed a gentleman. He was waiting for her at the restaurant with a champagne cocktail and a slightly nervous smile. He took her coat, kissed her cheek and told her that she looked lovely. As Laura sipped her drink, she began to relax. Well, as much as she could within the bondage of her dress. Perhaps it was going to be fine after all. The food was delicious and Laura ate as much of it as she could manage to squeeze in while Graham told her about his marriage break-up — the spark just fizzled out; they were still friends but no longer lovers; and his new interest in Nordic walking — 'a total body version of walking with the aid of fibreglass poles'. Laura resisted the urge to make a joke about him not looking old enough to need one walking stick, let alone two, but she had to concede that he did look fit. Forty-six next birthday, his torso was happily unencumbered by middle-aged spread, and his shoulders looked broad and hard-muscled beneath his well-pressed shirt.

In the ladies' room, Laura congratulated herself as she reapplied her lipstick. There's certainly nothing wrong with my date, she thought. And he had beautiful table manners. She pressed her lips together and dropped her lipstick back into her bag.

Graham insisted on accompanying Laura home in a taxi, and, relaxed by the wine and his easy company, Laura allowed her head to rest momentarily on his shoulder as she gave the driver directions to Padua. But she wasn't going to invite him in for coffee; the drink or the euphemism. She knew that she shouldn't let the gossip bother her, but she couldn't help it. And the 'tart' epithet was the slap that smarted most. She'd only slept with three men in her entire life, and one of them was Vince, so he didn't count. She wasn't proud of it; in fact she wished there had been more. Perhaps if she'd tried more men out, she might have found the right one for her. But not on a first date. And Graham was a gentleman. He wouldn't expect it.

Ten minutes later, a rather bewildered Graham was on his way home in the taxi. He hadn't even got past the front porch, let alone first base. Laura was in the bathroom gagging and gargling with antiseptic mouthwash. As she spat the stinging liquid into the basin, she glimpsed her still-startled expression in the mirror. Teary mascara was already dribbling black scribbles down her cheeks and her lipstick was smudged into a grotesque clown's mouth. She looked like a tart. She struggled furiously to escape from her dress, wrenching it over her head and viciously screwing it into a crumpled ball. In the kitchen, she flung it into the bin and yanked open the fridge door. The prosecco tasted rank after the mouthwash, but Laura persevered and gulped it down. She took the bottle through to the garden room and lit the fire in the grate, knocking over her glass and breaking it in the process.

'Shit! Bugger! Bollocks! Stupid sodding glass!' she addressed the sharp fragments which sparkled in the firelight. 'Stay there, broken then. See if I care!'

She wandered her way unsteadily back to the kitchen and found another glass. As she worked her way through the rest of the bottle, she stared into the flames wondering what the hell she'd been playing at.

Horribly drunk, and exhausted by sobbing and hiccupping, Laura fell asleep on the sofa, her tear-swollen face buried in her beautiful, newly burnished hair.

24

She slept for roughly ten hours, but when she woke, she looked like she'd been sleeping rough for several weeks. The thudding inside her head was soon echoed by a sharp tapping on the glass of the French windows. With considerable effort, Laura raised herself up just enough to see who it was that was making her already abominable headache even worse. Freddy. By the time Laura had struggled to a sitting position, he was standing over her, stony-faced, holding a mug of steaming black coffee. Laura clutched a blanket tightly around her aching body as Freddy registered the two wine glasses, the empty bottles and Laura's state of dishevelment.

'I see your date went well.' His tone was just a little more clipped than usual.

Laura took the coffee from him and muttered something unintelligible.

'Sunshine said that you were going out with your boyfriend.'

Laura sipped her coffee and shuddered. 'He's not my boyfriend,' she rasped.

Freddy raised his eyebrows at her. 'Well, it looks as though things got pretty *friendly* to me.'

Laura's eyes filled with tears but her belly filled with anger. 'What the hell's it got to do with you anyway?' she snapped.

Freddy shrugged. 'You're right. It's none of my business.' He turned to go. 'And thanks for the coffee, Fred,' he muttered.

'Oh, bugger off!' Laura replied, just about under her breath.

She took another sip from her mug. Why in God's name had she told Sunshine about her date?

Laura could feel the warning rush of saliva in her mouth. She knew she wouldn't make it to the bathroom, but it would be rude not to try. Halfway across the parquet floor she was sick. Very sick. As she stood cold and miserable with vomit-splashed legs, and still clutching the mug of coffee, she was glad that, at least, she'd missed the Persian rug.

An hour later, having cleared up the mess, been sick twice more, stood under the shower for ten minutes and dragged on some clothes, Laura sat at the kitchen table nursing a cup of tea and staring at a piece of dry toast. Her date had ended in disaster. The memory of Graham's tongue squirming lethargically in her mouth like the death throes of a particularly wet slug brought her out in a cold sweat. Well, that and the aftermath of two bottles of fizz. How could she have been such a fool? The sound of the doorbell pierced her mournful reverie. Sunshine. 'Oh God, no. Please not today,' she thought. There would be endless questions about last night and she just couldn't face it. She hid in the pantry. Sunshine would eventually come round to the back door if her ringing went unanswered, and if Laura stayed where she was, slumped at the table, Sunshine would see her. The ringing continued, patient and persistent, and then the back door opened and Freddy walked in.

'What on earth are you doing?'

Laura frantically shushed him and beckoned him over to the pantry. Even such a slight activity caused her temples to throb. She held onto one of the shelves loaded with ancient jars of pickles to steady herself.

'God, you look rough,' said Freddy helpfully. Again Laura put her finger to her lips.

'What?' He was beginning to lose his patience.

Laura sighed. 'Sunshine's at the front door and I really can't face her today. I know you probably think I'm being pathetic, but I just can't cope with all her questions. Not today.'

Freddy shook his head scornfully. 'I don't think it's pathetic. I think it's just plain mean. You're a grown woman hiding in a cupboard from a young girl who thinks you're great and loves your company, just because you've got a stonking and probably well-deserved hangover. At least have the guts to go and make your excuses to her face!'

Freddy's words stung like nettles on bare flesh, but before Laura could reply the mood at the front door suddenly turned nasty.

Sunshine had no idea who the blonde woman was marching up the path, but she looked pretty cross.

'Hello, I'm Sunshine. I'm the friend to Laura. Who are you?'

The woman narrowed her eyes as she looked Sunshine up and down, trying to decide whether or not she was obliged to answer.

'Is Freddo here?' she demanded.

'Nope,' said Sunshine.

'Are you sure? Because that's his fucking Land Rover on the drive.'

Sunshine watched with interest as the woman grew redder and crosser and began jabbing the doorbell with her immaculately manicured finger.

'That's *Freddy's* fucking Land Rover,' she replied calmly.

'So he *is* here then, the arsing arsehole!' the woman spat.

She jabbed at the doorbell again, and banged on the door with her fist.

'She won't answer,' said Sunshine. 'She's probably hiding.'

Felicity stopped banging for a moment. 'Who is?'

'Laura.'

'What, that funny housekeeping woman? Why in God's name would she be hiding?'

'From me,' Sunshine replied with a sad smile.

'Well, that bloody sodding shit of an arsehole Freddo better not be hiding from me!'

Sunshine decided to try and be helpful. The blonde woman was looking really furious now, and Sunshine was worried that she might break the doorbell.

'Perhaps he's hiding with Laura,' she suggested. 'He really likes her,' she added.

Sunshine's words didn't seem to help as much as she had hoped.

'You mean the bastard's probably humping the help?' The woman crouched down and began yelling through the letter box.

Freddy shoved his way into the pantry beside Laura and pulled the door to behind him. It was Laura's turn to raise her eyebrows.

'It's Felicity,' he hissed. The scorn had disappeared entirely from his voice to be replaced by an edge of desperation.

'And . . . ?'

It was Freddy's turn to sigh. 'We had a date last night, except I couldn't go, but I didn't exactly tell her until it was too late and I guess she's pretty pissed off . . .' He trailed off lamely.

Despite being cold, feeling sick and with a head that was about to explode, Laura couldn't help but smile. Her next words were delivered with as much relish as crammed the shelves that she was leaning against:

'Well, at least have the guts to go and make your excuses to her face.'

Freddy looked at her, astonished, and then his handsome face broke into a lopsided grin.

'I know you're in there, you bastard!' Felicity's voice shrieked through the letter box.

'You and that tart of a housekeeper! Well, if that dried-up, scruffy old bag lady is the best you can do, you were clearly punching well above your weight with me. You were crap in the sack anyway. She's welcome to you!'

Sunshine stood next to the incandescent Felicity, uncertain how to proceed. She had taken in all the words that had been spoken, or rather yelled, and was hoping to make some kind of sense of them later. Perhaps when Laura had stopped hiding, she would help her. Felicity appeared to have run out of steam.

156

She gave the front door a parting thump and strode off the way she'd come. Moments later, Sunshine heard a car door slam, an engine rev and tyres squeal as Felicity took her leave, in a foul temper, leaving a good deal of rubber on the tarmac. Just as Sunshine was about to go home, another visitor arrived. This woman was older, smartly dressed and smiling.

'Hello,' she said. 'Does Laura live here?'

Sunshine wondered what this one was going to do.

'Yes. But she's probably hiding.'

The woman didn't seem at all surprised. 'I'm Sarah,' she introduced herself. 'I'm an old friend of Laura's.'

Sunshine offered her a high five. 'I'm Sunshine. I'm the new friend to Laura.'

'Well, I'm sure she's very lucky to have you,' the woman replied.

Sunshine liked this new woman.

'Are you going to yell through the letter box too?' she asked her.

Sarah pondered a moment. 'Well, I thought I might just try the doorbell.'

Sunshine was hungry. It didn't look like she was going to get any lunch at Padua today.

'Good luck,' she wished Sarah, before setting off for home.

* * *

Freddy and Laura were still dithering in the pantry, straining their ears to hear if anyone remained at the front door. The doorbell rang

157

again. A single sound, followed by a polite pause. Laura retreated back into the pickles.

'You go,' she pleaded with Freddy. 'Please.'

Freddy relented, fuelled by remorse about the insults Felicity had aimed at Laura.

He opened the door to an attractive, middle-aged brunette with a confident smile and a firm handshake.

'Hello. I'm Sarah. Can I see Laura?'

Freddy stood back to let her in. 'You can, if she comes out from hiding in the pantry.'

At the sound of Sarah's voice, Laura hurried into the hall to meet her. 'You were hiding in there too!' she reminded Freddy.

Sarah looked at them both and winked at Laura.

'*Hiding in the pantry!* Now that's a euphemism if ever I heard one.'

'Not a chance!' Freddy's answer was a knee-jerk, but a kick in the teeth nonetheless for Laura.

Sarah, as usual, saw what was required. She took Laura by the arm.

'Why don't you make me a lovely cup of tea? And by the way, your hair looks gorgeous.'

25

Sarah Trouvay was a first-class barrister with a stellar career, two healthy, rumbustious young boys, and a rugged architect husband. She also had an unexpected talent for yodelling which had earned her extravagant plaudits as Maria in the school production of *The Sound of Music*. She and Laura had met at school and remained close friends ever since. Not close in terms of geography or frequent meetings; they rarely saw or spoke to each other more than two or three times a year. But the bond between them, formed at an early age and tempered over time by triumphs and tragedies, remained as durable as it was dependable. Sarah had witnessed the bright, sparky, dauntless young Laura gradually, relentlessly diluted by a bad marriage and a barrage of self-doubt. But she had never given up hope that one day, the real Laura would re-emerge victorious in glorious, shining Technicolor.

'What on earth are you doing here?' Laura asked as she filled the kettle.

'Well, the six very drunken and virtually unintelligible messages which you left on my voicemail in the early hours of this morning might have had something to do with it.'

'Oh God! I didn't, did I?' Laura hid her face in her hands.

'You most certainly did. And now I want to

hear all about it. Every last sordid detail. And I think we'll begin with 'Poor Graham'. Who the devil is 'Poor Graham'?'

Laura told her almost everything. Beginning with the dress, which was still hanging half out of the bin, and ending with the sinking of the second bottle of prosecco in front of the fire. The rest of the night — including the phone calls — had disappeared forever into alcohol-induced oblivion.

'Poor Graham,' Sarah was now able to agree. 'Whatever made you agree to go out with him in the first place?'

Laura looked a little embarrassed. 'Oh, I don't know. Maybe just because he asked. Nobody else has. He always seemed nice enough. Nothing obviously wrong with him.'

Sarah shook her head in disbelief. 'Nothing wrong doesn't make him Mr Right.'

Laura sighed. If only she could stop thinking about Mr Wrong as Mr Right. She hid her face in her hands again.

'Damn that ruddy gardener!' She had said it out loud, before she could stop herself.

'Who?'

Laura smiled ruefully. 'Oh, nothing. I'm just talking to myself.'

'That's the first sign, you know.'

'First sign of what?'

'The menopause!'

Laura threw a biscuit at her. 'I should have known it was never going to work when he started going on about Nordic walking.'

'He was trying to impress you with his pole!'

160

Sarah spluttered with laughter and even Laura couldn't stifle a guilty giggle.

And then she told her about the kiss in the porch. That dreadful, interminable kiss.

Sarah looked at her and shrugged her shoulders in exasperation.

'Well, what in God's name did you expect? You don't fancy him. You never have. It was always going to be like kissing cardboard!'

Laura shook her head emphatically. 'No. It was much, much worse. Cardboard would have been infinitely preferable.' She remembered the slug with disgust. 'And a lot less wet.'

'Honestly, Laura, why didn't you just offer your cheek, or failing that, pull away a bit quicker?'

Laura's cheeks were blotched with laughter and embarrassment.

'I didn't want to be rude. And anyway, his lips locked onto my face like a lunar module docking.'

Sarah was helpless with mirth. Laura felt bad. Poor Graham. He didn't deserve to be ridiculed. She remembered the bewildered look on his face when she finally broke the suction between them and garbled her good-bye before fleeing inside the house and slamming the door behind her. Poor Graham. But that didn't mean that she ever wanted to see him again.

'Poor Graham be damned!' Sarah always had the uncanny ability to know what Laura was thinking. 'Sounds more like 'Poor Laura' to me. He's a bad kisser with a dodgy pole. Swill your mouth out and move on!'

Laura couldn't help smiling, but just as her spirits were beginning to lift, a memory knocked them down like a rogue breaker toppling a tentative paddler.

'Shit!' She slumped forward in her chair and once again buried her head in her hands.

Sarah put down her cup of tea, ready for the next revelation.

'Freddy!' groaned Laura miserably. 'He found me this morning.'

'So?'

'He found me this morning, my face stuck to the sofa with dribble, wearing last night's smudged make-up and not much else, surrounded by empty bottles and two glasses. Two, Sarah! He'll think Graham 'came in for coffee'!'

'Well, however compelling the evidence might be, it is purely circumstantial. And anyway, what does it matter what Freddy thinks?'

'He'll think I'm a drunken harlot!'

Sarah smiled and spoke gently and slowly, as though to a small child. 'Well, if it matters that much, tell him what really happened.'

Laura sighed despondently. 'Then he'll think I *am* just a 'dried-up, scruffy old bag lady'.'

'Right!' Sarah slapped the palms of her hands down on the table. 'Enough of this moaning and wallowing. Upstairs, bag lady, and make yourself look presentable. After you've dragged me away from work to listen to your pathetic and tedious complaining, the least you can do is take me out to lunch. And I don't just mean a sandwich, I mean a proper hot meal. And a pudding!'

Laura clipped the top of Sarah's head playfully

as she passed her on the way out of the kitchen, mussing up her perfect cut and blow dry. Almost immediately, Freddy came in the back door.

Sarah stood up and offered him her hand and her brightest smile.

'Hello again. I'm afraid I didn't introduce myself properly. I'm Sarah Trouvay, an old friend of Laura's.'

Freddy shook her hand but refused to meet her gaze, turning instead to the sink to fill the kettle.

'Freddy. I've just come in to make a coffee. Can I get you one?'

'No thanks. We're just going out.'

The silence, deliberate on Sarah's part and embarrassed on Freddy's, was broken only by the rattle of water boiling in the kettle. Looking everywhere but at Sarah, Freddy caught sight of Laura's dress, hanging out of the bin. He fished it out and held it up.

'Hmm. Nice dress.'

'Yes. I bet Laura looked absolutely gorgeous in it.'

Freddy shifted uncomfortably in his muddy boots. 'I wouldn't know.'

At the sound of Laura's footsteps coming down the stairs, Sarah stood up.

'I know it's probably none of my business, but sometimes someone has to say something, even if they're the wrong person to do it. Last night: it wasn't what it seemed.'

She turned to leave the kitchen and over her shoulder added, 'Just *in case* you're interested.'

'None of my business either,' Freddy muttered

sulkily as he poured boiling water into his mug.

Liar, liar, pants on fire! thought Sarah.

★ ★ ★

The Moon is Missing was hosting a wake for a ninety-two-year-old former boxing coach and horse dealer called Eddy 'The Neddy' O'Regan. The mourners had clearly been toasting the dear departed enthusiastically for some time already, and the mood was cheerful, rowdy and sentimental. Laura and Sarah managed to squeeze into one of the booths, and over saucisse cassoulet and puréed potato, washed down with a glass of house red for Sarah and a Diet Coke for Laura, they caught up with each other's news. They had spoken briefly after Anthony died, but since then Sarah had been working on an important case that had only just been heard in court.

'Did you win?' Laura asked.

'Of course!' said Sarah, poking with her fork at the rather mushy-looking sausage and bean stew on the plate in front of her. 'But never mind about that. Tell me everything.'

Laura did. She told her about Anthony's will and the letter; the study full of things; hiding from Sunshine; and being the latest and juiciest subject of local gossip. And Felicity.

'I mean, it's lovely in one way; the house is beautiful, but the monumental lost property department that comes with it is another matter entirely. How the hell am I supposed to return all that stuff? It's madness. I have no idea what

164

to do about Sunshine, there's no guarantee that the website will work and most of the locals think I'm a money-grabbing slapper. I'll end up living in a house full of mice and cobwebs and other people's lost property until I'm one hundred and four, and when I do die, it'll be months before anyone notices and by the time they break in and find me, I'll be liquefying on the sofa.'

'And not for the first time,' Sarah replied with a wink. But then she put down her knife and fork and pushed away her plate.

'Laura. My dear, lovely, funny, clever, absolutely bloody infuriating Laura. You've been left a great big beautiful house, full of treasures with a dishy gardener thrown in. Anthony loved you like a daughter and trusted you with everything that was precious to him, and instead of turning cartwheels you sit here whingeing. He believed in you; I've always believed in you. It's not just Sunshine that you're hiding from; it's everything. And it's time to stop hiding and start kicking life up the arse. And to hell with what anyone else thinks,' she added, for good measure.

Laura took a sip of her Diet Coke. She wasn't convinced. And she was terrified of disappointing yet another person who loved her.

Sarah looked into her dearest friend's troubled face. She reached over and placed her hand over Laura's. It was time for some long-overdue home truths.

'Laura, you have to let go of the past. You deserve to be happy, but you have to make it

165

happen yourself. It's down to you. You were seventeen when you met Vince, still a child; but you're a grown woman now, so start behaving like one. Don't keep punishing yourself for things you did then, but don't use them as an excuse either. You have a chance now to make a really good life. Grab it by the balls and get on with it.'

Sarah sat back to see what impact her words were having. She was probably the only person in the world who could, and would, talk to Laura like that. She was determined to find the woman whom she knew was still in there and get her out. By force, if necessary.

'You do realise that we all fancied Vince, back then?'

Laura looked at her incredulously.

'Seriously. It wasn't just you. He was handsome, drove a flash car and smoked Sobranies. What more could a girl ask for? We all thought he was sex on legs. It was just bad luck that he chose you.'

Laura smiled. 'You always were an insufferable clever clogs.'

'Yes, but I'm right. Aren't I? Come on, Laura. You're better than this! When did you turn into such a wimp? This is a once-in-a-lifetime, twenty-four-carat-gold, fuck-off fantastic opportunity that most people can only dream about. If you chicken out of this one I'll never forgive you. But more importantly, you'll never forgive yourself!' Sarah raised her glass in a toast. 'And as for it being madness, well that should suit you perfectly. You always were a complete loony-tune!'

166

Laura smiled. It had been Sarah's nickname for her all those years ago at school, when life had still been exciting and full of possibilities.

'You complete arse . . . ' she muttered.

'I beg your pardon?' Even the normally imperturbable Sarah looked a little shocked.

Laura grinned. 'Me, not you.'

'I knew that.' Sarah grinned back at her.

It was slowly dawning on Laura that life was *still* exciting and full of possibilities; possibilities that she had wasted years of her life wishing for instead of chasing. She had some serious catching-up to do.

'What about Sunshine?' she asked. 'Any advice?'

'Talk to her. She has Down's Syndrome, she's not daft. Tell her how you feel. Work something out. And while you're at it, tell her what really happened on your date. If you won't tell Freddy, I'm pretty sure she will.'

Laura shook her head. 'Maybe, but he doesn't care anyway. You heard what he said when you suggested that we'd been up to no good in the pantry. 'Not a chance'.'

'Oh, Laura! Sometimes you can be really thick.'

Laura resisted the urge to stab her in the back of her hand with a fork.

'Do you remember Nicholas Barker from the boys' school?'

Laura remembered a tall, freckled boy with strong arms and scuffed shoes. 'He was always pulling my hair on the bus or ignoring me completely.'

Sarah grinned. 'He was shy. He did it because he fancied you!'

Laura groaned. 'Oh God. Don't say we're no further forward than we were in the fifth form.'

'You speak for yourself. But in my opinion, you've definitely got some serious ground to make up. Especially if you fancy Freddy as much as he obviously fancies you. And now I want some pudding!'

Sarah called a taxi from the pub to take her back to the station. As they stood waiting in the car park for it to arrive, Laura hugged her friend gratefully.

'Thanks so much for coming. I'm sorry I've been such a pain.'

'No change there,' quipped Sarah. 'But seriously, it's fine. You'd do the same for me.'

'Damn well wouldn't!'

That was Laura; always hiding behind a joke, shrugging away compliments. But Sarah would never forget that it was this Laura, eight years ago, who'd sat wiping away her tears in a side room of a hospital ward, while Sarah's shattered husband paced the car park chain-smoking and sobbing. It was Laura who'd held her hand while she delivered her first child, a precious daughter who died before they had a chance to meet. A daughter who would have been christened Laura-Jane.

Later that afternoon, Laura went and found Sunshine, who was sitting on the bench across the green from the house.

'May I sit down?' she asked.

Sunshine smiled. A warm, welcoming smile

which filled Laura with guilt and shame.

'I want to apologise,' she said.

'What for?'

'For not being a good friend back to you.'

Sunshine thought for a moment. 'Do you like me?'

'Yes, I do. Very much.'

'Then why do you hide?' she asked sadly.

Laura sighed. 'Because, Sunshine, this is all new to me; living in this house; the lost things; trying to do what Anthony would have wanted. Sometimes I get cross and muddled and I need to be by myself.'

'So why didn't you just tell me?'

Laura smiled at her. 'Because sometimes I'm just a silly arse.'

'Do you ever get scared?'

'Sometimes, yes.'

Sunshine took her hand and squeezed it in her own. Her soft, chubby fingers were freezing. Laura pulled her up from the bench.

'Let's go and have the lovely cup of tea,' she said.

26

'I think he needs the biscuit,' said Sunshine, tenderly stroking the bundle of fur and bones that ought to have been a lurcher. He watched her with frightened eyes that mirrored the beatings he had endured. Tired of their torture, his tormentors had kicked him out to fend for himself. Freddy had found him the previous evening lying on the grass verge outside Padua. It was raining hard and he was soaking wet and too exhausted to resist when Freddy had picked him up and brought him inside. He had been clipped by a car and had a superficial wound on his rump that Laura had cleaned and dressed while Freddy had held him shaking and wrapped in a towel. He refused to eat anything but drank a little water, and Laura stayed up with him all night, sleeping fitfully in an armchair while the dog lay inches from the fire, wrapped in a blanket and never moving. As the first wraithlike light of the winter dawn seeped through the lace panels of Anthony's study, Laura stirred. Her neck was cricked and complaining after a night spent folded awkwardly into a chair. The fire was reduced to a few struggling embers but the dog hadn't moved.

Please God, she thought as she leaned forward to check for the rise and fall of the blanket that would prove her prayer had been answered. Nothing. No movement. No sound. But before the tears that had filled her eyes could spill, the blanket suddenly twitched. There was a ragged intake of breath and the sonorous snoring that Laura had somehow managed to sleep through resumed.

Sunshine had been ecstatic when she had arrived that morning to find that they had a canine guest. It was the most animated that Laura had ever seen the normally rather solemn and serious girl. Between them they had coaxed him to eat a little cooked chicken and a slice of bread and butter. Sunshine had gently examined his skeletal frame and was determined to feed him everything she could.

'We mustn't feed him too much at once. His stomach will have shrunk and if we overdo it he'll be sick,' Laura warned.

Sunshine pulled a face which admirably communicated her disapproval of vomit.

'Maybe he needs another drink?' she suggested hopefully. Laura could understand her eagerness. She was desperate to do something to make the creature better, fatter, fitter. Happy. But sometimes not doing anything was what was needed, however hard that might be.

'I think he just needs to rest,' she told Sunshine. 'Just tuck the blanket round him and leave him in peace for a bit.'

Sunshine 'tucked him in' very carefully for about ten minutes before Laura finally persuaded her to come and help with the website. Freddy arrived earlier than usual and found them all in the study.

'How's the poor fella doing?'

Laura couldn't bring herself to look up from the screen. 'A bit better, I think.'

Since the episode in the pantry, the awkwardness between Freddy and Laura hung between them like smoke. Laura was desperate to clear the air and tell him what had really happened on her date, but somehow she could never find a way to begin the conversation. He went over to the fire and crouched down by the blanket. A pair of large, sorrowful eyes peered out at him. Freddy offered the back of his hand for the dog to smell but the dog's flinch was instinctive, born from bitter experience.

'Hey, hey, steady, lad. No one's going to hurt you here. I'm the one who found you.'

The dog listened to his gentle voice and poked his nose out warily from beneath the blanket to take a tentative sniff. Sunshine was watching their exchange closely. With an exaggerated sigh she placed both hands on her hips.

'He's supposed to be resting,' she said in a censorious tone.

Freddy held his hands up in surrender and came over to the table where Laura was in front of the laptop.

'So are you going to keep him?'

Sunshine replied before Laura could draw breath. 'That's for double damn sure, cross my heart and learn to fly we're going to keep him! He was lost and you found him. That's what we do,' she said, throwing her hands up in the air to underline and embolden her words. It took a little while for her thinking to catch up with her feelings, but when it did she added defiantly,

172

'But we're not giving him back.'

She looked to Freddy and Laura in turn for reassurance. Freddy winked at her and smiled.

'Don't worry, Sunshine. I don't think there's anyone to want him back.' But then he added, as though remembering his place, 'Of course, it's Laura's decision.'

Laura looked across at the blanketed bundle still roasting by the fire who was unaware that as soon as he had been carried over her threshold he was safe. From that moment he'd been hers.

'We'll have to give him a name,' she said.

Once again Sunshine was already on the next page.

'He's called Carrot.'

'Is that so?' said Freddy. 'And that's because . . . ?'

'Because he was hit by the car in the dark night because he didn't see it.'

'And?' continued Freddy with an interrogative tip of his head.

'Carrots help you see in the darkness.'

Sunshine delivered her denouement speaking loudly and slowly like an English tourist in a foreign country.

After the lovely cup of tea, which Sunshine permitted Laura to make while she stood guard over Carrot, Freddy went outside to work in the garden and Laura and Sunshine returned their attention to The Keeper of Lost Things. Laura had begun the Herculean task of entering the details of all the lost things onto a database that could be accessed via the website. Sunshine was selecting things from the shelves and drawers.

Once Laura had entered the details of a particular object it was marked with a sticky gold star that came in packets of fifty from the post office. They had bought ten packets, but now that they had made a start, Laura had a feeling they might need a good few more. Sunshine placed the objects in a neat line on the table: a pair of tweezers, a miniature playing card (the king of clubs) and a plastic model soldier. The friendship bracelet remained in her hand.

Knotted thread red and black bracelet. Found in the underpass between Fools Green and Maitland Road, 21 May . . .

Chloe felt her mouth water just before the first wave of vomit rose. The retching bent her double as she tried not to splash her new shoes. The concrete walls of the underpass reverberated with the sound of her shame and humiliation.

Everyone liked Mr Mitchell. He was the coolest teacher in school. 'The boys want to be him and the girls want to be with him,' her friend Claire had chanted only yesterday when he had passed them in the corridor. Chloe didn't. Not any more. She wanted to be any-where other than with him. Mr Mitchell ('Call me Mitch — I won't tell if you don't') taught music, and at first she too would have danced to any tune he chose to play. He had the ines-timable gift of plausibility. Coupled with a handsome face and slick charm, the adoration of Mr Mitchell was inevitable. Chloe had begged her mother for the private singing lessons she knew Mr Mitchell taught. From his home. Her mother was surprised. Her daughter was a quiet girl; happy to blend in with the chorus rather than take centre stage. She was a 'good' girl. A 'nice' girl. Money for singing lessons would be hard to come by, but perhaps her mother thought that they would be worth it if they gave Chloe a little more confidence. And Mr Mitchell was such a brilliant teacher. He really seemed to care about his pupils, not like some of them at the school who simply put in the hours, took the money and ran.

At first it had been exciting. The eye contact held just a little too long in class; the smile flashed in her direction. She was special to him, she was sure. On the way to that first singing lesson she was giddy with nerves. As she walked to his house she rubbed gloss onto her lips, pink and shiny: 'Passionate Pout'. And then she had rubbed it off again. During the third lesson, he had made her sit next to him at the piano. His hand on her thigh was thrilling, arousing. But wrong. It was like taking a shortcut down a dark alley late at night. You know you shouldn't. You know it's dangerous, but maybe just this once it will be all right. The next time he stood behind her and placed his hands on her chest; gently, caressingly. He said he needed to check that she was breathing correctly. The childish fantasy of romance had been rudely replaced by the sordid reality of his groping hands and hot, ragged breath in her ear. So why had she gone back? Even after

175

that, she had still gone back. How could she not? What would she tell her mother? She wanted it as much as he did. That's what he had told her, and she was shackled by the precarious truth in his words. She had at first, hadn't she?

The physical pain still echoed through her body, amplified by the action replays running through her mind. She had said no. She had screamed no. But perhaps just inside her head and not out loud. The body which had been hers alone was lost forever; taken or given, she still wasn't sure. She wiped her mouth again and as she did the friendship bracelet caught her eye. He had given it to her at the end of the first lesson because, he said, they were going to be very special friends. She ripped it from her wrist and threw it away. Taken. Now she was sure.

Sunshine squeezed the bracelet tight in her hand. Laura didn't see her wince. Her eyes were intent on the screen in front of her, her fingers rattling over the keyboard. Sunshine raised one warning finger to her lips for the benefit of Carrot and threw the bracelet onto the fire. She went back to the drawers to choose more things.

High on its shelf, the biscuit tin was still waiting for its gold star.

27

'Shall I make the lovely cup of tea when the bored van man comes?' Sunshine enquired helpfully.

Laura nodded distractedly, her mind preoccupied with where they were going to put the enormous Christmas tree that was currently languishing prone and prickly on most of the hall floor. Freddy was insisting that according to his measurements there would be a foot of clear daylight between the top of the tree and the ceiling once they had got it into position, and had gone to fetch the metal stand from the shed in order to prove his point before a full-scale argument broke out. Later that morning they were expecting a man who was coming to sort out broadband.

'We can't give you an exact time,' the customer services woman had told Laura, 'but we can give you a window of between 10.39 a.m. and 3.14 p.m.'

Sunshine had her eye on the clock in the hall, or at least as much of it as she could see beyond the branches. Laura had finally taught Sunshine to tell the time — more or less — and doing so at every opportunity had become her latest obsession. Curious about all the commotion, Carrot had left his comfortable bed by the fire to make tentative investigations.

One brief glance at the forestry lurking in the

hallway was enough to send him scurrying back to the study. Freddy returned with the stand, and having decided that perhaps the hall was the best place to accommodate both the prodigious height and girth of the tree, he and Laura were trying to manoeuvre it into position under Sunshine's rather erratic guidance when the doorbell rang and Sunshine skipped off to answer it, leaving Freddy and Laura in an awkward embrace with a giant conifer.

The man waiting on the doorstep had an air of superiority entirely unjustified by rank, appearance, education or ability. He was, in short, a supercilious git. A short, supercilious git. Sunshine didn't know that yet, but she could feel it.

'Are you the bored van man?' she enquired cautiously.

The man ignored her question. 'I'm here to see Laura.'

Sunshine checked her watch.

'You're too early. It's only ten o'clock. Your window doesn't open yet.'

The man looked at her the way the other kids had looked at her at school when they had called her names and pushed and shoved her in the playground.

'What the hell are you drivelling on about? I just want to see Laura.'

He pushed past her into the hall, where Laura and Freddy were still grappling with the tree. Sunshine followed him in, clearly upset.

'It's the bored van man,' she announced, 'and he's not very nice.'

Laura let go of the tree. Caught unawares, Freddy was almost toppled by its weight and let it fall. It missed the intruder by inches, causing him to yell angrily, 'Jesus Christ, Laura! What the bloody hell are you trying to do? Kill me?'

Laura faced him as she had never done before, with steady eyes and a steely composure.

'Now there's a thought.'

The man was clearly not expecting this new version of Laura, and she appeared to be enjoying his discomfort. Freddy was intrigued by this unexpected turn of events but trying hard to feign indifference, and Sunshine was wondering how it was that, if Laura actually knew the bored van man, she had asked him to come to Padua when he was so horrid. And she certainly wasn't going to make him the lovely cup of tea. Laura finally broke up the tense tableau.

'What do you want, Vince?' she sighed. 'You'd better come through to the kitchen.'

As he followed her out of the hall he was unable to resist giving Freddy the once-over, and Freddy returned his gaze with a hard stare. In the kitchen Laura didn't offer him anything other than a brief opportunity to explain his presence.

'Don't I even get a cup of tea?' he asked in a wheedling tone she'd heard him use so frequently in the bedroom when they were first married and it wasn't tea he had wanted. She shuddered at the thought. No doubt Selina from Servicing was horribly familiar with it too by now. She almost felt sorry for her.

'Vince, why are you here? What is it that you want?'

He flashed her a smile, intending seductive but executing sleazy.

'I want us to be friends.'

Laura laughed out loud.

'I do,' he continued, desperation beginning to whet the very edges of his words.

'What about Selina?'

He sat down and buried his head in his hands. It was so hammy that Laura was tempted to offer him the mustard.

'We broke up. I could never love her the way I loved you.'

'Lucky her. She left you, didn't she?'

Vince wasn't ready to give up just yet.

'Look, Laura, I never stopped loving you.'

'What, even while you were servicing Selina?'

Vince stood up and tried to take her hand. 'It was just a physical thing. Just sex. I never stopped thinking about you, missing you, and wanting you back.'

Laura shook her head in weary disbelief.

'So isn't it strange that you never thought to contact me before now? Not a birthday card, a Christmas card, a phone call. Tell me, Vince, why is that? Why now? Nothing to do with this big house that I happen to have inherited, I suppose?'

Vince sat back down, trying to marshal a coherent argument. Laura had always been too clever for him, even when she was just a girl. He *had* loved her then, in his own way, even though he knew that, really, she was out of his league, with her posh education and nice manners. Back then, though, he could still find ways to impress

180

her. Perhaps if their baby had lived, or they had managed to conceive again, things might have been different. He would have liked a son to play football with, or a little girl to take horse-riding, but it wasn't to be, and in the end their fruitless efforts to become parents became another of the things that drove them apart. Over the years, as Laura grew up, she became more of a match for him, and so less of a match in the marital sense. She noticed his faults and he, in turn, exaggerated them to annoy her. It was his only defence. At least Selina hadn't minded his elbows on the table or the toilet seat left up. Well, not at first.

Laura was still waiting calmly for his response. Her composure infuriated him and the mask of civility finally fell from his face, revealing the ugly truth.

'I heard about your date with Graham. You always were a frigid bitch,' he spat at her.

Before he came, he had promised himself that he would not lose his temper. He would show Miss Snooty-Pants that he was as good as her. But as usual, she rattled him, just by being herself. By being better than him.

Laura had finally had enough. She picked up the nearest thing to hand, an open carton of milk, which as luck would have it was on the turn, and hurled the contents at Vince's sneering face. She missed, but hit him squarely on the chest, splashing the rancid liquid all over his designer polo shirt and staining the dark suede of his expensive jacket. Laura was just looking round for further ammunition when the kitchen door opened. It was Freddy.

'Is everything okay?'

She rather reluctantly replaced the bottle of washing-up liquid on the draining board with a resounding thump.

'Yes, everything's fine. Vince is just leaving, aren't you?'

Vince barged past Freddy into the hall where Sunshine was hovering uncertainly. He turned to Laura in order to deliver his final insult with appropriate aplomb.

'I hope you'll be very happy in your big house with your little retard friend and your toyboy.'

Sunshine, no longer the child in the playground, answered him with admirable poise:

'I'm not the retard, I'm dancing drome.'

Freddy continued with rather more menace, 'And nobody talks to my girls like that, so sod off and don't come back.'

Vince had never known when to keep his mouth shut.

'Or else what?'

Seconds after the answer was delivered, Vince was nursing a bloody nose, lying on his back and struggling to extricate himself from the spiny clutches of the Christmas tree. When he finally managed to scramble to his feet, he lunged at the front door claiming grievous bodily harm and threatening to summon the police and his solicitor. As he slammed out of the house, Carrot's head appeared from behind the study door and he barked just once, but very sternly, at Vince's vapour trail. The three of them stared at the dog in astonishment. It was his first bark since coming to Padua.

'Well done, fella!' said Freddy, reaching down to stroke Carrot's ears. 'That certainly saw him off.'

The sound of the doorbell sent Carrot scuttling back to the study. Freddy charged across the hall and flung open the door to find a rather startled-looking young man with a plastic identity card strung around his neck and holding a black tool case.

'I'm Lee,' he said, flashing his card. 'I've come to sort out your broadband.'

Freddy stood aside to let him in and Laura guided him round the still prone Christmas tree and through to the study, which was immediately vacated by a supersonic Carrot. Sunshine trotted along behind them, thinking with all her might and still trying to work out exactly what was happening. Eventually she rolled her eyes and sighed loudly.

'You're the bored van man!' She checked her watch. 'You came in the window.'

Lee smiled, uncertain what to say. He'd been to some strange jobs before and this one was shaping up nicely to be right up there with them.

'Shall I make you the lovely cup of tea?'

The young man's smile broadened. Maybe things were looking up.

'I'd love a cup of coffee, if that's okay?'

Sunshine shook her head. 'I don't do coffee. I only do tea.'

Lee snapped open his tool case. It might be better to just get the job done and get out after all.

'Of course you can have coffee,' Laura intervened hastily. 'How do you take it? Come on, Sunshine — I'll make it and you can watch and then next time you'll know how to make it yourself.'

Sunshine considered for a moment and, remembering Vince's threats, she allowed herself to be persuaded.

'Then when the police get here I'll be able to make them the lovely cup of coffee too.'

28

The very thought of you.

The song broke Laura's sleep, although whether it was part of her dream or real music coming from the garden room downstairs she couldn't be sure. She lay still and listening, snuggled in her duvet cocoon. Silence. Reluctantly she crept out into the cold, rose-scented air, threw on her dressing gown and went over to the window to let the winter morning in.

And saw a ghost.

Laura peered out through the frosted pane, unwilling to trust what she saw: a shadow, perhaps a figure, pellucid as the rimy spiderwebs strung trembling in the icy breeze between the rose bushes. Laura shook her head. It was nothing. Customary common sense was temporarily out of service, and her imagination had cut loose, rampaging through reason with party poppers and a silly hat. That was all it was. Vince's visit had unsettled her. He had stomped dirty footprints all over her nice new life. But he was gone now, she told herself, and unlikely to return. She smiled, remembering with satisfaction the sour milk soaking into his shirt and the horror on his face as he squirmed like an upturned tortoise in the branches of the Christmas tree. But perhaps something else had unsettled her too. Freddy. He had called her 'his girl'. She had been ridiculously, dangerously

185

flattered. She had replayed the moment over and over in her head, but it was persistently and annoyingly accompanied by a warning voice telling her not to be so stupid. Now she didn't dare think about it at all. Time for the lovely cup of tea.

Downstairs the smell of Christmas tree cut through the air in every room. It was wonderful. The tree itself glittered and sparkled with tinsel and baubles and all manner of decorations that Laura had found in a box in the loft. Anthony had always put up a tree at Christmas, but his had usually been a much more modest affair and most of the decorations had hardly ever been used. Laura slotted two slices of bread into the toaster and poured herself a cup of tea. Noises in the kitchen had finally roused Carrot from his bed by the fire in the study, and he came and sat at Laura's feet waiting for his breakfast of toast and lightly scrambled eggs. In spite of their best efforts to fatten him up, he had barely 'thickened his skin' according to Freddy. But he did look much happier now, and was beginning to view life as a curious adventure rather than a terrifying ordeal. Today, Sunshine was going Christmas shopping with her mum, and Freddy was visiting his sister and her family in Slough. He had told Laura that his pre-Christmas visit was enough to keep his 'good big brother' certificate up to date, provided it was supplemented with generous (preferably cash) presents for his ungrateful niece and his surly nephew. Laura drained her teacup and brushed crumbs of toast from her fingers. Perhaps a day spent in her own company would do her good. Besides, she had Carrot, whose gentle head was resting in her lap. After a quick stroll around the frosty garden, which allowed Carrot to cock his leg up several trees and Laura to check that there were no spectres, wraiths or banshees loitering in the rose garden, she stoked up the fire in the study and Carrot settled himself back into his bed with a contented sigh. She fetched a box from one of the shelves and set out its contents on the table. The laptop bleeped and blinked into life and the vast virtual lost property department, of which she was now the Keeper, opened its doors. Laura picked up the first object in front of her.

Child's umbrella, white with red hearts. Found at the Alice in Wonderland sculpture, Central Park, New York, 17 April . . .

Marvin liked to keep busy. It stopped the bad thoughts creeping into his head, like black ants seething over the body of a dead songbird. The drugs from his doctor sometimes helped, but not always. When he had first fallen sick, he used to stuff his ears with cotton wads, hold his nose and keep his eyes and mouth clenched shut. He figured that if all the holes in his head were blocked, the thoughts couldn't get in. But he had to breathe. And no matter how teeny tiny he made the crack between his lips, the bad thoughts always managed to sneak in. But keeping very busy kept than away; and the voices too.

Marvin was the umbrella man. He would

take all the broken umbrellas that were thrown in the trash at the New York City Transit Lost Property Unit, and fix them up back in the dark and dingy room that was his only home.

It wasn't raining yet, but it was forecast. Marvin loved the rain. It washed the world clean and made everything shine; made the grass smell like heaven. Clouds the colour of gun smoke rolled in across the blue sky above. It wouldn't be long. Marvin was a giant of a man. He strode along Fifth Avenue, his heavy boots thudding on the sidewalk and his long, grey coat billowing behind him like a cloak. His wild black dreadlocks were frosted with grey and his eyes were never still; flashing whites like a frightened mustang.

'Free umbrellas!'

Central Park was his favourite place to work. He took the entrance on 72nd Street and headed for Conservatory Water. He liked to watch the pond yachts gliding across the water like swans. The boating season had only just begun, and despite the threat of rain a sizeable fleet had already set sail. Marvin's regular pitch was by the Alice in Wonderland sculpture. The children who played there didn't seem to mind him like some of the grown-ups did. Maybe they thought he looked like something out of a story too. There were no children today. Marvin set his bag of umbrellas down by the smallest mushroom on the sculpture, just as the first spots of rain began to polka-dot its smooth, bronze cap.

'Free umbrellas!'

His deep voice boomed like thunder through the rain. People scurried past but looked away when he offered them one of his gifts. He could never figure it out. He was just trying to be a good person. The umbrellas were free. Why did most people scaredy-cat away from him like he was the devil? Still, he stood his ground.

'Free umbrellas!'

A young guy on a skateboard skidded to a halt in front of him. Sopping wet in just a T-shirt, jeans and baseball boots, he was still grinning like the Cheshire Cat peeping over Alice's shoulder. He took the umbrella that Marvin was offering and high-fived his gratitude.

'Thanks, dude!'

He sped away, his board splashing through the puddles, holding a huge pink umbrella aloft. The rain slowed to a drizzle and the people in the park slowed to a stroll. Marvin didn't see her at first. A little girl in a red raincoat. She was missing one of her front teeth and had freckles across her nose.

'Hello,' she said. 'I'm Alice, like the statue.' She pointed to her namesake. Marvin hunkered down so he could see her better and offered her his hand.

'I'm Marvin. Pleased to meet you.'

She was British. Marvin recognised the accent from the TV. He always thought that Britain would be a good place for him, with his crooked teeth and fondness for rain.

'There you are, Alice! What have I told you

189

about talking to strangers?'

The woman who had joined them was looking at him as though he might bite.

'He's not a stranger. He's Marvin.'

Marvin smiled his best smile and offered the woman the best from his bag. 'Free umbrella?'

The woman ignored him. She snatched Alice's hand and tried to drag her away. Trash. That's how she was treating him; like he was trash. Marvin's face grew hot. The hairs on the back of his neck prickled and his ears began to ring. He was not trash.

'Take it!' he roared, thrusting the umbrella at her.

'Don't touch me, you moron,' she hissed as she turned on her heel, towing a tearful Alice behind her. As soon as her mother's grip slackened, Alice pulled free and ran back towards the sculpture.

'Marvin!' she yelled, desperately wanting to make things right. Their eyes met and before her mother could retrieve her Alice blew him a kiss. And he caught it. Before he went home he left a white umbrella with red hearts leaning against the White Rabbit. Just in case she came back.

* * *

Laura yawned and stretched back into her chair. She checked her watch. Three hours in front of the screen was more than enough for today. She needed some air.

'Come on, Carrot,' she said. 'Time for a walk.'

Outside the sky was marbled grey. 'Looks like rain,' she said to the reluctant dog. 'I think we might need an umbrella.'

29

The dining room looked like something out of a fairy tale. The table was laid with a snow white linen tablecloth and napkins. Silver cutlery framed each place setting and cut-crystal glasses winked and sparkled under the light from the chandelier. It was her first Christmas as mistress of Padua and Laura wanted to do the house justice. If she did, perhaps it would banish the unwelcome thoughts that crept into her head like black ants through a crack in the wall of a pantry. She just couldn't shake the feeling that the previous mistress still hadn't quite gone. She pulled the silver and white crackers from their cardboard box and set one on top of each precisely folded napkin.

That morning, even in the dark, she knew that something in the bedroom had changed. It was the same feeling that had told her, as a child on Christmas morning, that the stocking at the foot of her bed, empty when she had fallen asleep, was now full. She could sense, somehow, the alteration. As she padded over to the window in bare feet, she trod on things which were not the carpet: soft, hard, sharp, smooth. Daylight confirmed that the drawers of the dressing table had been pulled out and their contents strewn across the floor.

Laura picked up one of the wine glasses and polished away an imaginary smudge. Sunshine and her mum and dad were coming for Christmas dinner. Her brother had been invited, but he 'wasn't bovvered'. Freddy was coming too. She hadn't known whether to ask him or not, but a stern pep talk from Sarah had convinced her. He said 'yes', and since then Laura had wasted an inordinate amount of time trying to work out why. Her hypotheses were numerous and varied: she'd caught him by surprise; he was lonely; he wanted a roast turkey dinner but couldn't cook; he had nowhere else to go; he felt sorry for her. The one explanation she was most reluctant but also most excited to entertain was the simplest and most nerve-racking. He was coming because he wanted to.

Perhaps she had done it in her sleep, like sleep walking. Sleep trashing. It wasn't a burglary because nothing was missing. Yesterday she had found Sunshine in the garden room dancing to the A1 Bowlly song that had begun to haunt her, night and day.

'Did you put the music on?'

Sunshine shook her head. 'It was already on and when I heard it I came in for the dance.'

Laura had never known Sunshine to tell a lie.

'They're done!' Sunshine burst into the dining room, looking at her watch. She had been making mince pies and now the kitchen was dusty with flour and icing sugar. Laura followed Sunshine as she trotted purposefully back to the kitchen and hopped from foot to foot excitedly while Laura took the pies from the oven.

'They smell lovely,' she said, and Sunshine blushed proudly.

'Just in time,' said Freddy as he came in through the back door accompanied by a blast of freezing cold air. 'Time for the lovely cup of tea and an even lovelier mince pie.'

As they sat round the table, drinking tea and fanning mouthfuls of mince pies, which were still a little too hot, Freddy gazed thoughtfully at Laura.

'What's up?' he asked.

'Nothing.' It was a reflex rather than an answer.

Freddy raised his eyebrows. Sunshine shoved the rest of her mince pie in and then spoke with her mouth full.

'That's a lie.'

Freddy laughed out loud. 'Well, no points for tact there, but ten out of ten for honesty.'

They both looked at Laura expectantly. She told them. About the dressing table; the music; even about the shadow figure in the rose garden. Sunshine was unimpressed.

'It's just the lady,' she said, as though it ought to have been obvious.

'And what lady might that be?' Freddy asked, keeping his eyes firmly fixed on Laura.

'Saint Anthony's wedding wife. The Lady of the Flowers.' She reached for another mince pie and dropped it under the table for Carrot. Freddy winked at her and mouthed, 'I saw that.' Sunshine almost smiled.

'But why would she still be here, now that Anthony's gone?' Laura surprised herself by taking the idea seriously enough to ask.

'Yes. Why would she still be here making a

194

mess and disturbing the peace? And after we gave her such a lovely wedding, too?' Laura had no idea if Freddy was being serious or not.

Sunshine shrugged. 'She's upset.'

Despite her scepticism, Laura's stomach tipped like a tombola machine.

Christmas Day dawned bright and sunny, and as Laura ambled round the garden with Carrot, her spirits lifted. Christmas Eve had passed uneventfully, and she had even been to Midnight Mass at the local church. She'd had a few words with God and maybe that had helped. Laura and God didn't get together too often, but he was still on her Christmas card list.

Sunshine and her mum and dad arrived at twelve on the dot.

'Sunshine's been ready since eight,' her mum told Laura as she took their coats. 'She'd have been here for breakfast if we'd let her.'

Laura introduced them to Freddy. 'This is Stella and this is Stan.'

'We call ourselves 'The SS',' Stella chuckled. 'It's very kind of you to invite us.'

Stan grinned and thrust a poinsettia and a bottle of pink cava at Laura.

'There's nothing like a drop of pink fizz at Christmas,' said Stella, smoothing down the front of her best dress and checking her hair in the hall mirror. As Sunshine proudly gave them a guided tour of the house, Stella and Stan oohed and aahed appreciatively. Back in the kitchen Freddy was whisking gravy, basting roast potatoes, stabbing boiling brussels sprouts and drinking vodka martinis. And occasionally sneaking an appreciative glance at Laura. A couple of times, their eyes met, and he refused to look away. Laura was beginning to feel rather warm. He had insisted on helping, to show his appreciation for the invitation. He raised his glass to Laura.

'If they're The SS, then I'm 007.'

Christmas dinner was every bit as glorious as it ought to be. In the fairy-tale setting of silver and white and sparkle, they ate too much, drank too much, pulled crackers and told terrible jokes. Carrot camped out under the table taking tit-bits from whichever hand offered them. Laura discovered that Stella was in a book club and did flamenco, and Stan was in the darts team at his local pub. They were currently second in the league, and with three more matches in hand, they were hoping to take the championship. But Stan's real passion was music. Much to Freddy's delight, they shared a broad and eclectic taste, from David Bowie to Art Pepper to The Proclaimers to Etta James. It was easy to see where Sunshine's love of music and dancing came from.

While Laura, Sunshine and Stella cleared the table and then set about tackling the bombsite that had once been the kitchen, Freddy and Stan slumped back in their chairs like a pair of deflated souffles.

'That was the best Christmas dinner I've had in years.' Stan rubbed his belly affectionately. 'Only don't tell the missus,' he added, winking at Freddy.

Carrot had ventured out from under the table

and was sleeping contentedly at Freddy's side. Freddy poured Stan a glass of whisky.

'So is it as great as it sounds being a train driver? Every schoolboy's dream?'

Stan swirled the amber-coloured liquid in his glass and sniffed it approvingly.

'For the most part,' he replied. 'Some days I feel like I'm the luckiest man alive. But I nearly packed it in before I really got started.'

He sipped his whisky, reaching back for once to the memories he had struggled so hard to forget.

'I'd only been driving solo for a couple of weeks. It was my last run of the day; cold and dark outside and I was looking forward to my dinner. I didn't even see her until she hit the cab. After that, there wasn't much left of her to see.'

He took another sip of his whisky, bigger this time.

'It was in the local paper. She was ill, they said; bad nerves. Stood waiting in the cold. Waiting for my train. Terrible shame it was. She had a nipper; a girl. Dear little thing. They put her picture in the paper.'

Freddy shook his head and whistled through his teeth. 'Jesus, Stan, I'm sorry.'

Stan drained his glass and thumped it down on the table.

'It's the whisky,' he said. 'It makes me maudlin. It was a long time ago. Thank God, Stella drummed some sense into me and persuaded me to carry on driving.' They sat in silence for a moment and then Stan added, 'Not a word to Sunshine, though. I never told her.'

197

'Of course.'

Carrot's ears flicked at the sound of footsteps in the hall. Sunshine came in carrying a tray, followed by Laura and Stella. She set the tray down on the table.

'Now it's time for the lovely cup of tea and the even lovelier mince pies,' she said, pointing at the plate, piled high. 'And then we're going to play 'Conveniences'.'

Halfway through the first round, Sunshine remembered something that she had been meaning to tell her parents.

'Freddy's crap in the sack.'

Freddy nearly choked on his whisky, but Stella responded with admirable composure.

'What on earth makes you think that?'

'Felicity told me. She's Freddy's girlfriend.'

'Not any more,' growled Freddy.

Stan was shaking with laughter and Freddy was clearly mortified, but Sunshine was undeterred.

'What does it mean — crap in the sack?'

'It means not very good at kissing.' It was the first thing that came into Laura's head.

'Perhaps you should do more practice, then,' said Sunshine kindly, patting Freddy's hand.

When Sunshine and 'The SS' went home, the house fell silent. Laura was left alone with Carrot. And Freddy. But where was he? He'd disappeared while she had been seeing Sunshine and 'The SS' out and waving them off. She felt like a giddy teenager, uncertain if she was excited or afraid. It was the wine, she told herself. Freddy came out of the garden room

198

and took her by the hand.

'Come.'

The garden room was lit with dozens of candles and there was a bottle of champagne chilling in an ice bucket, flanked by two glasses.

'Will you dance with me?' Freddy asked.

As he placed the needle on the record, Laura spoke silently, to God for the second time in as many days. *Please, please let it not be Al Bowlly.*

In Freddy's arms she wished that Ella Fitzgerald would improvise a few more verses for 'Someone to Watch Over Me'. Freddy looked up and Laura followed his gaze to the bunch of mistletoe that he had attached to the chandelier above their heads.

'Practice makes perfect,' he whispered.

As they kissed, the photograph of Therese shattered silently into a starburst of splintered glass.

30

Eunice

1989

The photographs on the sideboard were supposed to help Godfrey remember who people were, but they didn't always work. As Bomber, Eunice and Baby Jane came into the sunny sitting room, Godfrey reached for his wallet.

'I'll have a tenner on My Bill in the 2.45 at Kempton Park.'

Grace patted him affectionately on the hand. 'Godfrey, darling, it's Bomber — your son.'

Godfrey peered at Bomber over the top of his spectacles and shook his head.

'Rubbish! Don't you think that I'd know my own son? Can't remember this chap's name, but he's definitely my bookie.'

Eunice could see the tears welling up in Bomber's eyes as he remembered the countless times he had placed bets for his father under the strict instruction, 'Don't tell your mother.' She took Godfrey gently by the arm.

'It's a beautiful place you have here, and it's a lovely day. I wonder if you'd be kind enough to show me round the gardens?'

Godfrey smiled at her, delighted.

'It will be my pleasure, young lady. I expect my dog could do with a walk too,' he said, looking at Baby Jane with a slightly puzzled air. 'Although, I must confess, I'd almost forgotten I had him.'

Godfrey put on the hat that Grace passed to him.

'Come along, Bomber,' he said to Baby Jane, 'time to stretch our legs.'

However offended Baby Jane might have been about being mistaken for a boy dog with her master's name, she hid it well. Better than Bomber managed to hide his sadness at being mistaken for his father's bookie. Grace put her hand to his face.

'Chin up, darling. I know it's tough. Yesterday morning he sat bolt upright in bed and accused me of being Marianne Faithfull.'

Bomber smiled in spite of himself. 'Come on, Ma. We'd best follow them before they get into mischief.'

Outside, the vapour trail of a plane was scrawled across the blue sky like the knobbled spine of a prehistoric animal. Folly's End House sadly had no folly, but it did have very beautiful and extensive gardens for its residents to enjoy. Grace and Godfrey had moved in just over three months ago, when it became clear that Godfrey's reason had set sail for faraway climes, and Grace could no longer cope with him alone. He occasionally took a brief shore leave in reality, but for the most part the old Godfrey had jumped ship. Folly's End was the perfect harbour. They had their own rooms, but help was on hand when they needed it.

Godfrey strolled arm in arm with Eunice in

the sunshine, greeting everyone they met with a smile. Baby Jane ran ahead. When she stopped for a wee, Godfrey shook his head and tutted.

'I do wish that dog would learn to cock his leg. Next thing we know, he'll be wearing lilac and singing show tunes.'

They stopped at a wooden bench by an ornamental fish pond and sat down. Baby Jane stood right at the edge of the pond, fascinated by the flashes and swirls of silver and gold as the koi carp gathered in hope of food.

'Don't even think about it,' Eunice warned. 'It's not sushi.'

As Grace and Bomber caught up with them, Godfrey was telling Eunice all about the other residents.

'We've got Mick Jagger, Peter Ustinov, Harold Wilson, Angela Rippon, Elvis Presley, Googie Withers and Mrs Johnson who used to run the launderette in Stanley Street. And you'll never guess who I woke up in bed with the other morning.'

Eunice shook her head, agog. Godfrey paused for a moment and then shook his head sadly.

'No, and neither will I. I had it a moment ago, and now it's gone.'

'You told me it was Marianne Faithfull,' said Grace, trying to be helpful. Godfrey laughed out loud.

'Now that, I think I would remember,' he said, winking at Bomber. 'By the by, have you placed my bet yet?'

Before Bomber could answer, Eunice directed his attention to a distant figure wearing enormous sunglasses and vertiginous heels, teetering in their direction.

'Oh God!' moaned Bomber. 'What on earth does she want?'

It took Portia some while to reach them across the lawn, and Eunice watched her precarious progress with quiet amusement. Baby Jane had jumped, unbidden, into Godfrey's lap and was warming up her growl. Godfrey watched Portia's approach with only mild curiosity and no sign of recognition whatsoever.

'Hello, Mummy! Hello, Daddy!' Portia crowed without enthusiasm. Godfrey looked behind himself to see who she was talking to.

'Portia,' began Bomber gently, 'he doesn't always remember . . . ' Before he could finish she had squashed herself next to Godfrey on the bench and tried to take his hand. Baby Jane growled a warning and Portia leapt to her feet.

'Oh, for pity's sake. Not that vicious dog again!'

Godfrey clutched Baby Jane protectively. 'Don't you speak about my dog like that, young woman. Who are you anyway? Go away at once, and leave us in peace!'

Portia was livid. She had driven twenty miles from London with a banging hangover and got lost three times on the way. And she was missing Charlotte's 'designer bags and belts' brunch.

'Don't be so bloody ridiculous, Daddy. You know damn well that I'm your daughter. Just because I'm not here every five minutes sucking up to you like your precious bloody son and his pathetic, lovelorn sidekick. You know bloody well

203

who I am!' she fumed.

Godfrey was unmoved.

'Young woman,' he said, looking at her scarlet face, 'you have clearly been out in the sun without a hat for far too long and have taken leave of your senses. No daughter of mine would use such language or behave in such an abhorrent manner. And this man is my bookie.'

'And what about her?' Portia sneered, pointing at Eunice.

Godfrey smiled. 'This is Marianne Faithfull.'

Grace managed to persuade Portia to go inside with her for a drink. Bomber, Eunice, Godfrey and Baby Jane continued on their stroll around the gardens. Under one of the apple trees, a small table was laid for tea and an elegant elderly lady sat drinking from a cup and saucer with a younger woman who was eating a lemon curd tart.

'They're my favourite,' she announced, as they said 'hello' in passing. 'Would you like one?' She offered them the glass cake stand. Bomber and Eunice declined, but Godfrey helped himself. Baby Jane personified dejection. The elderly lady smiled and said to her companion, 'Eliza, I think you have forgotten someone.' Baby Jane got two.

Back in the main house, they found Grace alone.

'Where's Portia?' Bomber asked.

'Taken herself back to London in high dudgeon, I shouldn't wonder,' said Grace. 'I tried to reason with her, but . . . ' She shrugged sadly.

'I don't understand how she can behave so

appallingly,' said Bomber.

Grace glanced over to where Godfrey was chatting to Eunice, to make sure that he was out of earshot.

'I think I can.' Grace took Bomber's arm and led him over to the sofa.

'I remember when she was very young.' She sighed sadly, summoning the memory of her small daughter with a gap-toothed smile and uneven pigtails. 'She always was her daddy's little girl.'

Bomber took her hand and squeezed it.

'And now she's losing him,' Grace continued, 'and perhaps for the first time in her adult life, she's faced with something that her money can't fix. Her heart is breaking and she can do nothing about it.'

'Except hurt those who love her,' replied Bomber crossly.

Grace patted his knee. 'She simply doesn't know how to cope. She left here in floods of tears, having called her darling daddy a wicked old trout.'

Bomber gave his mother a hug. 'Never mind, Ma, you've always got your 'precious bloody son'.'

Just as they were leaving, Godfrey beckoned Eunice over to his side.

'A word in your ear,' he winked conspiratorially at her and lowered his voice. 'Pretty damn sure that woman *was* my daughter. But there have to be some consolations for having this ruddy awful disease.'

31

According to Sunshine, Laura had had Freddy on a 'sleepover'. But Laura had not *had* Freddy on a 'sleepover'. She had slept with him, in the same bed, but she had not *slept* with him. Laura smiled to herself at how peculiarly British it was, using the same words for different meanings but still not actually saying what you mean. Sex. She had not had sex with Freddy. Yet. There. In the space of a few sentences she had gone from innuendo to intercourse!

On Christmas night, she and Freddy had danced and drunk champagne and talked. And talked and talked. She had told him all about school and tray cloths and Vince. She told him about the baby she had lost, and he had held her close, and she told him about the short stories that she had written for *Feathers, Lace and Fantasy Fiction* and he laughed until he cried. He had told her about his ex-fiancée, Heather — a recruitment consultant who wanted marriage and children, and he didn't. At least, not with her. He had also told her why he'd sold his small IT consultancy (much to Heather's consternation and the final wheel to fall off their relationship) to become a gardener. He'd got sick of watching the world through a window instead of living outside in it. Laura finally told him about Graham and their disastrous date, and after some hesitation and another glass of champagne, she even told him about the kiss.

He grinned. 'Well at least you haven't rushed upstairs yet to swill your mouth out, so I'll take that as a good sign. And I hope you kept that dress!'

He was quiet for a moment. 'I was too embarrassed to kiss a girl until I was seventeen because of this,' he said, lightly touching the scar that ran onto his mouth. 'I was born with a cleft lip, and the surgeon's needlework wasn't the neatest . . . '

Laura leaned forward and kissed him softly on the mouth.

'Well, it certainly doesn't seem to hamper your technique now.'

Freddy told her all about Felicity, a blind date set up by a woman whose garden he'd been working on for several years. She swore they'd get on 'like a house on fire'. They didn't, but Felicity was one of the woman's closest friends, so Freddy carried on seeing her whilst trying to work out a dignified escape route.

'One night, I couldn't face any more of her bragging and braying and calling me bloody Freddo, so I just stood her up. Not very dignified, I know, but damned effective as it turned out. I lost my client, but it was worth it.'

Finally, when Freddy and Laura had run out of words, they took comfort in each other's arms, sleeping furled around one another like petals in a bud.

They slept in the guest bedroom next to Therese's old room. The day Laura woke to find the drawers emptied onto the floor, she had moved her things into the room next door. She wasn't afraid, exactly. Or perhaps she was, a little. She had a horrible feeling that there was, if not a spectre, then an uninvited guest at her feast. A soup spoon was missing; one of the table legs was too short; one of the champagne cocktails was flat; one of the second violins was sharp. A sliver of disharmony jangled Padua and Laura had no idea what she should do to restore peace. Carrot would never go into Therese's bedroom, but he was perfectly happy to abandon his place by the fire on Christmas night to nestle at their feet on the bed where Freddy and Laura slept.

When Sunshine found out about the 'sleep-over' she wanted to know all the details. Whose pyjamas did Freddy wear; how did he clean his teeth without his toothbrush; did he snore? And did they kiss? Freddy told her that he had borrowed one of Laura's nighties, cleaned his teeth with soap and a flannel, and no, he didn't snore, but Laura did — enough to rattle the windows. And yes. They had kissed. Sunshine wanted to know if Freddy was any better at kissing now and he told her that he'd been having lessons. Laura had never seen Sunshine laugh so hard, but how much of it she believed was difficult to guess. How much of it she would repeat when she got home wasn't.

It was New Year's Eve and still very early. The guest room also had a view of the rose garden, but this morning it was barely visible through the driving rain. Freddy would be here later. They were going out this evening to join the celebrations at the local pub. But in the meantime, Laura was drawn inexorably to the study. Armed with enough toast for both of them and a pot of tea, Laura went into the study followed by Carrot and lit the fire. She took a small box down from its shelf and laid the contents on the table. Outside, it was raining harder than ever, and the sound of running water played counterpoint to the spit and crackle of the fire. For the first time Laura held in her hand an object she could not name, and even after reading its label, she was no wiser as to its purpose or origin.

Wooden house, painted door
and windows, no. 32.
Found in a skip outside no. 32 Marley Sheet,
23 October . . .

Edna peered at the young man's identity card. He said he was from the Water Board, come to check all the plumbing and the pipes. It was just a courtesy call. They were doing it for all their customers over seventy before the winter set in, he said. Edna was seventy-eight and she needed her reading glasses to see what was on the card. Her son, David, was always telling her to be extra careful about opening the door to strangers. 'Always keep the chain on until you know who they are,' he warned. The trouble was that with the chain on she could only open the door a crack, and then she was too far away from it to read the card. Even with her reading glasses on. The young man smiled patiently. He looked right. He was wearing a smart pair of overalls with a badge on the right-hand chest pocket, and was carrying a black plastic tool box. The identity card had a photo that looked like him, and she thought that she could just about make out the words 'Thames' and 'Water'. She let him in. She didn't want him thinking that she was a foolish, helpless old woman.

'Would you like a cup of tea?' she asked.

He smiled gratefully. 'You're a diamond and no mistake. I'm proper parched. The last brew I had was at seven o'clock this morning. Milk and two sugars and I'm a happy man.'

She directed him to the downstairs lavatory and then upstairs to the bathroom and airing cupboard on the landing which housed the water tank. In the kitchen, she put the kettle on and as she waited for it to boil, she looked out at the long strip of back garden. Edna had lived in her east London terrace for nearly sixty years. She and Ted had moved in when they got married. They had brought up their kids here, and by the time David and his sister Diane had grown up and left home, it was bought and paid for. Of course, they could never have afforded it now. Edna was the only one left from the old days. One by one, the houses had been bought up, tarted up and their prices hiked up as high as a tom's skirt, as her Ted would have said. These days, the street was full of young professionals with flash cars, fondue sets and more money than they knew what to waste it on. Not like the old days,

when kids played in the street and you knew all
your neighbours and their business.

The young man found his way back into the
kitchen just as Edna was pouring the tea.

'Just how I like it,' he said, gulping it down.
He seemed to be in a hurry. 'Everything's ship-
shape upstairs.'

He took a quick look under the sink in the
kitchen and then rinsed his mug under the tap.
Edna was impressed. He was a good boy like
her David. His mum had obviously brought
him up well.

Early that afternoon, the doorbell rang again.
Two visitors in one day was almost unheard of.
The crack revealed a small, smartly dressed
black woman who appeared to be somewhere
in her sixties. She was wearing a navy-blue suit
with a blouse so white it dazzled. Perched on
her concrete-set coiffure of brandy snap curls
sat a navy-blue hat with a wisp of spotted net
that just covered the top half of her face.
Before either of them could speak, the woman
appeared to buckle at the knees and clutched at
the door frame to prevent herself from falling.
Moments later, she was sitting in Edna's
kitchen, fanning her face with her hand and
apologising profusely in a rich Jamaican accent.

'I'm so sorry, my dear. It's just one of my
funny turns. The doctor says it's to do with my
sugars.' She lurched forward in her chair and
almost fell off it before recovering herself.

'I feel so bad imposing myself on you like
this.'

Edna flapped away her apologies.

'What you need is a hot, sweet cup of tea,' she said, filling the kettle once again. To be honest, she was glad of the company. The woman introduced herself as Sister Ruby. She was knocking on doors offering her skills as a spiritual healer, reader and advisor. She told Edna that she could read palms, cards and crystals, and was a practitioner of Obeah, Jadoo and Juju. Edna had no idea about Obadiah, Jedi or Judy, but she had always been fascinated by fortune tellers and the like, and was deeply superstitious. Hers was a house where new shoes were never put on the table, umbrellas were never opened indoors and nobody crossed on the stairs. Her Irish grandmother had read tea leaves for all the neighbours, and one of her aunts made her living as Madame Petulengra, giving crystal ball readings on Brighton Pier. When Sister Ruby, revived by her tea, offered to read Edna's palm, she was only too willing. Sister Ruby took Edna's hand, palm upwards, in her own, and passed her other hand over it several times. She then spent a full minute studying the crinkled topography of Edna's palm.

'You have two children,' she said, at last. 'A boy and a girl.'

Edna nodded.

'Your husband passed . . . eight years ago. He had a pain, here.' Sister Ruby clutched at her chest with her free hand. Ted had died of a heart attack on the way home from the pub. Family flowers only, but donations, if desired, to the British Heart Foundation. Sister Ruby

212

tipped Edna's hand this way and that, as though she were trying to decipher a particularly complex message.

'You are worried about your home,' she finally announced.

'You want to stay, but someone wants you to leave. It's a man. Is it your son? No.' She peered closely at Edna's hand and then leaned back and closed her eyes as though trying to picture the man in question. Suddenly she sat bolt upright and slapped her hands flat on the table.

'He is a businessman! He wants to buy your house!'

Over a second cup of tea and a newly opened packet of Bourbons, Edna told Sister Ruby all about Julius Winsgrave, property developer, entrepreneur and sleazy, greedy gobshite (except she didn't use the word 'gobshite' what with Ruby being a Sister and all). He had been trying to get her to sell for years, having bought most of the other houses in the street and made a killing on them. In the end, his bully-boy tactics had forced David to consult his solicitor and take out an injunction against Julius to prevent any further harassment. But Edna always felt the threat of him circling above like a vulture, waiting for her to die.

Sister Ruby listened carefully. 'He sounds like a bad and dangerous man.'

She reached down and picked up her capacious, well-used handbag and began rifling through its contents.

'I have something here that can definitely help you.'

She placed on the table a small, flat piece of wood in the shape of the front of a house. It was crudely painted with four windows and a blue front door. The same colour as Edna's.

'What number is your house, please?' Sister Ruby asked.

'Thirty-two.'

Sister Ruby took a pen from her bag and drew a large '32' on the front door of the house.

'Now,' she said, 'this is the most powerful Juju and it will protect you as long as you do exactly as I say.'

She held the house tightly in both hands and closed her eyes. Her lips worked furiously in silent incantation for several minutes before she finally placed the house in the centre of the kitchen table.

'Here it must stay,' she said decisively. 'This is the centre of your home and from here it will protect you. But you must know that now this house,' she said, pointing to the wooden model, 'has become your house. All the while you keep it safe, so too will your house be safe. But if you allow harm to come to it, the same and more will come to the bricks and mortar around you; whether it be fire, water, breaking, whatever. Nothing can undo the magic and nothing can undo the curse.'

Edna looked at the little wooden house and wondered if it could really protect her from Julius Winsgrave. Well, it certainly couldn't do any harm to try it. Sister Ruby took her cup and saucer to the sink, and despite Edna's protests, washed them thoroughly before setting them on the draining board to dry. As Edna turned her back to put the biscuits in their tin, Sister Ruby shook a wet hand over the wooden house and three drops of water splashed onto its painted facade.

'There now,' she said, picking up her bag. 'I've taken up quite enough of your time.'

Edna was searching for her purse, but Sister Ruby refused to take any payment for her services.

'It was a pleasure chatting with you,' she said, as she made her way towards the front door.

As the make-up came off, the face in the mirror grew younger. Under the fat curls of the wig was black hair, ironed straight. In jeans, boots and a leopard-print coat, Sister Ruby disappeared into Simone La Salle. She checked her designer watch and grabbed her designer bag. At the restaurant, Julius was already waiting; drumming his fingers impatiently on the immaculate linen tablecloth.

'Champagne, please,' she told the passing waiter in confident Estuary English.

Julius raised his eyebrows. 'Do you deserve it?'

Simone smiled. 'What do you think?' she said. 'It went like clockwork. My boy went this morning and sorted the stopcock. As luck would have it, the bathroom was directly above

215

the kitchen.' She checked her watch again. 'The kitchen ceiling should be down by now.'

Julius smiled. 'Mother and son make a good team.'

He pushed a fat brown envelope across the table. Simone checked the contents and then slid it into her bag. The waiter brought the champagne and filled both their glasses. Julius made the toast.

'It's been a pleasure doing business with you.'

After seeing Sister Ruby out, Edna went for a little lie-down on the sofa. Two visitors in one day were lovely but a little tiring. When she woke about an hour later it was raining. In the kitchen. The wooden house on the table was soaked. The paint had run and the windows had all but washed away, but the number 32 was still plainly visible. Edna looked up and saw a dark patch creeping horribly across the ceiling. The last thing she heard was the groan of lathe and plaster surrendering.

'Okay! Okay! I surrender.' Laura stroked the warm head that had been gently butting her knee for the last five minutes. Carrot was hungry and he needed a wee. It was long past lunchtime. Laura surveyed the sea of objects dotted with gold stars in front of her on the table and then checked her watch. It was nearly three o'clock.

'Poor Carrot,' she said. 'I bet you've been keeping your legs crossed.'

It was still pouring with rain, but fortunately

Carrot had been given (amongst a great many other things) a waterproof coat for Christmas. He trotted out into the garden whilst Laura made their lunch. He was soon back, padding a pattern of wet paw prints across the floor tiles. After lunch, Laura went upstairs to decide on her outfit for that evening. She embarrassed herself with how long it took to choose appropriate underwear. Appropriately inappropriate. Searching for a favourite pair of earrings, she wondered if she might have left them in Therese's bedroom and went to look. She turned the cold brass doorknob. The door was locked. From the inside.

32

Freddy poked Carrot with his toe from underneath the bedcovers.

'Get up, you lazy hound, and go and make us a cup of tea.'

Carrot snuggled deeper into his duvet nest and groaned contentedly. Freddy looked at Laura pleadingly and she promptly hid her head under the pillow.

'I suppose it's down to me then,' he said, hopping out of bed and searching for something to put on for the sake of warmth rather than modesty. Laura's dressing gown was hardly fit for purpose but conveniently to hand. Freddy threw open the curtains onto a new year and a blue sky and sunshine day. Laura stretched out, naked under the warm covers, and wondered if she had time to nip to the bathroom and make herself look a little more presentable, a little less middle-aged. But then, what was the point? Freddy had already seen her. Laura raked through her hair with her fingers and checked in the small mirror on the bedside table to see if she had any of last night's mascara smudged underneath her eyes. At least she had nice teeth.

It was a full two hours later before they were up, dressed and eating beans on toast when Sunshine arrived. They had promised her that if it was a nice day, they would all take Carrot for a walk on the nearby common. Laura and Freddy strolled arm in arm as Sunshine ran ahead with Carrot, throwing a ball-on-a-rope (another Christmas present) for him to retrieve.

'I get the distinct impression that young Carrot is only going along with this for Sunshine's amusement rather than his own,' said Freddy.

Laura watched as Carrot dutifully returned the ball to Sunshine only to have her fling it away in a random direction and command that he 'fetch!'

'I suspect that he'll only play along for so long before he finds something more interesting to do.'

Sure enough, after the very next throw, Carrot watched as the ball descended into a gorse bush and then wandered off to look for rabbits. Poor Freddy was designated by Sunshine as Carrot's second and was soon elbow deep in gorse spines.

'Leave it,' said Laura, as Freddy risked multiple puncture wounds. 'We'll get him another one.'

'No!' wailed Sunshine. 'It was the Christmas present to him. He'll be really upsetted and he'll hate me because I can't throw straight in a line because I'm a ming-mong.'

Sunshine was close to tears.

'You most certainly are not a ming-mong!' said Freddy, finally surfacing from the depths of the gorse bush, triumphantly waving the ball-on-a-rope. 'Who on earth called you that?'

'That's what Nicola Crow used to call me at school when I dropped the ball in rounders.'

'Well, Nicola Crow was an ignoramus and you, young lady, are dancing drome. And don't you forget it.'

He handed her the toy, smoothing away the pain from her face. But a smile was still too much to hope for. Tired of rabbits and having missed all the drama, Carrot wandered back and sniffed at his toy. Then he licked Sunshine's hand. The price of a smile.

As they walked on, Laura now holding Carrot's toy for safekeeping and Freddy inspecting his wounds, Sunshine pounced on a small, shiny object trodden into the grass.

'Look,' she said, digging it out of the mud with her fingers.

'What is it?' Freddy took it from her and rubbed the dirt away. It was a brass key ring in the shape of a baby elephant.

'We should take it home,' said Sunshine. 'We should write it a label and put it on the webside.'

'Don't you think that we've got more than enough lost things already?' said Laura, picturing the study crammed with things still waiting on shelves or in boxes for their gold stars. But Freddy agreed with Sunshine.

'Listen, I've been thinking about how we get people interested in the website. Putting all the stuff on there is only half the job. Getting the right people to look at it is the other. Now, Anthony's is a great story, and I'm sure we'll be able to get the local press, maybe even radio and television interested, but if we have some really recent things that have been lost and found as well as all the old stuff, I think it could really help.'

And what really helped Laura was that Freddy had said 'we'. She was no longer facing

Anthony's daunting legacy alone; she had help. Help that she had been too proud or too afraid to ask for.

Back at Padua Sunshine went straight to the study to find a label for the key ring. They had all been invited to tea by Sunshine's mum and dad, but she was determined to have the label written and the key ring on a shelf or in a box before they left. Laura went upstairs to get changed and Freddy rubbed the worst of the mud from Carrot's feet and legs with an old towel in the kitchen. On the way past, Laura tried the door handle of Therese's room. It was still locked. Back in the kitchen, she wrote a label for the key ring under Sunshine's watchful eye.

'Sunshine?'

'Umm?' She was concentrating hard to make out what Laura was writing.

'You know the other day when you said that The Lady of the Flowers was upset?'

'Yep.'

Laura put the pen down and blew on the wet ink. As soon as she put the label down, Sunshine picked it up and blew on it some more. Just to be sure.

'Well, do you think that she's upset with me?'

Sunshine adopted her 'how can you be so stupid?' expression and stance, which involved rolling her eyes, huffing and jamming her hands onto her hips.

'She's not upsetted with just you' — the 'of course' was understood — 'she's upsetted with everyone.'

That was not an answer that Laura was

221

expecting. If she believed what Sunshine was saying (and the jury were still having a latte break on that one), then she was relieved not to be the sole target of Therese's anger, but was still absolutely none the wiser as to what she could do to appease her.

'But why is she angry?'

Sunshine shrugged. She had lost interest in Therese for the moment and was looking forward to her tea. She studied her watch. She could do all of the 'o'clocks' and most of the 'half pasts', and anything in between became a 'nearly'.

'It's nearly four o'clock,' she said, 'and tea's at four o'clock on the spot.' She went and stood by the door. 'This morning I made fairy cakes, scones, the even lovelier mince pies and prawn folly fonts. For our tea.'

Freddy grinned. 'Which explains why you didn't get here until nearly half past eleven.' He winked at Laura and mouthed, 'Luckily for me.'

'And Dad made sausage rollovers,' said Sunshine, pulling on her coat.

33

Eunice

1991

'These sausage rolls are not a patch on Mrs Doyle's,' said Bomber, bravely soldiering on through his second. Since Mrs Doyle's retirement to a seafront flat in Margate, the bakery had been taken over by a franchise, and the handmade cakes and patisseries had been replaced with ready-made, mass-produced imitations. Eunice passed him a paper napkin as flakes of pastry fluttered down his front and into his lap.

'I'm sure Baby Jane will happily help with any leftovers,' she said, glancing across at the little pug's eager face. Baby Jane was out of luck. Despite its inferior quality, Bomber finished his lunch and did his best to redistribute the flakes of pastry he was wearing in the general direction of the wastepaper bin. Eunice had bought him two sausage rolls as a special treat, for once forsaking her concern for his health and waistline. They were going to see Grace and Godfrey later and visits to Folly's End had become increasingly difficult over the past year. She wished that there was something, anything, she could do to lessen Bomber's pain as he watched the man he once knew as his father recede inexorably towards some far distant, inaccessible horizon. Godfrey's physical health was a bitter irony cruelly yoked, as it was, to his mental fragility, leaving him like an overgrown, frightened and angry child. 'Body like a buffalo, mind like a moth' was how Grace described him. His plight was a dreadful punishment to those who loved him. To Godfrey, his friends and family were now strangers to be feared and, if possible, avoided. Any attempts at physical affection — a touch, a kiss, a hug — were met with a fist or a kick. Grace and Bomber both had the bruises to prove it. Grace was stoical as ever, but now, almost two years after they had moved to Folly's End, she no longer shared a room with her husband. These days it was only safe to love him from a distance. Portia kept her distance entirely. Her visits had stopped when the violence began.

Bomber shook his head in disbelief as he slipped a heavy manuscript from a brown envelope that had arrived with that morning's post.

'I'm sure she only does it to wind me up.'

It was his sister's latest manuscript.

'Does she send them to anyone else?' Eunice peered over his shoulder and helped herself to the synopsis sheets.

'I'm sure she does. I'm beyond embarrassment now. She definitely sent the last one to Bruce. He said he was almost tempted to publish it just to see the look on my face.'

Eunice was already engrossed in the pages she was holding, shaking with silent mirth. Bomber leaned back in his chair and tucked his hands behind his head.

'Well, come on then. Put me out of my misery.'

Eunice wagged her finger at him, grinning. 'It's funny you should say that, but I was just thinking that maybe we could get Kathy Bates to kidnap Portia, tie her to a bed in a remote woodland cabin, break both her legs thoroughly with a lump hammer, and then give her some top tips on how to write a novel.'

When they had first seen the film *Misery*, they had amused themselves over dinner afterwards by compiling a list of writers who might benefit from a term at the Kathy Bates school of creative writing. Eunice couldn't believe that they had forgotten Portia.

'Might be simpler if she just broke all her fingers, and then she wouldn't be able to write at all.'

Eunice shook her head at Bomber in mock disapproval.

'But then we would be deprived of such literary gems as this,' she said, waving the synopsis in the air. She cleared her throat and paused for dramatic effect. Baby Jane yapped at her to get on with it.

'Janine Ear is a young orphan being raised by her cruel, wealthy aunt, Mrs Weed. She is a strange child who sees ghosts, and her aunt tells everyone that she is 'on drugs' and sends her to a private rehab clinic called High Wood. The owner of High Wood, Mr Bratwurst, spends all the fees on heroin, and only feeds the girls bread and lard. Janine makes friends with a kind and sensible girl called Ellen Scalding, who dies when she chokes on a crust of dry bread because there is no nominated first aider on duty and Janine doesn't know how to do the Heimlich manoeuvre.'

Eunice paused to check that Bomber wasn't in need of such assistance himself. He was convulsed with silent laughter and Baby Jane was sitting at his feet looking vaguely puzzled. Eunice waited for him to compose himself a little before continuing.

'Mr Bratwurst is sent to prison for failing to meet the requirements of the health and safety legislation, and Janine accepts the position of au pair at a stately home called Pricklefields in Pontefract, where her charge is a lively little French girl named Belle, and her employer is a dark, brooding man with hidden troubles called Mr Manchester, who shouts a lot but is kind to the servants. Janine falls in love with him. One evening, he wakes up to find that his hair is on fire and she saves his life. He proposes. The wedding day is a disaster.'

'It's not the only thing,' spluttered Bomber.

Eunice went on.

'Just as they are about to exchange their vows, a man called Mr Mason turns up claiming that Mr Manchester is already married to his sister, Bunty. Mr Manchester drags them back to Pricklefields where they witness Bunty, out of her brains on crack cocaine, crawling round the attic on all fours, snarling and growling and trying to bite their ankles, chased by her carer

226

brandishing a syringe of ketamine. Janine packs her bag. Just as she is about to die from hypothermia wandering round on the moors, a kind, born-again Christian vicar and his two sisters find her and take her home. As luck would have it, they turn out to be her cousins, and even luckier than that, a long-lost uncle has died and left her all his money. Janine kindly shares her inheritance, but refuses to marry the vicar and join him as a missionary in Lewisham, because she now realises that Mr Manchester will always be the love of her life. She returns to Pricklefields to find that it has been burned to the ground. An old lady passing by tells her that the 'junkie bitch Bunty' started the fire and died dancing on the roof while it burned. Mr Manchester bravely rescued all the servants and the kitten, but was blinded by a falling beam and lost one of his ears. Now he is single again, Janine decides to give their relationship another chance, but explains to Mr Manchester that they will have to take things slowly, as she still has 'trust issues'. Six weeks later they marry and when their first son is born, Mr Manchester miraculously regains the sight in one eye.'

'It's comedy genius!' announced Eunice, grinning as she handed the pages back to Bomber. 'Are you sure you're not tempted to publish?'

Bomber threw a rubber which just missed her head as she ducked.

Eunice sat down at her desk and cupped her chin in her hands, lost in thought.

'Why do you think she does it?' she asked

227

Bomber. 'I mean, she can't just do it to wind you up. It's too much effort. And anyway, knowing Portia, the joke would have worn thin by now. There has to be more to it than that. And if she wanted to, she could self-publish. She could certainly afford it.'

Bomber shook his head sadly. 'I think that she genuinely wants to be good at something. Unfortunately, she's just picked the wrong thing. For all her money and so-called friends, I expect that hers is a pretty empty life sometimes.'

'I think, perhaps, that it's all about you.' Eunice stood up again and strolled over to the window. She could order her thoughts better when she was moving.

'I think she wants her big brother's approval — praise, love, validation, whatever you want to call it — and she's trying to earn it through writing. She's painted herself into a corner in every other way: she's rude, selfish, shallow and sometimes downright cruel, and she'd never admit that she cares a flying fortress what you think of her, but she does. Deep down, your little sister just wants you to be proud of her, and she's chosen to write, not because she has any talent or because it gives her any joy. It's a means to an end. You are a publisher and she wants to write a book that you think good enough to publish. That's why she always 'borrows' her plotlines from the classic greats.'

'But I do love her. I can't approve of the way she behaves — the way she treats Ma and Pa and the way she talks to you. But she's my sister. I'll always love her.'

228

Eunice came and stood behind him, and placed her hands gently on his shoulders.

1 know that. But I don't think Portia does. Poor Portia.' And for once, she meant it.

34

Laura sat on the bed, her fists clenched so tightly that her fingernails bit crescents into the flesh of her palms. She didn't know whether to be frightened or furious. Al Bowlly's voice drifted up from the garden room below, and his seductive tones were like fingernails scraping relentlessly down a blackboard.

'Well, I'm sick at the very thought of you!' she exploded and launched the book from her bedside table violently across the room. It hit one of the glass candlesticks on the dressing table, which fell to the floor and smashed.

'Bugger!'

Laura made a silent apology to Anthony. She got up and went downstairs to fetch a dustpan and brush, and to check what she knew already to be absolutely, unarguably, indubitably true. The Al Bowlly record was still in its faded paper cover, in the middle of the table in the study. She had put it there herself only yesterday, sick of hearing the tune which now haunted her, quite literally, day and night. She had hoped, rather foolishly now it seemed, that if she physically removed the record from the vicinity of the gramophone player it would stop. But Therese didn't have to play by those rules; physical rules. Her death had seemingly dispensed with such prosaic constraints, and she was free to make mischief in many more imaginative ways. And who or what else could it be? Anthony had been unfailingly kind to her while he was alive, so it was unlikely that he would take up such petty persecutions now he was dead. After all, Laura had done or was trying to do everything that he had asked of her. She picked up the record and looked at the smiling face of the man on the cover, with his slick black hair and his sultry dark eyes.

'You have no idea,' she told him, shaking her head. She put the record in a drawer and leaned back against it with all her weight as though to emphasise its closing. As if that would make any difference. She had told Freddy about the door to Therese's room and asked him to see if he could get it open. He had tried the handle and declared the door to be locked, but then said that he didn't think they should do anything about it.

'She'll unlock it when she's ready,' he had said, as though he were talking about a naughty child being left to exhaust a tantrum. Both Freddy and Sunshine seemed to accept Therese with an equanimity that Laura found infuriating. The troublesome presence of someone who was definitely dead and scattered in the garden should surely cause some consternation? Particularly as she should, by now, and thanks to their efforts, be existing somewhere in a state of postnuptial — although admittedly post-mortem — bliss. It was damned ungrateful. Laura smiled to herself ruefully. But who else could it be except Therese? Where reason fails, chimera flourishes. Just as she was finishing sweeping up the shards of broken glass, she heard Freddy and Carrot coming in from their walk.

Downstairs in the kitchen over tea and toast, she told Freddy about the music.

'Oh, that,' he said, feeding bits of buttered toast to Carrot. 'I've heard it too, but I never take much notice. I never know whether it's Sunshine or not.'

'I took the record away, but it made no difference, so now I've put it in a drawer in the study.'

'Why?' said Freddy, stirring sugar into his tea.

'Why did I take it away, or why did I put it in the drawer?'

'Both.'

'Because it's driving me mad. I took it away so that she couldn't play it any more.'

'Who? Sunshine?'

'No.' Laura paused for a moment, reluctant to say it out loud. 'Therese.'

'Ah. Our resident ghost. So, you took it away, which didn't work, and you thought that shutting it in a drawer might?'

'Not really. But it made me feel better. I keep wondering what else she might do. Why is she being such a bloody prima donna? She's got Anthony now, so what's the problem with me having the house? It's what he wanted.'

Freddy sipped his tea, frowning as he mulled over her question. 'Remember what Sunshine said. She said that Therese wasn't cross with you, she was cross with everyone. Her ire is indiscriminate. So it isn't about the house. Did anything like this ever happen while Anthony was still alive?'

'Not as far as I know. There's always been that scent of roses in the house, and a vague sense that Therese was still about, but I never saw or heard anything definite. And Anthony didn't mention anything.'

'So it's only since Anthony died that madam's started playing up?'

'Yes. But that's what's so wrong about it. I always assumed that she'd been waiting for him somewhere in the ether or wherever for all these years, practising her foxtrot or painting her nails . . . '

Freddy wagged his finger at her, gently admonishing the catty tone that had crept into her voice.

'I know, I know. I'm being horrid,' Laura laughed at herself. 'But honestly, what more does she want? She should be happy now she's got him back. Instead she's hanging around here misbehaving, like a disgruntled diva; deceased.'

Freddy put his hand over hers and squeezed it. 'I know it's unsettling. She's certainly a bit of a live wire — '

'Especially for someone who's supposed to be dead,' interrupted Laura.

Freddy grinned. 'I think you two might have got on rather well. From what Anthony told me about her, I reckon you're more alike than you realise.'

'He talked to you about Therese?'

'Sometimes, yes. Especially towards the end.' He drained his mug and refilled it from the teapot. 'But maybe we're missing something here. We're assuming that, just because Anthony's dead and we scattered him in the same place where he scattered Therese, they must be together. But are the ashes really what matters? Aren't they just 'remains'; what's left behind when the person is gone? Anthony and Therese are both dead, but maybe they're not together and that's the problem. If you and I both went to London separately and didn't arrange a place to meet, what would be the likelihood of us ever finding one another? And let's face it, wherever it is that they've gone has to be a whole hell of a lot bigger than London, bearing in mind all the dead people who will have pitched up there since . . . well, since people started dying.'

Freddy leaned back in his chair, looking rather pleased with himself and his explanation. Laura sighed and slumped back in her own chair despondently.

'So what you're saying is that Therese is actually worse off now than before he died, because at least then she knew where he was? Well that's just marvellous. We could be stuck with her for years. Forever. Bugger!'

Freddy came and stood behind her and placed his hands gently on her shoulders. 'Poor Therese. I think you should put the record back in the garden room.'

He kissed the top of her head and went out to work in the garden. Suddenly Laura felt guilty. It was probably all nonsense, but just supposing it wasn't? She had Freddy now, but what if, after all this time, Therese still didn't have Anthony?

Poor Therese.

Laura got up and went to the study. She fetched the record from the drawer and took it back to the garden room, where she placed it on the table next to the gramophone player. Picking up the photograph of Therese, she gazed at the woman, now blurred and distant behind splintered glass. She saw, perhaps for the first time, the person behind the paper picture. Freddy might think that they were alike, but Laura could see the differences. She had already lived fifteen years longer than Therese, but she had no doubt that Therese had lived her short life harder, brighter, faster than Laura ever had. What a waste.

Laura gently ran her fingertips over the face behind the cruel mosaic. What was it that Sarah had said? 'It's time to stop hiding and start kicking life up the arse.'

'I'll get you fixed,' she promised Therese.

Then she took up the record again and placed it on the turntable. 'Play nicely,' she said out loud to the room. 'I'm trying to be on your side.'

35

Eunice

1994

Eunice would never forget the scent of sun-warmed roses wafting in through the open window as she sat with Bomber and Grace watching Godfrey die. He was almost gone now. Just a worn-out body remained, barely ticking over, breaths too shallow to lift even a butterfly's wings. The fear and anger and confusion that had racked his last years had finally relinquished their tyranny over Godfrey and left him in peace. Grace and Bomber were able, at last, to hold his hands, and Baby Jane snuggled in close to him with her head gently resting on his chest. They had long since stopped trying to make conversation to fill the uncomfortable space between dying and death itself. Every now and then, a nurse would knock softly on the door, bringing tea and unspoken sympathy to a closing scene she had witnessed countless times before.

Eunice got up and went over to the window. Outside, the afternoon was passing by without them. People were strolling in the gardens or snoozing in the shade, and a group of children were chasing one another across the lawns, squealing with delight. Somewhere, high in one of the trees, a thrush was scatting against the

236

metronome tick of a sprinkler. Now would be a good time, she thought. To slip away on the coat-tails of a perfect English summer's afternoon. It seemed that Grace was in accord. She leaned back in her chair and exhaled a long sigh of resignation. Keeping hold of Godfrey's hand she struggled to her feet, grudging joints stiff from too long sitting. She kissed Godfrey on the mouth and stroked his hair with a frail but steady hand.

'It's time, my love. It's time to let go.'

Godfrey stirred, but just barely. Translucent eyelids fluttered and his weary chest rose for one final ragged breath. And then he was gone. Nobody moved except Baby Jane. The little dog stood and with infinite care, she sniffed every inch of Godfrey's face. Finally satisfied that her friend was gone, she jumped down from the bed, shook herself thoroughly and sat down at Bomber's feet, looking up at him beseechingly with an expression that clearly said, 'And now I really need a wee.'

An hour later they were sitting in what was called the 'relatives' room' drinking yet more tea. The relatives' room was the place where the Folly's End staff gently shepherded people once they were ready to leave the newly deceased. Its walls were the colour of faded primroses and the light was soft through muslin curtains, hung as a veil from prying eyes. With sofas plush and deep, fresh flowers and boxes of tissues, it was a room designed to cushion the sharp edges of raw grief.

After a few initial tears, Grace had rallied and

was ready to talk. In truth, she had lost the man she married long ago, and now, with his death, at least she could begin to mourn. Bomber was pale but composed, dabbing at the tears that occasionally leaked silently down his face. Before they had left Godfrey's room he had kissed his father's cheek for the final time. He had then removed Godfrey's wedding ring from his finger for the first time since Grace had placed it there a lifetime ago. The gold was scratched and worn, the circle a little misshapen; a testament to a long and robust marriage where love was rarely voiced, but manifest every day. Bomber had handed the ring to his mother who slipped it onto her middle finger without a word. Then he had telephoned Portia.

Grace came and sat next to Bomber and took his hand.

'Now, son, while we wait for your sister, I have something to say. You probably won't want me to talk about this, but I'm your mother and I have to say my piece.'

Eunice had no idea what was coming, but offered to leave them in private.

'No, no, my dear. I'm sure Bomber won't mind you hearing this, and I'd rather like you to back me up on this one if you don't mind.'

Eunice sat back down, intrigued. Baby Jane, who was sitting on the sofa next to Bomber, crawled onto his lap, as though to lend moral support.

'Right-ho. Here goes.' Grace squeezed her son's hand and gave it a little shake.

'Darling, I've always known since you were a

little boy that you were never going to be the sort of chap who got married and provided me with any grandchildren. I think that, secretly, your father knew that too, but of course we never spoke about it. Now, I want you to know that I don't give a jot about any of that. I've always been proud to have you as my son, and as long as you're happy and leading a decent life, well, that's all that matters.'

Bomber's cheeks were growing very pink, although whether it was his tears or Grace's words that were to blame Eunice couldn't tell. She was deeply moved by Grace's sentiments, but fighting a fit of the giggles at her peculiarly British way of trying to say something without *actually* saying it.

'Last week, Jocelyn took me to the cinema. It was supposed to be a little treat, to take my mind off your father for a bit.' There was the tiniest catch in Grace's voice, but she swallowed hard and carried on.

'We didn't pay too much attention to what was on; just bought the tickets and some mint imperials and went and sat down.'

Baby Jane wriggled in Bomber's lap to get comfortable. This was taking a little longer than she had expected.

'The film was *Philadelphia* with that nice Tom Hanks, Paul Newman's wife and that Spanish fellow.'

She thought carefully about her next words and finally settled upon: 'It wasn't very cheerful.'

She paused, hoping perhaps that she had said enough, but the puzzled expression on Bomber's face forced her to continue. She sighed.

'I just want you to promise me that you'll be careful. If you find a 'special friend' or' — the thought clearly just occurring to her — 'you have one already, just promise me that you won't get Hives.'

Eunice bit down hard on her lip, but Bomber couldn't hold back a smile.

'It's HIV, Ma.'

But Grace wasn't listening. She just wanted to hear him promise.

'I couldn't bear to lose you as well.'

Bomber promised. 'Cross my heart and hope to die.'

36

'It wasn't me, I promise,' said Sunshine.

They had come into the study to put some more things onto the website, and had found Anthony's treasured fountain pen lying in a pool of black ink in the middle of the table. It was a handsome Conway Stewart and Sunshine had admired it many times, lovingly stroking its shiny scarlet and black surface before reluctantly returning it to its drawer.

Laura saw the worried look on Sunshine's serious face and gave her a reassuring hug.

'I know it wasn't, sweetheart.'

She asked Sunshine to rinse the pen carefully under the tap and then put it back where it belonged while she cleaned up the mess on the table. When Laura returned to the study after washing her ink-stained hands, Sunshine was busy choosing more things from the shelves.

'It was The Lady of the Flowers, wasn't it?' she asked Laura.

'Oh, I don't know about that,' Laura bluffed. 'Perhaps I left it there and forgot about it, and somehow it leaked.'

She knew how unlikely it sounded, and the expression on Sunshine's face confirmed that she was completely unconvinced. Laura had been thinking about what Freddy had said, and the more she thought about it, the more concerned she became. If all these things were

Therese's doing, and a physical demonstration of her pain at still being apart from Anthony, then surely the longer it went on, the worse it would get? She remembered Robert Quintan's description of Therese as having 'a wild streak, and a fiery temper when roused'. Good God, at this rate she'd soon be setting fires and smashing up the place, and Laura was already a little tired of clearing up after a grumpy ghost.

'We should try and help her,' said Sunshine.

Laura sighed, slightly shamed by Sunshine's generosity of spirit. 'I agree. But how on earth do we do that?'

Sunshine shrugged her shoulders, her face crumpling into a perplexed frown. 'Why don't we ask her?' she eventually suggested.

Laura didn't want to be unkind, but it was hardly a practical suggestion. She wasn't about to hold a séance or buy a Ouija board on eBay. They spent the rest of the morning adding things to the website while Carrot snored contentedly in front of the fire.

After lunch, Sunshine and Freddy took Carrot for a walk, but Laura stayed behind. She was thoroughly unsettled. Normally the task of entering data onto the website was a therapeutic distraction, but not today. She could only think about Therese. Like a creature whose fur has been brushed against the nap, her skin prickled and her thoughts skimmed and zigzagged like a water boatman across the surface of a pond. She needed to do something about Therese. There had to be what Jerry Springer and his fellow reality TV ringmasters called 'an intervention'. If only she knew what the hell it ought to be.

Outside, gauzy sunlight seeped through clear patches in a grey marbled sky. Laura took her jacket from the hall and went out into the garden for some air. In the shed, she found Freddy's 'secret' packet of cigarettes and helped herself to one. She was only a high days and holidays smoker, really, but today she thought it might help. She wondered if Therese had smoked.

As Laura strolled aimlessly round the rose garden, puffing like a guilty schoolgirl, Sunshine's words slipped back into her head.

'Why don't we ask her?' It might not be very practical, but nothing about this whole situation was exactly run-of-the-mill and there was no point in Laura trying to deal with it as though it were. So maybe Sunshine was right. If it was Therese doing all these things — and some days Laura clung on to that 'if' like a passenger on the *Titanic* to a life jacket — then leaving her to her own devices would only mean more and more trouble.

'Why don't we ask her?' Laura was embarrassed even to be considering it. But what else could she do? Put up or shut up until . . . Laura didn't want to think about the possible endings to that sentence. She took a final puff on her cigarette and then, glancing round furtively to make sure that she couldn't be seen or heard, she let her words escape out loud into the chill of the afternoon air.

'Therese,' she began, just to clarify to whom she was talking — and just in case any other ghosts happened to be listening, she joked to herself — 'you and I need to have a serious chat. Anthony was my friend, and I know how desperately he longed to be with you again. I want to help, and if I possibly can I will, but wrecking the house, locking me out of my bedroom, and keeping me awake all night with your music isn't exactly appealing to my better nature. Clearly ghostbusting isn't my area of expertise, so if you know how I can help, then you'll have to try and find a way of sharing that with me.'

Laura paused, not expecting an answer, but feeling somehow that she should leave a gap for one anyway.

'I don't have the patience for puzzles and riddles, and I'm hopeless at Cluedo,' she continued, 'so you'll have to try and make it as clear and simple as you can. Preferably without breaking or setting fire to anything . . . or anyone,' she added, under her breath.

Once again, she waited. Nothing. Except for the cooing and canoodling of two amorous pigeons on the shed roof, practising for spring. She shivered. It was getting colder.

'I meant what I said, Therese. I'll do whatever I can.'

She marched back down the garden, feeling a little foolish and in need of a cup of tea and a consoling chocolate biscuit. Back in the kitchen, she put the kettle on and opened the biscuit tin. Inside was Anthony's pen.

37

'Well, if that's her idea of 'clear and simple', I dread to think what her 'cryptic' would be like.'

Laura was walking hand in hand with Freddy and they were mulling over the mystery of Anthony's pen. Carrot was trotting along in front of them, sniffing and marking his territory at alternate lamp posts. They had been to The Moon is Missing for a few drinks. Freddy had thought it might take Laura's mind off Therese for a bit, but the entire cast of *Blithe Spirit* was reliving the triumph of their first night in the bar. Marjory Wadscallop was still in full Madame Arcati hair and make-up and wasted no time in pointing out to Winnie the arrival of Laura and Freddy *together*. It had hardly been the quiet drink that Freddy had been hoping for.

'Are you sure that Sunshine put the pen back in the drawer?'

'Well, I didn't actually see her do it, but I'm sure she would have. Why? You don't think she's playing games, do you?'

Freddy smiled and shook his head.

'No, I don't. I really don't. Sunshine's probably the most honest out of all of us, including you,' he said to Carrot as he clipped the lead to his collar, ready to cross the road.

Back at Padua Laura poured them both another drink and Freddy livened up the fire that was barely smouldering in the garden room.

'Now,' said Freddy, snuggling up to Laura on the sofa, 'let's see if the wine has aroused our deductive juices.'

Laura giggled. 'That sounds positively smutty.'

Freddy raised his eyes in feigned surprise and took a swig from his glass.

'Right. Let's look at the clue again — a pen in a biscuit tin.'

'Not just any pen — Anthony's best, beloved Conway Stewart fountain pen; red and black marbled shaft with an 18-carat gold nib,' Laura added.

'Thank you, Miss Marple, but does that really help our investigation?'

'Well, it was the pen that Anthony used to write his stories.'

They sat in contemplative silence, listening to the spit and crackle of the fire. Carrot groaned blissfully as he stretched his spindly legs nearer to the hearth. Freddy nudged him with his toe.

'Watch it, mister. If you get any closer, you'll roast your toes.'

Carrot ignored him and wriggled infinitesimally nearer.

'Have you read all of Anthony's stories? Maybe the clue is in one of them.'

Laura shook her head. 'I told her I wasn't any good at clues. I specifically asked her to make it clear and simple.'

Freddy drained his glass and set it down on the floor. 'Well, maybe it *is* clear and simple to her.'

Laura resisted the temptation to point out that

of course it was, because Therese already knew the answer.

'I read everything he asked me to type, obviously, and certainly all of the short stories. But that was years ago now. I can't possibly remember all of them.'

'What about that book you showed me? The collection of short stories?'

'That was only the first of several that were published. I suppose he must have kept copies of the others somewhere, but I don't remember seeing them.'

Freddy grinned. 'I bet they're in the attic.'

'Why?'

Freddy pulled the face that Sunshine always pulled when she thought that they were being particularly obtuse.

'Because that's where everyone always puts the stuff they don't know what else to do with,' he said triumphantly. 'Although if I'd had a book published, I'd have it on my bookshelf in pride of place.'

Laura thought about it for a moment.

'But he wasn't proud of all the short stories that were published. Remember, I told you? His publisher wanted insipid, simple, happy ever afters and they fell out over it in the end.'

Freddy nodded. 'I do remember. Bruce wanted lemonade and Anthony gave him absinthe.'

Laura smiled. 'You would remember that. Anything to do with alcohol . . . ' she teased. 'But I suppose it's worth a try. I haven't really had a proper look in the attic, and even if the books aren't there, there might be something else.'

'Tomorrow,' said Freddy, standing up and dragging her to her feet. 'We'll look tomorrow.'

He kissed her firmly on the lips.

'Now what was that you said about being smutty . . . ?'

★ ★ ★

Laura woke with a jolt that broke her fall. Was she dreaming about falling or falling out of the dream? She could never tell. It was still dark and the silence was barely rippled by the hushed duet of Freddy and Carrot's breathing. The back of Freddy's warm hand rested on the outside of her thigh, and as her eyes grew accustomed to the dark, she could just about make out the rise and fall of his chest. She wondered what Anthony would think. She hoped he would approve; be pleased for her. After all, he had told her to be happy and she was. Mostly. She still worried about returning the lost things. The website was coming along nicely, thanks to Freddy, and though her fear of failing Anthony was deeply rooted in the fertile tract of her self-doubt, now courage grew alongside. Finally, she had found the guts to try. Therese was a constant shadow, but the general sweep of her life, the day-to-day at Padua was definitely happy. Oh, and of course she worried about Freddy. But surely that was an occupational hazard in a new relationship, particularly at her age? She worried that he hadn't yet seen the full horror of her treacherous stretch marks and her crow's feet in the unforgiving glare of the midday sun. She worried that he might not yet have noticed the insidious creep of cellulite crumpling her once pert bottom and threatening her thighs. And she was sorry, too, that Freddy had not seen her bottom at the peak of its pertness. Instead, it had been wasted on Vince. If only she had met Freddy when she was young. Younger, even. If only she had married Freddy. She smiled to herself at her foolishness and then stopped, mindful of the crow's feet, and vowed to wear enormous sunglasses and a wide-brimmed hat should she ever be foolish enough to venture outside in the sunlight again. And she wasn't even going to think about the menopause. The clue was in the name, wasn't it? But not so much a pause as a bloody great full stop as far as being remotely attractive to men was concerned. She was even breaking out in a sweat *not* thinking about it. She turned her pillow over and buried her face in the cool, fresh cotton. 'Get a grip, Laura!' she told herself. She reached for Freddy's hand and took it in her own. Instinctively he squeezed it, and Laura lay there in the darkness, blinking away the tears until eventually she drifted back to sleep.

Things always look better in the morning. It wasn't the sunlight that poked fun at Laura's imperfections, but the darkness with its looming doubts that mocked her in the sleepless spells that broke the night. After breakfast, she went out into the garden, hatless, and squinted into the morning sun. Freddy had gone into town and she was going up into the attic. She fetched the step-ladder from the shed and carted it upstairs with some difficulty. Carrot had decided to help by running up and down the stairs, barking excitedly in an attempt to ward off the invasion of the clanking, rattling metal legs that were clearly an instrument of the devil. As Laura propped the fully extended ladder against the wall, she could already hear Freddy scolding her for not waiting.

'We'll do it when I get back,' he had said.

But she was too impatient to wait. Besides, Sunshine would be here soon, and she was perfectly capable of calling an ambulance. As she pushed open the hatch into the attic, the musty smell of warm dirt and dust wafted out to greet her. She flicked on the light switch and, at once, her hand was sticky with cobwebs. Where to start? There were a few bits of old furniture, a large rug rolled into a sausage and a variety of boxes. She lifted the lids on those closest to her. They contained general house-hold flotsam and jetsam: an unused tea service, a canteen of silver-plated cutlery and various pieces of useless but decorative china. One contained books, but as far as she could see, none had been written by Anthony. Laura made her way cautiously across the joists, stooping awkwardly under the pitch of the rafters. A child's push-along horse on wheels stood lonely in a corner next to a large brown cardboard suitcase and a box from a dressmaker in London. Laura stroked the soft teddy-bear fur of the horse's nose.

'Well, you're not staying up here,' she promised him.

The suitcase was thick with dust, but not locked, and a quick peek inside told Laura that it was probably her best hope of finding something useful or interesting. She clipped its rust-freckled fasteners shut and dragged it over to the hatch. How on earth was she going to get it down? It was heavy, and she doubted if she could manage its weight and the ladder at the same time. The answer, of course, was to wait for Freddy, but if she did that, she might just as well have waited for him before going up there. Perhaps she could just let it slide down the ladder on its own. It looked pretty robust, and from what she had seen, it didn't appear to contain anything breakable. The 'slide down the ladder' turned out to be more of a sheer drop. As Laura let it go, it crashed onto the landing with an almighty thump and an explosion of dust. Laura went back for the horse, which was light enough for her to carry down the ladder. Having given him a softer landing than the suitcase, she went back up and fetched the box from the London dressmaker.

By the time Freddy returned, the ladder was back in the shed, Sunshine was in the garden brushing the dust out of the horse, and Laura had the suitcase open on the table in the study and was going through the contents. There were several old photograph albums, with thick pages the colour of dark chocolate interleaved with crispy embossed tissue papers; a couple of typed manuscripts, and some letters and assorted paperwork. The albums contained the first years of Anthony's life, long before Therese. A curly-haired toddler sat, legs splayed, on a tartan rug in a summer garden. A sturdy little boy rode astride a push-along horse on a neatly clipped lawn. A gangling youth with a shy grin wore oversized shin pads and wielded a cricket bat. It was all there: a parade of seaside holidays, country picnics, birthdays, christenings, weddings and Christmases. At first they were three; but then only two. The tall, dark man, so often in uniform, disappeared from their pictures as he did from their lives. Laura carefully unhooked one of the photographs from the brown paper corners that fixed it into the album. The man stood straight-backed and proud; so very handsome in his dress uniform. His arm was wrapped fondly round the shoulder of the woman, soignee in a Schiaparelli evening gown. And between them was a little boy wearing his pyjamas. A picture-perfect happy family.

The very thought of you.

Laura could hear the music playing in her head, or perhaps it was in the garden room. She wasn't always sure these days that she could tell the difference. This was the photograph; the evening that Robert Quinlan had described when he had come to read the will. This was the last time that Anthony had seen his father. The last dance, the last kiss, the last photograph. She would put it in a silver frame beside the photograph of Therese in the garden room.

'Found anything interesting yet?'

Freddy had brought her a cup of coffee and a

sandwich. He rummaged around in the suitcase beneath the papers and took out a small, velvet-covered box.

'Ah-ha! What's this? Hidden treasure?'

He flipped open the lid to reveal a white-gold ring set with an exquisite star sapphire and sparkling diamonds. He set it down in front of Laura who took it out of the box and held it up to the light. The star across the cabochon of cornflower blue was clearly visible.

'It was hers. Her engagement ring.'

'How do you know?' Freddy took it from her to inspect it more closely. 'It could have been Anthony's mother's.'

'No. It was hers, I'm sure. Therese wasn't a humdrum diamond solitaire type of woman,' she said, smiling ruefully at the thought of her own half-carat set in 9-carat gold. 'She was, by all accounts, extraordinary, like this ring.'

Freddy slipped it back into the velvet box and handed it to Laura.

'Well, it's yours now.'

Laura shook her head.

'It will never be mine.'

Freddy went outside to help Sunshine. He had promised to give the horse's wooden hooves a fresh coat of varnish. Laura continued emptying the contents of the suitcase onto the table. She found a bill of sale for fifty rose bushes: 'Albertine' × 4, 'Grand Prix' × 6, 'Marcia Stanhope', 'Mrs Henry Morse', 'Etoile de Hollande', 'Lady Gay' — the list went on — and a pamphlet on how to plant and care for them. The manuscripts were collections of Anthony's short stories that Laura had typed. As she flicked through the pages, she recognised them. Attached to the front was a harsh rejection letter from Bruce, the publisher.

' . . . entirely inappropriate for our readership . . . unnecessarily complex and self-indulgently ambiguous . . . dark and depressing subject matter . . . '

Someone had scribbled across the insulting comments with a red pen, and written 'Arse!' over Bruce's extravagant signature. It was Anthony's handwriting. 'Quite right too,' Laura agreed. She would re-read the manuscripts thoroughly later, but somehow she didn't think they would contain the answer she was looking for.

There was a rattle of metal wheels across the hall floor and Sunshine entered the study pushing the horse, followed by Freddy and a curious Carrot.

'He looks like a different horse!' Laura exclaimed, and Sunshine grinned proudly.

'He's called Sue.'

Laura looked at Freddy to see if he could provide an explanation, but he simply shrugged his shoulders. 'Sue' it was, then. Sunshine was eager to examine the contents of the suitcase and was spellbound by the ring. As she slipped it onto her middle finger, turning it this way and that to 'catch the sparkles', Laura had an idea.

'Perhaps it's the ring Therese wants us to find. Maybe that's what it's all about.'

Freddy was uncertain. 'Hmm, but what's the connection with the pen?'

Laura ignored the flaw in her argument; instead, warming to her theory, she said, 'It was her engagement ring. Don't you see? It's all about their connection, the bond between them. That's what an engagement is.'

Freddy was still doubtful. 'But so is a wedding, and that didn't work when we gave them one.'

The face that Sunshine was pulling clearly showed that not only was she totally unconvinced, but she thought that they were both being particularly obtuse once again.

'The pen was for the clue. That means writing,' she said.

She picked up the photograph of Anthony and his parents.

'That's why she plays the music,' she said, handing Freddy the picture. It was his turn to look to Laura for an explanation.

'It's Anthony and his parents. Robert Quinlan told us about it. His parents were going out one evening while his father was home on leave, and he came down to say goodnight and found them dancing to the Al Bowlly song. It was the last time he saw his father before he was killed.'

'And then when Saint Anthony met The Lady of the Flowers,' Sunshine was eager to tell the rest of the story, 'he told her all about it and so she danced with him in the Convent Gardens to stop him being sad.' She twisted the ring, which was still on her finger, and added, 'And now we have to find a way to stop her being sad.'

'Well, I think the ring's worth a try,' said

Laura, holding out her hand to Sunshine, who reluctantly took it off and gave it to her. 'We'll put it in the garden room next to her photograph. Now, where shall we put this splendid steed?' she added in an attempt to distract Sunshine. But Sunshine had seen the box from the dressmaker and carefully removed the lid. Her gasp of astonishment drew both Laura and Freddy to her side. Laura lifted from the box a stunning dress made of cornflower blue silk chiffon. It had clearly never been worn. Sunshine stroked the delicate fabric lovingly.

'It was her wedding dress,' she said, almost in a whisper. 'It was The Lady of the Flowers' wedding dress.'

Freddy was still holding the photograph. 'What I don't understand is why all these things were shoved into a suitcase and hidden away in the attic? It seems to me these were some of the things that must have been most precious to him: the ring, the photo, the dress, the beginnings of the rose garden. Even the manuscripts. He stood by them, refusing to change them, and so he must have been proud of them.'

Sunshine traced circles in the dust on the lid of the suitcase.

'They made him hurt too much,' she said simply.

Carrot poked his head round the door of the study and whined. It was time for his tea.

'Come on,' said Laura, 'let's put the ring and the dress in the garden room and find a home for this horse.'

'Sue,' said Sunshine, following behind Laura and Freddy. 'And it's not the ring, it's the letter.' But Laura and Freddy had already gone.

38

Eunice

1997

'I'm damn sure the ruddy man's just doing it to be bloody awkward!'

Bruce flounced across the office and flung himself into a chair like the tragic heroine of a silent black and white film. Eunice quite expected him to raise the back of his hand to his forehead to better illustrate his anguish and frustration. He had arrived, uninvited, and begun his rant before he had even reached the top of the stairs.

'Steady the Buffs, old chap,' said Bomber, fighting to keep his amusement from contaminating his platitudes. 'You'll do yourself an unpleasantness.'

Baby Jane, perched majestically on a new faux fur cushion, gazed at Bruce and concluded that his presence was unworthy of any acknowledgement.

'Would you like a cup of tea?' Eunice asked him, through gritted teeth.

'Only if it's accompanied by a large whisky,' Bruce retorted rudely.

Eunice went to put the kettle on anyway.

'Now what's brought all this on?' Bomber was genuinely interested to find out who had managed to infuriate Bruce so thoroughly. Bruce's hair, in the style of Barbara Cartland but the colour and consistency of cobwebs, quivered his indignation.

'Damn that Anthony Peardew! Damn and blast the man to hell.'

Bomber shook his head. 'I say — that's a bit harsh, isn't it? Unless, of course, he's passed the port to the right or ravished your only daughter.'

When first confronted by a man as camp as Bruce, Eunice had assumed that he was gay. But Bruce was married to a large German woman with Zeppelin breasts and the suggestion of a moustache who bred fancy mice and entered them into mouse shows. Astonishingly, Bruce and Brunhilde had managed to produce offspring: two boys and a girl. It was one of life's great mysteries, but not one upon which Eunice was inclined to dwell.

'He's gone completely round the bend,' expostulated Bruce, 'deliberately writing the kind of subversive codswallop he knows I won't publish, full of dark deeds and weird endings, or no proper endings at all. I suppose he thinks it's clever or fashionable or some sort of catharsis for his personal grief. But I'm not having any of it. I know what normal, decent people like, and that's good, straightforward stories with a happy ending where the baddies get their comeuppance, the guy gets the girl and the sex isn't too outré.'

Eunice plonked a cup of tea down in front of him, deliberately sploshing some of the dishwater-coloured liquid from the cup into the saucer.

'So you don't think that any of your readers might like to be challenged at all? Flex their intellectual muscles, so to speak? Form their own opinions or extrapolate their own conclusions for once?'

Bruce lifted the cup to his lips and then, seeing its contents close up, changed his mind and set it down again with an irritated clatter.

'My dear, the readers like what we tell them they will like. It's as simple as that.'

'Then why can't you tell them to like Anthony Peardew's new stories?'

Bomber kept the 'touché' under his breath. Just. 'Anthony Peardew. Wasn't he the chap whose collection of stories did rather well for you?'

Bruce raised his eyebrows so high in exasperation that they disappeared into his cobweb coiffure.

'For God's sake, Bomber! Do try and keep up. That's what I've been saying. The first lot did really well; happy stories, happy endings, happy bank balances all round. But not any more. He's gone from *The Sound of Music* to *The Midwich Cuckoos*. But I've drawn the line. I've told him: it's either 'Doe a deer' or out on your ear!'

Bruce had once worked from offices in the same building as Bomber, and still visited for a free cup of tea and a gossip if he was passing. However, failure to enlist Bomber in his condemnation of the villainous Anthony Peardew, and scant sympathy from Eunice meant that, on this occasion, Bruce's visit was a short one.

'I wish we'd managed to sign poor Anthony

before Bruce did,' sighed Bomber. 'I liked his first collection but his new stories sound intriguing. I wonder if I should try a spot of poaching . . . '

Eunice took a small parcel from the drawer in her desk and handed it to Bomber. It was wrapped in thick, charcoal grey paper and tied with a bright pink ribbon.

'I know it's not your birthday until next week' — Bomber's face lit up like a small boy's; he loved surprises — 'but I thought that after a visit from Bruce the Bogeyman, you could do with cheering up.'

It was a copy of *The Birdcage*. They had been to see it on Bomber's birthday the previous year, and he had laughed so hard that he had almost choked on his popcorn.

'I wish Ma could have seen it,' he had said. 'It's a damn sight more cheerful than *Philadelphia*.' Grace had been dead for eighteen months now. She had survived Godfrey by just over a year, and then died suddenly but peacefully in her sleep at Folly's End. She had been buried next to Godfrey in the grounds of the church where they had been members of the congregation and stalwarts of the flower-arranging team and the summer fete and harvest supper committees for almost half a century. As Bomber and Eunice had stood side by side in the sun-and-shade-dappled churchyard on the day of Grace's funeral, their thoughts had turned to their own leaving ceremonies.

'I'm for burning not burial,' declared Bomber. 'Less room for error,' he added. 'And then I

261

want you to mix my ashes with Douglas's and Baby Jane's — providing, of course, that I outlive her — and scatter us somewhere fabulous.'

Eunice watched as the funeral party wandered slowly back to their cars.

'What makes you so sure that you'll die before me?'

Bomber took her arm as they too began to make their way out of the churchyard.

'Because you're a good few years younger than me, and you've led a purer life.'

Eunice snorted her contention, but Bomber continued, 'And because you're my faithful assistant and you must do as I command.'

Eunice laughed. ' 'Somewhere fabulous' isn't a very specific command.'

'When I think of somewhere specific, I'll let you know.'

Just before they reached the lychgate, Bomber had stopped and squeezed her arm.

'And one more thing.' He had held her in his gaze with eyes that shone with unspilled tears. 'Promise me that if I ever end up like Pa, mad as a box of frogs and stuck away in a home, that you'll find a way to . . . you know what. Get. Me. Out.'

Eunice had forced a smile, though at that moment someone walked across her grave.

'Cross my heart and hope to die,' she had told him.

Now Bomber showed his present to Baby Jane, but once she had ascertained that it was inedible and didn't squeak or bounce, she lost what little interest she had mustered.

'So, what do you want to do for your birthday?' Eunice asked, twirling the pink ribbon around her fingers.

'Well,' said Bomber, 'how about combining my birthday with our usual annual outing?'

Eunice grinned. 'Brighton it is!'

39

'It's not the ring, and now Therese is sulking.'

Laura kicked one of Carrot's many tennis balls across the lawn in frustration. Freddy stopped digging and leaned on his spade, ready to commiserate as required. Laura had come out into the garden, where Freddy was digging compost into the rose garden, with little purpose other than to vent her frustration. Freddy grinned at her.

'Never mind. We'll sort it out eventually.'

Laura was in no mood for platitudes. Therese and Sunshine were both sulking; no doubt for very different, but for the moment, equally unfathomable reasons; she was running behind with the data input for the website, and Carrot had got completely over-excited when the new postwoman had called to deliver a parcel and had weed on the Chinese rug in the hall. She took another petulant swing at a tennis ball, missed and nearly fell over. Freddy resumed his digging in order to disguise his laughter. Laura had had high hopes that the sapphire ring might be the perfect panacea. She had replaced the broken glass in Therese's photograph, placed the picture of Anthony and his parents beside it, and the ring in its box in front of her. She had even tried to play the Al Bowlly song for her.

'How do you know that Therese is sulking?'

Freddy had recovered himself sufficiently by

now to try to be helpful.

'Because the bedroom door's still locked and because of that damn record!'

Freddy frowned. 'But I can't remember hearing it for days now.'

Laura raised her eyebrows in exasperation. 'For God's sake, Freddy! Do try and keep up. That's what I've been saying.'

Freddy ditched the spade and came and gave her a hug.

'Well, not very clearly, I'm afraid. I'm not very good at clues. You'll have to make it 'clear and simple',' he said, bracketing the phrase in the air with his fingers.

'Touché.' Laura grinned in spite of herself.

'Right,' said Freddy. 'How does Therese *not* playing dear old Al signify that she's sulking?'

'Because now, instead of playing it morning, noon and night, she won't allow it to be played at all.'

Freddy looked sceptical. 'I'm not sure I understand.'

Laura sighed. 'I've tried to play it over and over, but it simply won't. At first, I did it to be nice. I set up the photographs and the ring, and then, as a finishing touch, I thought I'd play the music; their song. But it won't play. She won't let it.'

Freddy chose his next words very carefully.

'Well, it is an old record and an old player. Maybe the needle needs changing or the record has been scratched . . . '

One look at Laura's face was enough to derail his argument.

'Okay, okay. You've checked. Of course you have. They're both fine.'

Laura picked up yet another tennis ball and threw it at him. But this time with a laugh.

'Oh God, I'm sorry. I'm such a grumpy cow, but I'm doing my best to help her and now she's just being bloody awkward. Come on, I'll make you a cup of tea. There might even be a chocolate biscuit if Sunshine hasn't finished them.'

Freddy took her hand. 'I shan't raise my hopes.'

In the kitchen, Sunshine had just put the kettle on.

'Perfect timing!' said Freddy. 'We just came in for the lovely cup of tea.'

Sunshine set out two more cups and saucers in ominous silence as Freddy washed his hands at the sink.

'Are there any chocolate biscuits left?' he asked her with a wink.

An unsmiling Sunshine placed the biscuit tin in front of him without a word, and then turned away to watch the kettle boil. Freddy and Laura exchanged puzzled glances and then began discussing the progress of the website. They had decided that in order to create more interest, people who claimed back their lost possessions could post their stories on the website if they wanted to. Freddy had come up with an online form people had to complete, giving very specific details of where and when they lost whatever it was that they were claiming. The website simply displayed a photograph of each item, the month

266

and year, and the general location where it had been found. The specific details on Anthony's labels were withheld in order for them to be sure that the people who came forward were the legitimate owners. Laura still had hundreds more items to photograph and post on the website, but enough had been completed to justify the site going live. It was, in any case, always going to be a work in progress, if they continued to gather things that other people had lost. There was going to be an item in the local newspaper that week, and Laura had already given an interview to the local radio station. There were now only days to go before the website went live.

'What if no one comes forward to claim anything?' worried Laura, chewing nervously on her fingernail. Freddy playfully slapped her hand away from her mouth.

'Of course they will!' he said. 'Won't they, Sunshine?'

Sunshine shrugged her shoulders dramatically, her bottom lip pouting like a ship's prow. She poured the tea and plonked the cups and saucers down in front of them hard. Freddy raised his hands in surrender.

'Okay, okay. I give up. What's up, kid?'

Sunshine put her hands on her hips and treated them both to her sternest look.

'No one ever listens to me,' she said quietly.

They were now. Her words dropped into the air and hung there, expectantly, waiting for a response. Neither Freddy nor Laura knew what to say. Each felt a prickle of guilt that Sunshine might actually have a point. With her diminutive stature and ingenuous features, it was easy to slip into the habit of treating her like a child and weighting her opinions and ideas accordingly. But Sunshine was a young woman — albeit 'dancing drome' — and perhaps it was about time that they started treating her as such.

'We're sorry,' said Laura.

Freddy nodded, for once without a trace of a smile on his face.

'We're sorry if you've tried to talk to us and we haven't listened.'

'Yes,' said Freddy, 'and if we do it again, just bash us.'

Sunshine thought about it for a moment and then clipped him round the ear, just for good measure. Then, serious again, she addressed them both.

'It's not the ring. It's the letter.'

'Which letter?' said Freddy.

'Saint Anthony's dead letter,' she replied. 'Come on,' she added.

They followed her from the kitchen into the garden room, where she picked up the Al Bowlly record and placed it on the turntable.

'It's the letter,' she said again, and with that she set the needle down onto the disc and the music began to play.

40

Eunice

2005

'The thought of you publishing that . . . ' Eunice consulted her inner omnibus of obscenities and, finding nothing suitably disparaging, expostulated her final word like a poisonous blow dart: 'thing!'

The hardback floozy of a book, with its trashy red and gold cover, languished half undressed in its brown paper wrappings alongside a bottle of champagne that Bruce had sent with it, according to the card, 'as some consolation for not having the wit to publish it yourself'.

Bomber shook his head in bewildered disbelief. 'I haven't even read it. Have you?'

Portia's latest book had topped the bestseller lists for the past three weeks, and as its publisher, Bruce's swaggering peacockery knew no restraint. His self-importance was index-linked to his bank balance which, thanks to Portia, now warranted a platinum credit card and first name terms with the branch manager.

'Of course I've read it!' Eunice exclaimed. 'I had to in order to slander it from an informed perspective. I've also read all the reviews. You do realise that your sister's book is being hailed as 'a searing satire on the saccharine clichés of contemporary commercial fiction'? One critic called it 'a razor-sharp deconstruction of the sexual balance of power in modern relationships, pushing the boundaries of popular literature to exhilarating extremes and giving the finger to those luminaries of the literary establishment who habitually kowtow to the conventions of Man Booker and its staid stablemates'.'

Despite her fury, Eunice couldn't keep a straight face, and Bomber was in stitches. He eventually composed himself sufficiently to ask, 'But what's it about?'

Eunice sighed. 'Do you really want to know? It's so much worse than anything else she's ever done.'

'I think I can cope.'

'Well, as you are already painfully aware, it goes by the intriguing title of *Harriet Hotter and the Gobstopper Phone*.'

Eunice paused for effect.

'Harriet, orphaned at an early age and raised by a dreadful aunt and a clinically obese and very sweaty uncle, vows to leave their home as soon as she can and make her own way in the world. After her A levels she gets a job in a pizza and kebab shop, Pizzbab, near King's Cross, where she is constantly mocked for her posh voice and her bifocal spectacles. One day, an old man with a very long beard and a funny hat comes into the shop to buy a kebab and chips, and tells her that she is 'very special'. He hands her a business card and tells her to call him. Fast forward six months and Harriet is earning a small fortune from phone sex. Her customers love her because she has a posh voice, 'as though her cheeks were stuffed with gobstoppers' — and so the ingenious title is explained. Our heroine, not satisfied with mere financial reward, seeks self-fulfilment and enhanced job satisfaction. In partnership with the beardy old man, aka Chester Fumblefore, she sets up a training school for aspiring phone sex workers called Snogwarts, so called because Harriet teaches her students to speak to every customer as though he were a handsome prince, even though most of them are more likely to be warty toads. Among her first pupils are Persephone Danger and Donna Sleazy who become her best friends and training assistants. Between them, they set up a vast call centre where their pupils can earn an honest living while they are training. Harriet invents a game called Quids In to increase productivity and raise morale in the workplace. The winner, who receives a cash bonus and a month's supply of gobstoppers, is the worker who satisfies the most customers in one hour whilst cunningly introducing the words 'brothel', 'todger' (twice) and 'golden snatch' into each phone sex liaison.'

Bomber laughed out loud.

'It's not funny, Bomber!' exploded Eunice. 'It's an absolute bloody disgrace. How can anybody give such utter drivel shelf room? Millions of people are paying hard-earned money for this excrement! It's not even well-written excrement. It's execrable excrement. And if it's not enough that Portia's being interviewed on every poxy chat show that's aired, there's a horribly tenacious rumour doing the rounds about her being invited to speak at the Hay festival this year.'

Bomber clapped his hands in glee. 'Now *that* I should gladly pay good money to see.'

Eunice shot him a warning look and he shrugged his shoulders in reply.

'How could I resist? I'm just thankful that Ma and Pa aren't around to witness the whole ruddy circus. Especially with Ma having been the chairwoman of the local WI.'

Bomber chuckled to himself at the thought of it, but then donned a more appropriately serious expression for his next question.

'Now, I'm almost afraid to ask, but I probably need to know. Is it terribly . . . explicit?'

Eunice let out a hoot of derision.

'Explicit?! Remember that time when Bruce was here ranting on about that Peardew chap and lecturing us on the key components of a bestseller?'

Bomber nodded.

'And he told us, and I quote, that the sex should never be too *outré*?'

Bomber nodded again, more slowly this time.

'Well, unless his definition of *outré* is informed by a far more adventurous carnal relationship with Brunhilde than we ever gave them credit for, I think he's changed his mind.'

Bomber placed his hands on the small wooden box that stood next to Douglas's on his desk and warned, 'Cover your ears and don't listen to this, Baby Jane.'

Eunice smiled a little sadly and continued.

'One of Harriet's customers has sex with a bread-making machine, another lusts after women with beards, hairy backs and ingrowing toenails, and yet another has his testicles bathed in surgical spirit and then stroked with the mane of a My Little Pony. And that's only chapter two.'

Bomber picked up the book from its wrappings and opened the front cover to be greeted by a glossy photograph of his sister wearing a self-satisfied smile and a silk negligee. He snapped it shut again with a resounding thump.

'Well at least she didn't simply steal someone else's plot wholesale this time. She did make some of it up herself.'

'Let's hope so,' said Eunice.

★   ★   ★

The next day all thoughts of Portia were purged by the glittering aquamarine waves and warm, salty wind of Brighton seafront. It was the 'annual outing', and this was the first without Douglas or Baby Jane. They had been coming every year since Eunice's twenty-first birthday trip with Bomber, and the day followed a familiar pattern that had been fine-tuned over the years to provide enjoyment and entertainment to all members of their small party. First they walked along the promenade. In the past, when Douglas and then Baby Jane had accompanied them, the dogs had gloried in the compliments and cosseting of passers-by that they inevitably attracted. Then there was the visit to the pier and an hour frittered away on the flashing, clanging, jangling slot machines. Then lunch of fish and chips and a bottle of pink fizz, and finally the Royal Pavilion. But as they strolled towards the pier, worry was washing away Eunice's happiness. Bomber had asked her twice in the space of ten minutes if they'd been there before. The first time, she'd hoped he was joking, but the second time she looked at his face and her world tipped sharply on its axis when she saw an expression of innocence and genuine enquiry. It was horribly, gut-wrenchingly famil-iar. Godfrey. He was following his father's painful footsteps to a destination Eunice couldn't bear to think about. So far, it was barely noticeable; a hairline crack in his solid, dependable sanity. But Eunice knew that in time he would be as vulnerable as a name written in the sand at the mercy of an incoming tide. As yet, Bomber seemed unaware of his gentle unraveilings. Like a man with petit mals, he passed through them blithely oblivious. But Eunice lived them all, second by second, and her heart was already breaking.

The coloured lights and bells and buzzers of the pier's amusement arcade welcomed them in to waste their money. Eunice left Bomber standing by a two-penny slot machine, watching lanes of tightly packed coins shunting back and forth to see which would tip over the edge, while she went to fetch some change. When she returned, she found him, like a lost child, coin in hand staring at the coin slot on the machine but completely unable to fathom the connection between the two. Gently, she took the coin from him and dropped it into the slot, and his face lit up as he watched a pile of coins tip and fall, rattling into the metal tray beneath.

The rest of the day passed happily and uneventfully. For the first time, as they were without a canine companion, they were able to sample the exotic delights of the Pavilion interior together, where they 'oohed' and 'aahed' their amazement at the chandeliers and clucked their disgust at the spit-roaster in the kitchen, which was originally driven by an unfortunate dog. As they sat on a bench in the gardens, basking in the coral light of the late-afternoon sun, Bomber took Eunice's hand and let out a sigh of blissful contentment Eunice remembered to treasure.

'This place is utterly fabulous.'

41

The navy-blue leather glove belonged to a dead woman. Not the most promising of starts for The Keeper of Lost Things. The day after the website launched a retired reporter had emailed. For many years she had worked for the local newspaper and she remembered it well. It was the first proper news item she had covered.

It made the front page. The poor woman was only in her thirties. She threw herself in front of a train. The train driver was in a terrible state, poor bloke. He was new to his job too. He'd only been driving solo for a couple of weeks. Her name was Rose. She was ill; what they called 'bad nerves' back then. I remember she had a little girl; such a pretty little thing. Rose had a picture of her in her coat pocket. They printed it in the paper with the story. I wasn't very comfortable with that, but I was overruled by the editor. I went to her funeral. It was a gruesome business altogether; not much of a body left to bury. But the photo was still in the pocket of her coat and she was wearing only one glove. It's such a small detail, but it seemed so poignant. And it was so cold that night. That must be why I've remembered it for all these years.

It was the glove Sunshine had dropped in horror when it had fallen out of the drawer. She had said at the time 'the lady died' and 'she loved her little girl'. Laura was dumbfounded. It seemed that Sunshine was right and once again they had been guilty of underestimating her. She had a very special gift and they would do well to listen to her a bit more carefully. Sunshine had read the email impassively. Her only comment had been, 'Perhaps her little girl will want it back.'

Sunshine was out with Carrot. She went out most days now to gather more lost things for the website, carrying a small notebook and pencil so that she could jot down the details for the labels before she forgot. Freddy was out laying a new lawn for one of his customers, so Laura was alone. Except for Therese.

'I know, I know!' she said out loud. 'I'm going to look for it today, I promise.'

Since Sunshine's revelation that Anthony's letter was the clue they needed, Laura had been trying to remember where she had put it. At first she thought that she might have left it in the dressing table in Therese's room, but the door remained locked, so she hadn't been able to check. In any case, it hardly seemed likely that Therese would be preventing her from finding the very thing that she wanted her to find. Even she couldn't be *that* awkward. Laura went into the study. She would just check the emails first. The website was proving popular, with hundreds of hits already. There were two emails. One was from an elderly lady who said that she was eighty-nine years of age and a silver surfer of two

277

years thanks to her local retirement centre. She had heard about the website on the radio and decided to take a look. She thought that a jigsaw puzzle piece found years ago in Copper Street might be hers. Or rather, her sister's. They hadn't got on, and one day when her sister had been particularly vicious she had taken a piece from the puzzle her sister was working on. She went for a walk to get out of the house, and threw the piece into the gutter. 'Childish, I expect,' she said, 'but she could be the very devil. And she was livid when she found that it was missing.' The old lady didn't want it back. Her sister was long dead anyway. But it was nice, she said, to have something to practise her emails on.

The second was from a young woman claiming a lime-green hair bobble. Her mum had bought the bobbles for her to cheer her up, the day before she started a new school she was feeling nervous about. She'd lost one in the park on the way home from a day out with her mum, and it would be nice to have it back as a memento.

Laura replied to both emails and then set about searching for Anthony's letter. By the time Sunshine returned with Carrot, Laura was poring over the letter at the kitchen table. She had found it tucked away in the writing desk in the garden room. As soon as she had found it, she had helpfully remembered that, of course, that was where she had placed it for safekeeping. Sunshine made the lovely cup of tea for them and then sat down next to Laura.

'What does it say?' she asked.

'What does what say?' said Freddy, bursting through the back door, his boots covered in mud. Laura and Sunshine both looked at his feet and commanded in unison, 'Off!'

Freddy laughed as he struggled out of his boots and left them outside on the doormat.

'Talk about henpecked!' he exclaimed. 'Now, what's all this?'

'It's Saint Anthony's dead letter and now we're going to find the clue,' Sunshine exclaimed with far more confidence than Laura felt. She began to read out loud, but resurgent grief choked his generous words in her throat before she could even finish the first line. Sunshine took the letter gently from her and began again, reading slowly and deliberately, helped by Freddy with some of the more difficult words. When she reached the final paragraph, where Anthony asked Laura to befriend her, her face lit up with a smile.

'But I asked you first!' she said.

Laura took her hand. 'And I'm very glad you did,' she replied.

Freddy slapped his palms on the table.

'Enough with the mushy stuff, you girls,' he said, rocking his chair backwards on two legs. 'What's the clue?'

Sunshine looked at him with dutiful amusement which quickly withered into undisguised scorn when she realised that he wasn't joking.

'You cannot be serious,' she said, looking to Laura for support.

'Well, it could be anything . . . ' Laura ventured uncertainly.

Freddy was studying the letter again.

'Well, come on, John McEnroe,' he said to Sunshine. 'Enlighten us.'

Sunshine sighed and like a schoolteacher sorely disappointed with her class she shook her head slowly before announcing, 'It's so obvious.'

And when she explained, they realised that, of course, it was.

42

Eunice

2011

Today was a good day. But the term was only relative. No day now was truly good. The best that Eunice could hope for were a few bewildered smiles, an occasional recollection of who she was and, most of all, no tears from the man she had spent most of her adult life in love with. She strolled arm in arm with Bomber around the bleak patchwork of bare earth and concrete paving slabs that the officer-in-charge of the Happy Haven care home grandiosely termed 'the rose garden'. The only trace of the roses were a few bent, brown sticks poking out of the earth like the detritus of a bush fire. Eunice could easily have wept. And this was a good day.

Bomber had wanted to go to Folly's End. Before he was too often lost in random bouts of oblivion, but knew that to be his inevitable fate, he had made his wishes clear. He had always intended to give Eunice his power of attorney when the time came, and thus salvage whatever scraps of dignity and security that could be wrung from a future as bleak as the one he faced. He could trust Eunice with his life, however worthless it might become. She would always do the right thing. But Portia got there first. Armed with ridiculous but omnipotent wealth and next-of-kin affiliation if not affection, she tricked Bomber into seeing a 'specialist', who, no doubt with her financial encouragement, legally declared him to be 'no longer capable of making rational decisions' and turned his future welfare over to his sister.

The following week Bomber was installed at Happy Haven.

Eunice had fought his corner as hard as she could; she had argued ferociously for Folly's End, but Portia was unmoved. Folly's End was 'too far away' for her to conveniently visit, and in any case, she claimed with astonishing callousness, it was only a matter of time before Bomber wouldn't have a clue where he was anyway. But for now, he did. And it was killing him.

Surprisingly, Portia did visit him. But they were strained, uncomfortable encounters. She veered wildly between bossing him about and cowering fearfully away from him. His reaction to both approaches was the same: painful bewilderment. Having deprived him of the one thing he wanted, she showered him with expensive, often pointless gifts. He had no idea what the espresso machine was, let alone how to work it. He poured the designer aftershave down the toilet and used the fancy camera as a doorstop. In the end, Portia spent most of the time during her visits drinking tea with Sylvia, the sycophantic officer-in-charge, who was a devoted fan of the Harriet Hotter books, of which there was now, regrettably, a trilogy.

Eunice did her best to make Bomber's room a

little piece of home. She brought things from his flat, and put photographs of Douglas and Baby Jane on every shelf and table. But it wasn't enough. He was drifting away. Giving up.

Eunice and Bomber were not alone in the garden. Eulalia was feeding a magpie with bits of toast she'd saved from her breakfast. She was an ancient, wizened husk of a woman with skin the colour of stewed prunes, wild eyes and an alarming cackle. Her twisted hands clutched knobbled walking sticks that she used to anchor and propel herself in a jerky, shuffling gait. Most of the other residents avoided her, but Bomber always greeted her with a friendly wave. Round and round they walked, mindlessly, like prisoners in an exercise yard. Eunice, because she couldn't bear to think, and Bomber just because, most of the time, he couldn't. Eulalia threw her last piece of toast at the black and white bird who snatched it from the ground and gobbled it down, never taking his bright, elderberry eyes off Eulalia. She shook her stick at him and squawked, 'Off with you, now! Away, before they put you in a pot for dinner! They would, you know,' she said, turning to Eunice and screwing one of her eyes into a grotesque wink. 'They feeds us all kinds of shit in here.'

Judging by the smell from the kitchen, which was wafting into the garden through an open window, Eunice had to concede that she might have a point.

'Him nuts, that one,' said Eulalia, waggling a hooked claw at Bomber, whilst somehow still managing to keep hold of the walking stick.

'Mad as an ant with his arse on fire.' She planted her sticks onto the concrete and began her painful, awkward shuffle back to the house.

'But him a lovely man inside,' she said to Eunice as she passed. 'Lovely, but dying.'

Back in Bomber's room, Eunice threw back the curtains to let in what little light the pale winter sun could spare. It was a nice room on the second floor; clean and spacious with rather grand French windows and a pretty balcony. Which Bomber wasn't allowed to use.

Eunice had opened them the first time that she had visited Bomber. It was a sultry summer day and the room was hot and stuffy. The key had been left in the lock, but an officious care assistant who had come in to check on Bomber banged the windows shut and locked the key in the medicine cabinet on the wall in Bomber's room. 'Health and safety,' she had spat at Eunice. After that day, Eunice never saw the key again.

'Let's watch a film, shall we?'

Bomber smiled. For him, now, his own life story was like an unbound manuscript, badly edited. Some of the pages were in the wrong order, some torn, some rewritten or missing altogether. The original version was lost to him forever. But he still found pleasure in the familiar stories told in the old films that they had watched so many times together. There were more days, now, when he didn't know his own name or what he'd just eaten for breakfast. But he could still quote, word for word, from *The Great Escape*, *Brief Encounter*, *Top Gun* and scores of other films.

'What about this one?' said Eunice, holding up a copy of *The Birdcage*.

He looked up and smiled and, for a precious, fleeting moment, the mists cleared.

'My birthday present,' he said, and Eunice knew that her Bomber was still in there.

43

'He's still in there,' said Sunshine in a worried voice. Carrot had taken up a sentinel post in the shed, having caught a whiff of a resident rodent, and Sunshine was growing increasingly anxious that Carrot's lunch might have mouse on the menu. Laura was in the study retrieving an item someone had contacted the website about and was coming to collect that afternoon.

'Don't worry, Sunshine. I'm sure the mouse will have the good sense not to show a single whisker while Carrot's in there.'

Sunshine was unconvinced.

'But he might. And then Carrot would kill him and be a murderinger.'

Laura smiled. She knew Sunshine well enough by now to know that she wouldn't give up until something was done. Two minutes later, Laura was back, towing a recalcitrant Carrot on his lead. In the kitchen she gave him a sausage from the fridge and unclipped his lead. Before Sunshine could raise an objection Laura pacified her.

'Mickey or Minnie will be quite safe now. I've shut the shed door, and now he's had a sausage, Carrot won't be hungry anyway.'

'He's always hungry,' muttered Sunshine, as she watched Carrot slope out of the room with mischief still clearly on his mind. 'When's the lady coming?' she asked.

Laura checked her watch.

'Any time now. She's called Alice and I thought you might like to make the lovely cup of tea when she gets here.'

As if on cue, the bell rang and Sunshine was at the front door before Laura was out of the starting blocks.

'Good afternoon, Lady Alice,' Sunshine greeted the rather taken-aback teenager at the door. 'I'm Sunshine. Please do come in.'

'What a great name.'

The girl who followed Sunshine into the hall was tall and slim, with long fair hair and a splatter of freckles across her nose. Laura held out her hand.

'Hi, I'm Laura. Lovely to meet you.'

Sunshine deftly commandeered Alice and took her through to the garden while Laura was left to make the tea. When she came out with the tray of tea things, she found Alice and Sunshine swapping musical heroes.

'We both love David Bowie,' Sunshine announced proudly to Laura as she began to pour the tea.

'I'm sure he'll be delighted,' said Laura, smiling. 'How do you take it?' she asked Alice.

'Builder's for me, please.'

Sunshine looked worried.

'I don't know if we've got any of that, have we?' she asked Laura.

'Don't worry, Sunshine,' said Alice, quick to spot her discomfort, 'it's just me being silly. I meant nice and strong with milk and two sugars.'

Alice had come to collect an umbrella; a

child's umbrella, white with red hearts.

'I didn't actually lose it,' she explained, 'and I can't be absolutely certain that it was meant for me . . . '

Sunshine picked up the umbrella that was already on the table and handed it to her.

'It was,' she said simply. Although, judging by the look of undisguised adoration on Sunshine's face, Laura reckoned she would have given Alice the family silver without a second thought and thrown in the deeds to Padua for good measure.

Alice took the umbrella from her and stroked its folded ruffles.

'It was my first time in America,' she told them. 'Mum took me to New York. It was more of a working holiday for her. She was an editor of a fashion magazine and she'd bagged an interview with a hotshot new designer who was tipped to be the next big thing on the New York fashion scene. He was, as it turned out. But all I remember about him then was that he looked at me like I'd escaped from a leper colony or something. Apparently he didn't 'do' children.'

'What's a leopard colony?' Sunshine asked.

Alice looked over to Laura, but then decided to wing it anyway.

'It's a place where, in olden times, they used to put people who had a terrible illness that made their fingers and toes drop off.'

Laura would have bet money that Sunshine spent the next five minutes surreptitiously counting Alice's digits. Thank goodness she was wearing sandals.

'There wasn't much time for sightseeing,'

Alice continued, 'but she promised to take me to see the sculpture of Alice in Wonderland in Central Park. I remember being utterly thrilled. I thought that the statue was named after me.'

She slipped off her sandals and wriggled her toes in the cool grass. Sunshine studiously followed suit.

'It was raining that afternoon and Mum was already running late for her next appointment, so she wasn't in the best of tempers, but I was beyond excited. I ran off ahead of her and when I got to the sculpture, there was this huge, strange-looking black guy with dreadlocks and big boots giving away umbrellas. He bent down and shook hands with me and I can still remember his face. It was a mixture of kind and sad, and he was called Marvin.'

Alice drained her cup and helped herself to another from the pot with confident teenage ease.

'My favourite story at the time was 'The Selfish Giant' by Oscar Wilde, and to me Marvin looked like a giant. But he wasn't selfish. He was giving things away. Free umbrellas. Anyway, when Mum caught up with me she dragged me away. But it wasn't just that. She was rude to him. Really horrible. He tried to give her an umbrella and she was an absolute bitch.'

Sunshine's eyebrows hiccupped in astonishment at the casual use of an expletive, but her expression was one of admiration.

'I only met him for a moment, but I've never been able to forget the look on his face as she dragged me away.' She sighed heavily, but then smiled as another memory eclipsed the last. 'I blew him a kiss,' she said, 'and he caught it.'

The date on the umbrella's label matched the exact day of Alice's visit to Central Park and the umbrella was found on the sculpture. Laura was delighted.

1 think it must have been meant for you.'

'I really hope so,' said Alice.

For the rest of the day Carrot lay guarding the door of the shed, and Sunshine talked about her new friend Alice. Alice was at university studying English Litter Tour and Drama. Alice liked David Bowie, Marc Bolan and Jon Bon Hovis. And 'the lovely cup of tea' had been summarily supplanted by the builder's variety.

That evening over a late supper of spaghetti bolognese, Laura told Freddy all about their visitor.

'It's working, then,' said Freddy. 'The website. It's doing what Anthony wanted you to do.'

Laura shook her head. 'No. Not really. Not yet, anyway. Remember what the letter said? 'If you can make just one person happy, mend one broken heart by restoring to them what they have lost . . . ' And I haven't done that yet. Of course Alice was pleased to find the umbrella, but we can't be absolutely sure that it was meant for her. And the girl with the hair bobble; her heart wasn't exactly broken when she lost it.'

'Well, at least it's a start,' said Freddy, pushing back his chair and getting up to take Carrot for a final stroll around the garden before bed. 'We'll get there in the end.'

But it wasn't just about the lost things. There

was the clue; the one that was so obvious once Sunshine had pointed it out. The thing that had started all this. Anthony had called it 'the last remaining thread' that had bound him to Therese, and when he lost it on the day she died that final thread was broken. If her communion medal really was the key to reuniting Therese with Anthony, how on earth were they supposed to find it? Freddy had suggested that they post it on the website as a lost item needing to be found, but as they had no idea what it looked like or where Anthony had lost it, there was very little useful information that they could share.

Laura cleared the plates from the table. It had been a long day and she was tired. The satisfaction that she had felt after Alice's visit had gradually dissipated, only to be replaced by a familiar feeling of unease.

And in the garden room the music began again.

44

Eunice

2013

In the residents' lounge at Happy Haven the music began again. Mantovani's 'Charmaine'. Quietly at first and then louder and louder. Too loud. Edie turned the volume up as high as it would go. Soon she would be gliding round the ballroom to the strings' *glissandos* in a froth of net and sparkles. Her feet would spin and sweep in her best gold dancing sandals and the glittering lights would swirl around her like a snowstorm of rainbows.

As Eunice and Bomber passed through the lounge on the way to Bomber's room, they saw a ragged bundle of nightclothes barely inhabited by a thin, whiskery old woman with a greasy straggle of grey hair and tartan slippers. She was stumbling round the room with her eyes closed and her arms lovingly wrapped around some invisible partner. Suddenly there was an explosion of sticks and expletives from one of the armchairs.

'Not again! Jesus fucking Christ and Jehovah! Not again! Not again! Not again!'

Eulalia had burst out of her chair cursing and thrashing.

'Not a-fucking-gain, you stupid, crazy, dirty

bitch! Me just want a bit of peace!' she roared, flinging one of her sticks at the dancer, who had stopped in her tracks. The stick missed Edie by a mile, but she let out an anguished yowl as tears began to course down her cheeks and urine down her legs and into her slippers. Eulalia had struggled to her feet and was pointing with one of her claws.

'Now she piss herself! Piss her pants. Piss the floor,' she cackled furiously through spittle-flecked lips. Eunice tried to move Bomber on, but he was frozen to the spot. Some of the other residents had begun shouting or crying, and others stared into the distance, oblivious. Or pretending to be. It took two members of staff to restrain Eulalia as Sylvia led poor Edie away. She was trembling and snivelling and dripping piss from the hem of her nightgown as she shuffled out miserably, clinging to Sylvia's arm and wondering where on earth the ballroom had gone.

Back in the safety of Bomber's room, Eunice made him a cup of tea. As she drank her own, she took in the new additions to Bomber's growing collection of swag. He had begun stealing things; random items that he didn't need. A vase, a tea cosy, cutlery, rolls of plastic bin bags, umbrellas. He never stole from the rooms of other residents, just from the communal areas. It was a symptom of his disease apparently. Petty theft. But he was losing things too. Thick and fast now he was losing words like a tree loses leaves in the autumn. A bed might be 'a soft sleep square' and a pencil 'a stick with grey middle writing coming out'. Instead of words, he spoke in clues; or, more often, not at all. Eunice suggested that they watch a film. It was all that was left of them now. Eunice and Bomber, who for so long had been colleagues and best friends. Bomber's occasional boyfriends had come and gone, but Eunice was his constant. They were husband and wife without sex or certificate and these were the last paltry scraps of their once rich relationship: walking and watching films.

Bomber chose the film. *One Flew Over the Cuckoo's Nest.*

'Are you sure?' Eunice asked. She had been hoping for something a little more jolly, for her own sake and for his, after what they had just witnessed. Bomber was adamant. As they watched the patients at the state mental hospital walking in the chain-link-fenced exercise yard, Bomber pointed at the screen and winked at her.

'That's us,' he said.

Eunice looked into his eyes and was shocked to see the clarity reflected back at her. This was the Bomber of old speaking; sharp, funny, bright and back for a rare visit. But for how long? Even the briefest visit was precious, but heartbreaking. Heartbreaking because he must know that he would have to go back. And to what?

It was a film that they had watched many times before, but this time it was very different.

As the Chief placed the pillow over Mac's pitifully vacant face and tenderly suffocated him, Bomber gripped Eunice's hand and spoke his final three words.

'Get. Me. Out.'

He was calling in her promise. Eunice stared at the screen and held on tight to Bomber's hand as the giant Chief wrenched the marble water cooler from the tub-room floor, hurled it through the massive windows and then loped off towards the breaking dawn and freedom. As the credits rolled, Eunice couldn't move. Bomber took her other hand in his. His eyes were full of tears but he was smiling as he nodded and mouthed silently at her, 'Please.'

Before Eunice could say anything one of the nurses burst in without knocking.

'Time for your medication,' she bustled, rattling the keys to the medicine cabinet on the wall. She unlocked it and was just reaching for the tablets when there was a terrified scream from the corridor outside followed by Eulalia's unmistakable cackle.

'That damn woman!' cursed the nurse, rushing to the door to investigate and leaving the cabinet unlocked.

★   ★   ★

It was time for Eunice to go. She must leave, but until she did she still had Bomber, and so she couldn't bear to go. But every minute was just a marker between now and then, not time to be cherished. Because the decision had been made. Eunice knew that there would only be one chance; one moment when all the love she had ever felt for this man would crystallise into the inconceivable strength that she would need. It was time. The imprint of the key was embedded into the flesh of her palm where she had gripped it so tightly. Eunice unlocked the windows and opened them, leaving them just ajar. She wanted so desperately to hug him one last time; to hold his warmth and feel him breathing against her. But she knew that if she did her strength would desert her, so instead she placed the key in his hand and kissed his cheek.

'I'm not going without you, Bomber,' she whispered. 'I wouldn't leave you this way. You're coming with me. Let's go.'

And then she left.

45

ELDERLY MALE IN DEATH FALL AT CARE HOME

Police are investigating the death of an elderly male resident of the Happy Haven care home in Blackheath, who fell from a second-floor balcony early on Saturday evening. The man, who has not yet been named, was suffering from Alzheimer's and is believed to have been a retired publisher. A post-mortem is due to be carried out later this week and police enquiries into what they are calling 'an unexplained death' are ongoing.

London Evening Standard

46

'There's a dead person in the study,' Sunshine announced in a conversational tone. She had come to find Laura, who was in the garden cutting roses for the house, to tell her this piece of news and to chivvy her along into making lunch. Carrot was lolling lazily on his back in the sun, with his legs in the air, but as Sunshine approached he jumped up to greet her.

It had been a year now since the website had launched and it kept both Laura and Sunshine busy. Sunshine had learned how to take photographs, and post them and the details of objects onto the website, and Freddy had even shown her how to run a Keeper of Lost Things Instagram account. Laura dealt with the emails. They were still working their way through Anthony's collection, as well as adding the new things that Sunshine gathered on her walks with Carrot. Laura and Freddy had also got into the habit of picking up things they found wherever they went, and now people had begun to send them lost items as well. At this rate the shelves in the study would always be groaning.

'A dead person? Are you sure?'

Sunshine gave her one of her looks. Laura went inside to investigate. In the study, Sunshine showed her a sky blue Huntley & Palmers biscuit tin. Its label read:

Huntley & Palmers biscuit tin
containing cremation remains?
Found, sixth carriage from the front, 14.42
train from London Bridge to Brighton.
Deceased unknown.
God bless and rest in peace.

Lupin and Booth funeral directors (Est. 1927)
was on the corner of a busy street opposite a
fancy bakery. As she stood outside, Eunice
smiled to herself, remembering Mrs Doyle's
and thinking that this was an appropriate place
for Bomber to end up. He had been dead for
six weeks now, and Eunice still hadn't had any
details about his funeral. The coroner had
eventually returned a verdict of accidental
death, but the staff at Happy Haven had been
severely criticised for their cavalier approach to
health and safety procedures and had only nar-
rowly escaped prosecution. Portia had wanted
Sylvia's head in a bedpan. She had been
mourning extravagantly all over the press and
the media, but Eunice couldn't help wondering
whether it was fuelled by genuine grief or the
associated publicity it was bound to generate
for her forthcoming book tour. Portia was too
famous to talk to Eunice directly now. She had
assistants for that kind of trivial task. Which
was why Eunice found herself staring through
an immaculate plate-glass window at a scale
model of a horse-drawn hearse and a tasteful
display of arum lilies. The only information she
had been able to extract from the lowliest assistant twice removed was the name of the funeral

directors who were dealing with all enquiries. She could have telephoned, but the temptation to be in the same building as Bomber was too great.

The woman behind the reception desk looked up at the sound of the bell and gave Eunice a smile of genuine welcome. Pauline was a large lady, dressed in Marks & Spencer's finest, with an air of capability and kindness. She put Eunice in mind of a Brown Owl. Unfortunately, the news she had to deliver was the cruellest and most shocking that Eunice could possibly hear.

'It was very small. Family only at the crematorium. The sister organised it; the one who writes those mucky books.'

It was clear from the repugnance with which Pauline imbued the word 'sister' that she and Portia had not exactly bonded. Eunice felt her head go into a tailspin and the floor rise up to meet her. Not long afterwards she was sitting on a comfy sofa drinking hot sweet tea with a nip of brandy and Pauline was patting her hand.

'It was the shock, love,' she said. 'Your face went as white as a ghost.'

Fortified by tea, brandy and biscuits, Eunice was made party to the whole dreadful story by a very forthcoming Pauline. Portia had wanted it done and dusted as quickly and quietly as possible.

'She was off on her book tour, you see, and she didn't want her schedule disrupted.' Pauline took a sip of her own tea and shook her head vigorously in disapproval. 'But she's having a proper showy-offy shebang when she gets back; a memorial service and then a burial of the ashes. She's inviting 'everyone who is anyone, darling' and the music will be provided by choirs of angels with his Holiness the Pope presiding by the way she was talking. It'll knock Princess Diana's do into a cocked hat, apparently.'

Eunice listened in horror.

'But that wasn't what he wanted at all,' she whispered tearfully. 'He told me what he wanted. He was the love of my life.'

And now, right at the last, she was going to fail him.

Pauline was good at listening and mopping up tears. It was her job. But deep inside her sensible suit and her easy-iron blouse beat the brave heart of a maverick. Back in the day, her blonde bob had been a pink Mohican and her nose still bore the tiny scar of a safety-pin piercing. She handed Eunice another tissue.

'All the boys are out at a big funeral this afternoon. I wouldn't normally do this, but . . . Follow me!'

She led Eunice through from the reception area down a corridor past the staff kitchen, the chapel of rest and various other rooms to the place where the cremation remains were stored awaiting collection. From one of the shelves she took down an impressive wooden urn and checked the label.

'Here he is,' she said gently. She checked her watch. 'I'm going to leave you alone with him

301

for a bit to pay your respects. The boys won't be back for another hour, so you won't be disturbed.'

Less than an hour later, Eunice was sitting on a train with Bomber's ashes in a Huntley & Palmers biscuit tin on the seat beside her. She had had to think and act fast after Pauline had left her. She found a plastic carrier bag and a biscuit tin in the little kitchen where Pauline had made tea. She emptied the biscuits into the bag and then tipped Bomber into the biscuit tin. She refilled the urn with the biscuits but it was too light. Frantically searching for additional ballast, she found a box of decorative gravel samples in one of the other rooms. She threw in a couple of large handfuls and then screwed the lid back on as tightly as she could and returned the urn to its shelf. As she made her way out through the reception area clutching the biscuit tin, Pauline didn't look up from her desk, but raised her thumbs to Eunice in a good luck gesture. She hadn't seen a thing.

As the guard blew his whistle, Eunice patted the tin affectionately and smiled.

'Brighton it is.'

Laura was astonished. She picked up the tin and gave it a gentle shake. It was certainly heavy.

'Don't shake it!' said Sunshine. 'You'll wake him up.' And then she giggled at her own joke.

Laura was wondering what else might be lurking in the dark corners of the study.

'No wonder this place is haunted,' she said to Sunshine.

302

After lunch Laura helped her to post the details on the website, but this was one thing she was fairly certain no one would come forward to claim.

That evening Freddy, Laura, Sunshine, Carrot, Stella and Stan had a celebratory dinner in the garden of The Moon is Missing, to mark the birthday of the website. Sunshine was full of stories about all the things that were currently posted, but most especially about the biscuit tin.

'It's certainly a queer thing to lose,' said Stella, tucking into her crumb-dusted, sautéed crayfish tails with hand-cut chips. 'And why on earth would you put your loved one in a biscuit tin?'

'Perhaps that's just it, love,' said Stan. 'Perhaps the bloke in the tin wasn't particularly loved and someone was just trying to get rid of him.'

'Perhaps it's not human remains at all. Maybe it just the sweepings-out of somebody's fireplace. That's exactly what it looks like,' said Freddy, taking a long swig of his ice-cold beer.

Sunshine was about to remonstrate with him when he winked at her and she realised he was only joking.

'It is a dead person and he was the love of her life and she *will* come and get him,' she replied defiantly.

'Okay,' he replied. 'Let's have a bet. What do you want to bet me that someone will come and get the biscuit tin?'

Sunshine screwed up her face in concentration and fed Carrot a couple of chips while she was thinking about it. Suddenly a huge smile lit up her face and she leaned back in her chair and folded her arms across her chest with a sigh of victorious satisfaction.

'You have to marry Laura.'

Laura spilled her wine in shock.

'Steady on, old girl,' said Stan. 'Blimey, Sunshine, you certainly know how to frighten the horses.'

Laura could feel her face reddening. Stella and Stan were chuckling merrily and Sunshine was grinning from ear to ear. Laura wished that the ground would open up and swallow her, and so swallowed her wine too quickly and ordered another large glass. Freddy said nothing. He looked as though he was somewhere between annoyed and disappointed, but then when he saw Laura's face, he leapt to his feet and thrust his hand out to Sunshine.

'It's a bet!'

★   ★   ★

It was hot that night and the air was heavy with the warm velvet scent of roses as Freddy and Laura wandered round the garden, while Carrot searched the shrubbery for intruders. Laura was still fretting about the bet that Freddy had made. He had been very quiet on the way home from the pub. Although they had been together for a little over a year, and Freddy virtually lived at Padua now, they had never made any real plans for the future. She counted herself very lucky to have a second chance at both life and love, but she was still afraid that any attempt, however light-hearted, to tether their relationship might cause love to bolt. And she did love him. Not in the silly, girlish way that she had been infatuated with Vince. This had, for her, grown stealthily into an abiding love, sparked first by passion and then sustained by friendship and trust. But alongside her love for Freddy grew the fear of losing him; the two emotions cruelly shackled together, each feeding the other. Laura had to say something.

'That bet with Sunshine, it's just a joke. I don't expect you to . . . ' She was so uncomfortable that she didn't know how to continue. It suddenly dawned on her that marrying Freddy might be exactly what she wanted and that was why she was so upset. Her foolish hopes of a Happy Ever After had been turned into a joke, and she felt like a laughing stock.

Freddy took her hand and swung her round to face him. 'A bet's a bet, and I'm a man of my word!'

Laura pulled her hand away. In that moment, all the doubts about their relationship, all the fears of failure and all the frustrations at her own imperfection converged to create a perfect storm.

'Don't worry,' she snapped, 'you don't have to wait until you've worked out a dignified escape route! I'm fully aware that I'm the one who's hitting above my weight in this relationship!'

'Punching,' replied Freddy quietly. 'It's 'punching above your weight'.'

He was trying to find a way of breaking into the emotional vortex that Laura was whipping up, but she wouldn't listen.

'I'm not a charity case! Poor old Laura!

Couldn't keep her husband out of someone else's knickers and the only date she's had in years was an unmitigated disaster, so what did you think, Freddy? Take her out and make her feel like she's worth something and then let her down gently when someone better comes along?'

Like a songbird caught in a trapper's net, the harder she fought, the more entangled she became, but she couldn't help herself. She knew how unreasonable she was being, how hurtful, but she couldn't stop. The insults and accusations flew while Freddy stood silently waiting for her to burn herself out and when she turned to go back into the house he called after her.

'Laura! For God's sake, woman! You know how much I love you. I was going to ask you, anyway. To marry me.' He shook his head sadly. 'I had it all planned. But then Sunshine well and truly stole my thunder.'

Laura stopped, but couldn't face him — nor could she silence the desperate and completely untruthful coup de grâce with which she finally broke her own heart.

'I would have said 'no'.'

As she walked on to the house, silent tears ran down her face, but somewhere in the darkness of the rose garden there was the sound of someone else weeping.

47

Eunice

2013

Portia gave the biscuits a magnificent send-off. She had wanted St Paul's Cathedral or Westminster Abbey, but finding that even her obscene wealth couldn't buy them, she had settled for the ballroom of a swanky Mayfair hotel. Eunice sat at the back in her designated seat, which was bedecked, as were all the others, with an extravagant black silk chiffon bow, and took in the splendid surroundings. The room was truly stunning, with a sprung wooden floor, floor-to-ceiling antique mirrors and, judging by the acoustics breathing Mozart's 'Lacrimosa' into the rarefied air, a state-of-the-art sound system. Either that or Portia had the entire London Philharmonic Orchestra and London Symphony Chorus hidden behind a screen somewhere. The mirrors reflected the monstrous arrangements of exotic lilies and orchids that loomed from shelves and pedestals like albino triffids.

Eunice had come with Gavin, a long-term friend of Bomber's since their school days together, who now made a living cutting, colouring and cosseting the hair of both genuine and manufactured celebrities. His client list was one of the reasons that Portia had invited him.

'Bloody hell!' hissed Gavin, under his breath. Well, almost. 'Talk about rent-a-mob. Most of these people didn't know Bomber from Bardot.'

He smiled superciliously at the photographer who was prowling up and down the aisle between the rows of seats snapping any of the 'mourners' whom the public might recognise. Portia had sold the rights for the occasion to a glossy magazine that any intelligent woman would only ever admit to reading at the hairdresser. The seats were mostly filled with Portia's own friends, associates and hangers-on, with the occasional celebrity punctuating the populace like a sparse sequin on an otherwise dull dress. Bomber's friends were gathered at the back around Eunice and Gavin, like theatre-goers in the cheap seats.

At the front of the room, on a table festooned in yet more flowers, stood the urn. It was flanked on one side by an enormous framed photograph of Bomber ('He'd never have chosen that one,' whispered Gavin. 'His hair's a complete mess') and on the other by a photograph of Bomber and Portia as children, with Portia on the crossbar of Bomber's bike.

'She had to get her face in the frame, didn't she!' fumed Gavin. 'She can't even let him be the star at his own bloody memorial! But at least I managed to persuade her to invite some of Bomber's real friends and include something in this whole damn fiasco that Bomber might actually have liked.'

Eunice was impressed. 'How on earth did you manage that?'

Gavin grinned. 'Blackmail. I threatened to go to the press if she didn't. 'Selfish Sister Scorns Brother's Dying Wishes' wasn't the kind of headline her publisher would want to see and she knows it. Speaking of which, where is Bruce the Bouffant?' He scanned the rows of heads in front of him, searching for the offending barnet.

'Oh, I expect he'll come with Portia,' Eunice replied. 'What exactly are you doing?'

Gavin looked very pleased with himself.

'It's a surprise, but I'll give you a clue. You remember the wedding at the beginning of *Love Actually* where members of the band are hidden in the congregation?'

Before he could go any further the music changed and Portia and her entourage swept down the aisle to 'O Fortuna' from *Carmina Burana*. She was wearing a white Armani trouser suit and a hat with a brim the size of a tractor wheel swathed in black spotted net.

'Jesus Christ!' spluttered Gavin. 'You'd think she was marrying Mick Jagger!'

He clutched Eunice's arm, barely able to contain his hysteria. Eunice's eyes filled with tears. But they were tears of laughter. She only wished that Bomber were here to share the fun. In fact, she wished she knew where Bomber was at all. She hadn't told Gavin about it yet. She was waiting for the right moment. The service itself was strangely entertaining. A children's choir from a local school — private and very exclusive — sang 'Over the Rainbow', Bruce

309

read a eulogy on Portia's behalf as though he were delivering a soliloquy from *Hamlet,* and an actress from a minor soap opera read a poem by W. H. Auden. Prayers were said by a retired bishop whose daughter was apparently an old friend of Portia's. They were short and rather difficult to decipher on account of the whisky that he'd had with his breakfast. Or perhaps for his breakfast.

And then it was Gavin's turn.

He rose from his chair and stood in the aisle. Using the microphone he had concealed under his seat, he addressed the gathering with a theatrical flourish.

'Ladies and gentlemen, this one's for Bomber!'

He sat back down and a frisson of anticipation shivered through the assembly. Gavin looked at Eunice and winked.

'Show time!' he whispered.

There was a single, thrilling chord and then from somewhere at the back of the room, a man's voice singing softly, accompanied only by a piano. The voice came from a staggeringly handsome man wearing an immaculate dinner suit and a subtle sweep of eyeliner, who was indeed his own special creation. The opening bars of 'I Am What I Am' from *La Cage aux Folles* floated up into the hushed air and Gavin rubbed his hands together in delight.

As the singer made his way down the centre of the room and the tempo of the song picked up, he too picked up six showgirls seated strategically at the aisle end of their rows. Each one stood in turn and shed respectable coats to reveal risqué

310

costumes, lavish jewels and astonishing tail feathers. Eunice was amazed that they had been able to sit on them. By the time the gorgeous creature and his extraordinary entourage had reached the front of the room, the song was reaching its climax. He turned in front of the urn to face his audience and belted out the final lines while his chorus line high-kicked in unison behind him. With the final, defiant note, all but one person in the room erupted into a spontaneous standing ovation. Portia simply passed out.

Gavin basked unashamedly in his triumph all the way to the country churchyard in Kent where the biscuits were to be buried next to Grace and Godfrey. Portia had provided a cavalcade of black stretch limousines to transport everyone, but Eunice and Gavin chose to travel independently, listening to show tunes and eating salt and vinegar crisps in Gavin's Audi convertible. Eunice felt slightly guilty about Godfrey and Grace being forced to share their grave with an urn of assorted biscuits under false pretences, but she was hopeful that, given the circumstances, they would understand that it had been unavoidable. As they pulled into the very churchyard where Eunice had promised to carry out Bomber's final wishes, Eunice confessed everything to Gavin.

'Holy Mary mother of God and Danny La Rue in a shoe box!' he exclaimed. 'My poor darling girl, what on earth are you going to do now?'

Eunice checked her hat in the rear-view mirror and reached for the door handle.

'I have absolutely no bloody idea whatsoever.'

311

48

Shirley switched on the computer and checked the voicemail messages. It was Monday morning, and Mondays were always busy because of all the strays that were brought in over the weekend. She had worked at Battersea Dogs & Cats Home for fifteen years now and had seen a lot of changes. But one thing never changed; the strays kept coming. The post had already arrived and Shirley began sorting through the pile of envelopes. One envelope was addressed in fountain pen. The writing was in a sweeping, extravagant hand and Shirley was curious. Inside was a handwritten letter.

To whom it may concern,

Please find enclosed a donation in memory of my beloved brother who has recently died. He was very fond of dogs and adopted two from your establishment. The only condition that I attach to said donation is that you erect a plaque in his memory in some public place in your grounds. It should read:

'In loving memory of Bomber,

a precious son, an adored brother, a loyal friend and a devoted dog lover.

Rest in peace with Douglas and Baby Jane.'

I shall send my representative in due course to ensure that these instructions have

been carried out in a satisfactory manner.
Yours faithfully,
Portia Brockley

Shirley shook her head in disbelief. Damn cheek! It was true that all donations were gratefully received, but a plaque like that would cost a pretty penny. She turned her attention to the cheque that was attached, rather quaintly, by a paperclip to the letter and nearly fainted. There were so many noughts that it looked as though the '2' at the beginning of the figure had been blowing bubbles.

49

Laura felt as though she were poised on the brink of a precipice and didn't know whether she was going to fall or fly. She had made sure that she was going to be alone today. Sunshine was having a rare day out with her mum and she hadn't seen Freddy since her shameful outburst in the rose garden. She had tried ringing him, but his phone went straight to voicemail where she had left a grovelling and heartfelt apology, but it seemed it was too late. She had heard nothing in reply and Freddy had not been back to Padua since that night. She couldn't think what else to do. Sunshine kept telling her that Freddy would come back, but Laura knew now that he wouldn't. She had slept fitfully and woke stranded in a no-man's-land somewhere between excitement and foreboding. The house felt oppressive. Even Carrot was restless, pacing up and down, his nails clicking on the tiles. As Laura prepared for her visitor, she had a feeling that the storm was about to break. Padua had been very quiet for the past few days. The door to Therese's bedroom remained locked from the inside and there had been no music. But it was not the kind of quiet that came with peace and contentment. It was a bitter silence brought on by desolation and defeat. Laura had failed Therese and in so doing she had failed Anthony. His final wishes remained unfulfilled.

Someone was coming to collect the ashes in the biscuit tin. They had been claimed. Laura hadn't told Sunshine and it wasn't just because of the bet. She wanted to do this alone. She couldn't explain why, even to herself, but it was important. The doorbell rang at precisely two o'clock, the agreed hour of their appointment, and Laura opened the door to a small, slim woman in her sixties, stylishly dressed and wearing a cobalt-blue trilby.

'I'm Eunice,' she said.

As Laura took the hand she was offered, she felt the tension that had gripped her melt away.

'Would you like tea, or perhaps something stronger?' asked Laura. For some unfathomable reason it felt as though they had something to celebrate.

'Do you know, I'd actually love a stiff drink. I never dared to hope that I would ever get him back, and now I'm about to, frankly I feel a tad wobbly.'

They settled on gin and limes in Anthony's honour, and took them through to the garden, collecting the biscuit tin from the study on the way. As Eunice sat nursing her drink in one hand and the biscuit tin in the other, her eyes filled with tears.

'Oh my dear, I'm so sorry. I'm just being a complete silly arse. But you have no idea how much this means to me. You have just mended a foolish woman's broken heart.'

She took a sip from her drink and then a deep breath.

'Now, I expect you want to know what this is all about?'

Eunice and Laura had exchanged several emails via the website, but they had only covered sufficient details to establish that it was actually Eunice who had lost the ashes.

'Are you sitting comfortably?' she asked Laura. 'I'm afraid it's rather a long story.'

Eunice began at the beginning and told Laura everything. She was a natural storyteller and Laura was surprised that she had never written anything herself. The abduction of Bomber's ashes from the funeral directors had Laura in tears of laughter, laughter that Eunice could at last share, now that she had got Bomber back.

'It all went splendidly until I got on the train,' she explained. 'At the station after I got on, I was joined in the carriage by a woman with two small children, who had obviously overdosed on sweets and fizzy pop, judging by the tide marks around their mouths and their uncontrollable behaviour. Their poor mother could barely keep them in their seats, and when the little girl announced that she 'needed a wee right now!' the mother asked me if I could possibly keep an eye on her brother while she took the little girl to the toilet. I could hardly say no.'

Eunice took a sip of her drink and hugged the biscuit tin closer to her side as though she might lose it again.

'The little boy sat in his seat poking his tongue out at me just until his mother was out of sight and then leapt to his feet and made a run for it. Sod's law helpfully ensured that this was just as the train was pulling into a station, and I wasn't quick enough to stop him jumping off the train when the doors opened, and so I was forced to follow him. I had my bag over my arm, but by the time I realised I had left Bomber in his seat it was too late.' Eunice shuddered at the memory. 'I'm sure you can imagine the pandemonium that followed. The mother was beside herself, wildly accusing me of kidnapping her son. Frankly, I was only too glad to give the little bugger back. I was absolutely frantic about leaving Bomber on the train and reported it straight away, but by the time the train had reached Brighton he was gone.'

Laura topped up their glasses. 'It's an unusual name, Bomber.'

'Oh, that wasn't his real name. His real name was Charles Bramwell Brockley. But I never knew anyone call him that. He was always Bomber. And he would have loved you,' she said to Carrot, gently stroking his head, which was by now resting in her lap. 'He loved all dogs.'

'And he was a publisher, you say? I wonder if he ever crossed paths with Anthony. He was a writer; short stories in the main. Anthony Peardew.'

'Oh yes,' Eunice replied. 'That's a name I remember well. His is a great story, you know: Anthony and Therese, the study full of his collection, the website. There has to be a book in it.'

Laura thought about her schoolgirl dreams of being a writer and smiled wistfully. Too late for all that now.

Eunice was still hugging the biscuit tin tightly to her side.

'Do you still work in publishing?' Laura asked her.

Eunice shook her head. 'No, no. My heart wasn't in it after Bomber . . . ' Her voice trailed away. 'But if you're ever interested in giving the book a go, I'd be very happy to help. I still have contacts and I could recommend you to some agents.'

The two women sat in silence for a while, enjoying their drinks, the scent of the roses and the peace and quiet of a sunny afternoon.

'And what about you, Laura?' Eunice finally spoke. 'Do you have someone in your life — someone you love like I loved Bomber?'

Laura shook her head. 'I did, until a few days ago. But we had a fight.' She paused, thinking about what had *actually* happened.

'Okay — *I* started an argument; a pathetic, ridiculous, puerile argument. Well, it wasn't even an argument, because he didn't argue back. He just stood there listening to me rant on like a hysterical halfwit before I flounced off. I haven't seen him since.'

Laura was slightly surprised at the relief she felt from simply saying it out loud. 'My name is Laura and I've been a complete bloody idiot.'

'You're very hard on yourself, my dear.' Eunice squeezed her hand and smiled. 'But you love him?'

Laura nodded miserably.

'Then talk to him.'

'I've tried. But he never answers his phone and

318

I can't say I blame him. I was *spectacularly* horrible. I've left messages saying I'm sorry, but he obviously isn't interested any more.'

Eunice shook her head. 'No, that's not what I meant. Talk to *him*, not his phone. Find him and tell him to his face.'

Suddenly Eunice reached inside her bag and took out a small box.

'I almost forgot,' she said. 'I brought you something for the website. I found it all those years ago on the way to my interview with Bomber. I've always kept it as a sort of lucky charm. I never really gave a thought to the person who must have lost it. But now it seems only fair that you should have it. I know it's a long shot, but maybe you might be able to find whom it really belongs to.'

Laura smiled. 'Of course, I'll try. I just need to make a note of any details you can remember.'

Eunice didn't even need to think about it. She rattled off the day, date, time and location without hesitation. 'You see,' she said, 'it was one of the best days of my life.'

Laura took the box from Eunice.

'May I?' she asked.

'Of course.'

As Laura took the medallion from the box, she knew for just a moment what it felt like to be Sunshine. The object in her hand spoke to her just as surely as if it had a voice of its own.

'Are you all right?' Eunice sounded as though she was very far away, speaking down a bad phone line. Laura scrambled to her feet, unsteadily.

'Come with me,' she said to Eunice.

The door to Therese's bedroom swung easily open and Laura placed the communion medallion, with its tiny picture of St Therese of the Roses framed in gold, on the dressing table next to the photograph of Anthony and Therese. The little blue clock, which had stopped, as usual, began ticking again of its own accord. Laura held her breath, and for a moment the two women stood in silence. And then downstairs, in the garden room, the music began, softly at first and then louder and louder.

The very thought of you.

Eunice watched in astonishment as Laura punched the air with joy, and through the open window there blew a swirling shower of rose petals.

★ ★ ★

As Laura walked Eunice to the garden gate, Freddy pulled up outside the house in his battered Land Rover and jumped out. He greeted Eunice politely and then looked to Laura.

'We need to talk.'

Eunice kissed Laura on the cheek and winked at Freddy. 'That's exactly what I said.'

She closed the gate behind her and walked away, smiling.

50

The five of them walked together along the promenade, Eunice and Gavin arm in arm carrying Bomber, Douglas and Baby Jane in a striped canvas shopping bag. Eunice had been going to go alone, but Gavin wouldn't hear of it. When Bomber had first been forced into Happy Haven he had asked Gavin to keep a friendly lookout for Eunice, but Gavin hadn't known how to without offending Eunice's notoriously independent spirit. However, since the memorial service when Eunice had made her full and frank confession, Gavin had found a chink in her armour and was using it to keep his word to Bomber. It was a perfect seaside day: bright and breezy with a sky the colour of blue Curaçao. Gavin had left the Audi at home and they had travelled by train so that they could both toast soon-to-be absent friends thoroughly and with impunity.

Eunice wanted the entire day to be a proper memorial for Bomber, and so they were following the time-honoured itinerary. As they strolled towards the pier they met a young couple walking a pair of miniature pugs wearing his-and-hers diamanté collars. Eunice couldn't resist stopping to admire them. The two little dogs submitted to appropriate fuss and compliments before trotting happily on their way. Gavin looked at Eunice's downcast face and gave her arm a squeeze.

321

'Chin up, old girl. It won't be long before Bill Bailey comes home.'

Eunice was finally permitting herself to adopt a dog. She had always intended to after Bomber died, but then, when she had lost his ashes, she somehow felt she didn't deserve one. She had to honour her obligations to old friends before she could allow herself a new one. The black and white collie with a white blaze and black spots had been kept on the end of a chain outside a shed for most of his miserable life, and the staff at Battersea had not been optimistic about his chances of rehabilitation. But the little dog had a big, brave heart and was willing to give the world another chance. The staff named him Bill Bailey after the song for luck, in the hope that he would find the perfect person to come home to. And he had. Eunice. As soon as she saw him, she fell for his pointy ears and his big, dark eyes. He was wary at first, but after a couple of visits he had decided that Eunice was the one for him and deigned to lick her hand. Next week, he would be hers for good.

Eunice and Gavin took it in turns to carry the shopping bag. To start with, Eunice had been reluctant to part with it, but the combined remains of her three friends were surprisingly heavy and she was glad for Gavin to take a turn.

'Bloody hell!' he exclaimed. 'We should have put them in one of those tartan shopping trolley affairs that old ladies push instead of carrying a bag.'

Eunice shook her head emphatically.

'You must be joking! And make me look like

an old lady?' she retorted.

Gavin winked at her. 'Don't worry. You don't look a day over forty, old girl.'

Inside the amusement arcade it was hot and noisy and the air was thick with the smell of hotdogs, doughnuts and popcorn. By the expression on Gavin's face he thought Eunice had lured him into Babylon. The coloured lights spun and flashed in frantic synchronicity with the buzzers and bells. The money clinked into the machines and clattered out, although the former much more frequently than the latter. As one of Gavin's best brogues slipped on a squashed chip he looked ready to flee, but Eunice filled his hand with coins and nodded towards Bomber's favourite machine.

'Come on, you — get stuck in! Bomber loved this one.'

As Eunice posted a coin into the slot, she remembered the confusion on Bomber's face the last time they were there; but then how quickly it had been replaced with a smile when she had come to his rescue. Today was for happy memories, not sad ones. Eunice made Gavin stick it out for almost half an hour, by the end of which he was almost enjoying himself. Against all the (most likely fixed) odds, he won a small and very ugly teddy bear on a claw-game machine, which he proudly presented to Eunice as a gift. As she inspected the lopsided bear's comical face, she had an idea.

'We should buy a souvenir for each of them,' she said, holding up the striped bag.

In one of the kiosks on the pier, they found a

key ring in the shape of a doughnut for Douglas. In a shop in The Lanes Gavin spotted an antique Staffordshire china pug.

'He looks like a boy dog to me,' said Gavin, 'but perhaps Baby Jane would prefer that.'

They had fish and chips for lunch and Gavin ordered a bottle of champagne for them to toast the contents of the striped bag, which had its own chair. Eunice was determined not to let it out of her sight for a single moment. The champagne gave Eunice the courage to face what she had to do next. She had to let them go. The pavilion sparkled white in the sunlight and its domes and spires seemed to billow and prick the sky.

In Xanadu did Kubla Khan / A stately pleasure-dome decree . . .

It always put Eunice in mind of Coleridge's opium-inspired verse. They went inside first. It was to be Bomber's last tour and Douglas and Baby Jane's first. Eunice carefully bypassed the kitchen where the dog-powered spit-roast was exhibited. In the gift shop she bought a snow globe containing a model of the pavilion for Bomber's souvenir. Just as Eunice was about to pay, something else caught her eye.

'I'll take a tin of those biscuits too, please,' she told the woman behind the counter.

'Feeling peckish already?' asked Gavin, as he offered to carry them for her.

Eunice smiled. 'I owe a lady called Pauline a tin of biscuits.'

Outside in the grounds, by the pond, they found a bench and sat. The pavilion hung upside down in the water's reflection like a collection of Christmas tree baubles. Eunice took a pair of scissors from her pocket and cut a hole in one of the bottom corners of the striped bag. She had thought long and hard about how she could carry out Bomber's final wishes. Once she had decided on the 'where', she had to work out the 'how'. She didn't even know if it was allowed, but she hadn't asked in case the answer was 'no', so stealth was essential. Eventually, inspiration had come, as ever, from one of their favourite films: *The Great Escape*. If a dozen or so men could scatter the dirt excavated from three tunnels via their trouser legs in full view of armed guards, then surely Eunice would be able to scatter the ashes of three dear friends through the hole in the bottom of a shopping bag without drawing unwelcome attention. She was about to find out.

'Would you like me to come with you and keep a lookout? I could whistle the theme music if that would help.'

Eunice smiled. This part she really was going to do alone. Gavin watched as the small figure walked determinedly across the grass, back straight and head held high. At first, he took her path to be random, but it soon became apparent that it was anything but. When she rejoined him at the bench the striped bag was empty.

'Bomber was right about this place,' he said, staring at the reflection in the pond. 'It is utterly fabulous. By the way,' he added, 'what did you write?'

'Chocks away!' she replied.

51

The cursor on the screen in front of her winked encouragingly. The star sapphire ring on the third finger of Laura's left hand was still an unfamiliar weight as she lifted her hands to begin typing. Freddy, her fiancé of just three days, was in the kitchen making the lovely cup of tea with Sunshine, and Carrot lay sleeping at her feet. Laura was finally ready to chase her dream. She had found the perfect story and no one could describe it as being too 'quiet'. It was a sweeping story of love and loss, life and death, and, above all, redemption. It was the story of a grand passion that had endured for over forty years and finally found its happy ending. Smiling, she began to type. She had her perfect opening line . . .

The Keeper of Lost Things

Chapter 1

Charles Bramwell Brockley was travelling alone and without a ticket on the 14.42 from London Bridge to Brighton . . .

Acknowledgements

The fact that I am writing this means that my dream has finally come true and I am now a proper author. It has been a long journey and there have been some strange diversions, frustrating traffic jams and many bumps in the road. But here I am. There are so many people who have helped me to get here and if I were to mention all of you it would be a novel in itself, but you know who you are and I thank you all.

My parents are, of course, to blame. They taught me to read before I started school, enrolled me at the children's library and filled my childhood with books, for which I am eternally grateful.

Thank you to Laura Macdougall, my incredible agent at Tibor Jones, for believing in me and *Keeper* from the very beginning. We first met under the John Betjeman statue at St Pancras (it was definitely a sign) and within minutes I knew that I wanted to work with you. I thank you for your unstinting support and enthusiasm, your unfailing professionalism and determination, your expert guidance in my initial forays with Twitter and Instagram and your lemon curd.

Thank you Charlotte Maddox at Tibor Jones for all your work with my foreign rights deals and for being such an enthusiastic cheerleader for *Keeper*, and to the whole team at Tibor Jones — undoubtedly the coolest agency on the planet

— for making me feel so much at home with you guys. You rock!

Thank you to Fede Andornino, my editor at Two Roads and founder of Team Sunshine, for taking a risk on *Keeper*. Your humour, patience and boundless enthusiasm have made working with you an absolute joy. Yay! Thanks also to the whole team at Two Roads, especially Lisa Highton, Rosie Gailer and Ross Fraser for welcoming me so warmly and for all your hard work in turning *Keeper* into a real book. Thank you also to Amber Burlinson for her brilliant copyediting skills, Miren Lopategui for her careful proofread and Laura Oliver for actually *making* the book. Thank you to Sarah Christie and Diana Beltran Herrera for bringing Padua's rose garden to life and creating a beautiful cover.

Thank you to Rachel Kahan at William Morrow, another member of Team Sunshine, for your invaluable editorial input and for the humour with which it was imparted. Thanks also to all my foreign publishers for taking *Keeper* all over the world!

Huge thanks to Ajda Vucicevic. You were there at the start and your faith in me has never faltered.

Peter Budek at The Eagle Bookshop in Bedford has been my friend, mentor, and shoulder to cry on through good times and bad. He has also provided me with endless cups of tea, invaluable advice and heaps of wonderful research material. Pete, you are a legend. Now finish writing at least one of your books!

Tracey, my mad friend, you died while I was

writing *Keeper*, and I am so sad that you are not here to share this with me, but you inspired me to keep trying when I was sorely tempted to give up.

Thank you to the staff at Bedford and Addenbrookes Hospitals for all your care and kindness, and for making sure that I was still around to finish this book. Special thanks go to the staff at The Primrose Unit for your continued support and interest in my writing.

I should like to thank Paul for putting up with me. Whilst writing *Keeper* I have filled the house with all the lost things I found, left bits of paper covered in notes all over the place and generally allowed my 'stuff' to creep into every room. I have locked myself away for hours on end and then emerged grumpy and demanding dinner. And yet, you're still here!

Finally, I should like to thank my wonderful dogs. They have had to put up with 'We'll go for a walk as soon as I've finished this chapter' far too many times. Billy and Tilly both died while I was working on *Keeper* and I miss them every day, but Timothy Bear and Duke are asleep on the sofa as I write this. Snoring.

We do hope that you have enjoyed reading this large print book.

Did you know that all of our titles are available for purchase?

We publish a wide range of high quality large print books including:
Romances, Mysteries, Classics
General Fiction
Non Fiction and Westerns

Special interest titles available in large print are:
The Little Oxford Dictionary
Music Book
Song Book
Hymn Book
Service Book

Also available from us courtesy of Oxford University Press:
Young Readers' Dictionary
(large print edition)
Young Readers' Thesaurus
(large print edition)

For further information or a free brochure, please contact us at:
Ulverscroft Large Print Books Ltd.,
The Green, Bradgate Road, Anstey,
Leicester, LE7 7FU, England.
Tel: (00 44) 0116 236 4325
Fax: (00 44) 0116 234 0205

THE ST. TROPEZ LONELY HEARTS CLUB

Joan Collins

Contessa Carlotta Di Ponti, stunningly beautiful and sole heir to a vast fortune, has finally escaped her abusive marriage and is looking to find true love in Saint-Tropez. She soon meets the colourful jetsetters and hangers-on who populate the Mediterranean paradise every summer, including Fabrizio Bricconni, gigolo and long-suffering toyboy of an ageing socialite. The party season kicks off with a spectacular bash at billionaire Harry Silver's palatial mansion, but tragedy soon strikes and, amid the social glitz and the parties, a series of bizarre and increasingly dangerous incidents occurs. Could seemingly innocuous events — a bad oyster, a fatal wasp sting, a faulty funicular — mean something more sinister? It is up to glamorous detective Gabrielle Poulpe to solve the mystery, or life in Saint-Tropez could be over for ever . . .

HOLDING

Graham Norton

The remote Irish village of Duneen has known little drama, and yet its inhabitants are troubled. Sergeant PJ Collins hasn't always been this overweight; mother of two Brid Riordan hasn't always been an alcoholic; and elegant Evelyn Ross hasn't always felt that her life was a total waste. So when human remains are discovered on an old farm, suspected to be those of Tommy Burke — a former love of both Brid and Evelyn — the village's dark past begins to unravel. As the frustrated PJ struggles to solve a genuine case for the first time in his life, he unearths a community's worth of anger and resentment, secrets and regret.

MILLER'S VALLEY

Anna Quindlen

For generations, the Millers have lived in Miller's Valley, a small American town on the verge of enormous change. Mimi Miller describes her life, from the 1960s to the present, with intimacy and honesty, as though revealing it to the best friend she never had. As Mimi eavesdrops on her parents and quietly observes the people around her, she discovers more and more about the toxicity of family secrets, the dangers of gossip, the flaws of marriage, the inequalities of friendship, the risks of passion, loyalty and love. Home, as Mimi begins to realize, can be a place where it's just as easy to feel lost as it is to feel contented . . .

THE WOMAN WHO RAN

Sam Baker

Helen Graham is a new arrival in a tiny Yorkshire village, renting dilapidated Wildfell Hall. The villagers are intensely curious — what makes her so jumpy, and why is she so evasive? Their interest is Helen's worst nightmare. Looking over her shoulder every day, she tries to piece together her past before it can catch up with her. With everything she knows in fragments, from her marriage to her career as a war photographer, how can she work out who to trust and what to believe, when most days she can barely remember who she is?